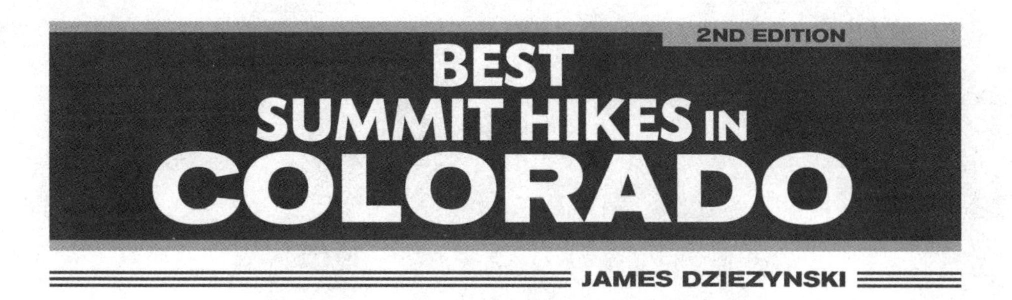
2ND EDITION
BEST
SUMMIT HIKES IN
COLORADO
JAMES DZIEZYNSKI

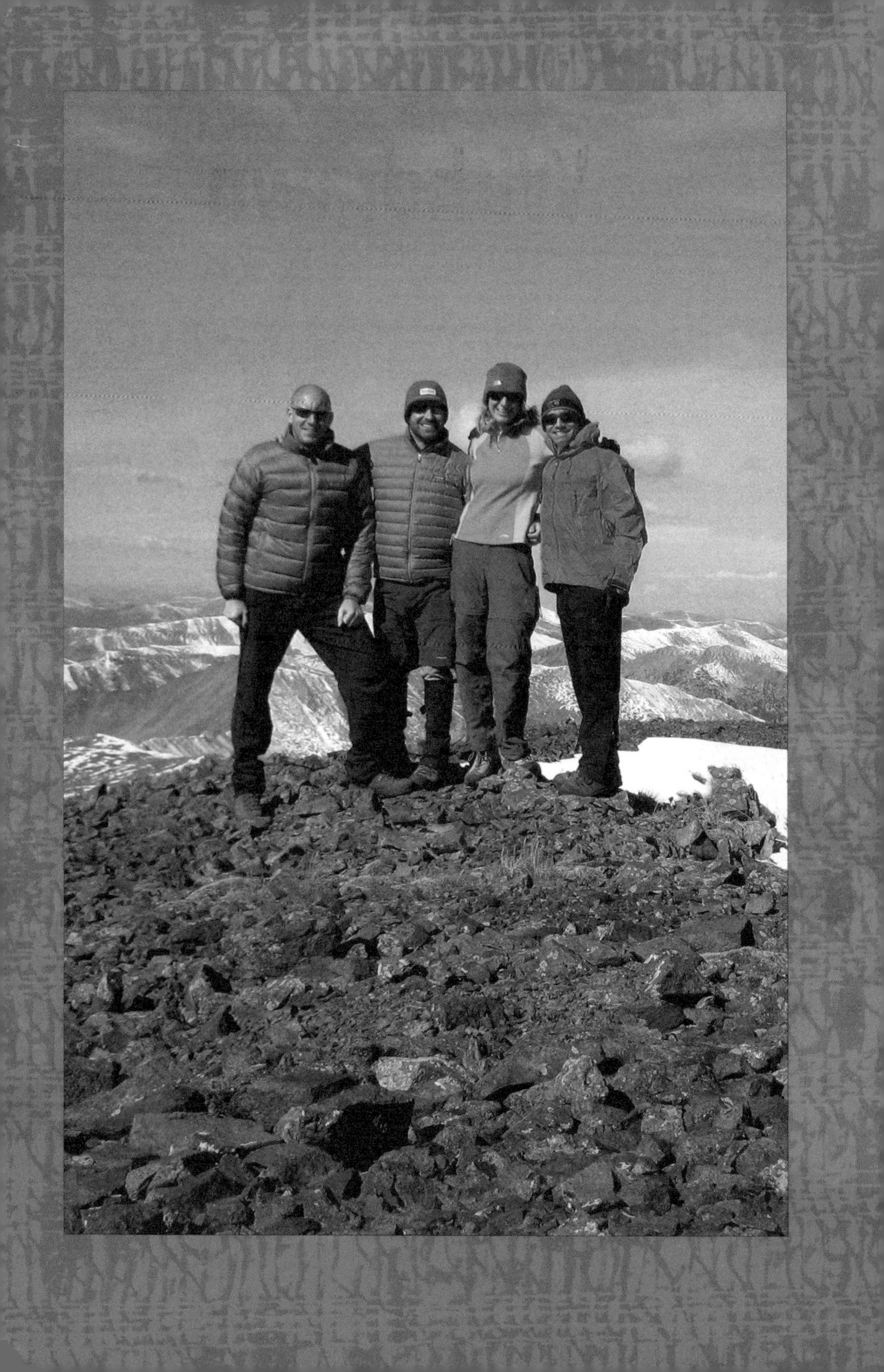

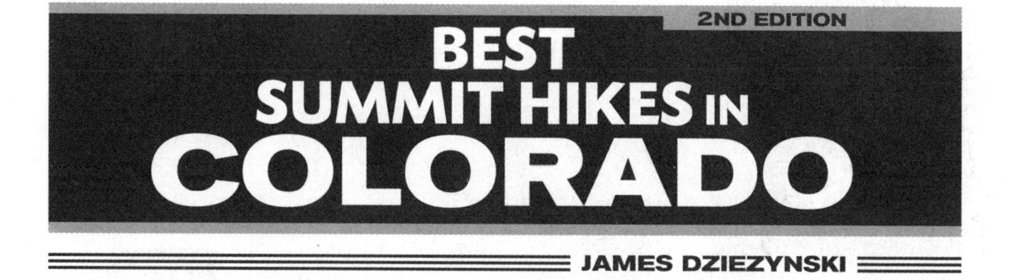

THE ONLY GUIDE YOU'LL EVER NEED
50 CLASSIC ROUTES AND 90+ SUMMITS

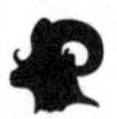 **WILDERNESS PRESS** . . . *on the trail since 1967*

Best Summit Hikes in Colorado:
The Only Guide You'll Ever Need—50 Classic Routes and 90+ Summits

2nd EDITION 2012
2nd printing 2014

All cover and interior photos, except where noted, by James Dziezynski
Auhtor photo by Katie Harwood
Maps: James Dziezynski and Scott McGrew
Cover design: Scott McGrew
Book design: Lisa Pletka
Book editor: Amber Kaye Henderson

ISBN-13: 978-0-89997-712-6

Manufactured in the United States of America

Published by: **Wilderness Press**
c/o Keen Communications
PO Box 43673
Birmingham, AL 35243
(800) 443-7227
info@wildernesspress.com
www.wildernesspress.com

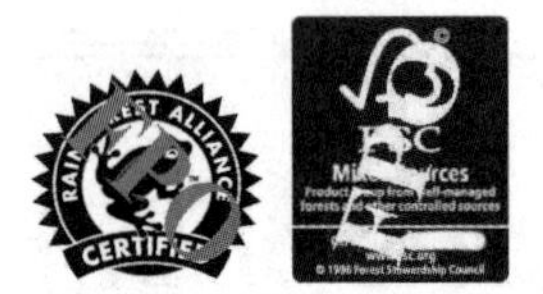

Visit our website for a complete listing of our books and for ordering information.
Distributed by Publishers Group West

Cover photos: *(front)* Top: 13,663-foot Carbonate Mountain, Leadville, Colorado
Bottom: Passing the Little Diamond on Mount Alice, Rocky Mountain National Park
Frontispiece: A summit party atop Carbonate Mountain

SAFETY NOTICE: Although Wilderness Press and the author have made every attempt to ensure that the information in this book is accurate at press time, they are not responsible for any loss, damage, injury, or inconvenience that may occur to anyone while using this book. You are responsible for your own safety and health while in the wilderness. The fact that a trail is described in this book does not mean that it will be safe for you. Be aware that trail conditions can change from day to day. Always check local conditions and know your own limitations.

Acknowledgments

Thanks to all the people (and animals) whose support and mountainous spirits encourage and inspire me.

Huge thanks: Sheila Powell, Jody Pratt, Marie Willson, John Dziezynski, Laura Keresty, Willie Scott, and border collies extraordinaire Fremont and Mystic.

On the mountain: Bart Deferme, Jenny Salentine, Arvind Mohanram, David and Daniela Tanguay, Katarina Stastny, Dani van Heerden, Merril Tydings, Kyle Sevits, Paul Lenhart, Paul Retrum, John Ragozzine, Christina Sheedy, and Seth Griffiths.

Behind the scenes: Doug Schnitzspahn, Jayme Moye, Susan Fecko, Heather Harrison, Emily White, Roslyn Bullas, Lindsey Tate, Emily Gillis, Valerie Soraci, Donald Martinson, Valerie Wimberly, Ron Pratt, Þóra Briem, David and Lynne Dziezynski, Amy and Michael Karls, Sharon and Pete Fuller, Nancy Coulter-Parker, and feline friends Xanadu and Zebedee.

Special thanks: Ingrid Niehaus and the team at Mountainsmith, Native Eyewear, Chris Dickey and Pro-Bar, Patagonia, and National Geographic Maps.

In memory of: Jonny Copp, James Baggett, Arthur Dziezynski, and Talus the border collie.

Peak Locator Map

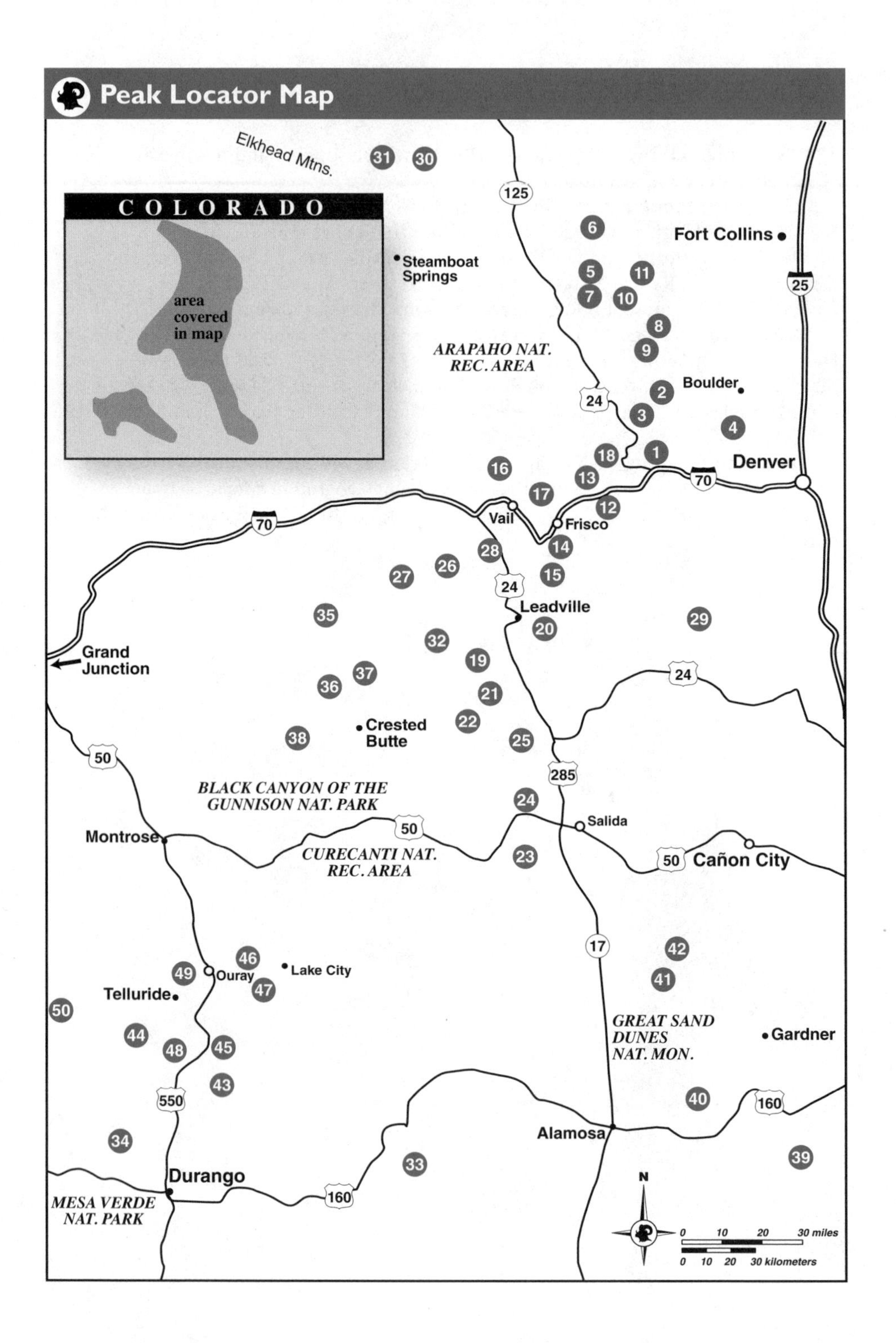

List of Peaks and Elevations

Contents

The Hikes

Preface

No Time Like the Present

It's hard to believe that *Best Summit Hikes in Colorado* has been in publication for five years now. I am humbled and grateful to all those who helped make the book a success and warrant a second edition.

The first edition of *Best Summit Hikes* was a lesson in tenacity and endurance. When I signed on to the project in the autumn of 2005, I had a flexible job, a decent 4x4 truck, and enough money to do the project right. I owed readers the authenticity of personally hiking every peak in the book. I was ready to rock.

When the business of actually hiking rolled around in May 2006, the flexible job had unexpectedly gone out of business, my once-mighty truck blew its engine, and my budget dissolved. Times were tough. Peanut butter *or* jelly tough.

I had a decision to make. I could delay the whole endeavor until things got better. If I went for it, it was an uncertain proposition. I scrambled to buy an 18-year-old Honda Accord, just to have something—not the ideal mountain vehicle. Though I desperately wanted a new camera, I was going to have to work with the humble digital in my possession. I couldn't eat out much nor gather my bearings at hotels. And I had to stay out in the field for extended periods since the price of gas had rocketed in 2006 to roughly $3 a gallon, an all-time high at the time. In other words, I had plenty of reasons to stop before I even started.

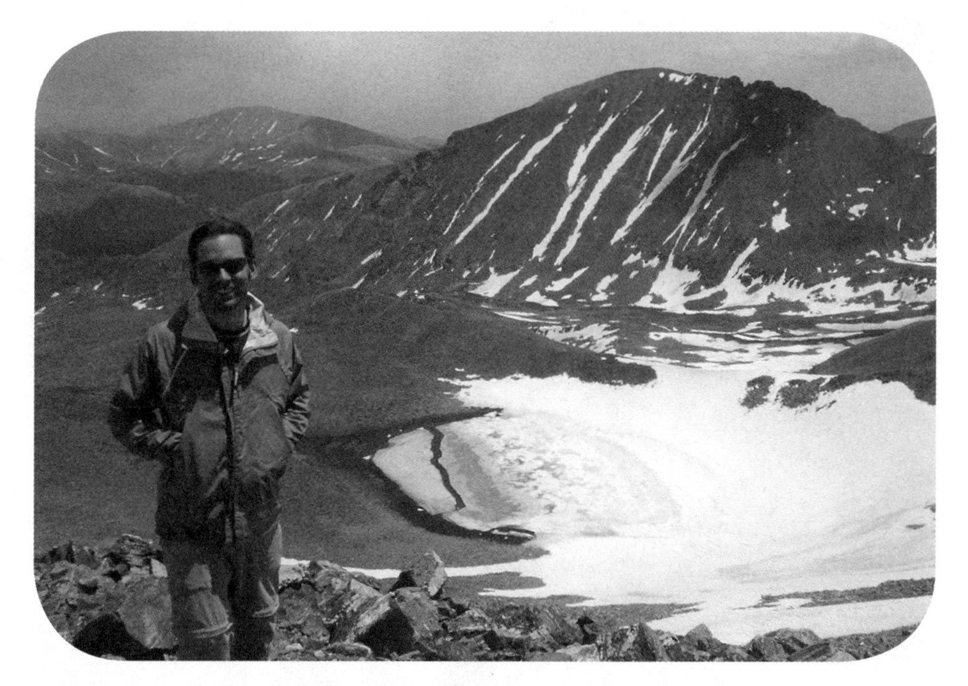

From the top of Pacific Peak, which is just shy of 14er status, it's easy to see why size doesn't always matter when it comes to deciding the best summits in Colorado.

It was fortunate that the subject matter happened to be a wonderful metaphor. We have every reason not to climb mountains. They are cold, barren places where exposure, rockfalls, avalanches, and thunderstorms batter the body and the spirit. You have to get up early to visit them, and for most of us, that means a rushed weekend of bleary-eyed driving between the actual business of wandering into brain-cell-dissolving thin air. As with many of the challenges of life, it's easier to sleep in.

Perhaps because the task was so grandiose and the end so far away, the entire process became very simple. Put one foot in front of the other. Walk uphill. Repeat.

From May to September, I adapted to a spartan but incredibly fulfilling existence, intimately connected with the spirit of the mountains. I wrapped up my final hike in a dance of golden aspen leaves on a crystal-blue September afternoon on East Beckwith Mountain. Somehow I had done it. All I really had to do was find a way to get started.

Mountains occupy a unique place in the human heart. They are gratuitous and essential. Every peak is flush with glory and peril, and they demand great things from us. Mountains haunt our dreams and engage our spirit. They will outlast us in every way, and when we are long forgotten, the connection we forged in those high reaches will silently sustain.

There's no time like the present to find your mountain.

James Dziezynski
July 2012
Boulder, Colorado

The Colorado Rocky Mountains

Overview

Wind, water, fire, ice, and earth are the artists responsible for shaping Colorado's mountains. These elemental influences have made the landscape regions distinct both in character and contour. While all major mountains in Colorado are considered part of the broad North American Rocky Mountain Range (which runs from New Mexico to British Columbia), subranges within the chain have undergone varying degrees of elemental influence. As a result, these geological deviations give each mountain region a unique flavor.

For example, the glacially carved Sawatch Range is known for its gentle slopes and great elevations, greeting hikers like a kindly old grandfather. Crumbling marine shale gives mountains in the Maroon Bells–Snowmass Wilderness the essence of a great manor house in disrepair; it's a place where seemingly solid rocks embedded in the earth can pop out like rotten teeth. Pods of pristine peaks can be found in the sporadic outcrops and dramatic profiles of the Sangre De Cristo Range. Incredible sculptures of imposing granite define the remote Grenadier Range, daring you to enter their impressive kingdom.

There are many more subranges in Colorado, not to mention sub-subranges, such as the Spanish Peaks in the Sangre De Cristo Range of the Rocky Mountains. Geology is the primary factor in defining ranges, though categorization can be influenced by other whims. One example is the group of high Sawatch Mountains known as the Collegiate Peaks. These well-known mountains bear the names of prestigious eastern US universities, a far cry from the mellifluous names that had been bestowed upon them by native people. They differ little from surrounding Sawatch mountains, though it is interesting to note that they were initially grouped (before being named) according to mining boundaries.

However they are grouped on the map, as you spend more time in the mountains, you will begin to unveil the "personalities" of individual peaks. Until one actually sets foot on the slopes, the objective data and raw facts serve merely to foster our curiosity. Experiencing the mountain with your own senses reveals the spirit of the peak. Each journey to the high country transforms that two-dimensional mark on the map into a vivid memory. And whether the mention of a mountain brings to mind warm memories or recollections of chilling close calls, every step of the way will have been an adventure. Such are the adventures hikers yearn to live.

Geology and Biology: A Very Brief History

The definitive characteristic of the Rocky Mountains can be found right under your boots. Eons of change have put the "rock" into the Rocky Mountains. How these mountains were built is an intriguing tale. Fossils abound in compressed chronicles of stone, each representative of a past ecosystem. Dynamic transformations over the years have yielded a wealth of information and, conversely, have contributed to new scientific mysteries.

To summarize all the geological mayhem, Colorado's rock has been shaped by three primary forces: plate tectonics, volcanic eruptions, and glacial polishing. Starting at the bottom of the pile are the Precambrian foundations of igneous and metamorphic rock, formed some 600 million years ago when most of planet Earth was a volatile, volcanic work in progress. Very little is known about this period. To put it in perspective, scientists believe the most advanced form of life at the time was a multicelled piece of slimy bacteria. (Similar life-forms can be found today in the back of my refrigerator.)

Then, 300 million years ago, the land began to rise up as continental plates collided. This created enormous sand dunes and other soft formations that served as a holding place for the mountains to come. Much of the trademark flagstone adorning the buildings at the University of Colorado in Boulder was formed in this era. Around 250 million years ago, the gnawing power of erosion had whittled down this sandstone, making space for great lakes of silty water and nearly uninhabitable swamps. Rising temperatures made life demanding for primitive creatures. If that wasn't bad enough, an event known as the Great Extermination, in which life was eradicated on a global scale, made survival for our prehistoric friends an incredible act of endurance. This period of unexplained catastrophe ushered out the old, slimy age and introduced a new explosion of diverse life across the globe.

Between 250 and 100 million years ago, Colorado's climate transformed flat, muddy swamps into great tropical forests. Incredibly dense and lush, these forests were ideal homesteads for a variety of dinosaurs. The really big boys called Colorado home, including the biologically enigmatic sauropods such as diplodocus and brontosaurus. These huge creatures had shockingly tiny brains, an anomaly that was offset by the fact that all they had to do was eat and grow bigger. Giant ferns grew in the verdant swamps, unchecked by dry weather or pollution. It was a great time for all. But, like all good things, it had to end.

Persistent erosion and changing temperatures began to have a profound effect on the landscape between 100 and 65 million years ago. Swampy basins lost their thickets of vegetation, resulting in marshy lakes that continued to expand onto flat tracts of land. All the hard work that plate tectonics had done to build up the land was nearly for naught. By the end of this era, most of Colorado was hundreds of feet underwater. This inland salty sea was host to incredible creatures, from gargantuan sea life to enormous flying reptiles. Seashells of ammonites and other critters from this period can be found today in several regions, notably the Elk and Gore Ranges.

From about 60 to 38 million years ago, the mountains began to rebound. An uplift of plates elevated mountains to modest heights: 3,000–4,000 feet higher than the seas below. Water rose with the land, pooling in isolated lakes or disappearing completely. Fearsome predators such as the jaw-some Tyrannosaurus rex roamed the land. As a whole, the animals and plants of this era show a gradual downsizing trend. The great giants found food sources vanishing or became snacks for smaller, more aggressive species. The times, they were a-changin', setting the stage for the huge alterations in the land. Scientists speculate that the famous "doom asteroid" struck Earth in this time period. (The asteroid theory is based on high levels of iridium found in rock/plant samples, suspected to be a direct result of a huge meteor slamming into Earth in the Yucatan Peninsula near the modern-day city of Cancun in Mexico.) This collision affected life-forms of all sizes and triggered volcanic flows throughout the region. The impact was felt on a global level, yet it was only the first act in a show that would take place over the next few million years. The greatest changes were just around the corner. . . .

Colorado's defining era was about to begin. Roughly 37 million years ago, massive continental plates were thrust into motion. This movement slid the North American Plate westward over the steadfast Pacific Plate, unleashing torrents of volcanic lava and ash. Incredible pressure pushed the land higher and higher, transforming those unassuming 3,000-foot hills into crowns atop enormous peaks. For millions of years, the land was altered as heavy rains washed away volcanic ash. Geologists are a bit puzzled that the mountains formed in the region that is present-day Colorado. Normally, tectonic-based ranges rise a mere 20–600 miles from the oceanic coast. These mountains rose up thousands of miles inland, possibly indicating a distinctive geologic event, which has never been repeated.

Dinosaurs too big (or perhaps too dull in the skull) for the new land to support disappeared. Smaller, smarter, and faster was the order of the day. The last titans gave way to more adaptable creatures. Mammoths, camels, bison, lions, and other warm-blooded creatures flourished, replacing the reptiles who had ruled this domain for millions of years. This golden era introduced the reign of the giant mammals, a tenure that was to be very short lived. Of all the creatures in this ancient mammalian menagerie, only a select few would survive into the modern day.

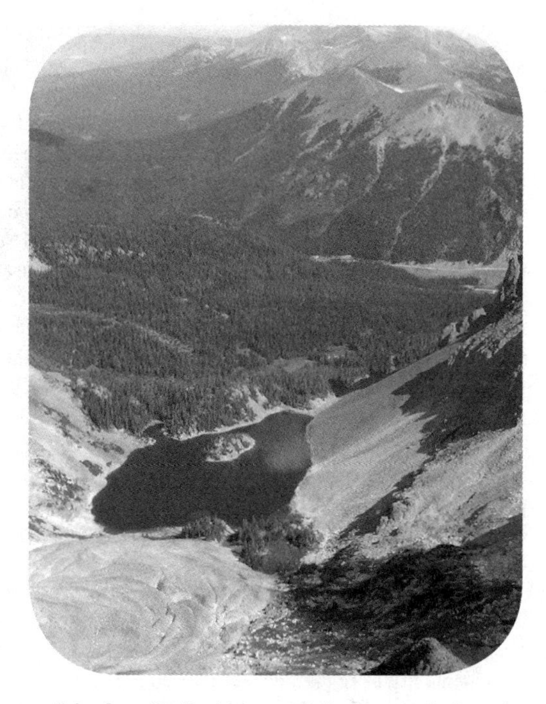

Talus flows like liquid down to Lake Agnes at the foot of Mount Richthofen.

About 1 million years ago, things began to calm down, and the Colorado we know today began to take shape. Rock that had lain for millions of years under seas was now sky high. The Colorado Plateau rose up from huge faults and rifts. Plate motions made mountains out of molehills; the Sangre De Cristo and Wet Mountains ranges in the east are direct results of this powerful subduction. Volcanic eruptions added to the artistry. One example: The striking, crumbling precipice of Lizard Head Peak just outside of Telluride is the durable throat of a long extinct volcano.

A mere 16,000 years ago, an ice age passed over the land. This was the last hurrah for the monster mammals, including the tusky mammoth. Only the hearty bison survived the advancing and receding glaciers, just to be hunted to near-extinction by white men in the 1800s. Glacial rivers smoothed and polished the land, carving deep cirques in the sides of mountains. In modern times, these glaciers are making their last stand as Colorado's mountains prepare for the next great geological event.

Poets would have us believe that mountains are static and permanent features, everlasting monuments that contrast with mankind's brief stint on Earth. The less romantic truth is that mountains are constantly changing. Discrete modifications in height occur every few years, though it takes precision instruments to sense most changes. Events such as the explosive eruption of Washington's Mount St. Helens in 1980 are business as usual for mountain ranges but have a long-lasting impact on humans when they occur in our lifetime. Mountains are no less subject than we are to the forces of nature, though they offer resilience that projects permanence.

Human History in the Colorado Rockies

After the most recent ice age (roughly 11,000 years ago), the first human inhabitants took up residency in the Rockies. These primitive people endured harsh winters in pursuit of the great mammals that roamed in the valleys. Mammoths were coveted for the amount of meat they would yield and for their sturdy bones and ivory tusks, which could be shaped into tools. People migrated with the animals, leaving few permanent settlements in their wake.

Laramide Orogeny

The Rocky Mountains owe their airy existence to a geological event known as the Laramide Orogeny. The word *orogeny* comes from the Greek language and means "mountain building." In context, orogenies specifically describe mountains that have risen as a result of plate tectonics. To simplify what is an incredibly complex process, think of Earth's continents as floating plates akin to shards of broken ice on a pond. The "pond" that our continents float upon is called the lithosphere. When these shards collide, whole continents are shaped by the plates driving into one another until one finally yields and slides beneath the dominant shard—a process known as subduction. As the "defeated" plate drifts under the "victorious" plate, the land of the upper plate is pushed higher and higher, and the raw forms of mountains appear. After centuries of refinement at the behest of the elements, the mountains begin to take on the dramatic shapes we identify with our greatest peaks. The collision that formed Colorado's mountains is known as the Laramide Orogeny.

The Laramide Orogeny (named for the Laramie Mountains in eastern Wyoming) began roughly 80 million years ago, though the start of such a slow-acting phenomenon is difficult to pinpoint. The process continued for nearly 40 million years. As the North American continental plate slid westward, it eventually converged with the oceanic Pacific Plate, also know as the Farallon Plate. The North American Plate was the dominant of the two and began to glide over the Pacific Plate, pushing it down.

Slowly, the Pacific Plate slid between the North American Plate and Earth's mantle—the last solid layer before the planet's molten core. Because of the relatively snug fit of these plates and the shallow angle of subduction, there was little volcanic activity. As the plates converged in fits and starts, the land from Alaska to Mexico grew increasingly higher.

Prototypes of the Rocky Mountains formed at this time. As the plates settled, cracks in the layers (called geologic faults) released high-pressure volcanic magma. These delayed eruptions occurred several million years after the start of the Laramide Orogeny. Major flows in the Sawatch and San Juan Ranges contributed to the formation of mountains. Eventually, the plates locked into place and the magma was sealed below the Earth, surfacing from time to time to heat a hot spring or to vent through fumaroles. The land stabilized over the centuries, making the Rocky Mountains a fixture on the continent, where they will continue to stand tall for generations to come.

Many of the tribes that formed over the years are familiar names: Apache, Arapahoe, Cheyenne, Crow, Shoshoni, Sioux, and Ute, to list a few. These people flourished as they mastered yearly patterns of migration. Autumn and winter were spent on the warmer, lower plains, while spring and summer were ideal times to hunt and forage in the mountains.

Undoubtedly lost in these annals of time are the first true ascents of the major mountains in Colorado. While most of these feats have gone undocumented, it is naive to assume that the native people were any more exempt from the lure of the mountains than we are today. Alas, history is written from the perspective of the conqueror and not the conquered, and the mystery of who first set foot atop these peaks will remain unknown.

Among the first meddling Europeans to explore the Rockies was Francisco Vásquez de Coronado, the fabled ambassador of Spain who was, unfortunately, very good at his job. His journeys to the southern Rocky Mountains (mostly in New Mexico) in 1540 introduced native people to the ways of the white man. While there were a few beneficial results for the indigenous peoples from these encounters, such as the introduction of the horse and metalworking, the downside was a near eradication of the natives' culture, habitat, and spirituality.

The Spanish influence on the southern Rockies is evident today, with many peaks in the San Juan Mountains (itself an obviously Spanish moniker) named after Spanish explorers and missionaries. A select few mountains have reverted back to their native names in modern times.

A slow stream of Western European men began to infiltrate the Colorado region, mostly in search of fur and timber, and an uneasy alliance between the natives and newcomers was reached. In the late 1700s, as the nation of America came into being, people grew more curious in what lay in the uncharted lands to the west. The Scottish Canadian explorer Sir Alexander Mackenzie crossed the Rockies in 1793, on his way to the first transcontinental navigation of North America. He would later go on to discover the Arctic Ocean. The turbulent river that runs from Great Slave Lake north to the Arctic is named in his honor. Following in his footsteps, bold miners and fur traders set up the first European settlements in Colorado.

Shortly after Mackenzie's exploration, the fabled Lewis and Clark Expedition (1804–1806) set about making detailed descriptions of the land along the Missouri and Columbia Rivers, which entailed crossing the Rocky Mountains. They encountered many of the native peoples on their journey, many of whom were peaceful, or at worst, ambivalent to the band of American explorers. Lewis and Clark opened the door for many famous explorers, whose names are on our maps today: Kit Carson, Jim Bridger, Zebulon Pike, John Fremont, Jedediah Smith, and John Colter. These mountain men became larger than life for their exploits in the Wild West.

Lewis and Clark opened the door for many explorers: Kit Carson, Jim Bridger, Zebulon Pike, John Fremont, Jedediah Smith, and John Colter. These mountain men became larger than life for their exploits in the Wild West.

Miners doggedly combed the land for precious minerals in the Rocky Mountains region and finally hit gold in Colorado in 1859. Gold deposits in the mineral-rich South Platte River region were the catalyst that led to an explosion in mining. "Pikes Peak or Bust" was the order of the day, as dreamy miners dug into the rocky earth in search of great wealth. William Green Russell, a native Georgian, was the first to establish a successful gold mine, just outside of the present-day city of Englewood. By the 1860s, Central City and Idaho Springs were major hubs of mining commerce, with cities on the plains such as Boulder, Golden, and Denver playing supporting roles.

Now that the land had tangible value, greed became a motivating factor in the extermination and relocation of the native people. Overpowered by the guns of the white man, the native tribes were hastily removed from the landscape as more and more settlers claimed legal ownership of the earth. Friction culminated in the disgraceful slaughter of peaceful Cheyenne and Arapahoe natives in Kiowa County, a horrible event later known as the Sand Creek Massacre. On November 29, 1864, a cowardly group of Colorado militiamen mercilessly slaughtered an encampment of mostly elderly men, women, and children, killing more than 200. This point marked the beginning of the end for the people who had called Colorado home for centuries.

As the gold mines in the high country began to sputter out, mining got a shot in the arm with the great silver discoveries outside of Leadville in 1879. More and more settlers stayed in Colorado after the lodes ran dry, moving to major cities and leaving ghost towns in their wake. The population grew as Colorado's agreeable climate, natural resources, and intrinsic beauty became widely known. Out-of-work miners turned to agriculture in the high country, and hundreds of ranches sprang up.

Colorado achieved statehood on August 1, 1876, becoming the 38th state of the United States. Since then, it has grown to become a major recreational and tourist destination. Mining experienced a modern boom during both World Wars. Molybdenum, an element crucial in strengthening the armor plating on tanks and warships, became a major resource. The Climax Molybdenum Mine, on Fremont Pass outside of Leadville, continues to carry out operations to this day.

In modern times, skiing and other outdoors recreation have given new life to the high country. With our newfangled horseless carriages and high-tech Gore-Tex jackets, the backcountry has never been more accessible. The value of Colorado's wilderness in an era of development and industry is priceless; we must ensure future generations will enjoy the mountains as we do today by honoring and respecting the land.

Wildlife

High-elevation critters are a hearty bunch. Despite the harsh conditions experienced at altitude, animals of many sizes flourish, all the way up to 14,000 feet. Survival depends on clever adaptations to the environment. These creatures employ a great bag of tricks to endure year after year. Hibernation, torpor, seasonal fur camouflage, ingenious den designs, and unique physiological adaptations are among the strategies that are proven winners in the alpine kingdom.

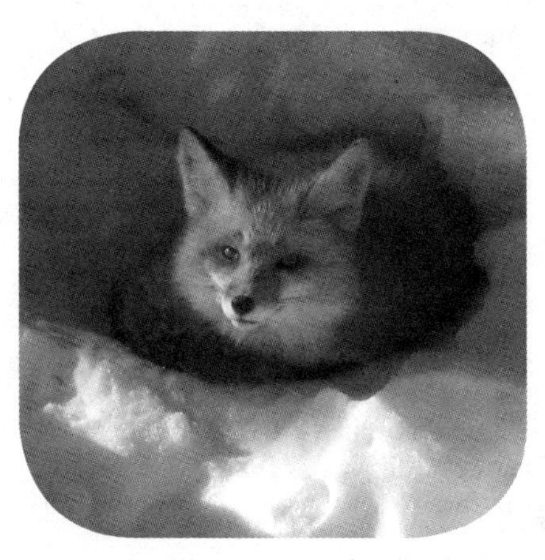

A sunny winter day warms up a foxy friend.

Hikers and backpackers entering the backcountry need to respect local wildlife. Once on their turf, we need to play by their rules. They experience the world through a different set of sense organs, oftentimes superior to our own eyes, ears, and noses. And since neither man nor animal is looking for trouble, reducing the chances of a bad encounter is essential for both.

By now you should know to never feed the wildlife, no matter how cute or hungry they look. Feeding animals can make them reliant on hikers as a food source. At high-traffic areas such as Rocky Mountain National Park, the pudgy jaybirds and ground squirrels begging at popular trailheads prove that many people disregard this rule. Wildlife must remain wild. An animal that retains the skills that have kept its kind alive for hundreds of years must not lose that proficiency by developing a craving for Cheetos.

Do not approach wild animals and never do anything that would frighten them. Animal behavior is unpredictable, and it is always best to give even the "friendly" animals their space. Slow-moving and less aggressive animals should not be stressed out by visitors trying to handle them. Take photographs from a safe distance.

To put it simply, be respectful, and acquiesce to them if you must. Life is hard enough in the high country; the last thing the animals that live there need is meddling humans to goof things up.

Mammal Roll Call

Furry friends are plentiful in the mountains. Largest of all are the impressive moose that live in pockets throughout marshy areas of the Rocky Mountains, notably in the Gore Range peaks outside of Vail. Moose are not native to Colorado. They were introduced in 1978 as a small group and have flourished, comprising about 600 animals today. With male bull moose averaging 1,100 pounds, they are not to be trifled with. Even the daintiest female moose can weigh 800 pounds when full grown. Moose are the largest members of the deer family (Cervidae), and their name comes from an Algonquin word meaning "twig eater." These muscular mammals are relatively rare in Colorado, so consider yourself lucky if you spot one. (Note that bison, which can weigh up to 2,000 pounds, are not considered wild animals in Colorado. The only native populations that exist are on ranches, where they are raised for meat or hides.)

More commonly found are the moose's cousins, the elk. Elk originally roamed the plains east of the Rockies, but they have since adapted to conditions in lower high-altitude regions. Don't be surprised if you happen to see them higher on the mountain, as they will wander to the very tops of peaks when summer weather is agreeable. Elk are by nature herd animals, though young bucks are known to be a bit more adventurous and may leave the comfort of the group for short periods of time. Like moose, they are generally peaceful but can get aggressive during the rut (mating season). The famous bugle of elk during the mating season is a haunting call, a distinct tone that must be heard to be appreciated.

Deer round up the major members of the ungulate order (ungulates are the hoofed mammals). Mule deer make up the largest subfamily in the mountains. Although their role in life is primarily serving as prey for larger carnivores, mule deer are scrappy and rugged. While still herd animals, they often band in much smaller groups than elk, sometimes in families of only four to six members. I've encountered mule deer above 14,000 feet and even on the summits of some fairly rugged peaks (such as Mount Zirkel). Keep your eyes open, and you may spot them, too.

Black bears are perhaps the most feared of the mountain mammals and among the most misunderstood. Most are shy and will avoid confrontations with humans. Because they are omnivores, black bears are perfectly content to munch on berries and vegetation, hunting for meat only when they have to. Remember, however, that they are still equipped with the finest in carnivore technology and are excellent swimmers and climbers. Unless you are Carl Lewis, you cannot outrun a black bear. Smaller black bears are often mistaken for large dogs, while larger black bears can easily be mistaken for bison. Some males can grow to weigh more than 800 pounds and reach 6 feet tall, from ground to shoulder. With a healthy, glossy coat and a face that shows a relaxed dominance, it is easy to get captivated in the presence of such an incredible beast. Note that bear's fur changes with the seasons, fluctuating from near black to light brown. For information on bear encounters, read the section "What to Do if You Encounter a Black Bear," on page 12.

Grizzly bears (also known as brown bears) are considered to be extinct in this area, but just to be safe, the Colorado Department of Natural Resources considers the grizz an endangered species. The last known grizzly was killed by hunters in the San Juan Mountains in 1979. There have been no confirmed sightings since, though reports come in every year of their existence. Wyoming does have confirmed grizzly populations however, and it is not far-fetched to think some of this group may wander into Colorado. Rumors persist of a small population in the Sawatch Range around Mount Elbert. While it may be easy for an inexperienced wildlife observer to confuse a grizzly and a black bear, they are quite different in both appearance and demeanor. Grizzly bears are brownish-yellow and are more muscular than black bears. Their enormous heads and muscular humps over the shoulders make them formidable and majestic animals. Grizzlies are more aggressive than black bears and are much more unpredictable. The good news in Colorado is that if there are any grizzlies in the state, they do well to stay out of sight.

Mountain lions (also known as cougars, pumas, or panthers) are the elusive kings of the mountain and the least predictable. Because they live as individuals, as opposed to in packs, their behavior can differ from cat to cat. Large felines are nature's perfect predators: fast, stealthy, smart, and equipped to win any battle. You may have never seen a mountain lion, but I guarantee they've seen you! Most lions have no need to attack humans and seem smart enough to avoid the trouble (not to mention expending the effort to attack a 200-pound human when that energy can be better used to take down a 400-pound elk). However, mountain lions have an instinct to pursue fast-moving creatures and several attacks on humans have occurred when people were running or biking. If presented with the opportunity of an easy kill, a hungry lion will stalk smaller people or children. Such tactics are generally thought to be acts of desperation by emaciated or older lions and are very rare, with the average being one attack per year over the past 120 years. The fact that lions have ample opportunity to attack oblivious hikers and normally choose not to indicates that we are not their favorite targets. With their high intelligence and reliance on stealth, it may benefit both the mountain lion and the hiker that they stay in the shadows. For more information, read the section "What to Do if You Encounter a Mountain Lion," on page 11.

✱ ✱ ✱ ✱ ✱ ✱ ✱

Large felines are nature's perfect predators: fast, stealthy, smart, and equipped to win any battle. You may have never seen a mountain lion, but I guarantee that they've seen you! Nonetheless, most lions have no need to attack humans.

✱ ✱ ✱ ✱ ✱ ✱ ✱

The lesser carnivores you may see include bobcats, badgers, coyotes, weasels, martens, red foxes, and if you're extra lucky, the recently reintroduced lynx. There may be traces of gray wolves in northern Colorado. Lynx were believed to be extinct in Colorado by 1973, but a successful reintroduction of 200 cats was initiated in 1999 in the San Juan Mountains. As of 2012, this population seems to be doing well. Wolverines were extirpated in Colorado by the early 1900s, but rare sightings have been reported in the mountains.

Weasels often surprise people by hanging out on the summits of peaks. While they tend to inhabit lower-elevation regions, they may venture high to prey on unsuspecting rodents sheltered in high talus fields. Badgers are low-slung animals that resemble superskunks. I spotted one outside the town of Mancos, an impressive fellow sporting a fashionable gray-and-white coat. Coyotes are masters of adaptation and can live anywhere, from the slums of Los Angeles to the alpine boreal forests of Alaska. It is a special treat to hear the lonesome howl of the coyote echoing in the night—and to hear that howl answered by his fellows far away.

Mountain goats and Rocky Mountain bighorn sheep are often confused. Bighorn sheep are masters of the mountain, moving about steep cliffs with fearless ease. These nondomesticated cousins of farm sheep should not be called rams, a term that denotes an uncastrated male sheep. Bighorn sheep are noted for their curled horns, which are used primarily in contests of strength between males during the mating season. By butting their heads with incredible force, they use the "Mike Tyson system" of wooing female mates—brute force. Bighorn sheep are the official state animal of Colorado and the mascot of Colorado State University.

Mountain goats are often snowy white (and keeping those coats clean is no easy task while cavorting on dirty mountaintops). Their name is a bit of a misnomer, as they are more closely related to antelopes than goats. Much like bighorn sheep, they are master rock climbers. On more than one occasion, I've seen lines of goats walk effortlessly across rock faces I would rate at least class 4 rock climbing (see section on class ratings on page 48). Adult mountain goats weighing 200 pounds can scale 60-degree slopes with ease. With their tufted beards and wise, expressive eyes, they are another species that can be gentle as a lamb or brazen as a bull. Be warned: An angry mountain goat can inflict some serious damage on an unassuming hiker, especially if said hiker is on a narrow ledge. Give them their space, and they will almost always peacefully pass on by.

Yellow-bellied marmots are among the most common critters in the mountains. These beaverlike rodents are charming and cute, but they do have a sinister side. Many have completely lost their fear of humans, boldly rummaging through backpacks or approaching hikers to beg for food. Many a tent has been gnawed through and many a food bag ripped asunder by marmots. Nighttime assaults on tents can be especially annoying, as the persistent pests not only threaten your food, but they can also rob you of precious sleep. Marmots are also quite curious about parked automobiles, and more than one has been known to chew clean through rubber hoses, lured by the sweet scent of brake fluid or antifreeze (both of which are obviously toxic). Marmots can be pesky at times, but the mountains wouldn't be the same without them.

Pikas are small, grayish, mouselike animals with large ears. They can be seen popping in and out of rocky talus fields, industriously gathering straw and flowers for their dens. No doubt you have heard their trademark "rubber ducky" squeak at one time or another. Their soft gray fur is indicative of their relation to rabbits; they are of the same family. Amazingly, pikas do not hibernate in the winter. Instead, they rely on densely insulated burrows and large reserves of stored food to get them through the cold months. This incredible system makes them one of the elite animals that can actually endure winters above 14,000 feet. Biologists fear pikas may be headed toward extinction as development and pollution encroach on their environment.

Beavers are always hard at work in high-elevation ponds. Beavers that live in higher elevations develop thick and luxuriant coats, a trait that made them appealing to early fur trappers. Salt-loving porcupines are the second-largest rodents in Colorado, behind beavers. River otters were believed extinct in Colorado by 1970, but efforts to reintroduce new populations have been successful, notably along the Dolores, South Platte, and Colorado Rivers. These playful members of the weasel family are a delight to watch as they frolic on riverbanks, tumbling and swimming just for the fun of it. The unmistakable stench of the skunk indicates that they too are out in the mountains. Mink and muskrats round out the smaller water-loving mammals. Like beavers and river otters, they are semiaquatic animals that live on the banks of rivers, ponds, and lakes.

Finally, how can we forget about the little guys? Uinta chipmunks are curious and bold, and too often their cuteness is rewarded with an ill-advised handout of pretzels or peanuts. They need to retain their foraging skills to get them through the winter, so please make a point of not sharing, even if they are agreeable to taking food from your hand. Golden-mantled ground squirrels are often mistaken for chipmunks because they share the same habitats, color schemes, and personalities. An easy way to tell the two apart: Chipmunks have stripes on their furry faces and squirrels do not. A variety of rabbits exist in Colorado. The mountain cottontail is the most common; as a result, these bunnies serve as a food source for coyotes, mountain lions, and other predators. Snowshoe hares are speedy animals whose coats change color with the seasons. The smallest of the mammals include field mice, pocket gophers, and shrews.

On the Wing: Major Birds of the Rocky Mountains

Bird-watching has gone mainstream in the past few years, proving that it's not only nerdy foreigners in giant Coke-bottle glasses who peep at the life in the sky (which is not to imply that I have ever subscribed to the stereotype that bird-watchers are necessarily nerdy, foreign, or visually impaired!). Birds in the Rocky Mountains are plentiful and come in a delightful array of colors. There are far too many to cover in this brief overview, but I'll note some of the most prevalent birds you'll encounter in the mountains. (Bird lovers should check out **birding.com/wheretobird/colorado.asp** or pick up a copy of *Birds of Colorado Field Guide* by Stan Tekiela, published by Adventure Publications).

No other bird conveys majesty on the wing quite like the bald eagle. Bald eagles were nearly extinct in the lower US by the early 20th century, but they have made a great comeback, thanks to conservation efforts. (The only American bald eagles born outside of North America in this century were hatched in European zoos.) Today, a healthy population flourishes in Colorado. Females may have a wingspan of 7 feet and are larger than their male counterparts. An interesting bit of eagle trivia: Native Americans are rumored to have set up eagle traps on the summit of Longs Peak, giving strength to the argument that John W. Powell wasn't the first person to stand atop that fabled 14er. Golden eagles are slightly smaller than bald eagles and have brownish-beige colorings. Incredibly agile in flight, these birds of prey mate for life and are one of the few threats to rodents living above 13,000 feet.

Peregrine falcons prefer cold mountain regions, migrating north to the Arctic and south to the Rockies and other northern American mountain regions. Because they are seasonal visitors, your best chance to see peregrine falcons is during spring and early summer. They are unrivaled as the fastest animals on earth, capable of unleashing a free fall, diving attack that regularly exceeds 200 miles per hour! In this incredible display, called a stoop, the falcon folds its wings, extends the razor-sharp talons on its feet, and plummets at mind-bending speeds toward an unsuspecting bird below. The aim is to damage or completely sheer off a wing (a direct impact would injure both birds). When the disabled prey hits the ground, the falcon descends to finish off the job. If you are fortunate enough to witness a peregrine falcon stoop, the awesome image will remain in your mind for years to come.

Red-tailed hawks are smaller simulacrums of the golden hawk. Whenever you hear the telltale screech of a bird in movies or on TV, chances are that you are hearing the distinct cry of the red-tailed hawk.

Ravens and crows can be found throughout Colorado. Both are large black birds with fancy ebony beaks. The two are difficult to differentiate. One major difference can be seen in their flying postures: crows tend to flap, flap, flap their wings, while ravens will flap a little and then soar through the air, similar to the way hawks fly.

Gray jays are friendly avian beggars with stylish gray and black markings. Jays relentlessly haunt campsites and picnic tables, looking for scraps of food. Mountain bluebirds are a striking electric-blue color, painted the same hue as the clear mountain sky. As you make your way along mountain trails, several varieties of swallows may gleefully zip by you with an audible *thwipp*. Appropriately named redwing blackbirds are distinguished by the bright red "armband" on the shoulders of their black wings. Robins, owls, ducks, cranes, herons, and woodpeckers are also common in the mountains.

Ground-patrolling birds are abundant. White-tailed ptarmigans are extremely likable, peaceful fellows. They amble about on the tundra, only mildly concerned when hikers approach. "Mumbling" ptarmigans often have broods of adorable chicks in tow. Ptarmigans are masters of camouflage, with brownish, speckled, ground-imitating feathers in the summer and pure snow-white plumage in the winter. On one occasion, I came across pockets of nearly invisible white ptarmigans huddled against the cold in a January subzero whiteout. Their hearty, stoic, stick-it-out approach to winter earns my respect. The more fidgety pheasant is equally good at camouflage but has a bad habit of abandoning its guise when hikers come too near. The loud and frantic flapping of startled pheasants has been scaring the living daylights out of hikers since time immemorial. There are other grouse species in Colorado, none of them as bizarre as the rarely seen Gunnison sage-grouse. Looking like a ruffled member of avian aristocracy, the male of this species has a distinctive white ring of feathers on its neck that it inflates with air sacs during mating rituals—what lady-grouse could resist such a display?

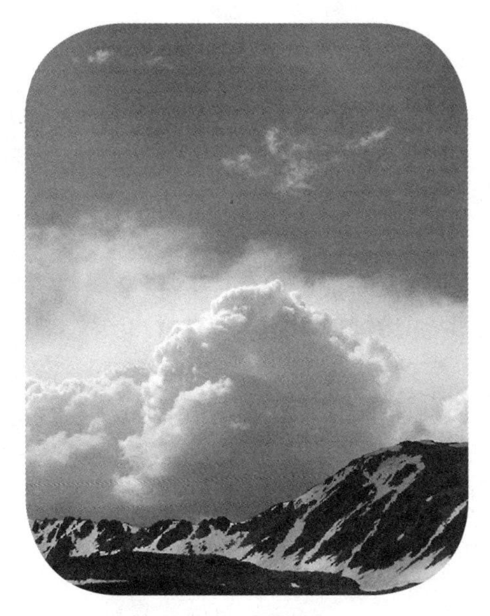

Storms roll into the Pacific Peak basin.

Last, but not least, are the iridescent hummingbirds that hover about in search of nectar. Usually blue-green or yellowish in color, hummingbirds are often mistaken for large bugs upon first sight. Despite their small size, they are curious creatures, prone to investigating bright-colored clothing and backpacks.

Something Fishy

Fish in the pure, cold mountain streams are the object of anglers' affections (and often the objects of their meals as well). The only trout truly native to Colorado's higher mountain lakes is the sleek cutthroat trout; other members of the trout family have been introduced. These include the speckled rainbow trout, brown trout, and brook trout. The mountain whitefish is another native species; it prefers to live in lower-elevation rivers. Introduced and stocked species include the landlocked Kokanee salmon and lake trout.

Fishing is a big industry in Colorado, and those hoping to participate need to acquire a license from the Colorado Department of Wildlife (**wildlife.state.co.us/fishing**; [303] 297-1192). Many high-altitude lakes are stocked by aerial drops in the spring, making for fine fishing throughout the summer and autumn months.

Animal Encounters

What to Do if You Encounter a Mountain Lion

Mountain lion encounters are rare, since the big cat is an elusive animal. In areas where human development infringes on habitat and territory (such as Boulder and Colorado Springs) the chance of seeing lions increases. Hikers are seldom bothered by mountain lions; attacks on humans usually happen as a result of the chase-and-kill reflex triggered by a runner, biker, or jogger.

Unlike bears and other predators, mountain lion behavior is highly unpredictable. Lions may quietly stalk unsuspecting passersby until they have exited the cat's territory without incident. Other times, lions will burst out of the woods for no apparent reason other than to attack. If you come across a mountain lion, do not run! Mountain lions (who can run close to 45 miles per hour) can easily chase down a human (who, on average, can run about 20 miles per hour). If you come upon a lion, look at it without directly gazing into its eyes (focus on the feet). Slowly back away; if the animal is focused on you, talk firmly but calmly.

✲ ✲ ✲ ✲ ✲ ✲ ✲

If you come across a mountain lion, do not run! Mountain lions (who can run close to 45 miles per hour) can easily chase down a human (who, on average, can run about 20 miles per hour).

✲ ✲ ✲ ✲ ✲ ✲ ✲

More extreme measures need to be taken if the lion has an active interest in you. When a lion perks up and begins stalking you, you must act. Do everything you can to make yourself look bigger, including opening your coat or waving around your hiking poles and arms. Groups of hikers should huddle together and make noise, throwing rocks or sticks at the lion. Try to pick up potential weapons without crouching down. Do not turn your back on a mountain lion. Children and smaller people, usually women, should get behind larger companions. If the confrontation has gotten to this stage, aggressive scare tactics should repel mountain lions (who aren't used to having their prey fight back).

In the worst-case scenario—an attack—fight back with all you have. Punch, kick, swing, bite, scratch, and aim for the eyes or nose. Try to stay on your feet and get back up if you get knocked over. Mountain lion attacks usually come in one or two powerful waves; these cats are not endurance fighters. This is not universally true, however, as emaciated lions may fight to the last. Never play dead with mountain lions. This apocryphal defense only applies to some grizzly bears. A mountain lion will seize the opportunity of passive prey by administering a deadly bite to the neck. Climbing trees is another bad idea. Mountain lions are proficient climbers, and you'll only end up out on a limb. If you successfully fend off the animal, leave the area immediately. You'll probably be roughed up if you've survived an attack. Keep your guard up; patient mountain lions are capable of regrouping and finishing off wounded prey. Report any attacks to the local sheriff or wildlife bureau.

What to Do if You Encounter a Black Bear

Feared, hated, and reviled for centuries, black bears have earned an unfair reputation as bloodthirsty killers. They are nowhere near as aggressive as grizzly bears, yet they carry the burden of being associated with their ferocious cousins. Many are shy and will run away at the first sight of humans. Most conflicts occur in areas where human and bear habitats overlap (even then, bears are more prone to raid a garbage can than attack a person). Most black bear attacks are defensive in nature, with the attacker usually defending a kill or protecting cubs.

Black bear attacks are rare, but they do happen, most often when a hiker surprises a bear or comes too near a den with cubs. If you encounter a black bear, give it space. If the bear does not go away, you need to leave the area—even if it means missing out on a coveted summit. Black bears aren't looking to pick a fight. If you see them stand up on their hind legs, it is not always an aggressive action; they are simply trying to get a better view of things. If a bear becomes uncomfortable, it will begin growling, slapping the ground, or clamping its jaws as a warning. This is your cue to leave. Back away slowly and do not turn your back on the bear; as with mountain lions, look at the animal but not directly into its eyes.

One thing to note is that most of the audible and visible displays of a black bear are defense mechanisms designed to scare you off. Even the "bluff charge" where a bear runs at you while growling is more often than not a (terrifying) warning, telling you to get lost. In most circumstances, there is no reason to intimidate the bear. Quietly leaving the area is the best decision for both of you.

While their habits are somewhat predictable, that does not mean that black bears will never assault humans. When they decide to attack, they will not bother with the defensive behavior noted above. An aggressive bear may casually walk over on all fours without barking or growling, giving the illusion of a harmless saunter. A seemingly calm bear coming toward you is a threat. At this point, you must take measures to fend it off, including making yourself look larger. Yell out loud and throw rocks, sticks, and whatever else is around at the bear. Do not run, but slowly back away. Bears are excellent runners, swimmers, and tree climbers. Again, research has shown that most black bear attacks are defensive in nature, usually by a sow protecting her cubs. Measured swats or light bites that do not break the skin are extremely effective in frightening off intrusive hikers.

In the rare case of an all-out attack, fight back. As with mountain lions, do not play dead. Most black bears only want you out of their territory, and playing dead leaves you in the danger zone with a greater chance of being killed. Bear spray may give you peace of mind, but its effectiveness in real life is marginal at best. A determined bear will continue to attack through the pain, and you may end up blinding yourself in the confusion.

The key to bear safety is to avoid confrontations that may turn ugly. Be smart and respect bears of all sizes.

Tips and Common Sense When Dealing with Wildlife

- Always give animals ample space and respect. Elk, deer, and other "gentle" wildlife can attack if frightened or threatened.
- Never attempt to feed any wildlife, period.
- When scaring away smaller animals, such as marmots, aim carefully when throwing sticks or stones. Your goal is to scare them, not injure them.
- A loud whistle is a good first-line defense against animals that get too close.
- Be especially cautious when in close company of mountain goats and bighorn sheep. These encounters often happen on high ledges or ridges, where a well-timed head-butt could create a nasty fall.
- Report any animal attacks to park rangers or to the Colorado Division of Wildlife.
- Stay alert during dusk and dawn, as these are prime hunting conditions for predators.
- When hiking in remote areas, make as much ambient noise as you can, such as conversations, singing, whistling, and so on. In situations such as these, that friend who is an endless chatterbox becomes a valuable commodity. You want to make yourself known, so as not to scare any animals in the area. Bear bells are encouraged.

Additional Tips for Those Who Hike Alone

- Use a bear bell or other noisemaking device. I have two when I go out solo, and I secure one to each of my hiking poles. The natural motion of the poles makes them loudly ring out.

- Avoid using an MP3 player, iPod, or Walkman, especially in tree line.
- Leave a detailed plan of where you'll be hiking with a friend or family member. Include your route, trailhead, what gear you'll be wearing, and what time you expect to be home. Include emergency phone numbers to contact for the person keeping an eye on you.
- Remember to keep your first-aid kit stocked; it goes without saying that you should bring one on every hike.
- Stay calm during one-on-one encounters with wild animals. Even if you're terrified, maintaining a confident demeanor and dominant posture will help in confrontations with predators.

Trees, Plants, Fungi, and Flowers

Alpine Flowers

Alpine flowers are among the most rugged and beautiful in the world. Wildflowers bloom in every hue, often together in a single meadow. Seeing natural bouquets in remote mountain meadows is a treat even for the most macho of hikers. Of the hundreds of purple, red, blue, yellow, pink, and orange flowers, there are a few that stand out. My personal favorite is the whimsical elephant's head, a pink specimen that grows in watery areas between 8,000 and 11,000 feet. Flowers on the stalk resemble a totem pole of miniature pachyderms, each with a gleefully raised trunk. Mountain columbine, the state flower of Colorado, comes in a variety of shades. Columbine alternates colored stripes (usually light blue, purple, or red) with white petals that spread out like a parasol. Monk's hood is a popular purple perennial that is a relative of the buttercup. Indian paintbrush is a red or white flower that looks like a tussled thistle. In years of heavy rainfall, the "paintbrush" part of the plant may bloom fiery red. Other flowers of note include lupines, cinquefoils, Parry's primroses, wild roses, buttercups, spring beauties, larkspurs, white phlox, king's crowns, and marsh marigolds. A good book to consider if you'd like to learn more about alpine flowers is the budget-friendly *Colorado Flowers and Trees* by James Kavanagh, published by Waterford Press.

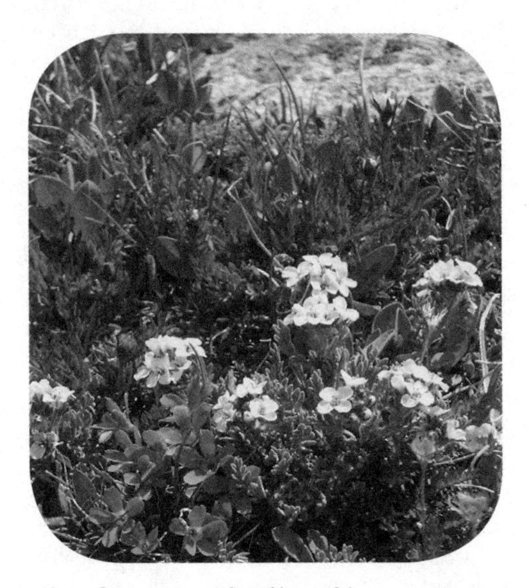

Alpine flowers are tough and beautiful.

One of the best surprises to be found in Colorado's backcountry are wild berries. Raspberries, blueberries, mountain strawberries, huckleberries, and blackberries are among the treats growing wild. Shrubs that produce such berries usually bloom in late summer, mostly in areas close to a steady water supply. Wild strawberries are a unique and succulent surprise, just edging out wild raspberries as my personal favorite.

Fungus among Us

Wild mushrooms are another mountain delicacy. Unless you are well-versed in mycology, however, never attempt to eat unknown fungus. Many mushrooms are poisonous and can make you very sick. For those who know what they are looking for, keep in mind that many wilderness areas require a permit to gather mushrooms. Permits are usually free and serve as a way for biologists to monitor the growth of certain mushrooms; call the park service ahead of time to find out more.

Areas with high precipitation, such as the central San Juans, host a variety of quirky mushrooms that make colorful decorations along the trail. The poisonous fly agaric is like a mushroom you'd find in a fairy tale, with its bright red dome speckled with white faux barnacles. Shaggy stems are yellow mushrooms that look like they were molded from fluffed custard. Giant boletuses resemble huge ground sponges in color and texture. Those in the know will keep an eye out for tasty morel mushrooms, prized culinary delicacies that proliferate in the wake of forest fires. (Connoisseurs will actually follow wildfires around the country, in hopes of scavenging a harvest of morels.)

If you are interested in learning more about Colorado's mushrooms, check out the Colorado Mycological Society's Web page at **cmsweb.org.** This comprehensive website has information on the different types of fungi and mushrooms growing in Colorado's mountains.

Notable Shrubs

Hikers have a love/hate relationship with the various mountain willows found in the high country. These are among the toughest plants on Earth and are the only widespread vegetation found in the high arctic regions. On the plus side, many willows color the landscape in autumn with tranquil reds and yellows. Occasionally they work well as emergency handholds, and dense thickets can provide shelter when fast-moving thunderstorms appear out of the blue. Their sturdy roots also help keep soil from being washed off steep slopes. On the negative side, many willows grow more than 6 feet tall and present a veritable obstacle course for bushwhackers. Besides being extremely difficult to navigate through in thick patches, the branches are scratchy, and their dense roots can disguise swampy holes just waiting to swallow your boots. Trying to navigate a willow patch in winter can make the most mild-mannered hiker explode in expletives, especially after postholing for an hour to hike half a mile.

As you ascend higher, you will encounter the group of thick, low-lying shrubs collectively known as the krumholtz, a German word meaning "twisted wood." The presence of these shrubs denotes the termination of tree line, which can happen anywhere between 10,400 and 12,200 feet in Colorado. Shrubs forming the krumholtz are incredibly tough; they had better be if they hope to withstand the fury of the elements on a daily basis. Versions of subalpine firs, Engelmann spruces, and limber pines are reconfigured in dwarfed proportions to better adapt to their harsh environment. They grow in dense outcrops, usually protected by rocks. Year after year, they endure weeks of subzero temperatures, hurricane-force winds, torrential downpours, and a very brief growing season. Although they may appear lifeless, many of the shrubs you'll encounter in the krumholtz are hundreds of years old. Be respectful of such wizened elders when you trek in alpine regions.

Topping out the list of high-altitude plants are the tiny alpine avens, a vital food source for resident pikas. Growing in small, dense patches, avens are surrounded by brawny, bright green stalks that resemble little ferns. Yellow or white flowers bloom in the summer and early autumn. Avens have developed amazing alpine adaptations: long taproots grow deep into the scarce alpine soil to suck up fleeting moisture, thick "hairs" protect stems and leaves from wind damage, and red pigmentation is used to filter out powerful ultraviolet rays and to efficiently convert sunlight into heat.

Major Trees

Conifers (trees whose seeds are encased in woody cones) dominate the mountainsides where conditions are favorable to growth. Engelmann spruces, Douglas firs, subalpine firs, and lodgepole pines grow in areas that are cool and have adequate water supplies. Drier regions (usually the sunnier south-facing hills and valleys) are more suited to ponderosa pines. Blue spruces and western hemlocks are other common trees growing between 8,000 and 12,000 feet.

Aspen trees are symbolic of Colorado's forests. They are deciduous (Latin for "temporary") trees, meaning they shed their leaves to conserve energy when cold weather arrives. Colorado's aspen trees are known as quaking or trembling aspens because of the way sunlight plays off their rounded leaves and because of the "shimmery" sound they make when the wind blows. Aspens are members of the willow family. Each stand of trees is actually one living unit, with every tree sharing a common network of roots. Trees that spawn from this network (known as clones, because they share identical genetic markers) live between 80 and 140 years before dying off and letting new trees generate from the root system. These roots go deep enough into the ground to resist the devastating effects of fire and avalanches; this is why you will see aspen stands rebound in areas affected by these phenomena, while other trees take years or decades to repopulate. Modern biologists have proposed the oldest living thing on Earth may be an enormous aspen stand in Utah known as Pando (see sidebar, below). The powdery film on the bark of aspen trees serves as a natural sunscreen; in a pinch, it can also work as a very basic sunblock for human skin.

Lower elevations find other deciduous trees: poplar, cottonwood, and balsam trees are common near rivers and lakes. Because of their fibrous makeup, these trees split poorly, rot easily, and are ill-suited for burning. If you are hunting for campfire wood, stick with the sappy (but burnable) evergreen trees or dried aspen logs.

All Hail Pando, King of All Living Things!

Pando is a fitting name for a great king; wouldn't you agree? Pando (Latin for "I spread") refers to an enormous quaking aspen colony located near Fish Lake in the Wasatch Range in southern Utah. Formed from a single seed, the "trembling giant" encompasses more than 107 acres and is estimated to be at least 80,000 years old. The trees that make up Pando are genetic clones that share a common, archaic network of roots. Trees that sprout from this matrix live approximately 140 years and are replaced by fresh saplings on a regular basis. Pando supports more than 40,000 trees!

Pando is considered to be a single organism; think of the individual trees that grow from the shared roots as being like hairs on a human head. They live, grow, and die—with the genesis of new trees from a single living source. While it is impossible to weigh such a massive growth, biologists say that Pando makes a great case for the heaviest living thing on Earth (in direct competition with the fabled redwood trees in California). Ideal climate conditions have helped the colony live for so long. Some biologists think Pando may be closer to a million years old. To put it into human terms: Modern man (*Homo sapiens*) came onto the scene about 40,000 years ago and migrated to the Americas about 10,000 years ago.

Pando's survival strategies have endured fire, ice, wind, and heat. Assuming water levels in Utah do not drastically change, Pando's reign could carry on for thousands of more years. Long live the king!

Safety in the Mountains

Altitude: This Is Your Brain on Thin Air; Any Questions?

Note: The following overview is not a substitute for attaining a deeper knowledge of altitude-related symptoms. Wilderness first-aid courses are great opportunities to learn more and are advised for those spending a great deal of time at altitude. Suggested reading includes *Altitude Illness: Prevention and Treatment* by Stephen Bezruchka, M.D., and *Going Higher* by Charles Houston, M.D., both published by The Mountaineers Books.

We humans have grown rather fond of oxygen. The air we breathe enables our intricate respiratory systems to relay oxygen to the vital organs of our bodies. At altitude, decreased oxygen levels cause the body to alter how it utilizes the invaluable gas. The series of adaptations that occur at high elevations are known as acclimatization. Simply put, acclimatizing allows your body to properly function when the concentration of oxygen in the air is reduced.

First off, it's important to know what happens to the air at altitude. "Thin air" is a layman's term used to describe the paucity of oxygen at higher elevations, due to lower atmospheric pressure. At sea level, oxygen levels are "compressed" by the weight of the atmosphere; therefore, at sea level, oxygen molecules are abundant. As you ascend higher, the weight of the atmosphere lessens, meaning the particles of air have more space to move around. As a result, less dense air will contain smaller concentrations of oxygen. Air circulating the summit of Colorado's highest peaks, 14,000 feet above sea level, will contain roughly one third of the oxygen found in the air at sea level.

People used to living at sea level begin to feel the effects of altitude around 5,000 feet. Journeys to higher elevations can provoke severe changes; life-threatening ailments associated with altitude have occurred as low as 8,000 feet. Knowing what is happening to your body is key to functioning well at altitude. A little understanding will aid in making each trip to altitude an enjoyable one. The most important thing to remember: Ascending slowly and avoiding overexertion are vital in adapting to altitude. And if you begin to feel bad—very bad—descent is the smartest decision and the easiest way to feel better.

How Our Bodies Adapt to Altitude

Our body has three major involuntary systems that change to cope with altitude, though how proficiently it does so is different for each individual. Rate of respiration, heart rate, and increased red blood cell production all work to bring oxygen levels to adequate levels when a person is confronted with decreased oxygen. Most obvious to the hiker is an increased rate of respiration. By breathing faster (even at rest), we are able to coax more oxygen out of the air. When respiration takes priority, simple tasks such as drinking from a water bottle or holding a conversation can leave one winded. Above 13,000 feet, it is normal to rest and catch your breath every few steps.

One's heart rate increases to efficiently pump each oxygen-reduced packet of blood through the body. Anyone who has felt the curious heart-pounding result from simple tasks at altitude knows that it doesn't take much to trigger the familiar throbbing sensation in the chest. Opening the wrapper of a candy bar or fighting with the stubborn cap on summit register tubes can leave one wheezing!

Red blood cell production is a much slower process than respiration and heart rate, taking approximately a month to fully adapt at a given altitude. For those spending weeks or months at altitude, this is the final step to being fully comfortable at high elevations. The more red blood cells present in the body, the more carriers there are for oxygen. Blood initially gets thicker at elevation due to dehydration. The blood remains thick as the body acclimates to the increased presence of red blood cells.

Other bodily functions are affected by these primary changes in body rhythms. Diuresis is inevitable; as the body speeds up, it needs to expel more extraneous fluid. Peeing a lot is not necessarily a bad thing. Urine color is a good indicator of hydration. Clear urine is a sign of proper hydration, while thicker yellow or foul-smelling urine is an indication that the body needs more water/fluids. It can be annoying if you're trying to get a good night's sleep, but not peeing a lot at altitude can be a sign that your body is not making the proper adjustments. (Don't be alarmed; just pay attention if this happens.)

Digestion can also be affected by altitude, as there is often not enough oxygenated blood in the digestive tract to break down fatty foods. As a result, appetites may diminish (though psychological factors may play a part in this too). Sour or acidic stomachs are common at altitude; regular antacids are helpful in making your tummy feel better. Increased flatulence is a comical (if you're a guy) side effect, though more discreet individuals (usually women) can find this a bit embarrassing. Hey, you're up in the mountains; let it rip! Farting can relieve pressure and actually make you feel better, so don't hold it in!

Along with digestion, you may need to go number two more than you would at home. This is normal; as things speed up in your body, so will your metabolism. Having to poop more is natural. Cheeky National Outdoors Leadership School (NOLS) instructors have dubbed the telltale light-brown piles of unacclimated hikers "NOLS gold." Lighter-colored feces are a result of nutrients passing through the body too quickly to be fully absorbed. A yucky side effect is the appeal of such nutrient rich piles to animals—that is why it is important to properly dispose of human waste. Make a hole at least 8 inches deep for human waste and cover it up; pack out any nonbiodegradable materials.

High-altitude edema or peripheral edema is a temporary swelling of the face, eyes, fingers, and ankles. This condition is more prevalent in women, though it will affect most people going up to 14,000 feet to some degree. A less scientific term for this condition is sausage fingers. By itself, it is not a threat, but an early indicator of other possible symptoms, notably acute mountain sickness (AMS). Again, there's no reason to be alarmed, but pay attention. Using hiking poles (which keep the fingers active in the act of gripping) can help reduce the possibility of peripheral edema in the hands. Prolonged peripheral edema can split the skin on the thumb and fingertips, sometimes below the fingernail. This can be a painful condition that makes some simple chores (such as priming a pump-pressure stove) difficult.

High-altitude edema or peripheral edema is a temporary swelling of the face, eyes, fingers, and ankles. Using hiking poles can help reduce the possibility of peripheral edema in the hands.

How Long Does It Take to Acclimate? How Long Do the Effects Last?

Full acclimatization takes about one month for most people, though most feel strong at high altitude (more than 5,000 feet) after three to four days. The rate of ascent is an important factor: acclimating from sea level to 8,000 feet is easier than adapting from 8,000 feet to 16,000 feet. If properly ascending, hikers in Colorado generally feel "normal" after two to three days above 10,000 feet. After approximately 6–10 days, your body will have completed most major high-altitude-related adjustments; it takes roughly 7–14 days to lose the major benefits of acclimatization.

Illnesses and Symptoms of Altitude Sickness

Just about everyone who ventures up to altitude gets a sampling of AMS at one time or another. In mild cases (which are most common), the condition is bearable, though a little uncomfortable. Slight headaches, nausea, loss of appetite, malaise (a vague lack of energy or ability to think clearly), and sleeplessness are common and can often be dealt with by using over-the-counter pain relievers. For fast relief (that has worked for me), Advil Liqui-Gels are tops—and I'm not just saying that because they gave me a free car! (I'm just kidding of course. My car, a mountain-beaten 1989 Honda Accord, looks like it was donated by Sanford and Son.) Aspirin, acetaminophen, or ibuprofen may work better for you. Mild AMS can occur anywhere between one and three days after arriving at altitude and usually lasts a few hours to two days, as symptoms gradually diminish. These conditions are generally harmless, but they do raise a yellow flag. If they do not subside, they could lead to more serious conditions.

Moderate cases of AMS are quite a bit worse. This is the worst condition I've experienced (read sidebar "The Bierstadt Incident," on page 24 for details), and even though it truly was a moderate case, I felt like I'd just gone 10 rounds with Mike Tyson in a room lit by 80,000-watt lightbulbs after eating a gallon of moldy mayonnaise. If you couldn't guess, moderate AMS is like a powerful hangover and is generally unaffected by most pain relievers (though antacids or Pepto-Bismol–type medicines may soothe your stomach). Moderate AMS is an amplified version of mild AMS: the headache is more intense, the nausea often results in vomiting, and even simple exertion can leave you out of breath. The only way to feel better is to descend. Going higher may be possible for stubborn souls, but it could cause the condition to worsen. Descending 1,000–3,000 feet will make a big difference and is recommended. (It may even rebalance the body enough for you to give the hike another go in a few hours.)

Severe AMS is no joke. This life-threatening condition cannot be ignored, as it may be a precursor to cerebral edema. All the conditions of moderate AMS are present, along with the following symptoms: lack of balance and muscle coordination, confusion, or severe mood changes. At this stage, people may become unaware of their surroundings and may become angry, hostile, or unintelligible. A good test is having them walk a straight line, similar to the sobriety test issued by the police. Rapid descent is your only choice; get the afflicted person down any way you can. Wait until the person is back to normal (which may take days, or not happen at all until you descend farther) to resume ascending, doing so with an eye on potential recurrence.

When diagnosing AMS, it is important to note that the symptoms may instead be signs of hypothermia (covered on page 31), fatigue, stress, dehydration, or nerves. A good rule of thumb: If the person isn't having fun (or can't tell you if they are or not), descend immediately.

HAPE and HACE are acronyms for altitude sickness in its most dangerous and deadly form. While both conditions are relatively rare in Colorado, both can happen as low as 8,000 feet above sea level. High-altitude pulmonary edema (HAPE) occurs when fluid from the blood leaks into the lungs. As blood struggles to adapt to altitude, pressure in the arteries (which is aggravated by exertion, dehydration, and cold) causes water and fluids to escape into the lungs. HAPE is a progressive condition. After several hours or days of undiminished AMS, the victim's condition may enter into HAPE. He or she will breathe rapidly, even when at rest. The smallest tasks will be exhausting and will leave the victim moody and tired. Often, even speaking becomes a laborious chore. If the condition is allowed to get worse, breathing becomes visibly frothy and audibly bubbly and is often accompanied by a dry cough that expels sputum from the lungs. The victim's lips turn permanently blue, due to the lack of oxygen traveling through the body. (Lips should be the same color as one's fingernail beds.)

HAPE is not a moderate condition; without immediate treatment at a medical facility, a victim can rapidly phase into unconsciousness and death. Descending will help, but professional medical treatment is paramount. Even with the best medicines, the decline is sometimes irreversible. It's serious business; luckily, it is fairly rare between 8,000 and 14,000 feet. In Colorado, most HAPE victims come from sea level and ascend to over 9,000 feet in a matter of hours (by plane or car), and stay there—or worse, go higher. Recovery from HAPE is normally a total return to the old self, though any occurrence may denote a propensity for HAPE.

High-altitude cerebral edema (HACE) is as scary and deadly as HAPE. HACE is a progression of severe AMS and is caused by excessive water swelling the brain. As cells dilate in a desperate effort to absorb more oxygen, the brain gets waterlogged. By the time your body is taking these extreme measures, it may be too late. HACE is characterized by severe confusion, inability to speak or function, inability to move, numbness or weakness on one side of the body, severe nausea, and severe headache. HACE shuts down a body at a terrifying rate: unconsciousness, coma, and death are the inevitable outcomes of untreated cases. Descent is imperative, and medical attention must be found for the victim. Even with treatment, permanent neurological damage may result. This is a rare condition for Colorado's modest heights, but people have died from HACE at as low as 10,000 feet. Don't be scared of it, but be aware of it.

The X-Factor at Altitude: Psychological Strength

Performing well at altitude is not all in the legs and lungs. One's mental state can enhance or impede the experience of being at high elevations. Hikers who are relaxed, strong, confident, happy, and positive experience few problems at altitude—and when trouble does occur, they calmly deal with it. Part of this comes from knowing one's body and how it reacts: experience in the mountains is a big plus. Fear, anger, and apprehension increase the body's overall stress level and can actually accelerate and magnify the symptoms of AMS (or even induce "phantom" symptoms such as migraines, nausea, or weakness). Because emotions are extremely personal and affect us in very individual ways, there's no way to universally prescribe how one should balance the competing needs of the body, the mind, and the psyche when making decisions. A few things to consider:

- Highly emotional people are likely to have difficulty finding the balance between smart hiking and overthinking things. Hiking partners can make or break a day in the mountains. My advice: When you find a good hiking partner, hold onto 'em for life!
- Whenever an unexpected stressor (bad weather, irritable companions, exposure, and so on) happens, I take five slow, deep breaths. It sounds corny, but it helps me center my mind and focus on what needs to be done.
- Though we often escape to the mountains to clear our heads, burdening and troublesome thoughts may make it difficult to perform well at altitude. High-altitude hiking, scrambling, and climbing require an elevated state of concentration, which is sometimes a pleasant distraction from these issues. Some days, however, even the mountains

can't purge these thoughts. Don't feel bad if you miss a summit because of a heavy heart; it happens to the best of us.

For some people, the mental side of hiking isn't an issue. For other more sensitive souls, a bad experience can make the prospect of returning to altitude an intimidating invitation. Take this into consideration when assessing why a hiking partner feels bad: sometimes a good joke or an encouraging comment can take the edge off and make reaching the summit that much easier.

Fitness and Altitude

Research on fitness and altitude is a mixed bag. Some sources insist that fitness has nothing to do with altitude sickness, though all agree obesity seems to be a catalyst for AMS. Fitness levels seem to have no impact on involuntary adjustments, so in a technical sense, it may be genetics or nutrition (or both) that determine the rate of acclimatization. That being said, stronger legs and lungs are undoubtedly a boon at altitude. Powerful muscles and leaner bodies will exert themselves less, thereby decelerating the effects brought on by tough physical efforts. Add in the psychological edge of knowing your body is mountain ready, and it's safe to say that fitness does play a part in adapting to altitude. The key for a newcomer to altitude is to keep a moderate pace, hydrate properly, and don't be a hero. Once you are adjusted, you can try all the pushups you want on the top of your favorite 14er. In the meantime, give your body the time it needs to adjust—no matter if you exercise infrequently or are an Olympic marathon runner.

Sleeping at Altitude

Oh, sweet sleep, how elusive you can be for those who seek slumber on high! A person's body continues to adjust to altitude, even if they're completely tuckered out. Even the most worn-out backcountry traveler may find sleep hard to come by. An increased rate of respiration inhibits deep sleep and promotes snoring—just ask your beleaguered tentmate. Also, having to urinate more will wake you from a sound sleep, often several times a night. In addition, you may feel your heart pounding for no good reason; other times you may feel as though you are suffocating for no reason. The strange, sometimes scary, irregular patterns of a companion's breathing may also keep you awake. An odd breathing cadence, known as periodic breathing, is normal at high altitudes and in most cases is nothing to worry about.

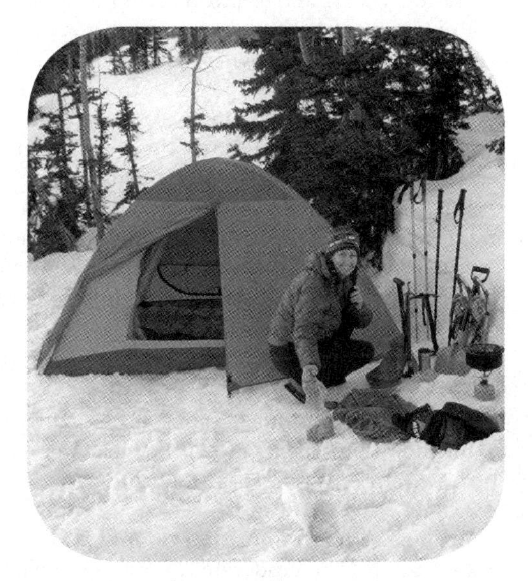

"Camp low, and climb high" is a good motto when acclimating.

The key to good sleep: Climb high, and sleep low. Don't attempt to sleep at elevations over 10,000 feet if you have just arrived from low elevation. Only increase sleeping elevation

It is my experience not to rely on prescription drugs—your body will naturally adjust and, perhaps, as is the case with muscle memory, get the knack of acclimating for the next time you visit high altitudes (this is a common belief among Russian mountaineers).

by 1,000 feet per night, once over 10,000 feet. Avoid caffeine and sugars before bed. As tempting as they may be, do not take sleeping pills. Over-the-counter pills decrease the rate of respiration and are detrimental to proper acclimatization. When you do fall asleep, you may have what the Sherpas of the Himalaya call the "sleep of the dead," a dreamless passing of time. More common are brief, incredibly vivid or erotic dreams, thought to be a result of rapid eye movement sleep while your body stays in a near-waking condition. Remember, a good night's sleep is essential to good performance in the mountains. You can get away with a day or two of bad sleep, but once your body is more comfortable at altitude, make the time to get a good night's rest.

Prevention and Treatment of Altitude Sickness

The golden rule for treatment of altitude-related illnesses: descend, descend, descend! In Colorado, a difference of 1,500–2,500 feet will usually alleviate any symptoms of AMS. If HAPE or HACE is present, descend as low as you possibly can. (For people living in high-altitude places such as Leadville—elevation, 10,000 feet—this may require leaving town.)

For mild cases, ibuprofen, acetaminophen, and aspirin can help relieve discomfort without having to descend. Antacids and Pepto-Bismol can help settle queasy and gassy stomachs. Energy drinks such as Gatorade and Cytomax can help prevent dehydration and restore sugars and electrolytes to the body.

Preventing altitude sickness is easier said than done. Ascend slowly and don't over-exert yourself. Out-of-towners should spend at least one to two full days above 8,000 feet before heading out to the peaks in this book. Locals in Colorado may be able to ascend and descend quickly enough to avoid any ill effects of altitude. Day hikes taken at a reasonable pace are often easier on the body than forcing a night's sleep at altitude. And one last axiom: Never take a headache higher.

It is my experience not to rely on prescription drugs—your body will naturally adjust and, perhaps, as is the case with muscle memory, get the knack of acclimating for the next time you visit high altitudes (this is a common belief among Russian mountaineers). However, for those pressed for time or hoping to bag that one special summit, there are some doctor-prescribed options.

Drugs for Altitude Adaptation

Always consult your doctor before trying prescription drugs. The medicines used for altitude adjustments affect the heart, blood vessels, and respiratory systems. Never "borrow" a friend's prescription unless the situation is life or death (HAPE or HACE, for example).

Acetazolamide is more commonly known by the brand name Diamox. It is taken to ward off mild to moderate AMS and to help facilitate sleep at altitude. Basically, this medicine helps the body balance pH levels in the blood that can help regulate respiration and aid in acclimatization. Acetazolamide is taken in advance of heading to altitude as well as while one is there; it may also be taken if AMS becomes apparent. In that sense, it is both a preventative and a cure. While it may not be useful in cases of severe AMS, it should be taken nonetheless to reduce the work the body has to do to get back to normal. For those coming to Colorado from lower elevations, acetazolamide is a good option that has proven to work well, especially at elevations of 12,000–14,000 feet.

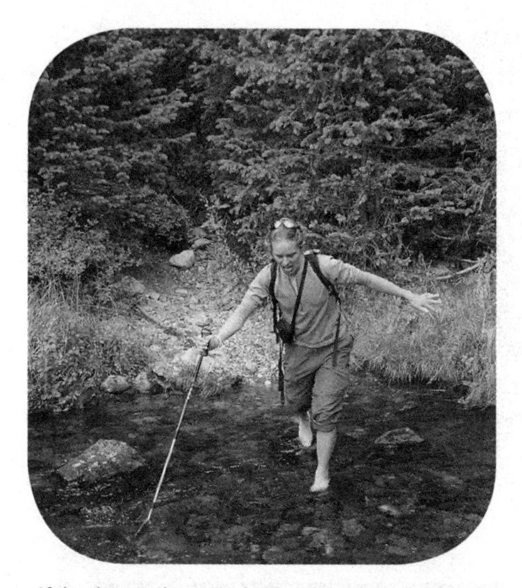

If the thin air doesn't take your breath away, the cold water might!

Dexamethasone is a steroid that is usually reserved for severe cases of AMS and HACE. It is often carried by mountain guides for use in emergency situations. If you are heading to the remote backcountry for a number of days with unproven or weaker companions, it may be wise to take along "dex" (available by prescription only) in case of extreme emergencies.

Nifedipine is used specifically to curb the affects of HAPE. This drug is rarely seen in Colorado, though it may be advised for hikers who have had previous bouts of HAPE at altitudes up to 14,000 feet.

Use of narcotics of any kind should absolutely be avoided. Speaking frankly, marijuana should never be used at altitude—besides impairing judgment, marijuana decreases respiration and can actually promote or worsen AMS.

There are other drugs prescribed for those with specific conditions, including issues with vision, digestion, or prior illnesses. The scope of this book does not cover individual cases—consult your doctor.

What the Locals Know: Eight Tips for You and Your Out-of-Town Friends

1) Even if your friend is a superman or superwoman back home, don't push them too hard at altitude. Chances are they won't let on how tired they are. Be tactful and make it seem like you are the one who needs the rest, extra drink, or snack break.

2) Pay attention to your friend's moods. A jovial pal who becomes quiet may be starting to feel lousy. Don't take an angry or edgy friend too personally; acclimatization can make anyone grumpy.

3) Ibuprofen is a good preventative for altitude sickness, for those who rarely hike or who may be trying a difficult climb in Colorado.

4) Offer to carry a little extra weight (or do so without your friend's knowledge).

5) Never downplay the accomplishment of climbing a Colorado mountain. It may be easy for you, but it may be a life-changing experience for your friend.

6) Likewise, if a friend gets sick, don't make them feel bad about it. As soon as it's apparent that going down is the best idea, concentrate on their well-being and try to get their mind on other things. Remind them that altitude sickness isn't a sign of weakness; it's a sign of too little oxygen.

7) Offer to take photos for your pal. Not only is it cool for your friend to see him- or herself on top of a mountain, it's one less thing they have to worry about if they are struggling with the thin air.

8) And one from personal experience: Don't ask them if they are OK 700 times on a single hike. They may be fine, and your insistent questioning may make them think they aren't. Most people will let you know if they aren't doing well, either by subtle hints or outright saying so.

Dogs at Altitude

Because animals are infinitely tougher than humans, it would be hard to tell if your dog was feeling bad at altitude. In general, dogs seem to be barely affected at altitude—many can be seen joyfully running up to the summits of Colorado's highest peaks. It's important to keep dogs hydrated and, of course, to keep an eye on their demeanor. If they become lethargic or struggle to keep up, it may be a good time to turn around. They aren't immune to altitude, but they are naturally better equipped to deal with it.

The Bierstadt Incident: A Personal Tale of Altitude Woe

Even though I've done extensive climbing over 14,000 feet, my one—and hopefully only—instance of mild AMS happened in Colorado. I was 22 at the time and chock-full of bravado. I had always fared well at altitude, so after spending more than three weeks at sea level in Maine, I figured that I'd be fine to go directly from my red-eye flight into the mountains. No problem.

I picked a mountain that has an easy standard route: 14,060-foot Mount Bierstadt. I made my first bad decision before even getting on the mountain. Instead of taking the easier standard route, I intended to climb an alternate way that started at 13,000-plus feet from the Mount Evans Road. It dropped down a gully, crossed a basin, and then ascended the mountain. My entire day would be spent over 12,500 feet.

It was indeed a fun route, well within my ability, and I felt fine until I was about 300 vertical feet from the summit. I felt my whole body go shaky and I became nauseous. I lost sensation in my fingertips and got very dizzy. I yelled to my hiking partner (who was about 50 feet from the summit) that I was going down. At the time, I felt he could have summited without me and then caught up with me on the way down; he decided to abandon the top and help me down.

We dropped into the low basin and I still felt OK; not great, but I was moving under my own power. Unfortunately, I had to climb 1,000 feet uphill via a loose gully to reach the truck. The turning point was when I tried to eat a handful of totally unappetizing imitation M&Ms. I threw up at the smell of them, and I bonked.

The hike up was no picnic; waves of nausea and spinning black fuzz in my peripheral vision enervated my every step. By the time I topped out of the gully, I had been dry heaving for over an hour and didn't have the strength to walk across a flat section to the truck. My hiking partner (who had already taken my backpack) went to the truck, dropped off the packs, and returned to piggyback me to the parking area. Grateful, but still feeling awful, I fell asleep on the drive home. When I awoke an hour or two later, I was back in Boulder and I felt fine. Not even a hint of the breakdown that previously incapacitated me was present.

I had learned my lesson. Even strong climbers need to respect altitude! From that day on, I was more aware of my body and took the time to reintroduce myself to altitude after visits to sea level. It was a rough lesson to learn (and it was only moderate AMS), but I'm a much wiser hiker, having learned it firsthand.

Weather: The Wild World above the Mountains

If one needs to be assured that mountain environments are untamed, simply look to the sky. Mountain weather is a powerful element of backcountry travel that must be respected. Predicting weather at high altitude is a difficult science. The factors that contribute to storms may not be evident until the clouds are already forming. This isn't to say that mountain weather is completely random. Storm trends tend to be good heralds of what to expect in a given mountain range or at a specific time of the year. While clouds can build up quickly, how they do so can offer clues to the oncoming weather.

(Note: If you want to be a storm expert, see Appendix D for more comprehensive resources on mountain weather.)

Why So Many Storms? How Mountain Weather Builds

From late spring to mid-autumn (prime hiking season), afternoon storms should be expected to roll in between 1 p.m. and 4 p.m. every day. Storms and lightning are daily threats during this time because of the temperature variations from night to day and the available moisture present. Nights are cool and promote condensation of water vapor in the air; after sunrise, heat from the sun initiates evaporation. As hot and cool air collide, electricity forms in the condensed clouds and continues to build throughout the day. At the hottest part of the day (often around 2–3 p.m. in the high country), the balance is tipped, and the storms unleash brief but formidable torrents of rain, sleet, snow, and hail.

If no larger fronts have been forecast, these storms usually run their course by late afternoon. Be warned: These storms often display the violent power of lightning, making exposed travel above tree line especially dangerous.

General Weather Advice

The proven best advice for safe hiking in Colorado: Start early! Beginning your hikes in the early morning (and in some cases, predawn) will ensure that you are back into the safety of tree line if storms hit. For hikes in this book, consider the estimated time and distance along with your own pace to formulate the best time to start, summit, and finish a hike. Being off summits by 11:30 a.m. or earlier is a good guideline. As you get better at reading weather, you'll be better able to tell if you can push it back a little later. As a side note, with almost all hikes, if I can't be on the trail by 8:30 a.m. at the latest, I'll change the summit from a goal to an optional bonus.

I'm not a big fan of dawdling on summits unless the weather is near perfect. Some people like to snack, nap, or recharge on top of mountains—even when storms are looming. If you have gotten a later-than-expected summit, snap a few pictures, and then descend to a safer locale to eat and rest—preferably in tree line.

You can use the children's rule of counting the time between lightning and thunder to determine storm distance: count the seconds between the sight of lightning and the crash of thunder and divide it by five; for example, a five-second count means that the storm is 1 mile away. Continue to count successive flashes and booms. If the time decreases, the storm is drawing near. If the time increases, the storm is moving away.

If you wake up the morning of a hike socked in by fog, it isn't necessarily a reason to call off the hike. If a cold front has moved in, it may rain and be foggy, but it can also ward off thunderstorms. If you are good at navigating in these conditions, it's worth giving it a try, but be warned: you run the risk of having storms build and having no real way of seeing them coming until that first flash and boom.

If you can feel or see electricity in your hair, the storm is forming right above you. This is an especially dangerous situation—if you're this close to the storm, it's advisable to drop metal items—such as hiking poles, snowshoes, ice axes, and so on—and recover them later.

Local forecasts are good general indicators, but they do not apply to the variable conditions at elevation. The following sections discuss such conditions in greater detail.

Be prepared for bad weather. I bring a sturdy Gore-Tex shell and light rain pants on every hike, even when the weather looks clear.

Reading the Clouds

Many of Colorado's days start off sunny and clear, often with a small smattering of clouds harmlessly hanging in the sky. As the sun begins to heat up the atmosphere, radiation and wind cause moisture to evaporate and rise. Air becomes less dense as it warms, creating lower air pressure—the perfect canvas for storms. Moisture that rises with the warm air eventually cools and forms clouds.

The clouds that form over the course of a typical Colorado day can cue you into developing weather. Cumulus clouds look like puffy, cottony towers that initially form as individual mounds. Their presence indicates that the cycle of weather has been set in motion, with moisture cooling on high. As long as they remain spaced out and their bottoms remain fluffy and white, you are in no immediate danger. When cumulus clouds begin to build and fuse together, the sky will become dense, with individual clouds being less distinct.

Be very wary of cumulus clouds if they begin to have dark, flattened bottoms and start to grow into towering pillars that reach high into the sky. When this happens, cumulus clouds transform into cumulonimbus clouds, which most people recognize as thunderheads. These powerful clouds are the bringers of lightning, rain, snow, thunder, and hail—it is very important to pay attention to cumulonimbus clouds, especially if it is after noon. A wise safety rule: When puffy white clouds begin to turn an angry shade of gray, it's a good time to assess your position on the mountain—cumulus clouds can build very quickly, forming storms from clear skies in less than an hour.

Be very wary of cumulus clouds if they begin to have dark, flattened bottoms and start to grow into towering pillars that reach high into the sky. A wise safety rule: When puffy white clouds begin to turn an angry shade of gray, it's a good time to assess your position on the mountain.

Other clouds you may see in Colorado include:

- **Stratocumulus** clouds resemble darkened cumulus clouds lumped together. Unlike the epic, storm-nurturing cumulonimbus, stratocumulus clouds indicate a cold front and precipitation, often free of lightning and thunder (but not always). These clouds are common in winter and during colder days.
- **Lenticular** clouds are the sleek, smooth clouds that arc like the bubbles in a lava lamp. These high-altitude clouds are indicators of strong winds and changing fronts; they often precede bad weather, which will generally arrive within 48 hours.

- **Nimbostratus** clouds form a uniform, gray cloud cover below 8,000 feet that creates fog and rain. It is often possible to climb above these moisture-laden systems to clear weather above.
- **Cirrocumulus** clouds are wispy, white, distant clouds that often form in flat sheets (such as the mackerel sky). These high-altitude dwellers form above 20,000 feet and are stabilizing clouds, meaning they carry no precipitation.
- Similar in form to cirrocumulus clouds are **altocumulus** clouds, which form from 8,000 to 20,000 feet. Altocumulus clouds have the same globular, wavy appearance as cirrocumulus clouds, but the white is interwoven with darker gray patches, indicating an oncoming cold front and potential storms later in the day.

Barometers Many people who venture into the outdoors have barometers built into their watches, GPS units, or other electronics. Barometers measure atmospheric pressure; as a general rule, lower atmospheric pressure indicates bad weather, while higher pressure is a sign of clearing weather. Keep in mind that atmospheric pressure drops as you ascend, even on the clearest of days. I've learned to pay close attention to the fluctuations in my barometer when sketchy weather begins to blow in—a fast drop in pressure nearly always means storms are coming. Barometers aren't perfect in predicting storms, but they do give you one more clue in predicting mountain weather.

Lightning Pressing your tongue against the terminals of a standard nine-volt battery creates a mildly uncomfortable shock that indicates how much charge is left in the battery. Multiply that voltage roughly 5,555 times and you have the power behind a normal lightning bolt! Anyone who has ever been caught in one of Colorado's brief but violent storms knows the fearful helplessness one feels when at the mercy of such a powerful and unpredictable adversary.

Lightning travels far too fast for a person to outrun and may strike several miles away from the visible center of a storm, even under clear blue skies. Many people only think about the most obvious danger from lightning: getting hit by a thunderbolt. While a direct strike is the worst thing that can happen, it's not the only threat. Splash strikes occur when lightning jumps from the initial strike target to surrounding areas. Ground strikes (or step voltage) hit the hiker from below as lightning dissipates into the surrounding ground. Contact strikes occur when a person is holding something that absorbs a direct strike, such as an ice ax or tent pole. Finally, shock wave strikes happen when a nearby bolt is powerful enough to generate a shock wave that can easily knock a large man off his feet.

Safety in Lightning Storms

Obviously, avoiding storms is the best practice in the mountains. Weather forecasts should always be referenced before heading out. However, even the most prepared and knowledgeable hiker can be caught in fast-building storms. I've seen storms metastasize from clear blue skies directly overhead in less than 15 minutes (and at all times of the day).

If you are caught in a storm, stay calm. You must assess the danger quickly and act accordingly. Storms don't give you time to factor in all the variables: if you need to seek shelter, it must be done without hesitation. Following are a few rules for finding relatively safe places in lightning storms:

- Stay away from water, including the faux safety in gullies and streambeds.

- Always try to get as low as safely possible, hopefully back into tree line or the lowest areas in open meadows. Never stand under trees in open areas—keep moving to safer areas.
- Immediately get off summits and ridges, even if it means diverting to an off-trail pocket of safety.
- If you smell, hear, or feel electricity in the air (examples: your hair stands up or your snowshoes start to hum), move down quickly! Even if your lungs are burning, move as fast as you can to safer places. Sometimes you have to suck up the pain and just keep moving.

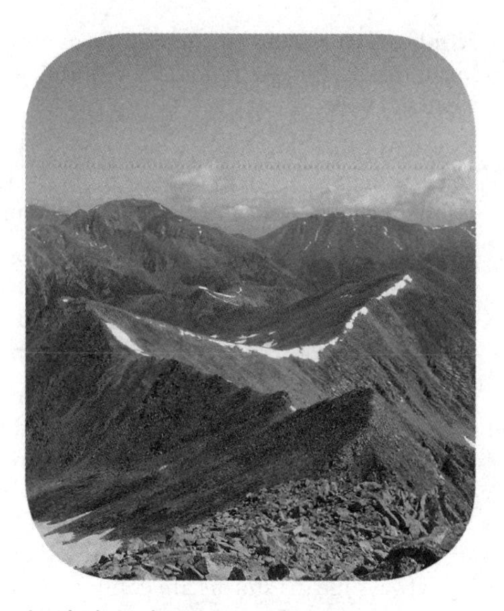

Avoid ridges when storms are brewing.

- Space out a minimum of 60 feet from your companions (think of this as the distance between a pitcher and catcher on a baseball field). If one member should get injured by lightning, maintaining this distance will keep other party members from being hurt.
- Stay away from metal objects such as hiking poles, ice axes, and climbing gear. Tent poles are especially dangerous—if you are stuck in your tent, make sure that you are not in contact with the poles and you are insulated from the ground on a foam pad or backpack.
- If you are stuck in the storm with nowhere to go, assume the safety position. Sit on a backpack or foam pad to protect yourself from ground-traveling electricity. Crouch down, but do not lie down (the idea is to minimize your surface area with the ground). If in the heart of a storm, sit on your pack and pull your knees close to you. Interlock your hands and put them over your head, resting your elbows on your knees. This last resort is known as the "Oh, s***!" position in most circles. Should lighting strike, it will course through your hands and into your legs, terminating in the ground. It sounds painful, but this position channels electricity through your body without it coursing through your vital organs. Lightning is especially prone to exit through the eyes or ears . . . not pretty stuff. For additional safety, feel free to consult the god of your choice while in this posture.
- The best shelter can be found in low-lying shrubs or trees. Avoid the highest patches or trees, and assume the crouched position while sitting on a backpack or foam pad. Stay a safe distance from companions. Pay attention to the progress of the storm and wait until it has passed for at least 20 minutes to proceed up or down.
- Caves obviously make great shelters, but be wary of "spark plug gaps" (gapped rocks that have an exposed or open top). These gaps actually attract lightning—look for better shelter if you can.

Lightning Strike First Aid

In the awful instance a companion is struck by lightning, it is imperative to act quickly. A body hit by lightning is not holding an electrical charge, so it will be safe to touch them. Any type of strike will often induce cardiopulmonary arrest—quickly check the ABCs of first aid: airway, breathing, and circulation. Cardiopulmonary resuscitation (CPR) should be performed if the victim has stopped breathing or has no pulse. CPR is an invaluable technique that should be known by anyone heading into the backcountry.

In a case of a "light" strike, in which the victim does not lose consciousness or vital functions, there will still be extensive burning that may not show up for many hours after the initial injury. Any tangle with lightning requires an immediate exit from the mountain and a visit to a hospital or medical facility. Call for help if possible, and evacuate the victim from the area as soon as you can.

Weather Trends by Season

Weather can blow in from any direction, any time of the year. I've seen lightning in January, snow in July, and hail on 80°F days. While anything is possible, there are some general patterns Colorado weather follows each season. These patterns can help you assess weather trends and make an informed decision when field forecasting.

Spring conditions (March–early to mid-June) Spring weather is often cool, bright, and free of thunderstorms. Days start cold and only warm up slightly, making early spring less prone to lightning storms. A bigger threat in spring is the danger of avalanche and rotten snowpack. As the sun heats up the snow, cornices become especially vulnerable to breaking off and triggering snowslides. Hiking conditions in spring often require winter mountaineering gear such as crampons, ice axes, helmets, and ropes. This is also the ideal time to attempt couloirs and other steep snow routes, depending on the stability of the snowpack. Late spring is a great time to hike, as many of the mountain flowers and trees are in bloom.

Start early (predawn on longer hikes) and be off summits by 11:30 a.m. There are only a few multiday storm fronts that hit Colorado each summer, so you should have a weather window most mornings to reach your summit.

Summer conditions (mid-June–September) Summer is the season of storms—but also of the best mountainside conditions. Nearly every day is punctuated by thunderstorms that roll in from approximately 1–4 p.m. Trails will be clear of most snow and the days are long. Start early (predawn on longer hikes) and be off summits by 11:30 a.m. There are only a few multiday storm fronts that hit Colorado each summer, so you should have a weather window most mornings to reach your summit. Night hiking is also a nice option in the summer.

Autumn conditions (late September–late October) Autumn is a very brief season in Colorado. As the weather cools off, storms become less common. Another benefit of cool air: It does wonders to keep a hard-working hiker from overheating. Beautiful colors emerge in the foliage during this season. There is less daylight and a better potential of snow (and of the rare but dreaded snow-thunderstorm). Autumn is perhaps Colorado's most enjoyable and safest time of the year to climb mountains.

Winter conditions (late October–March) Winter in Colorado is a beautiful and dangerous world. Summits are hard-fought prizes that require in-depth mountaineering experience to attain. Trailheads often require a monumental effort to reach. The skills required for winter conditions take years to develop and demand a hearty constitution. Avalanches, hypothermia, frostbite, and fatigue are constant threats. Personally, I love winter adventures, but they must be undertaken with caution and courage. This book mentions a few good starter peaks for winter hiking in Appendix A. For those robust enough to challenge the outdoors in the harsh months, a unique and hidden world is yours to discover.

General First Aid

Mountains in Colorado, even the "easy" ones, are rife with natural booby traps and hidden hazards. Seemingly stable talus fields roll under your feet when you least expect it; solid-looking snow patches will swallow your legs in shin-bruising postholes; rocks will careen down from above like Randy Johnson fastballs. Bumps and bruises are part of the game in the mountains. Minimizing your risks and beefing up your knowledge in case of injury are important factors to safely enjoying the mountains.

Note: This overview is not a substitution for outdoors-related first-aid training. I would highly recommend all backcountry hikers take a wilderness first-aid course and be certified in CPR.

Blisters

Nothing ruins a good hike quite like painful blisters (or a hiking companion who won't shut up about their blisters). Ill-fitting boots are the primary blister-causing culprits, especially new boots that have not been properly broken in. It's a good idea to wear your new boots around town before setting out into the backcountry. Leather boots in particular require a suitable break-in time to mold to the shape of your foot.

Water and moisture also play a role in blister formation. When feet are wet, the skin is softer and easier to blister. Bulky or bunched socks can cause friction blisters. Irritants such as pebbles, twigs, or debris in your boots can also be to blame.

Blister prevention starts with well-fitting boots. The toes should be a little less than half an inch from the end of the boot. Many blisters occur in boots that are too loose or improperly laced during descents. A single-layer, lightweight noncotton sock (such as Smartwool light hiking socks) helps keep feet cool and dry. Wool and wool-synthetic blends will wick moisture away from the feet. Cotton acts like a sponge, keeping moisture in the fibers and against the skin. I like to bring an extra pair of socks and a small towel in case I splash into an unexpected puddle. For hikes where there will be river crossings, I make sure to bring sandals or water shoes so my boots don't get soaked. For swampy or muddy hikes, a pair of Gore-Tex (or similar waterproof material) gaiters will prevent water/rain from seeping in above the top of your boots. If you are prone to blisters in a specific spot on your foot, adding a piece of moleskin or Molefoam can prevent abrasion before it generates a blister.

Blister treatment should be administered at the first sign of discomfort. Most blisters start off as hot spots, which are pink or red disks of irritation on the skin. Applying moleskin or waterproof, plastic tape can ward off blister formation. Avoid using

Band-Aids, as the non-adhesive part of the bandage will continue to rub against the skin. If a blister has already developed, do not pop or drain it. Ruptured blisters are breeding grounds for infection. Keep the blister intact; as long as it is not punctured, you will not risk infection. Cut a small circle out of moleskin and pad the area around the blister, leaving the actual blister exposed but below the level of the moleskin material (in other words, make the blister the middle of a moleskin doughnut). Tape the moleskin in place (covering the blister hole if you wish) with medical tape.

Only if the blister has already ruptured or is too large to comfortably continue hiking should you try to drain it. This should be a last resort. Clean the area thoroughly. Heat a needle with a match or stove flame to sterilize it. Once you have done so, poke a small hole in the bottom of the blister and gently squeeze the fluid out, top to bottom. Immediately clean the wound and apply a sterile pad. Wash the area out several times a day to ward off infection.

Dehydration/Overhydration

Dehydration is the most common ailment suffered in the mountains. Because hikers often don't drink until they feel thirsty, dehydration may not be apparent until the individual feels excessively tired or cranky. It is important to drink before a hike—about 8–10 ounces—and continue to drink roughly 8 ounces every half hour.

Dehydration is a catalyst for other more serious problems, such as cramping, hypothermia, and AMS. Signs of dehydration include a loss of energy, dark urine, and moodiness. A well-hydrated hiker should urinate frequently in the mountains, and the liquid should be clear and copious.

Sports drinks such as Gatorade, Cytomax, and Endurox will help replace salts and electrolytes; adding in a mildly salty snack such as pretzels or nuts can help replace salts, which in turn help the body process water. (Electrolytes are electrically conductive ions that help balance fluid levels on the cellular level in the body. This not only means feeding the cells water but also preventing overhydration.)

I like to bring 70–100 ounces of water in a hydration pack along with 32 ounces of Gatorade when I hike. I sip from the hydration pack all day and enjoy the Gatorade as a treat on layer breaks, summits, or snack breaks.

Overhydration is rare but something to look out for. Humans cannot process much more than 1 liter (32 ounces) of water per hour; excess water will usually be filtered out through the body. This process can dilute the nutritional absorption of food in the intestines. In other words, if you are dehydrated, there is no need to chug two bottles of water in five minutes; 8–16 ounces will be adequate. In extreme cases (usually during marathons or other high-endurance sports) water intoxication can occur. For most hikers, this isn't a threat.

Hypothermia

Hypothermia is a dangerous condition that results from a loss of body heat to the extent that core temperatures fall below 95°F. Prolonged exposure to wind, rain, snow, and chilly temps can bring about hypothermia. Many cases of hypothermia occur on rainy days, when the temperatures can be anywhere between 35°F and 55°F—so this is not just a winter weather malady.

Dehydration can speed up the onset of hypothermia. The initial signs of mild hypothermia include uncontrollable shivering, loss of coordination, and change in mood. Hypothermic hikers may not be able to zipper a coat or put on gloves, and they may not realize where they are. In their confusion, hypothermic victims may insist on continuing

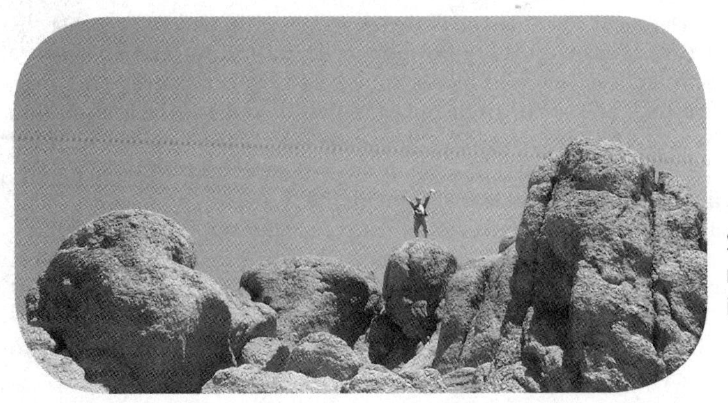

Storm-free days are a reason to celebrate in Colorado.

to hike or will agree to wait for other members of the party. Never leave a hiker who you suspect is hypothermic alone. In severe cases, the victim may become completely disoriented and collapse, unconscious. If core temperatures continue to drop, the victim may lapse into a coma, which can cause permanent damage or death.

Hypothermia must be assessed and dealt with immediately. First priority is to get the victim out of wet clothes and, if possible, out of the wind and weather. Often, layers of dry clothing, adequate shelter, and warmer settings will be enough to reverse mild hypothermia. The victim should consume liquids, preferably those with a sugar base. The liquid does not need to be heated, though a warm mug may feel good in the person's hands. The important thing is to get water into the body. If camping, get the victim into a sleeping bag and heat up water in watertight bottles to place in the bag. In an emergency, body-to-body contact will help, but care must be taken that it doesn't chill the person helping to a state of hypothermia. Warming should be done gradually.

Remember, hypothermia affects judgment and coordination—do not climb higher until you and your partner are certain the effects are gone. On a personal note, I once got mild hypothermia on a 60°F, sunny and windy day, thanks to a very steep snow slope and a poorly wicking first layer (which was brand-new). My hiking partner noticed that I was shivering, and moreover, that I was complaining—which is not characteristic of me in the mountains. When I peeled off the offending layer, it was soaked with sweat. Before the condition got worse, I put on dry layers and drank Gatorade until I felt better. We finished the day without further incident, but it goes to show, hypothermia can occur in unlikely conditions.

Intestinal Ailments, Giardia, and the Importance of Water Filtration

As the body adjusts to altitude, it often produces more acids in the stomach. Most stomachaches and nausea in the mountains are a direct result of the body responding to changes in elevation. Nerves can also play a role in upset stomachs. For these instances, it is wise to bring along antacids and to avoid fatty foods and alcohol on hikes. More severe nausea that does not respond to antacids can be a sign of AMS; if these are accompanied by vomiting, head down.

Diarrhea may occur if a person is overhydrated, nervous, or experiencing mild AMS. It is important to drink enough to replace liquids in cases of diarrhea; sports drinks and salty snacks will help replenish the body's balance. Because energy bars can be hard to digest (or enjoy) at altitude, I suggest bringing along palatable gels (I prefer chocolate Gu) to help replenish lost electrolytes and sodium.

All water in Colorado should be treated with a filter, purification tablets, or by boiling. That seemingly fresh mountain stream is prime habitat for the pesky protozoan *Giardia lamblia,* more commonly known as giardia. Giardia has a long incubation period, anywhere between one week and one month. Once infected, an individual will experience awful bouts of explosive diarrhea, flatulence, cramps, vomiting, and dehydration. These symptoms will settle down but still be apparent after an initial period of flulike symptoms. Giardia will continue to cause trouble until it is properly treated by a medical doctor.

Hygiene and Sanitation

Keeping clean in the outdoors can be a challenge, but staying hygienic is imperative. Good Leave No Trace practices (covered a bit more in the next section) mean you'll have to pack out any nonbiodegradable hygiene products, but staying clean is worth it. Alcohol-based hand-cleaning gels should be used after going to the bathroom, as well as before eating any snacks or preparing meals. Keep those hands clean!

On camping trips, I always bring along baby wipes (such as Wet Ones) to keep myself clean and avoid that "crusty" feeling. These wipes have to be packed out, but they can keep your butt cleaner than wiping with leaves or snow. Women may also want to bring similar wipes for staying clean during their menstrual cycle.

Be cautious when accepting snacks or drinks from strangers; the food is probably safe, but the hands of your new friend may not be.

When brushing your teeth, bathing, or washing your hair, make sure to use eco-friendly toothpastes, soaps, and shampoos.

Sunburn/Snow Blindness

At high elevation, radiation from the sun is extra powerful and needs to be taken seriously. High in the mountains is not the place to work on your tan. Ultraviolet rays from the sun are more concentrated the closer you are to the atmosphere, causing untreated skin to burn quickly. Avoid sunburn by applying sunblock with a minimum UV rating of 15 every 90 minutes. In real life, hardly anyone keeps to this schedule while hiking. I like to use a less precise but equally effective system. I keep a small bottle of sunblock in my pocket and put it on every time I stop for snacks, to pee, or to adjust my layers of clothing. Sometimes I'll end up putting it on three times in an hour, but it's better than getting burnt. Keep in mind that even cloudy days shower your body with UV rays.

Although you may not have an obvious lobster-red sunburn, even a subtle burn will make sleeping difficult, keep you from hydrating (as the body is repairing the damage), and make you feel achy all over.

Wearing a wide-brimmed hat, visor, or baseball cap will help keep the sun off your face. Although you may not have an obvious lobster-red sunburn, even a subtle burn will make sleeping difficult, keep you from hydrating (as the body is repairing the damage), and make you feel achy all over. Pain relievers will help you feel better and make sleep come a little easier when a sunburn is keeping you awake. Drink enough liquids to help your body heal. Lotions will help soothe burns and relieve the infernal itching that comes with peeling sunburn.

Note that hiking on snow doubles the amount of radiation being aimed at your body. It's not unusual to get burns on your palms, the roof of your mouth, under your chin, or other less noticeable places from reflected light. Make sure to apply sunscreen everywhere vulnerable.

Snow blindness is a painful, often debilitating condition where the cornea of the eye becomes inflamed; put simply, it is sunburn of the eyes. Once afflicted, the condition takes several days to go away. The victim will experience severe headaches, sleeplessness, and general fatigue. There's not much one can do to expedite healing, other than staying in a dark room and keeping up a steady dose of ibuprofen. I will say this several times in this book: do not skimp on good eye protection. Make sure your glasses are large enough to cover the entire area around your eyes, including the sides and bottom. Lenses must block out 95%–100% of all UVA and UVB radiation. Prevention of snow blindness is easy; recovery is not.

Heat Exhaustion

Heat exhaustion occurs when the body works up excessive heat that it cannot effectively dissipate. Dehydration is the first symptom of heat exhaustion; most cases are triggered by exertion in hot, dry environments. A victim will have cool and clammy skin, weakness, nausea, and may even faint. In extreme cases (known as heat stroke), the pulse will be rapid and the victim may become seriously disoriented.

Cooling the victim down and providing fluids are important steps in reversing this condition. Cease any strenuous activity, and rest, preferably with the feet elevated. Work on cooling the face, head, and body. Find shelter in the shade, or set up a tent (with the doors open) to provide shade if you are above tree line. Many cases of heat exhaustion occur when there is snow on the ground; use it to your advantage to help cool the victim. Once the person feels better and can hold down liquids, assess the situation. Unless the person is feeling 100%, descend and try for your summit another day.

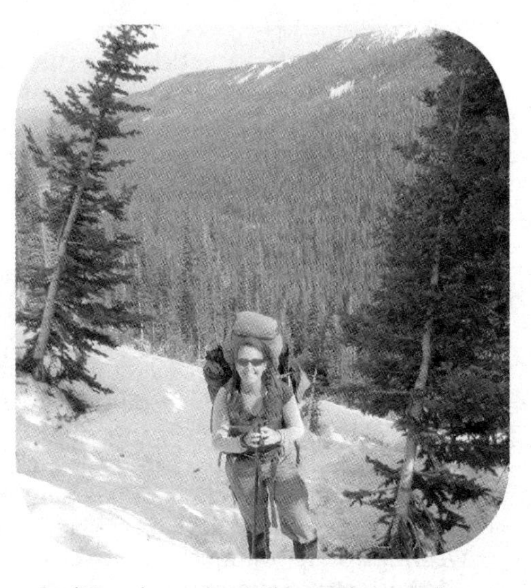

Conditions change drastically once above tree line.

Frostbite

Frostbite is a painful and serious condition in which the blood vessels in the body freeze and crystallize, causing damage to body tissue and circulation. Injury from frostbite can cause permanent impairments and, in severe cases, loss of appendages. Most frostbite will occur on the nose, ears, fingers, and toes. When the body gets cold, it prioritizes the areas close to the heart, leaving body regions distant from the core vulnerable to the cold. Initial symptoms include a bluish discoloration of the skin, sharp pain, numbness, and a burning sensation. If caught in the early stages (considered frostnip), warming the injured body part will prevent further damage. Note that frostbite rarely appears without hypothermia, so make sure to treat your victim for all conditions.

In severe cases, the skin will become blue or black, and hideous blisters may swell up. Never rub or try to massage frostbitten skin; this will only further damage tissue. Only a slow and painful thawing of the injury in lukewarm water will regain sensation. In these cases, evacuate the victim and seek medical attention. If the foot is severely frostbitten, do not attempt to thaw it in the field; once rewarmed, it will be too painful to walk on.

Note that women are more prone to frostbite than men. Poor circulation, diabetes, or overly tight clothing and footwear can also promote frostbite. Alcohol should also be avoided in cold conditions, as it can dehydrate a body and make the limbs less sensitive to the warning signs of frostbite as it develops.

Fractures, Sprains, and Broken Bones

Twisted ankles and sprained wrists are among the most common injuries in the mountains. Any swollen or bruised limb should be tended to immediately. SAM splints (soft aluminum splints lined with foam) or inflatable splints are lightweight and can be used to set and immobilize injuries. In a pinch, you can use hiking poles, sleeping pads, or an ice ax to set an injured limb. Anti-inflammatory medicines should be taken by the injured hiker, and evacuation should begin as soon as possible.

Shock

Shock occurs whenever the body experiences a sudden loss of blood pressure. Normally, blood loss from an injury causes this sensation, but people can incur shock (in the medical term) from witnessing a disturbing event or from sheer panic. Loss of blood pressure can disrupt the circulatory system and, if prolonged, can cause permanent damage to vital organs or death. A victim of shock may display any of the following symptoms: confusion, rapid pulse, clammy skin, dull or distant eyes, and rapid breathing. Additionally, the victim may feel nauseous, weak, and frightened. If shock occurs, do everything you can to keep the person warm. If they are conscious, provide liquids. Talk to the victims and reassure them that they are not alone. Be calm and help ease them by tactfully apprising them of the situation. Seek medical attention if victims experience shock—and always in the case of blood loss.

Panic

Mountains can be intimidating places, and for good reasons. No matter how experienced the hiker, the bottom line is that Mother Nature holds the trump card when it comes to control. Storms, stress, exposure to heights, witnessing an accident, or unexpected illnesses can induce panic. A panicked individual can "lock up," both physically and mentally. Fear can literally make one weak in the knees and impair balance and judgment, often in the places where concentration and focus are imperative. If you begin to panic, focus on taking at least five deep breaths. Remember, your body is reacting to a perceived risk—one that must be dealt with using logical thought. If you are on tricky terrain, breathe deeply and flex your fingers slowly a few times—assure your body that your mind still has control. Figure out your safest option and follow through with confidence. This advice is easy to dispense from the comfort of my warm office, but it's a bit more difficult to execute in the heat of the moment. My own experience has been that when you control your breathing, you control your mind, and thus control your body.

If you are with companions who begin to panic, talk to them calmly and reassure them of their options in simple, supportive language. Offer suggestions in a positive tone. Once the moment of panic is over (for example, a tricky move has been accomplished), continue to be reassuring and positive. Panic is one of those ailments that is really all in the head—which proves that mountain climbing is just as much about mental strength as it is powerful legs and lungs.

Suggested First-Aid Kit

Every hiker should carry an individual first-aid kit. In addition, groups heading into the backcountry should also carry a group kit with extra supplies or individual-specific drugs. Keep in mind that preexisting conditions should be known before heading into the backcountry and appropriate medical treatments should be included in your kit. Here is sample list of what every basic first-aid kit should have:

- ☐ Adhesive bandages (Band-Aids or similar brand): Minimum of 10 standard 1-inch bandages
- ☐ Butterfly bandages: to serve as temporary stitches for minor wounds
- ☐ Sterile pads: at least two medium and two large pads for larger wounds
- ☐ Antibiotic ointment packets or tubes (Neosporin or similar brand): to help wounds heal
- ☐ Roller bandages: to wrap around wounds and hold dressings in place
- ☐ Medical tape: to secure dressings or to tape up fingers and hands when climbing
- ☐ Moleskin: used to pad blisters or as a blister preventative
- ☐ Alcohol pads: used to clean small wounds. For large wounds, use soap and water with a syringe (alcohol will damage exposed tissues). Make sure to replace these pads in your kit every six months, as they can dry out even when left in the package.
- ☐ Iodine: used as antiseptic to clean out wounds
- ☐ Thermometer: used to gauge body temperature
- ☐ Medical scissors: used to cut medical tape or dressings
- ☐ Aspirin: used as a painkiller and also as a blood thinner (which may help with altitude adjustment). Avoid giving aspirin to children; instead administer acetaminophen-based pain relievers such as Tylenol.
- ☐ Ibuprofen: good old "vitamin I." Ibuprofen is an anti-inflammatory that is available under brand names such as Advil, Motrin, and Nuprin.
- ☐ Sugar packets or sugar candies: used for low blood sugar, notably when diabetes is present
- ☐ Elastic bandage (Ace or similar brand): used to compress sprains or similar injuries
- ☐ Sanitary pads: not only useful for female hygiene, but they also serve to absorb blood in larger wounds
- ☐ Rubber gloves: used to prevent infection from body fluids or wounds
- ☐ Sterile tweezers: used to remove debris, slivers, ticks, or glass from skin
- ☐ Syringe: used to wash out wounds
- ☐ Safety pins: various uses, including holding dressings in place
- ☐ Resealable plastic bags (Ziploc or similar brand): used to pack out contaminated materials
- ☐ Foam-lined aluminum splint (SAM or similar brand): used to mobilize a broken or fractured limb

- Antacids (Tums or similar products): used to neutralize stomach acids
- Laxatives: used to help with bowel movements
- Pen and paper to record accident vitals

Besides these things, I keep a small LED light in my first-aid kit; these lights are inexpensive and can come in handy when fumbling through your kit at night. Make sure you get one that doesn't require squeezing to light up—it's hard to dress a wound while keeping a squeeze light on. I keep two packets of energy gels for instances when a body needs fast, easy-to-digest energy. I bring an emergency reflective blanket to keep myself or a victim warm. I also leave two to four extra batteries of the appropriate size to fit my headlamps or GPS units in my first-aid kit.

A few other items to consider:

- Sunscreen
- Lip balm with sunblock (such as ChapStick)
- Hand warmers
- CPR mask/shield
- Small backup knife or multitool (such as a Leatherman)

People who have allergies to bee stings should carry epinephrine pens, which are available through your doctor. Other prescriptions drugs such as Diamox (to deal with altitude) should be acquired as needed from your doctor. Note that sleeping pills are not tolerated well at altitude and should be avoided.

Nutrition: Eating Smart

Most outings into the mountains will take several hours, so you'll need an extended form of energy to perform well throughout the day. Carbohydrates are vital for extended energy, while simple sugars can give you a boost of short-term energy. Fatty foods are difficult for the body to digest and should be avoided at altitude. Snacks should be eaten throughout the day to keep from bonking, a term usually used to describe the effects of low blood sugar or lack of fuel for the body.

What Works

Easy-to-digest foods—such as bananas, granola, nuts, dried fruits, peanut butter, and simple sandwiches on wheat/grain breads—are all good energy sources.

Eat what tastes good to you. If you like a turkey and mustard sandwich in normal life, it's a good idea to take it on your hike with you. Palatable foods are just as important as healthy foods.

Pasta and potatoes give a good boost of carbohydrates and serve well as a meal the night before a big hike. Breads, crackers, and dried fruits (raisins, for example) are good sources of carbohydrates the day of the hike.

Breakfast can be a tricky issue for hikers. Because your body is probably not used to getting up at the early hours required to get a safe start on the trail, breakfast may be unappealing. My trick for such mornings: If I am driving to the trailhead and my stomach doesn't feel like eating when I awake, I'll make a point to eat a peanut butter and jelly sandwich when I am 45 minutes or so from the trailhead. Delaying breakfast gives me time to wake up and actually enjoy the food instead of forcing it down.

Fruits are always good choices at altitude. Many have natural ingredients that help active bodies; for example, bananas have high potassium levels that help ward off cramps. Besides tasting good, they are good sources of natural sugars and there is even speculation that some fruits, such as pineapple, may help bodies adjust to altitude.

What to Avoid

As previously mentioned, fatty foods are tough to digest at altitude. Most junk food won't seem palatable at higher elevations because saturated fats and oils won't be prioritized by your body. Not only can fatty foods make your stomach churn, but they can also slow active hikers down by providing inefficient energy sources.

Coffee is a diuretic that can promote dehydration, though the psychological boost (not to mention the caffeine) makes a cup of joe a morning ritual for many hikers. Don't drink too much coffee on the morning of a hike. One cup should do the trick.

Alcohol is an obvious no-no during the hike, as it not only promotes dehydration but can also impair judgment. Save those celebratory beers for after the hike. In general, the effects of alcohol at altitude, both good and bad, are amplified. Consider this before partying too hard the night before a big hike—if you get a hangover, it's going to feel twice as bad at altitude and last twice as long.

Note that you may come across delicious wild berries on your hikes. These are generally safe to eat, but it's a good idea to wash them off with filtered water if you are unsure of their cleanliness. Remember, however, you may be doing yourself more harm than good if you rinse them off in rivers or lakes, as such water can carry giardia.

Gear

As much as I appreciate a good pair of lederhosen, I can't blame modern hikers for outfitting themselves in more practical (if less stylish) attire. Modern mountain fashion has evolved to be both functional and fashionable. Gone are the days when your average alpinist resembled a threatening, grizzled version of Jim Henson (with fewer teeth). Advances in gear technology are a big reason why more and more people keep heading to the hills.

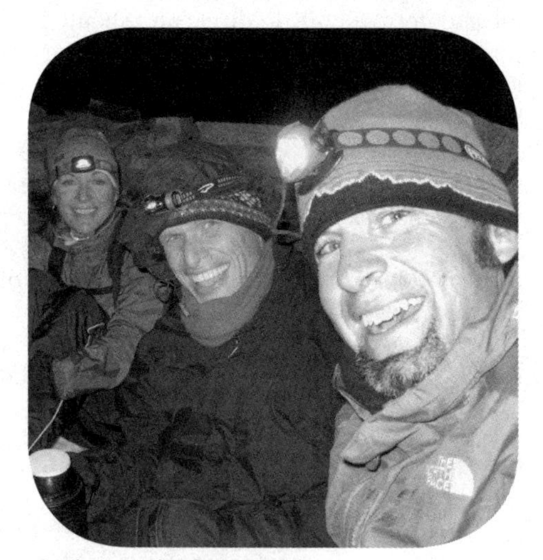
Good gear makes for happy hikers.

You don't need to have the latest and greatest in everything to enjoy the mountains, but I highly recommend not skimping on two vital items: boots and sunglasses. Boots are going to be what physically connect you with the mountain. Because you will be on your feet for many hours, you owe it yourself to get the most comfortable and functional footwear you can. Likewise, high-quality sunglasses will keep your eyes safe in the optically hostile environment of high-altitude sunlight. As a hiker on a budget, I'm reluctant to spend big bucks on trendy new gear, but keeping my eyes and feet in top shape is worth every last dollar.

Footwear/Boots/Gaiters

Boots are the most important pieces of gear for hikers. Proper fit, durability, and "grippy" outsoles (the tread) are essential qualities in a good boot. Different boots perform well in different settings, though with enough time on the trail, you'll begin to develop a penchant for a particular type of boot. Here's a rundown of mountain footwear.

Trail Runners Pros: Trail runners are running shoes that have been beefed up to handle trail duty. These shoes are lightweight and offer a bit more foot control, thanks to their lack of bulk. Many hikers (including me) like to use trail runners on mountains where there are established trails, dry terrain, or semitechnical scrambling. Cons: Trail shoes fare poorly in snow, mud, or other wet conditions. Avoid off-trail hiking and bushwhacking in trail runners. Talus fields and rocky gullies can awkwardly twist ankles; trail runners do not provide good support on such uneven and loose terrain.

Light Hiking Boots Pros: Light hikers are the perfect all-around boot: light enough to keep your feet from getting fatigued, tough enough to stand up to burly mountain conditions. A good light hiking boot starts with a solid outsole (such as Vibram or similar rubber blends) and is flexible yet supportive. Some brands use a Gore-Tex lining to make the boot waterproof without adding excess weight. Cons: Many light hiking boots compromise on outsoles; imitation or cheap outsoles wear out quickly and slip on rocks. Look for good outsoles and you'll be in good shape. Light hikers lack support when you're carrying a heavy backpack, and like trail runners, they may not be adequately protective on rocky scree slopes or in snowy conditions.

Backpacking Boots Pros: Backpacking boots are obviously great when you're lugging heavy loads; their sturdy design is intended to offer superb durability and excellent support. Traditional backpacking boots are made of hard-wearing leather, though newer models have cut off a few ounces by using ultraresilient synthetics such as Kevlar. Backpacking boots have great ankle support and are perfect for off-trail terrain as well as loose rock slopes and talus fields. Cons: Backpacking boots can be heavy, slow to dry, and tough to break in. Some hikers feel clumsy when trying to scramble or climb in bulkier boots, though climbing rock in boots is a skill that comes with practice. Ventilation is compromised, and hikers with hot feet may feel uncomfortable as their little piggies roast on long trails.

Mountaineering Boots Pros: These specialized boots are made for the harshest conditions. Most models are leather, leather blends, or plastic. They are extremely stiff and protective, thanks to sturdy shanks that reinforce the foot bed. Nearly all models have notches to accept crampons. Their rigidity is essential when climbing ice or technical snow with crampons. Plastic boots include insulated liners, and many leather boots have built-in insulation to keep feet warm. Cons: Mountaineering boots are made for snow, ice, prolonged mixed routes, and cold weather. As a result, they are very bulky, heavy, and require extended break-in periods. They are also quite expensive. These specialized boots are only required if you plan to attempt winter or early-spring ascents. Note that many backpacking boots and even some light hiking boots will accept certain crampons for basic snow travel. Ask at your local outdoors store if you'd like to try a lighter solution for simple snowfield travel.

Along with good boots, you're going to need a high-quality pair of socks. Your socks should fit without bunching and have padding in high-friction areas, such as the toes. Avoid cotton socks because they absorb moisture and keep sweat against your skin. Most hiking socks are made of high-quality wool such as merino wool or a wool/synthetic blend. There is no need to layer socks—modern socks wick moisture from the feet and dry relatively quickly, eliminating the need for a liner. As a hot-footed hiker, I use thin wool running socks for most hikes.

A neglected piece of "footwear" is a useful pair of gaiters. Gaiters are knee-high leggings that fit over boots and keep snow, water, and debris from leaking in above the cuff of the boot. Gaiters are ideal in muddy or snowy conditions, which are typical in early spring. The ever-stylish shorts-with-gaiters look is a telltale sign of a transplanted New England hiker.

Because I am often asked about the footwear I use, here are the facts, current as of the writing of this book. I wear Salomon XA Pro trail runners, Tecnica Vento Mids as my light hikers, and a pair of beautifully crafted, all-leather, lined-with-Gore-Tex Aku Utah Lite GTX backpacking boots.

Eyewear

High-altitude sun is especially harmful to our eyes, which is why I highly recommend tossing that adorable pair of Hello Kitty shades for something a bit more mountain worthy. Good mountain sunglasses will have lenses that block out 95%–100% of UVA and UVB rays. Make sure that your lenses don't distort your depth perception, a common feature of cheap sunglasses. Also ensure that peripheral light is adequately shielded. Frames should fit comfortably on your head; glasses that are too tight can form friction sores behind the ears (ouch!). Finally, secure your glasses with a tether (such as Croakies) to prevent them from falling off in case of a slip.

Layers

Dressing in layers instead of a single garment is standard practice in the mountains. Temperatures fluctuate at various points in a single hike, from the hot sun in the parking lot to the chilly gusts on summit ridges. A simple system of layers will help keep you comfortable in every weather condition.

Technical hiking clothes aim to keep you dry and warm. The ability of fabrics to wick and draw moisture away from the skin allows garments to dry quickly and prevent chills from your own sweat. Here's a rundown of a good layering system:

First layer: Thin, lightweight, and nice to the touch. Your first layer rests against your skin, so it should fit well and dry quickly. Cotton is a no-no for the upper body (read the sidebar "Cotton Kills?" opposite); it does not wick and can make you very cold. An adequate quick-drying shirt is usually made of synthetic fibers, such as polypropylene or Capilene. Old-school hikers may prefer silk, which is functional but gets very smelly after a few uses. For the lower body, go with underwear that is comfortable. Synthetic, wicking underwear is available in both short and long versions. If you are not donning long underwear, cotton briefs are acceptable (especially for women, who find that cotton ventilates better). Or you can always go commando and not wear any undies at all.

Second layer: This is your insulating layer. Fleece jackets are a great choice, especially microfleece and Windstopper garments. Vests can help keep your core warm and are easy to stuff in your backpack. For the lower body, nylon or synthetic fabric shorts or pants will do just fine. Zip-off pants that convert into shorts are popular and practical. Avoid cotton jeans and other cotton pants, as they will keep moisture next to you body.

Third layer: In colder weather, bringing along a down or thick fleece jacket is a good idea. Keep in mind that it can snow in any month in Colorado, so if there are storms forecasted, it's not a bad idea to bring an extra layer of warmth any time of year.

Outer shell layers: Complement your layering system with a waterproof, windproof shell. Gore-Tex or equivalent shell fabrics will keep you dry while allowing heat and water vapor from the inside to vent. For pants, lightweight, water-resistant garments are acceptable unless you intend to glissade on snow, in which case, you'll want something tougher. Gore-Tex pants with reinforced knees and butts are perfect for glissading.

Cotton Kills?

Perhaps "cotton kills" is a bit overdramatic, but it's not entirely off the mark. Cotton is hydrophilic, meaning it loves to absorb water. This makes it a poor choice to wear when you're working up a sweat in the mountains. Heat loss is rapid when moisture is present, and cotton garments keep sweat against your skin, making your body work harder to heat up and stay warm. Cotton garments that get saturated can chill a body, even in mild temperatures, bringing on dangerous hypothermia. In this regard, cotton can indeed be a catalyst to life-threatening conditions.

Cotton should be avoided as an upper-body layer in all cases, especially against the skin. The same goes for cotton jeans, pants, and shorts. The only place cotton is acceptable on a hiker's body is over your naughty bits. Cotton briefs and panties are fine because you won't be sweating excessively in these areas. (Or, as many hikers prefer, don't wear underwear at all.) Finally, avoid wearing the classic cotton waffle weave long underwear so popular in the Midwest; you'll essentially be wearing a skintight sponge.

Backpacks

Backpacks for day hikes should be able to carry all your gear and food. A volume of 1,800–2,500 cubic inches will give you enough room to stuff everything in. A good pack will fit comfortably on the back. Most will have adjustable shoulder straps, a waist belt, and a chest strap. Another good feature of many packs: an inner hydration sleeve to hold a water bladder (such as a CamelBak). A backpack made of high-quality, abrasion-resistant material will be more wear-resistant and may even give curious marmots a challenge when they try to gnaw their way to your M&Ms.

Hydration Systems

I'm a big fan of hydration systems. CamelBaks and similar systems let you hydrate without stopping, meaning you can take small sips throughout the day without much effort. Water bladders of 70–100 ounces should suffice for day hikes in Colorado. The one drawback with hydration systems is that they freeze easily. When hiking in temps at or near freezing, blow water from your straw back into the bladder to keep the tube from freezing solid. Tube and bladder insulators are available, but for extremely cold weather, you're better off using water bottles and insulated holders.

Headwear/Neck Gaiters

Baseball caps, visors, and wide-brimmed hats are great for keeping sun off your face and are recommended at elevation. Cotton baseball caps and visors are OK, but for winter-style caps, go for fleece, wool, or wool blends. Soft fleece neck gaiters are a secret weapon in staying warm. While it's true that you lose a great deal of heat through your head, you also lose a good percentage of warmth through your neck. Keep it warm with a neck gaiter.

Gloves

Gloves can be layered for effective warmth. Thin liner gloves are often warm enough to keep your hands comfortable on windy days. Shell gloves are needed for colder weather or when traveling on snowfields. For really chilly conditions, use a mitt instead of a glove (keeping the fingers together keeps them warmer), along with a waterproof, windproof shell. Convertible mitts that pull back to allow the fingers to perform dexterous tasks are useful as well.

Navigation and GPS

Paper maps are a must for every hike, as well as basic knowledge in using a compass. Because electronics can fail, you need to have a reliable manual system to navigate vast landscapes. Dense forests and barren tundra are prime venues for people to become disoriented. That said, I am a huge proponent of GPS navigation. Today's GPS systems are accurate and affordable, and most have improved battery life and satellite locking. Integrating a GPS with your computer can help you track out hikes or examine your stats when you are finished. This book is very GPS-centric. For tracking the hikes in this book, I used two Magellan eXplorist 600 units, an older Magellan Meridian Platinum for backup, and a basic Magellan eXplorist 100 for super backup. When fully equipped, I resembled a deranged, bird-watching cyborg. More detailed explanations on using GPS with this book are given on page 47.

Besides triangulating your position on Earth, many GPS units offer additional helpful information such as elevation, distance traveled, barometric pressure, time of day, elevation maps and contours, temperature, bearing, and heading. More advanced units also have accurate compasses and storm-warning features. GPS units are fun and functional, and they add a margin of safety to the hiker who knows how to use them.

Watches

Keeping track of the time is important to ensure that you elude the inevitable afternoon thunderstorms. Most watches will function perfectly fine at altitude. If you are using a watch that measures altitude and barometric pressure (most watches use barometric pressures to determine altitude, so you will probably have both functions), make sure to calibrate your watch at the beginning of your hike. All hikes in this book have an accurate starting elevation that you can use to set your watch's altimeter.

Useful Extras

Here's a short list of a few additional items you may find helpful in the outdoors:

Trekking poles: Amazingly, the most-asked question I've gotten on hikes is whether or not I like using my trekking poles. I love 'em! I know they aren't for everyone, but they suit me well. Besides stabilizing my hiking, they help me set a good cadence. I use them to test snow and water depths, and in a pinch, I've used them to scare away animals. Some people find them cumbersome, but I recommend giving them a try—I rarely hike without mine.

Cell phones: We are all aware of the egregious faux pas of calling your friends and family from the summit—"Guess where I am!"—right? OK, maybe I'm being a bit harsh. Actually, cell phones are good to have in case of emergencies, though getting signals in the backcountry can be spotty. For solo hikers, calling to report you are safely off a mountain will alleviate the worry of your anxious friends.

Sandals or water shoes: Bring these along if you anticipate water crossings. The last thing you want is to slog around for hours in waterlogged boots.

Minitripods: For exquisite mountain photography, tripods are the way to go. Small, inexpensive, and lightweight tripods are perfect for summit shots. These smaller 'pods fit easily into the side pouches of backpacks.

Extra cords/straps: I like to carry a small length of cord on the topmost loop strap on my backpack. In scrambling situations on sketchy terrain, I'll use it to lower my backpack. It can be unnerving when an outcrop of rock nudges you outward while you're attempting a tricky move. Taking off the pack and sending it down first is a safe and smart idea.

There are countless other situations where extra cord is useful, especially when camping in the backcountry.

Cameras

When the first edition of *Best Summit Hikes* came out in 2007, the transition from film to digital cameras was just about complete. In the years since, digital has fully taken over, and mountain photography has never been easier. It won't be long before the dedicated digital camera is replaced by high-quality smart phones, many of which already take excellent photos.

There will always be a place for high-end photography in the mountains, but for most of us, a decent point-and-shoot will do the trick (most of the photos in this book were taken with point-and-shoot cameras). I suggest buying an extra battery/batteries for your camera when spending time in the mountains. Portable, small, and lightweight solar rechargers are perfect for multiday outings, and you can pick up a decent one for around $100.

Hiking Ethics

The 10 Essentials

This long-standing list has withstood the test of time. These survival items should be in your pack every time you head into the backcountry:

1) Complete basic first-aid kit, with items updated every six months
2) Map and compass
3) Pocketknife and emergency whistle
4) Matches and fire starter
5) Emergency bivy sack/blanket/shelter
6) Flashlight or headlamp
7) Clothing for warmth and for rain protection
8) Extra food
9) Extra water
10) Sun protection

The ever-important "11th essential" is a hiking companion, though I don't recommend trying to stuff him or her into your backpack—unless the person is really tired.

Leave No Trace

Leave No Trace ethics promote a system of keeping wilderness areas pristine by minimizing human impact. There are eight basic tenets in Leave No Trace travel:

1) Plan ahead and prepare.
2) Travel and camp on durable surfaces.
3) Dispose of waste properly.
4) Leave what you find.
5) Minimize campfire impact.
6) Respect wildlife.
7) Be considerate of other visitors.
8) Pack out what you pack in.

In addition to these rules, I would suggest picking up any trash you find along the trail and pack it out.

Trail Ethics

When out on the trail, you'll meet all manner of man and beast. It's important to be respectful of the land, the wildlife, and other hikers. Here's a simple list of 10 things you can do to maintain courtesy in the backcountry:

1) Greet other hikers with at least a smile. On crowded peaks, you may be smiling a lot, but there's nothing wrong with that, is there?

2) Be tactful before offering unsolicited advice. Most people will ask for help if they need it when in the mountains.

3) No matter how friendly your dog is, if he jumps on strangers or insists on thrusting his snout into their groins, keep him on a leash!

4) If someone needs help, help them. It sounds logical, but I've seen many people refuse to help others in need for whatever reason. Of course, if you are traveling solo (especially if you're a woman), use your best judgment before committing to helping others. Unfortunately, that's the way of the world.

5) Always yield to uphill hikers and don't be offended if they don't say hi. It's tough work climbing at altitude—give them room to maintain their pace.

6) Yield to horses and bikers. And don't step aside with a scowl; they will pass in a few seconds.

7) Don't be afraid to tell new trail friends that you would like to hike alone (or with your partner). Likewise, respect the wishes of others you may meet on the trail. Remember, many people embrace the solitude found in the mountains.

8) Encourage other hikers and keep a positive tone.

9) Never downplay other hikers' accomplishments, and never speak in condescending tones. Boasting that you hike Mount Elbert as a warm-up is obviously going to deflate the hiker who trained all winter to reach the top. We all climb for different reasons.

10) Finally, don't take out your frustrations on your hiking partners. If you don't feel good, or if it's not your day, say so. Alert your partners if you are starting to feel off or ill. Good communication will make every outing a better experience.

Using This Book

My goal in writing this book was simple: provide accurate information for the best summit hikes in Colorado in an enjoyable-to-read format. All of the standard routes in this book are nontechnical and may be climbed without ropes or protection, though some sections may require scrambling and exposed moves. Although I provide a difficulty rating system, I always say there are no "easy" mountains in Colorado. Because of the variable nature of weather and the influence of altitude, even a short hike with mild terrain can be difficult for the uninitiated hiker. Likewise, a technical scramble may be less taxing on your legs and therefore be easier on your body. Be ready to sweat, no matter where you hike . . . and bring your camera. These are truly the best summit hikes in Colorado!

Driving Directions

I find clear, concise driving directions of the utmost importance—starting a day late and frustrated because you couldn't find the trailhead is not only annoying, but it can also take you out of a safe weather window. I put extra time and effort into writing my directions, and I hope they will get you to the trailhead with ease. Because backcountry roads can change, I encourage readers to call ahead to see if conditions are suitable for your vehicle.

Vehicle Recommendations

In describing the types of vehicles that can reach certain trailheads, I've added notes for those of us who don't have 4x4, high-clearance trucks (48 of the 50 hikes in this book were driven to in a front-wheel drive Honda Accord). When I mention the types of vehicles needed to reach the trailheads, here is what I mean:

Passenger Car (PC): Passenger cars are any vehicle with low clearance and without off-road modifications. In this regard, minivans are often included in this class. Trailheads that have easy access via a paved road or well-maintained dirt roads are perfect for cars.

Tough Passenger Car (TPC): This is a politically correct way to describe a beater, a vehicle you aren't afraid to sacrifice a few parts of to reach a trailhead. My car fits this bill perfectly. Trailheads that TPCs can reach are generally passable but may have a few areas where your car will bottom out or have to blast through mud and water. My Honda Accord made it up some wild roads during the research for this book, including the access roads to Pacific Peak and the "shelf of horror" on Mount Sneffels. I'm not saying that you should drive your car as if it were a TPC, but the odds of reaching the trailhead are in your favor if you have the guts (and don't mind a few bangs and bumps). Good luck and Godspeed!

Sport Utility Car (SUC): Sport utility cars describe any light-duty, off-road vehicle with decent clearance. All-wheel drive (AWD) or 4x4 transmissions are standard for most of these vehicles. (Note that AWD drive is inferior to true 4x4. AWD uses power transfers to relegate a certain amount of available torque to whatever wheel can best use it, while 4x4 spreads an even amount of torque over all four wheels, giving them each power and traction at all times.) SUCs can handle mildly rutted roads, relatively steep terrain, and some rocky roads, though those without a "low" 4x4 option may have trouble. I've seen SUCs at trailheads where I am convinced that they must have been dropped off by helicopter (such as on Uncompahgre Peak). Examples of this type include Subaru Outback, Toyota RAV4, Honda CRV, Honda Element, Ford Escape, and small pickup trucks.

Sport Utility Vehicle (SUV): It may be odd to see these lawyer-pleasing behemoths beyond the familiar confines of the Starbucks parking lot, but most SUVs actually perform well in the backcountry. SUVs can tackle most rugged terrain, though many lack the high clearance to navigate tougher or more remote roads. Examples include Ford Explorer, Honda Ridgeline, Jeep Grand Cherokee, Nissan Pathfinder, and Chevy Blazer.

4x4 High-Clearance Trucks (4x4): These are vehicles specifically designed for the rigors of rocky, rough, and steep roads. These trucks or Jeeps have high ground clearance, true 4x4 transmissions (usually with both four high and four low settings), rugged suspension, tough tires, and strong engines. These vehicles can make it up almost every road and are required for one of the best hikes in this book, Storm King Peak in the Grenadiers (Hike 45). (There is only one hike in this book for which a 4x4 would not be able to get to the end of the road: Mount Blanca.) Examples include Toyota Tacoma, Jeeps of the CJ series (Wrangler, Rubicon, and so on), Dodge Ram trucks, Nissan Frontier, Nissan Xterra, and Chevy Silverado.

Modified 4x4: These amazing machines have been customized with huge tires, reworked suspensions, powerful engines, roll cages, and increased torque to get over anything in their way. Clever adaptations such as winches and independent tire-control mechanisms help these modified monsters succeed on 4x4 roads. Most of these vehicles are purely recreational, and very few are street legal. They are the only vehicles that have a shot of making it up the awesome test piece road that leads up to Mount Blanca.

GPS

Just thinking about the complexity of satellites in space beaming information down to a cool little handheld receiver makes me feel like James Bond. While Global Positioning System (GPS) units are undoubtedly valuable tools for tracking eclectic supervillains, I tend to use mine purely for wilderness navigation.

The hikes in this book have all been tracked and mapped using GPS. You don't need a GPS to use this book, but you will find it a nice complement to the information provided in each chapter. One thing to consider: Even the best GPS units have a slight margin of error that may conflict with the data collected on your personal GPS. (Note that this same margin of error is noted in many traditional cartographic techniques as well.) When using GPS, it's important to give the technology leeway for slight differences. Government standards on GPS satellites create an intentional margin of error for commercial units, though this discrepancy has been reduced in most modern receivers to plus or minus 30 feet.

Ratings

Round-Trip Distance: This is the total mileage you will be hiking over the entire route. Remember, hike distance is not an indicator of how easy or difficult your trip will be—some of the hikes in this book that are a mere 5.0 miles are many times more difficult than those double that length.

Hiking Time: The low end of estimated hiking times (for round-trip distances) are my personal hike times, including time taken for photography, snack breaks, and bathroom breaks. My estimates are meant to provide a good idea of what the average hiker can expect as a time investment: they are not meant to judge ability or fitness. Less experienced hikers should expect to complete the hikes in the upper range of the times given, while strong hikers will probably complete the hikes in less time than the estimates.

Difficulty: I have rated the hikes on a scale of 1–10, with 1 being the easiest. None of the hikes in this book requires ropes, so the difficulty is relatively based on the challenge of nontechnical scrambles and hikes. Elements that contribute to the difficulty include steepness, route finding, distance, terrain, on-trail/off-trail, scrambling difficulty, and exposure. Not included in difficulty ratings are seasonal tribulations such as ice, snow, and high-river crossings (though such conditions are noted when the prime hiking time is during a specific season).

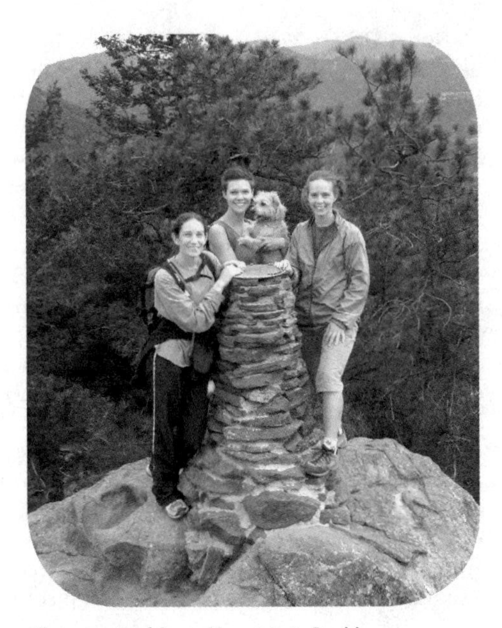

The summit of Green Mountain in Boulder

Class: I'm not a huge fan of the class rating system due to variations of opinion on what defines a particular type of terrain (not to mention the structure of these ratings is more beneficial to technical rock climbers than hikers). Class ratings were first introduced by the Sierra Club in the 1930s to offer a relative scale for gauging hikes in the Sierra Nevada Range; rock climbers' influence has since changed the title of the system to the Yosemite Decimal System. While the system has been universally adopted, it is most useful when defined in relation to the region it covers.

To make this system useful for Colorado's hikes, I've modified the ratings to accommodate Colorado's varied terrain. Here's how the class system works for this book:

Class 1: Easy, on-trail hiking terrain with few obstacles and minimal exposure. Class 1 trails are well-maintained and easy to follow (they may even be dirt roads). Many hikes begin with class 1 terrain that gradually gives way to sections with more difficult ratings.

Class 2: This is your standard hiking trail. Terrain may be rocky or muddy and may require the use of hands for very short segments. On-trail class 2 routes are festooned with rocks and may be steep, with minimal exposure. Off-trail class 2 includes stable rock and talus fields, wide open tundra, stable ridgelines, and easy-to-navigate fields.

Class 2+: This designation defines class 2 terrain that has sustained, simple scrambling or steep, strenuous trails that offer low-technical challenges. A 2+ rating may also cover off-trail terrain that is rife with obstacles such as fallen trees, swamps, and river crossings. Additionally, 2+ covers loose talus fields, rocky ridges, and off-camber paths.

Class 3: This is the fun stuff! Class 3 terrain utilizes handholds and is often steep; in other words, class 3 is true scrambling. Route finding is important on class 3 terrain, as a majority of it is off-trail or on rocky ridges. Exposure is more noticeable, though under normal conditions, you shouldn't need ropes (though if you're climbing off-season, they might be a good idea). Helmets are a good idea on class 3 terrain.

Class 3+: The hardest hikes in this book are 3+; these are advanced routes that require skilled scrambling and difficult route finding and may require tricky moves in highly exposed areas. Class 3+ routes have solid handholds, but you will need to commit to your moves. Some moves on class 3+ routes may be unnerving, though fall potential is low (think high-risk moves with a very low probability of failure). Helmets are recommended on 3+ terrain.

Class 4: None of the standard routes in this book are class 4, though by some definitions, the class 3+ routes may be considered low class 4 in other regions. Class 4 goes beyond scrambling and gets into low-level climbing; slipping or falling on class 4 terrain may be fatal, so the stakes are fairly high. Often, class 4 routes are found on rock that is too loose to be protected, or on ridges that have sustained, highly exposed sections with good handholds.

Class 5 and up: Used to designate technical rock climbing utilizing protection, ropes, harnesses, and belay devices.

Examples of class designations for hikes on some familiar Colorado peaks:

Class 1: Bison Peak, Longs Peak (from standard trailhead to the boulder field), Mount Thomas

Class 2: Mount Elbert, James Peak, Uncompahgre Peak

Class 2+: Mount Sneffels, Windom Peak, Blanca Peak

Class 3: Longs Peak (from boulder field to summit), Mount Eolus, Mount Richthofen

Class 3+: Mount Lead, Fools Peak, Storm King Peak

Class 4: The finishing move on Mount Sunlight Peak, North Maroon Peak

Class 5: The Diamond on Longs Peak, bolted climbs, vertical routes

Start Elevation: This one is obvious: it's the elevation above sea level at the beginning of your hike.

Peak Elevation: Also obvious: this is the elevation of the summit.

Total Elevation Gain: This is the total amount of elevation you will gain on both your ascent and descent; it is not the difference between start and summit elevations. Elevation gain is graphically displayed in the elevation profile graphs provided for each hike.

Terrain: Terrain features may not be obvious on maps. Knowing what will be under your boots lets you equip yourself accordingly.

Best Time to Climb: Almost all of the hikes will be most enjoyable from late June to mid-September, though some peaks are best scaled in early spring, when snowfields provide optimal terrain. A few peaks are great to climb year-round.

Gear Advisor: These are suggestions about gear that I found very helpful for a given hike. This includes footwear suggestions and terrain-specific gear such as helmets, ice axes, gaiters, crampons, or sandals for water crossings.

Crowd Level: If you're looking for solitude, check the crowd level. Traffic levels will always be higher on weekends during hiking season. Following are definitions for the four levels of crowds.

High: This designation refers to popular trails that see a lot of traffic. Such trails are good for social hikers or those wanting the comfort of others on the mountain—a very common occurrence on 14ers, since they are Colorado's "glory peaks."

Moderate: You probably won't be alone on hikes with a moderate crowd level, but you won't be overwhelmed by the masses. Such hikes are often somewhat well known. A moderate crowd level can be expected on the easier-to-access 13ers.

Low: You'll probably have the summit to yourself, but you'll likely see a few others out and about on low-traffic peaks. You can expect low traffic on hidden gems or on mountains with remote trailheads.

Hermit: These are peaks where you have a great chance of being all alone, save for a few resident animals. These are the true secrets of Colorado (though some of these peaks may have initial access areas where you'll encounter hikers headed to alternate destinations).

Don't expect summit registers; if there are logbooks, expect them to have a short list of exclusive signatures. These hikes are great for solitude, but I'd still highly recommend bringing along a companion for hermit hikes.

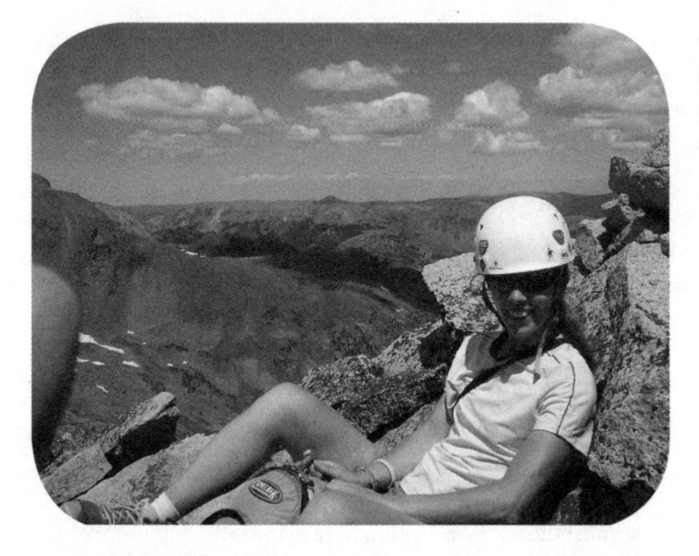

There's nothing better than a good day in the mountains!

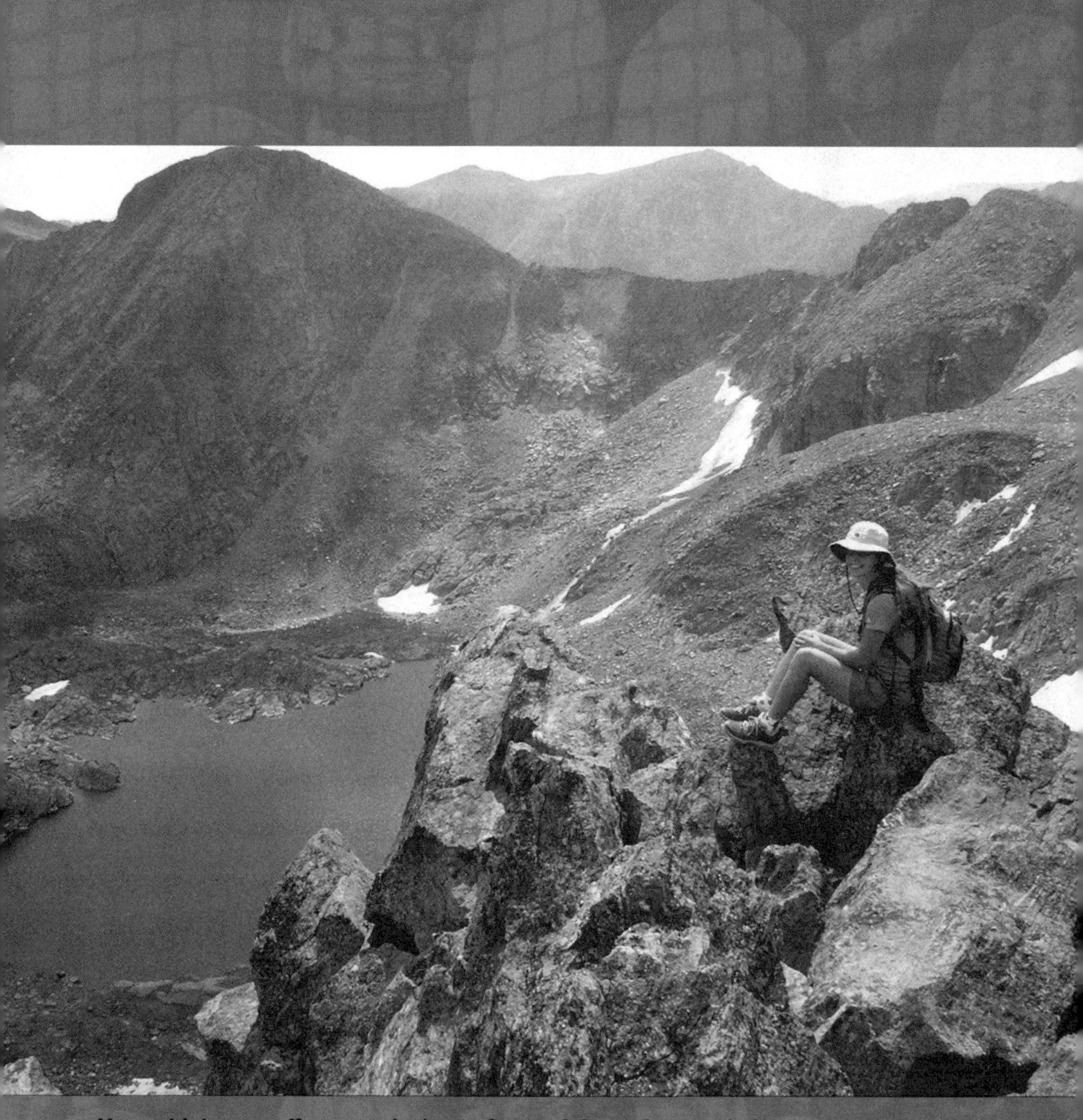

Mount Ida's apex offers superb views of peaceful meadows and alpine lakes. Herds of elk can often be seen grazing in the distance from Ida's spacious summit.

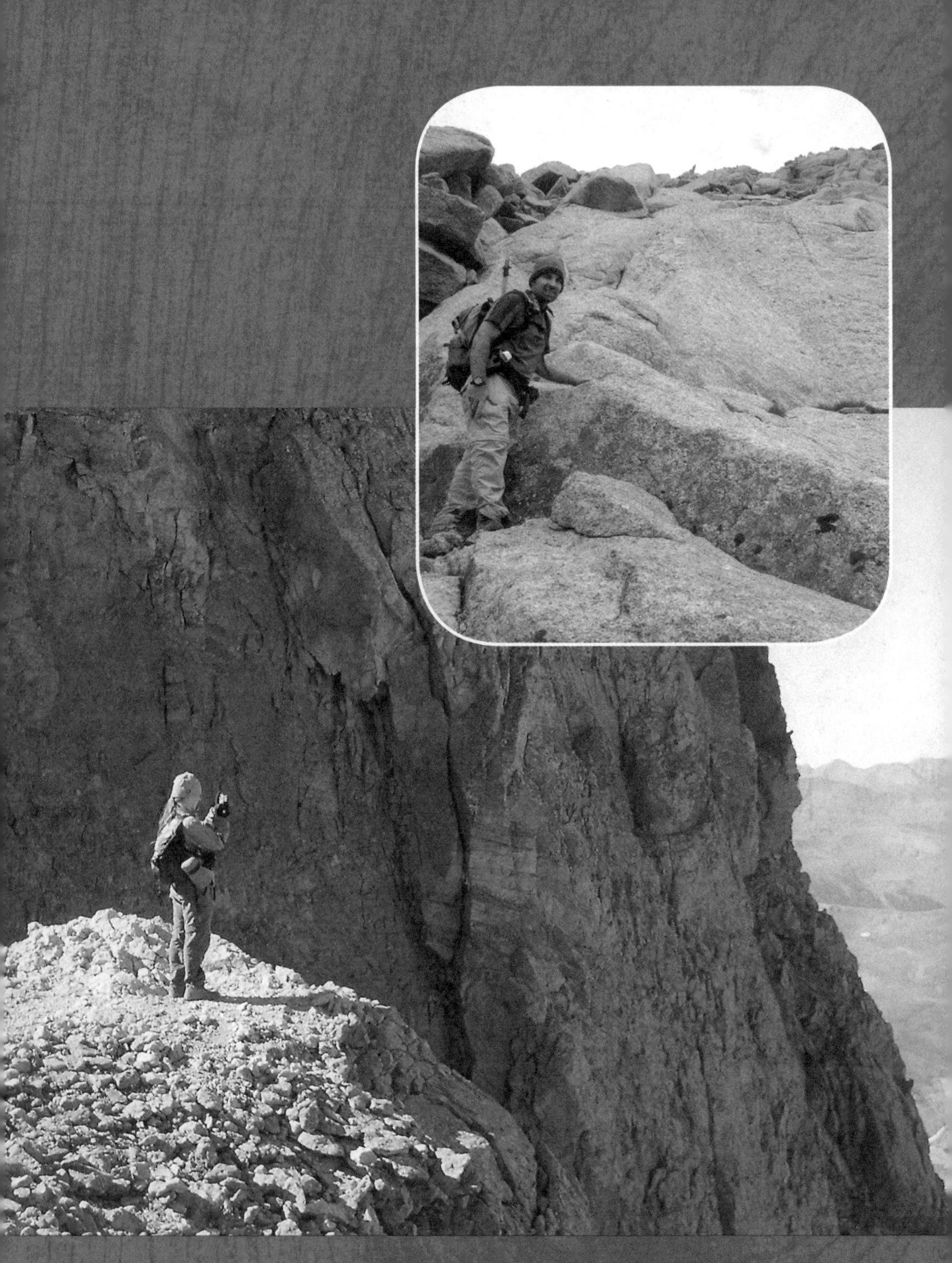

Top: **Scrambles on Sunlight Peak**
Bottom: **Lining up the perfect photo on Uncompahgre Peak**

Trip Outtakes

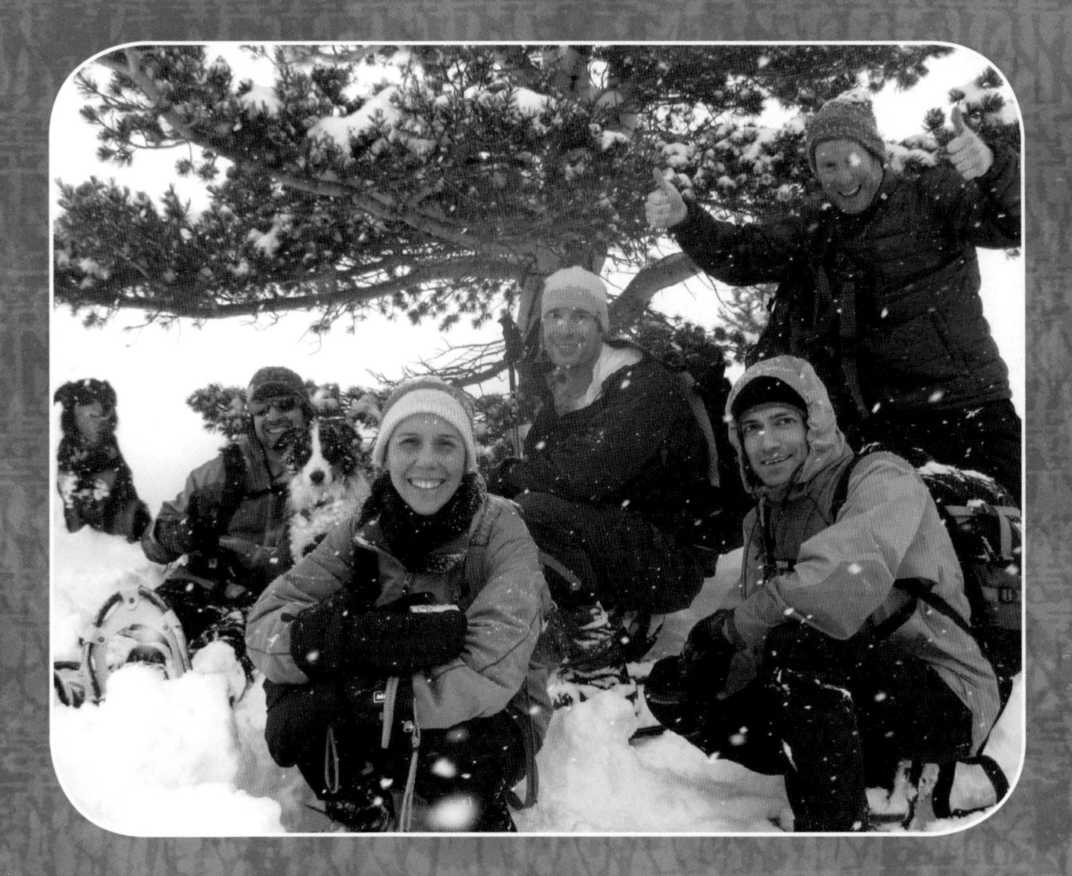

All photos by James Dziezynski unless otherwise noted

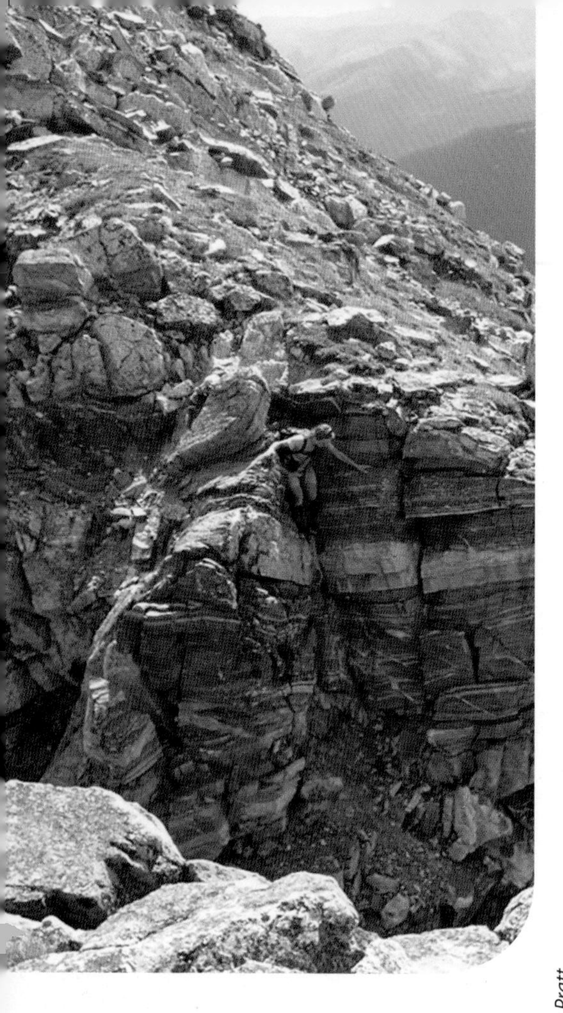

The **Citadel's** twin summits offer fun scrambling to reach their lofty pinnacles. This slot is the easiest way to descend the east summit (photo taken from the west summit).

This mountain goat means business! Remember to respect wildlife, especially those who have a propensity for head-butting hikers off narrow ridges.

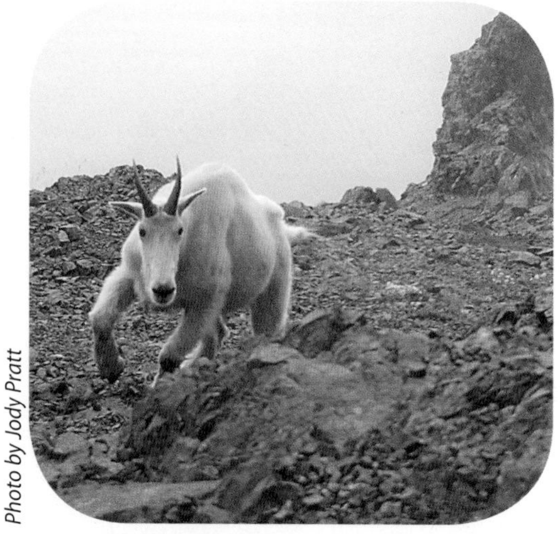

Photo by Jody Pratt

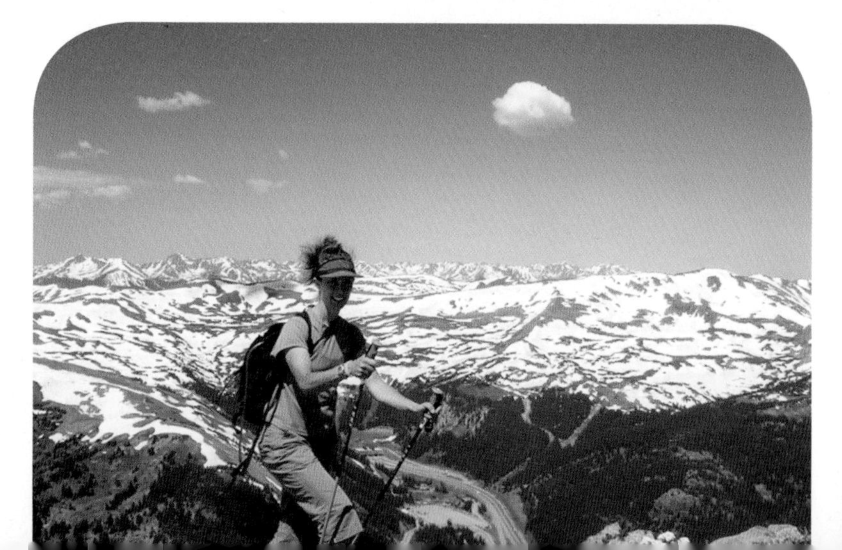

Mount Sniktau starts from the high point of Loveland Pass and offers great views for not a lot of work, relatively speaking!

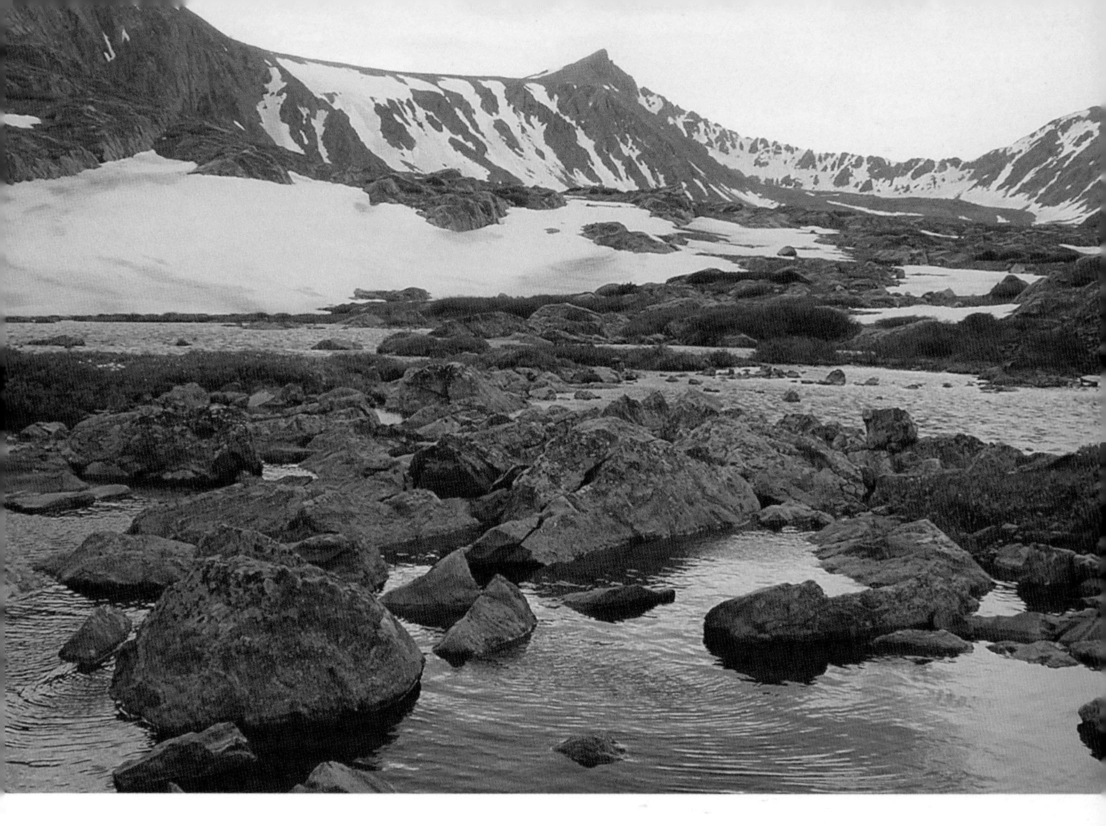

Spring thaw comes to the Mohawk Lake Basin with 13,950-foot **Pacific Peak** looming in the distance.

This inflatable clown suit was the perfect way to celebrate the summit of 14,309-foot **Uncompahgre Peak** and a fine homage to Billy and Benny McCrary of *Guinness Book of World Records* fame.

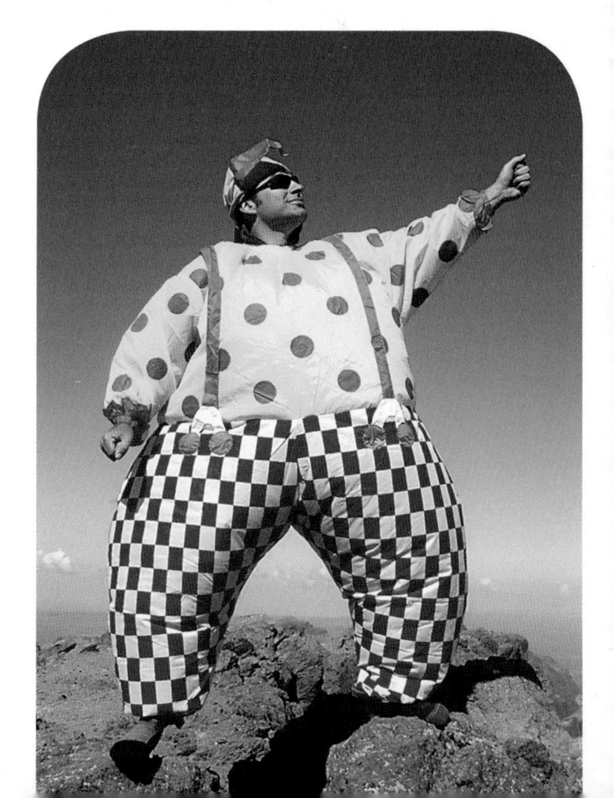

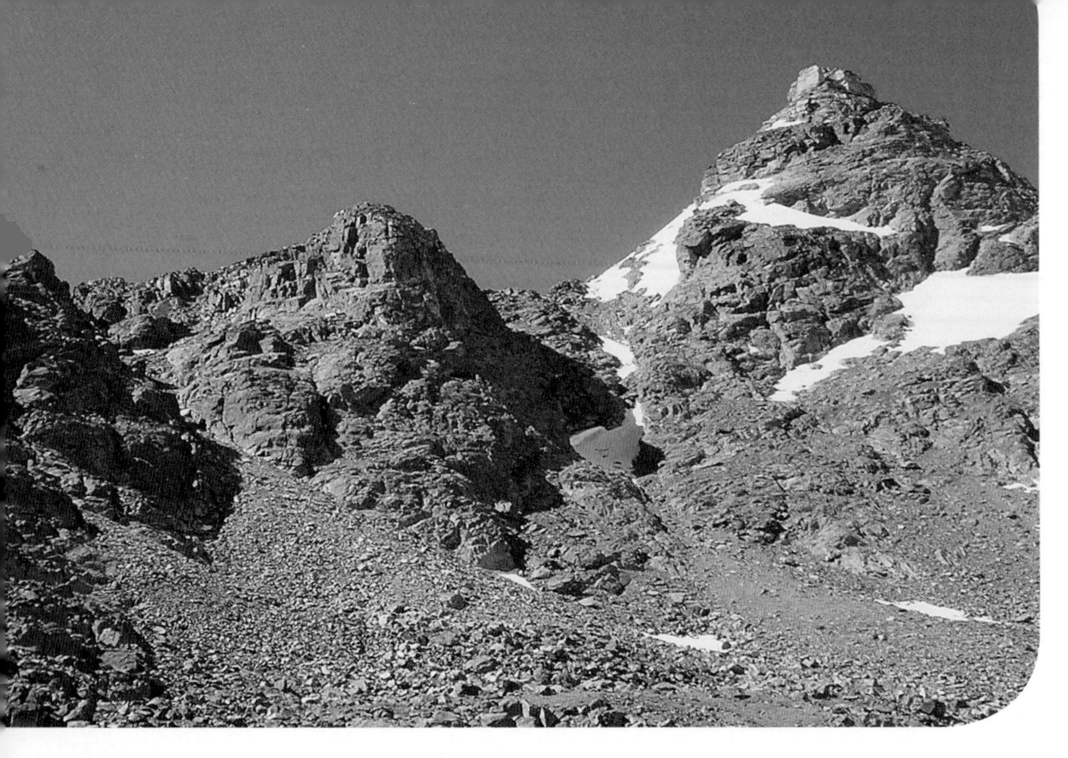

Navajo Peak's classic pyramid resembles an ancient Mayan temple. Airplane Gully is located to the right of the shadow from the pinnacle on the far left.

Classic class 3 terrain on **Pyramid Peak,** a possible side trip when hiking Belleview Mountain

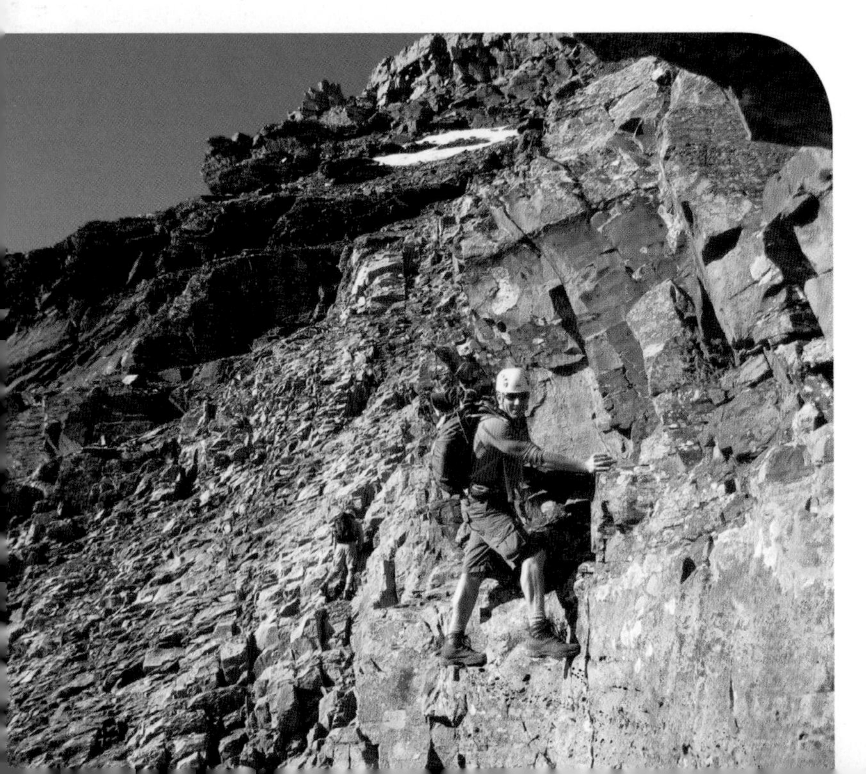

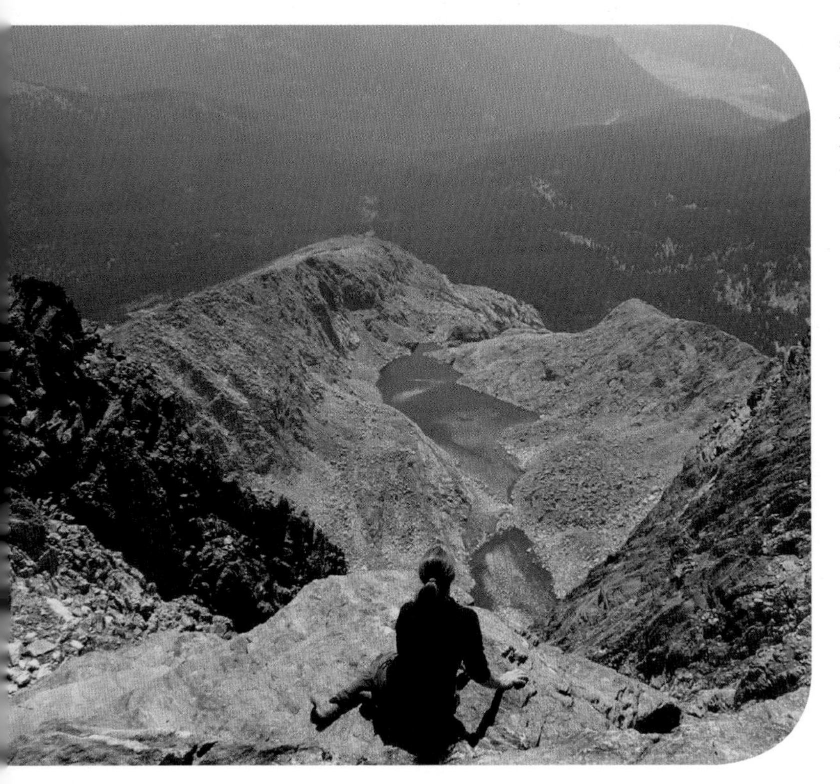
An amazing look at the aptly named Spectacle Lakes from just below the summit of **Ypsilon Mountain** in Rocky Mountain National Park

Neva Peak looms on the traverse back to **Jasper Peak.**

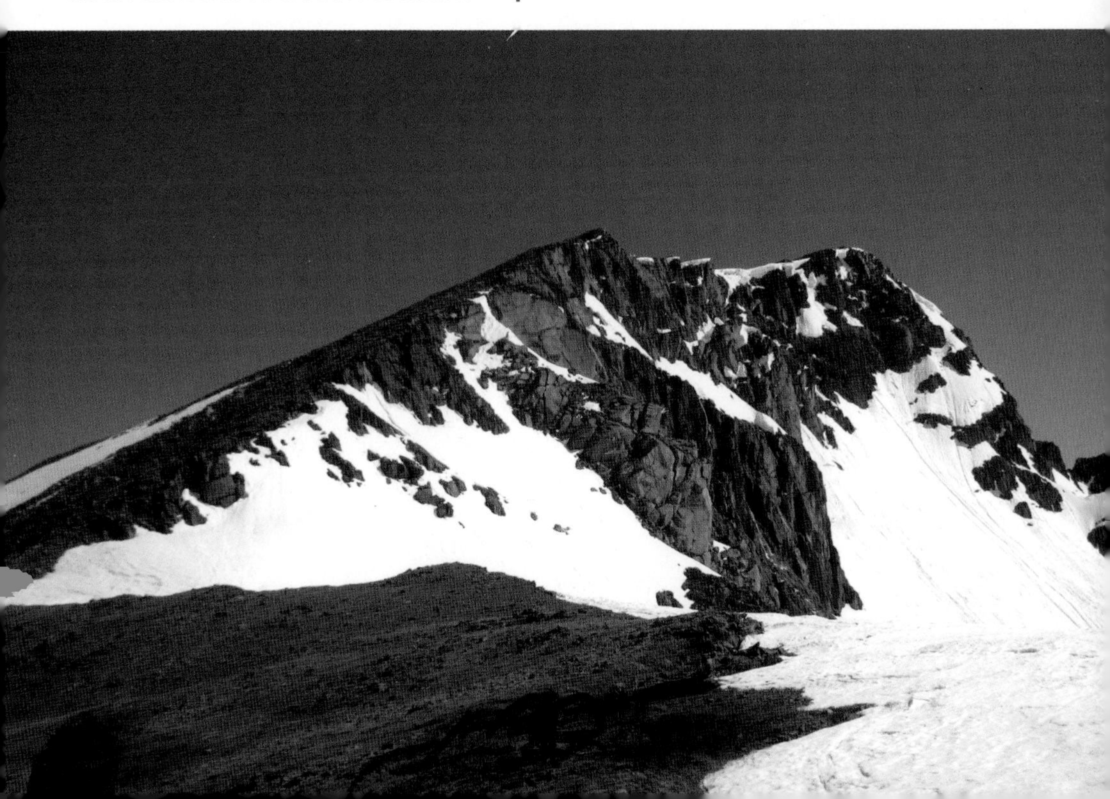

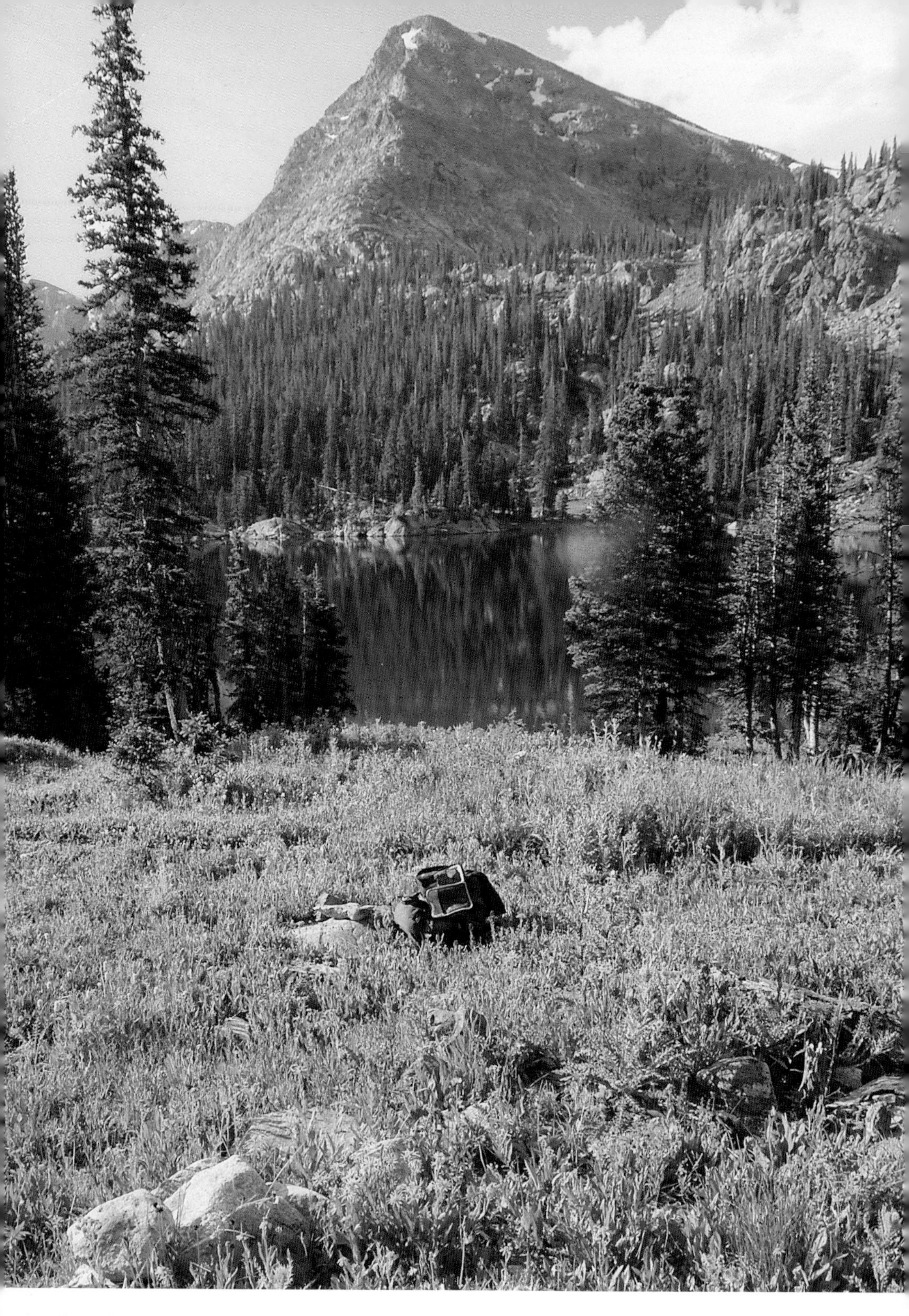

Fools Peak is one of Colorado's best seldom-climbed mountains, and an aesthetically pleasing picture when viewed from Lower Lake Charles.

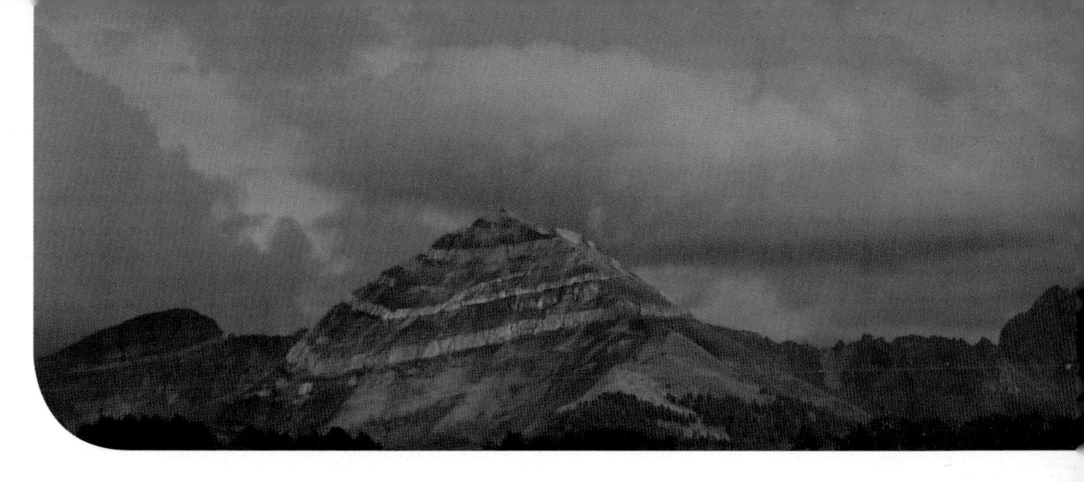

Storm clouds create an ominous portrait of **Hesperus Mountain.**

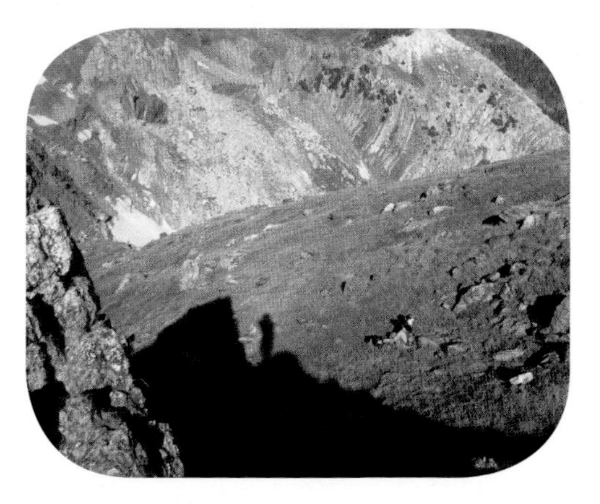

A sneaky photographer is caught in the shadows capturing a peaceful moment on **"Medium Agnes."**

The gully up to the summit of **Mount Sneffels** offers a great look at the colorful palette of the San Juan Mountains—and yes, that's a Hartford Whalers baseball cap on my head.

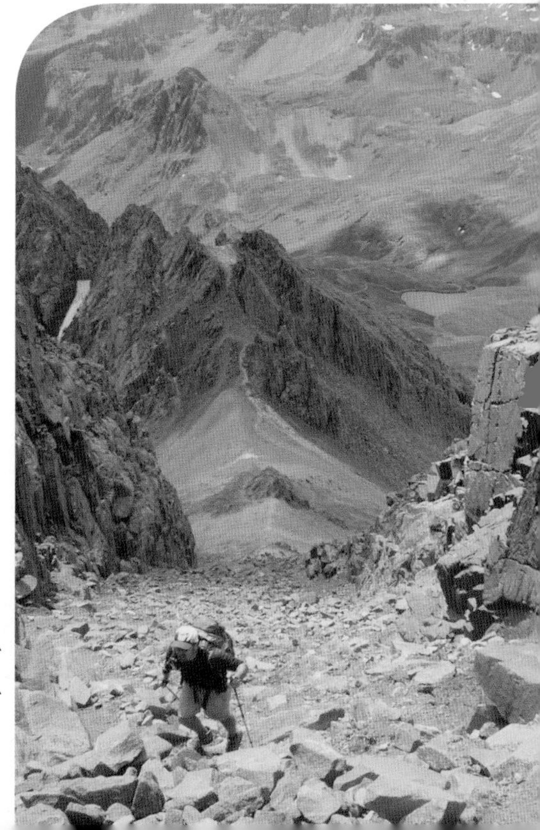

Photo by Jody Pratt

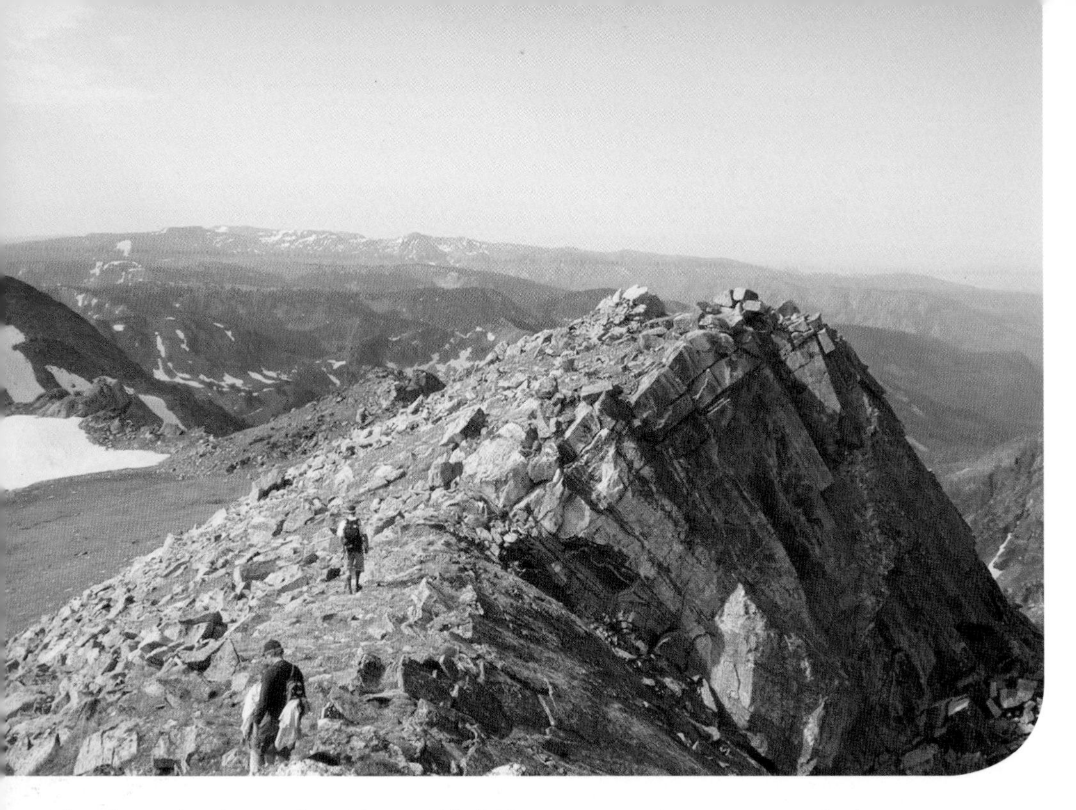

Hikers begin the descent from **Mount Zirkel.** This unique northern panorama looks out onto Steamboat Springs on the horizon.

Bobblehead Goofy is looking the wrong way on the summit of **Eureka Mountain**—he's missing a stunning view of the Sangre De Cristo Mountains!

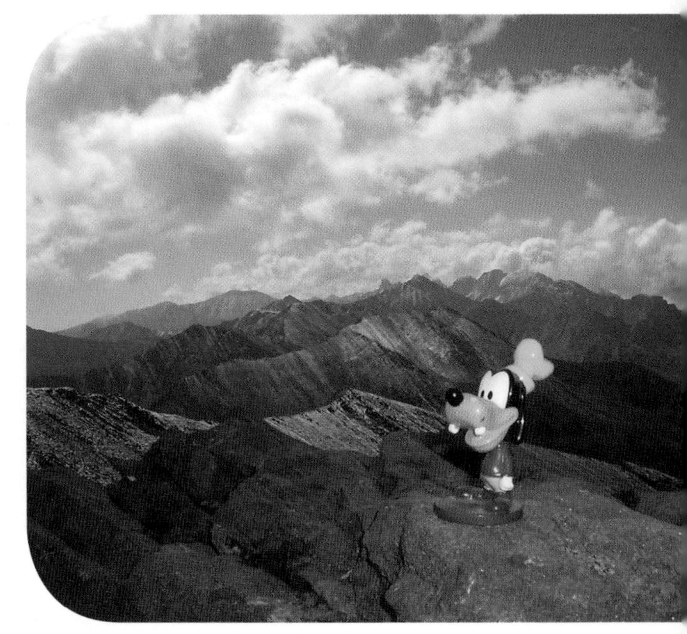

Windy and clear on the summit of **Engelmann Peak**

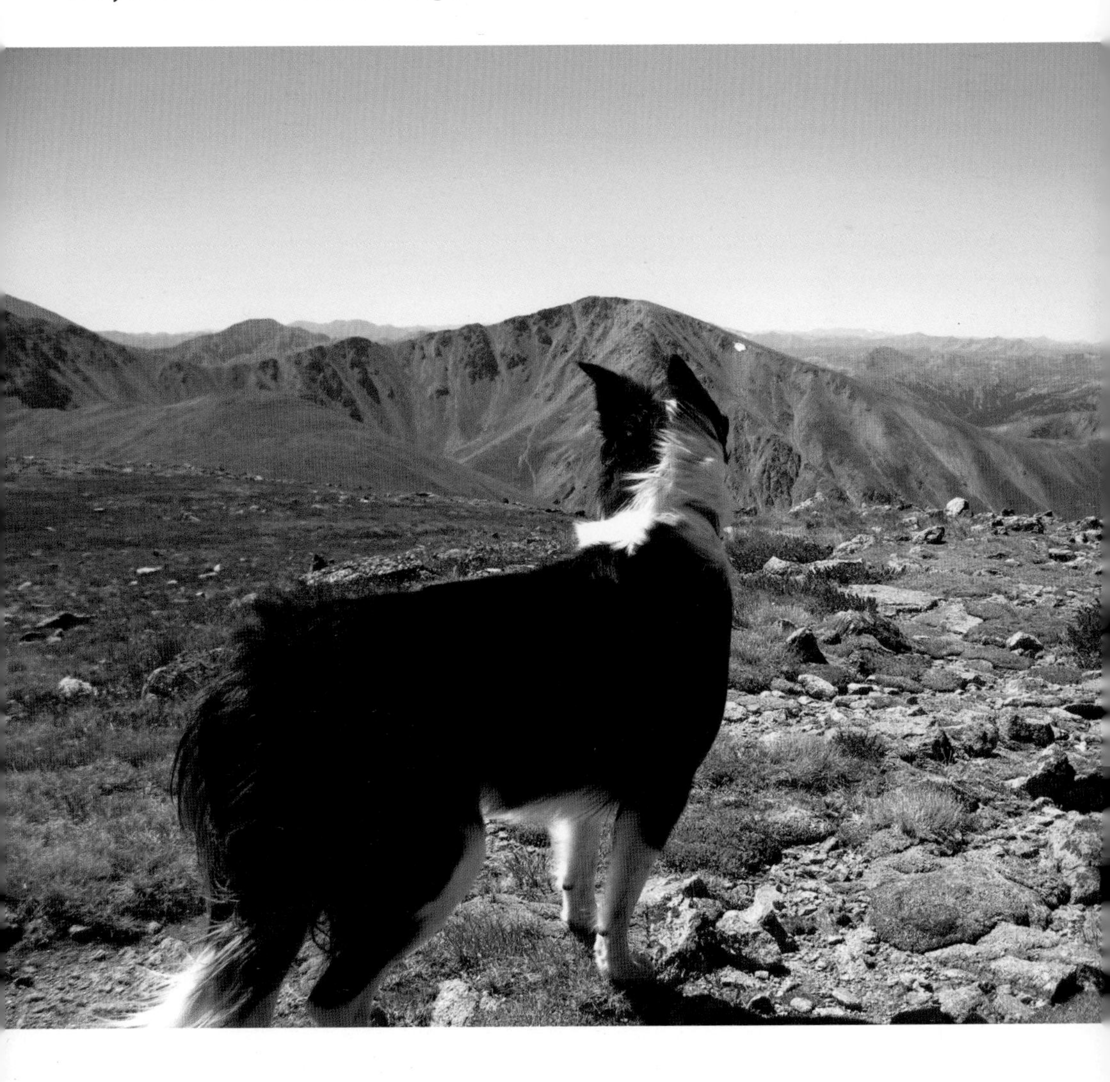

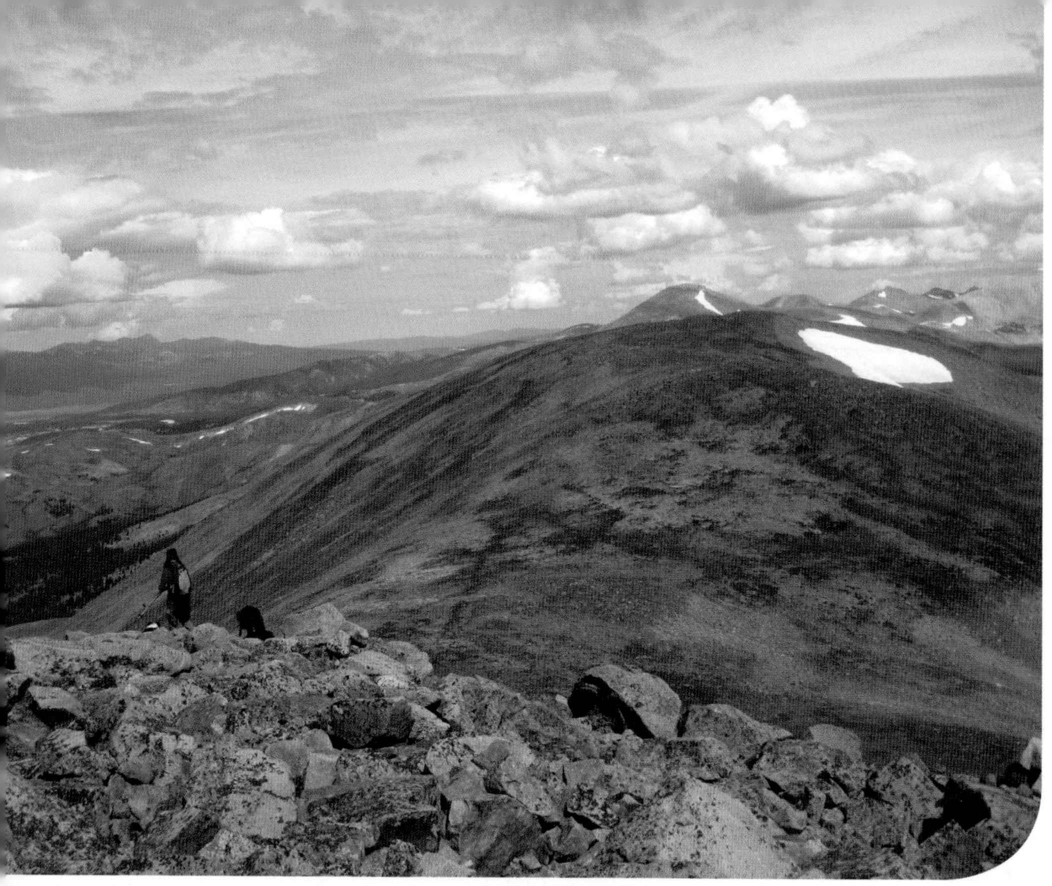

The rolling peaks that connect Weston Peak to **Mount Sherman**

Stunning views of 13,189-foot Red Peak from Eccles Pass en route to **Deming Mountain**

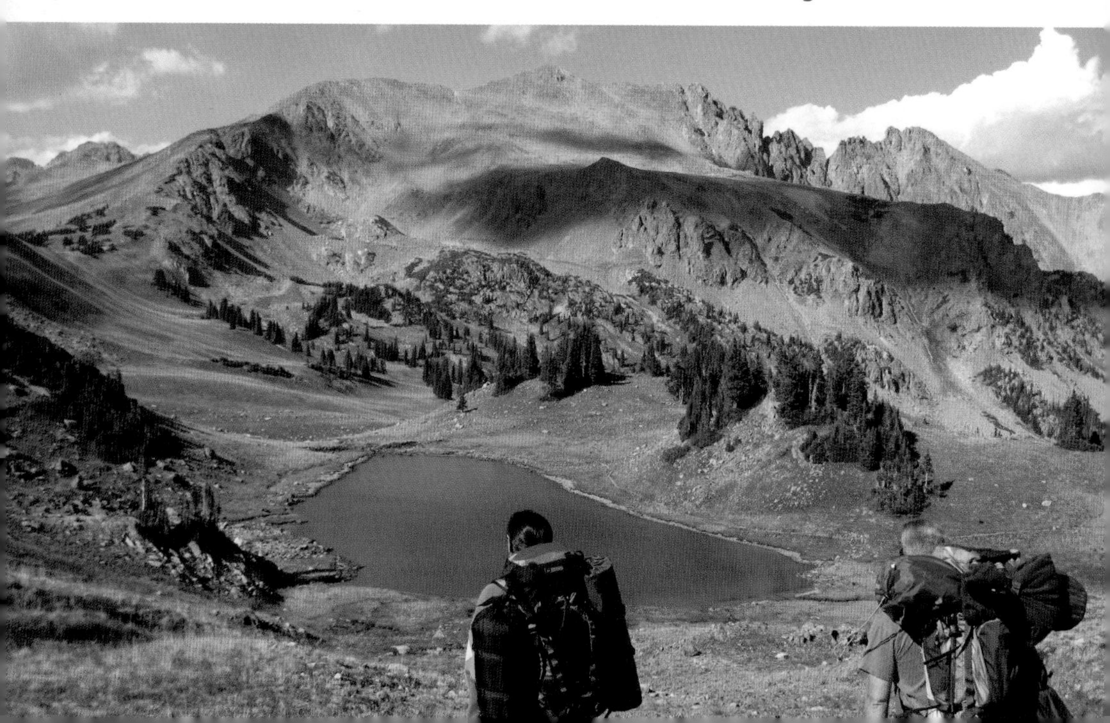

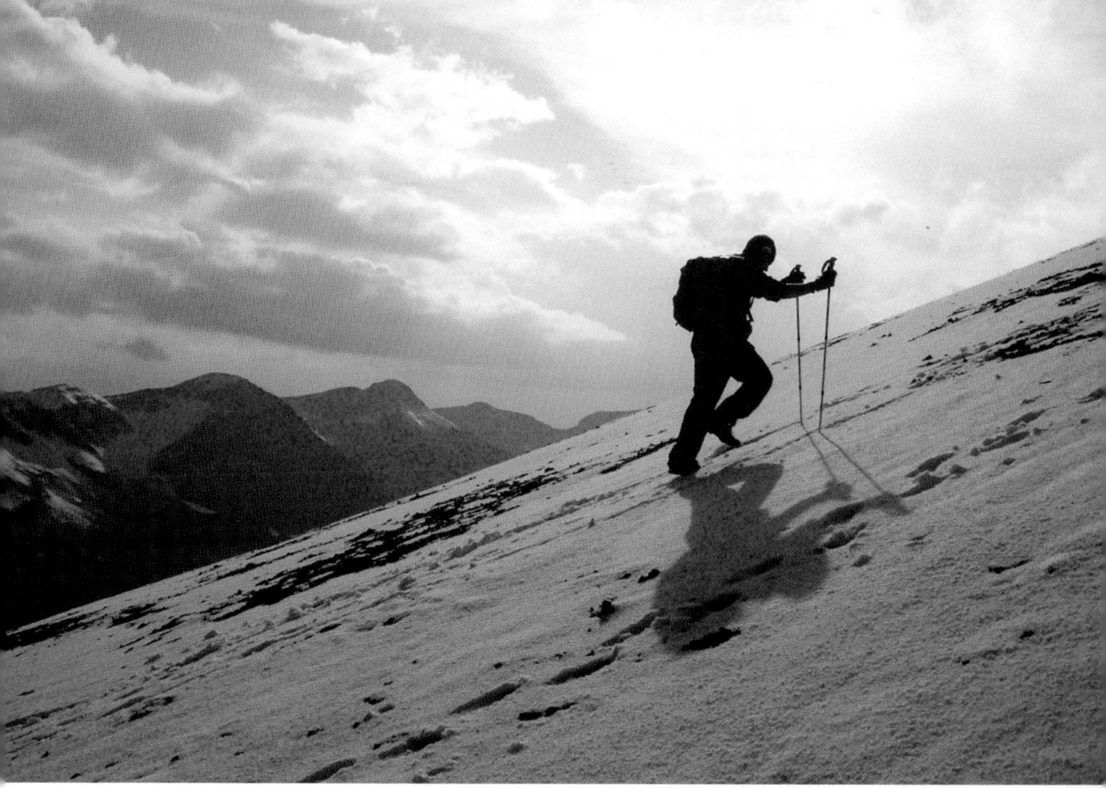

Photo by Jody Pratt

An ephemeral dreamscape of colors following a barrage of storms during the push up **Treasury Mountain,** just outside of Crested Butte

Lead Mountain's exciting ridge is a little-known gem in the Never Summer Range. Bring a helmet and sturdy boots for this airy class 3 ascent.

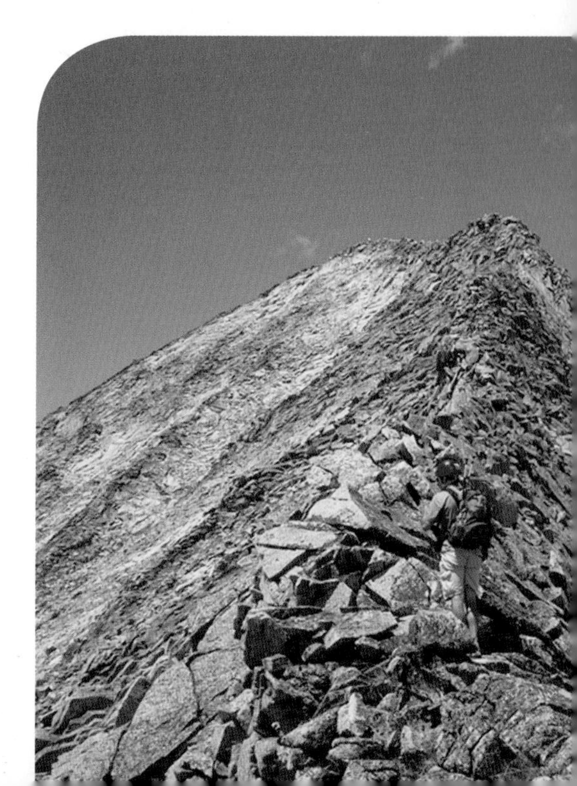

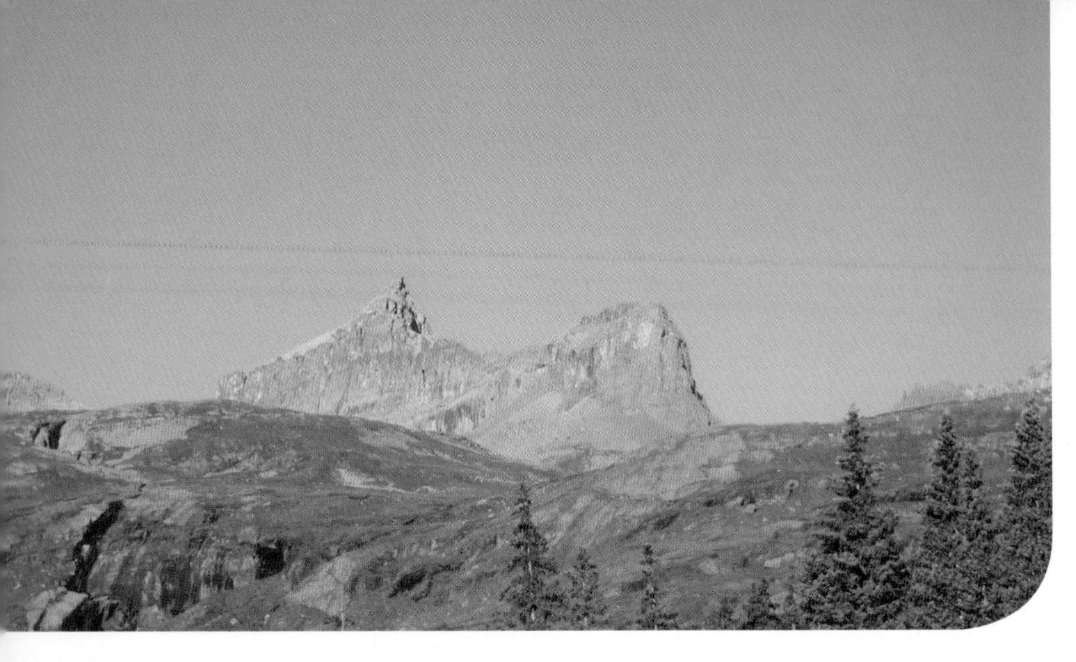

Golden Horn's impressive summit spire rises from the ebony-streaked walls of the Ice Lakes Basin.

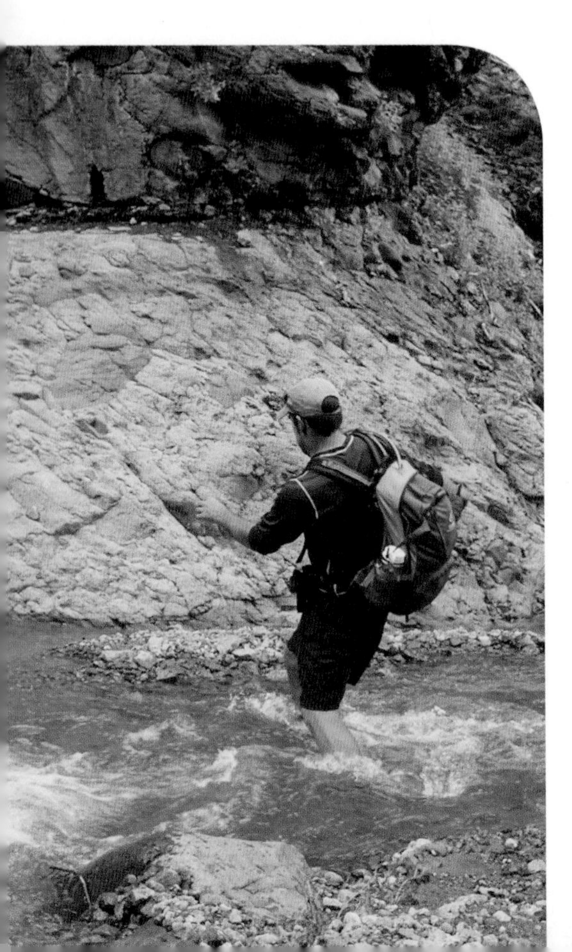

The trickiest part about getting to **Summit Peak** is this chilly stream crossing at Confusion Rock. The hard-to-spot trail goes uphill to the right of the light gray rock.

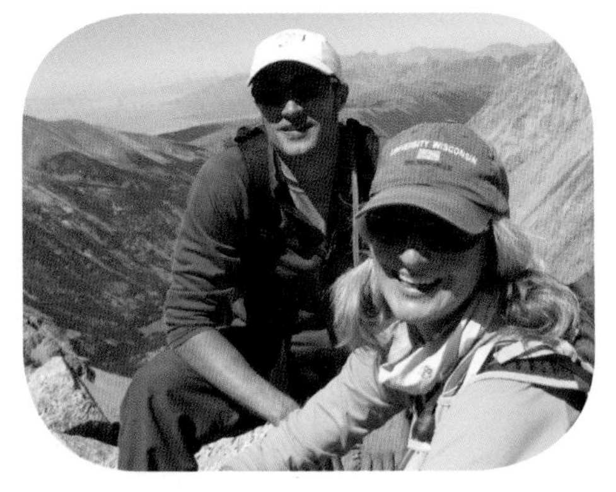

A beautiful **Sangre De Cristo** autumn summit day

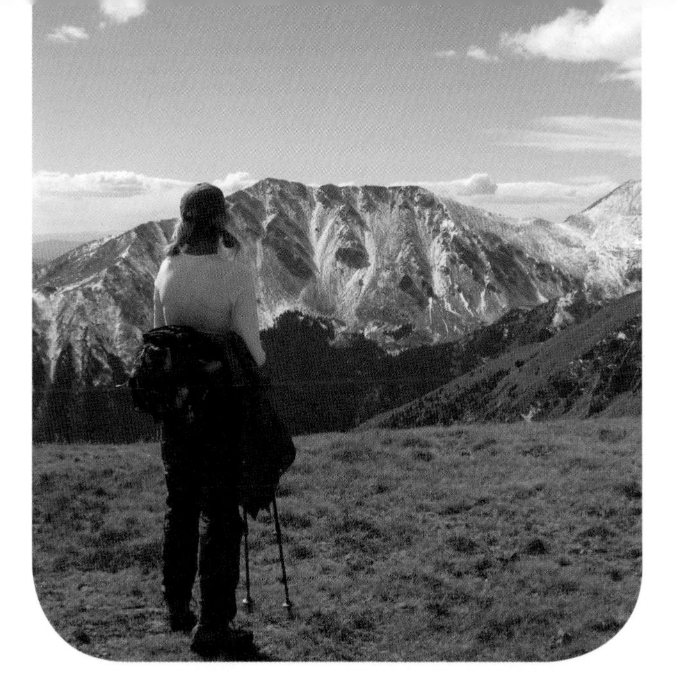

Incredible views on the flats between Carbonate Mountain and **Tabeguache Peak**

Untouched photo showing the natural sepia light at sunrise at the Boulder Field on **Longs Peak**

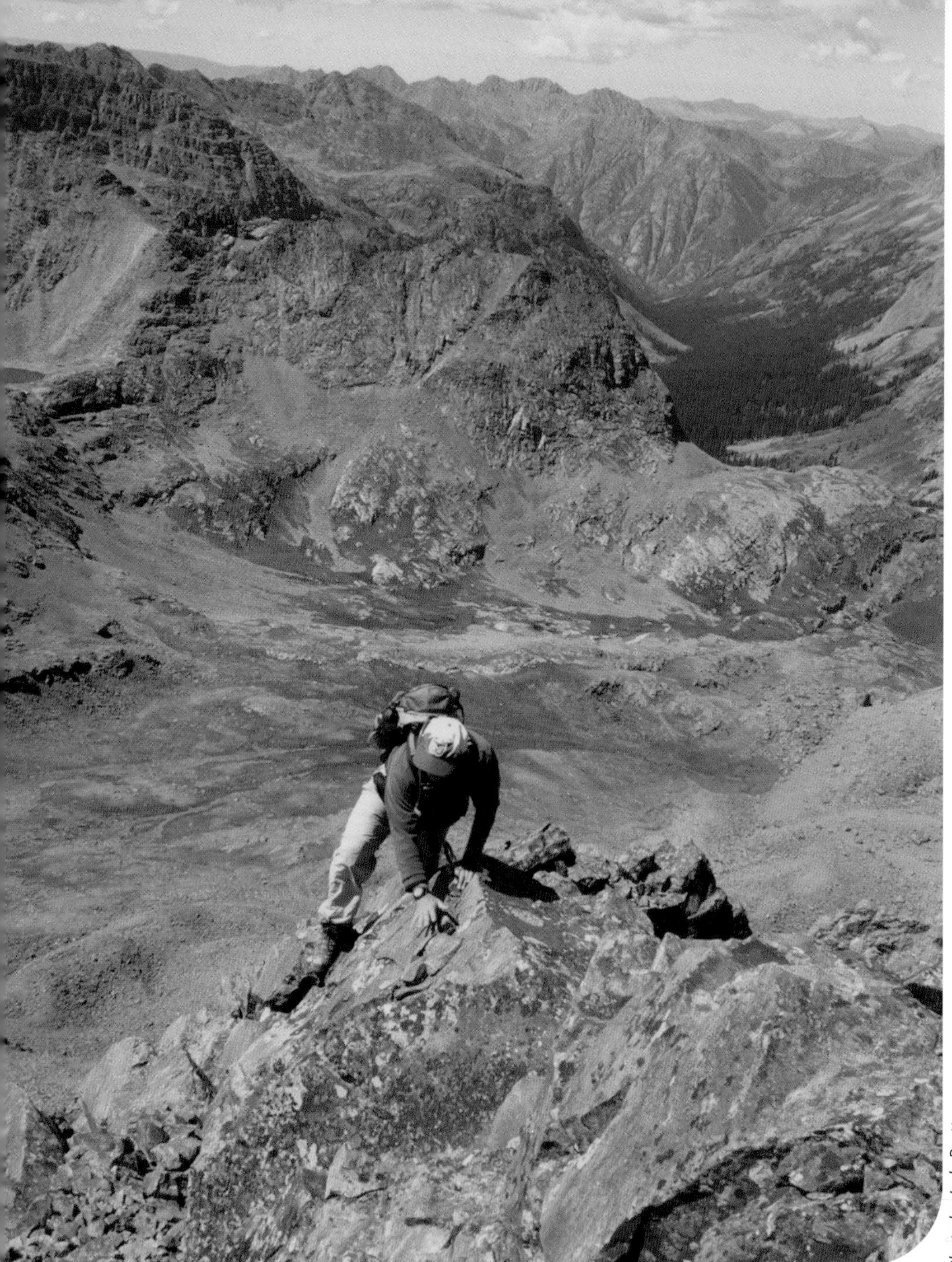

Photo by Jody Pratt

Scrambling high on the shoulder of **Storm King Peak**

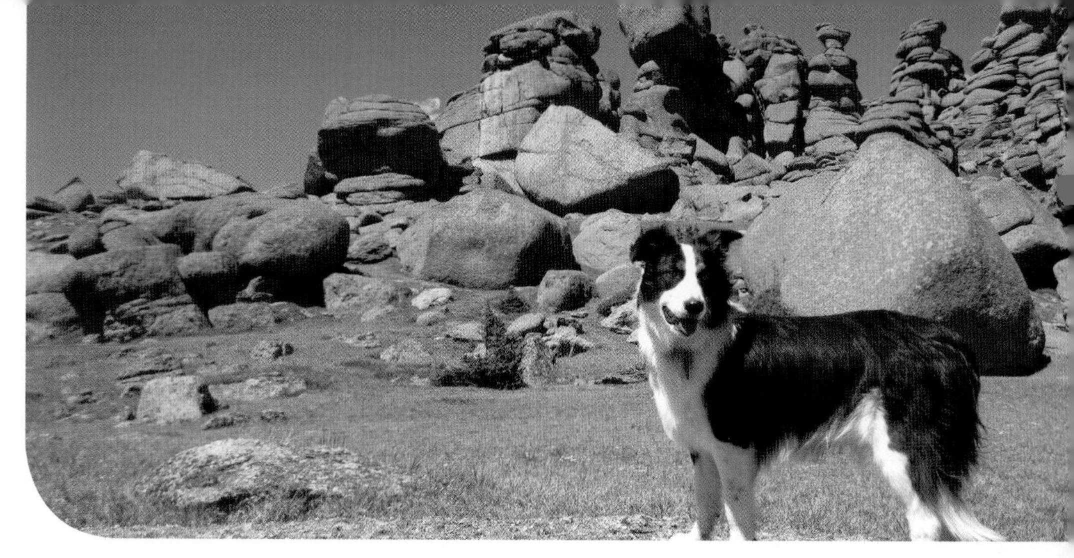

Fremont the border collie about to enter the maze of pillars en route to the summit of **Bison Peak**

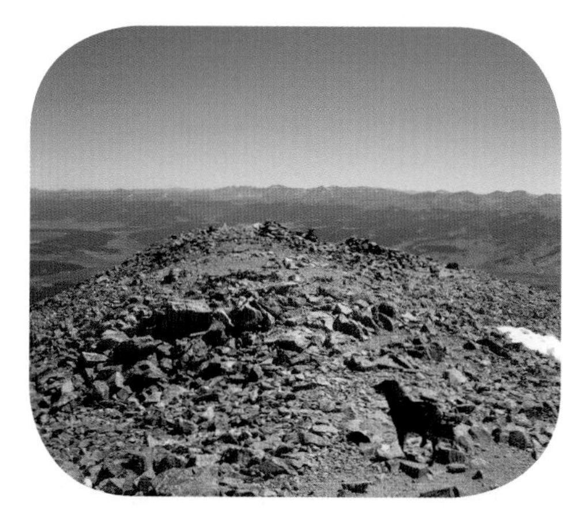

Mystic begins the descent from Colorado's highest peak, 14,433-foot **Mount Elbert.**

On the saddle of **Mount Richthofen**

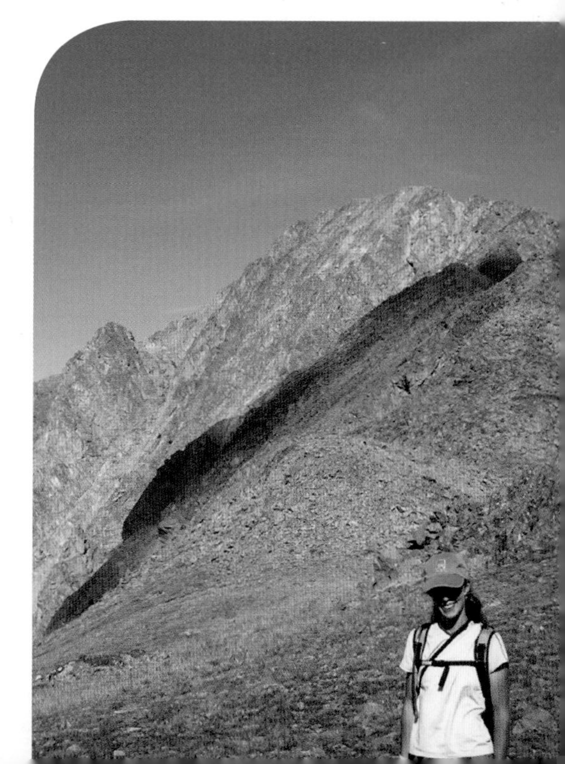

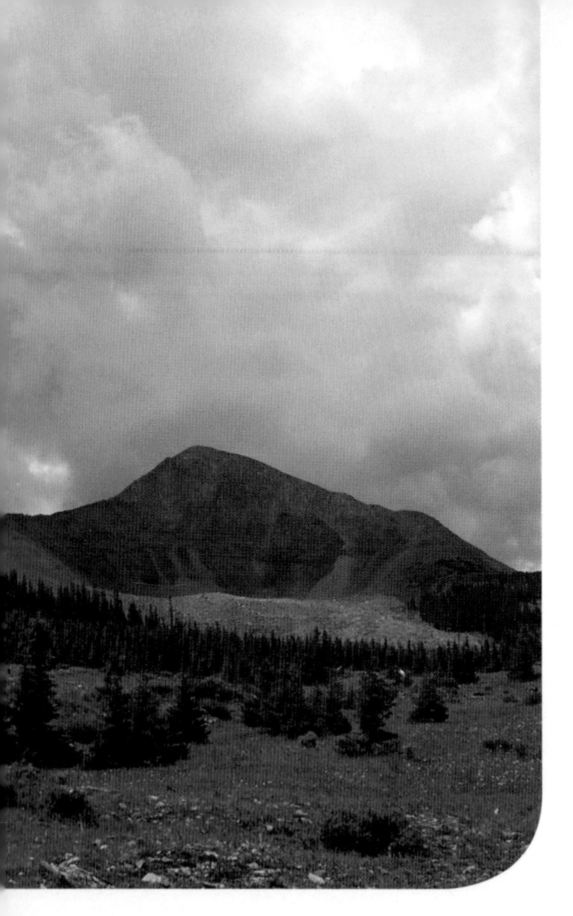

Lone Cone may be Colorado's most remote peak, but it's a worthy climb.

Beginning the wild class 3 scramble to the summit of **Belleview Mountain**

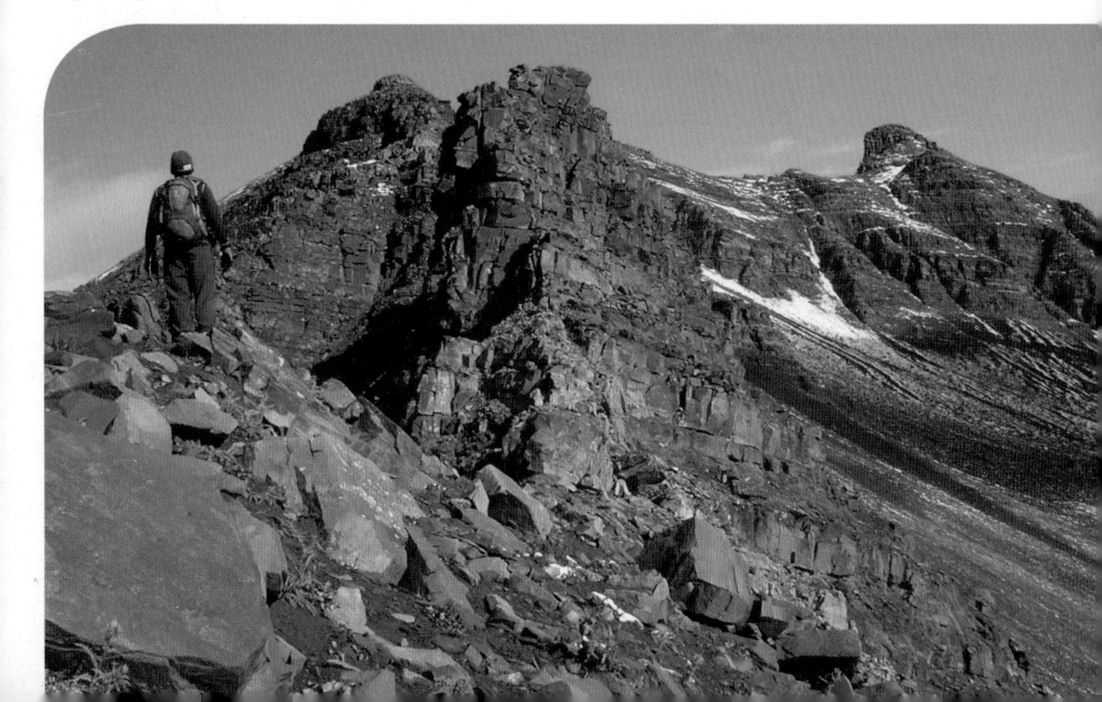

The Hikes

Looking out on a mountainous world

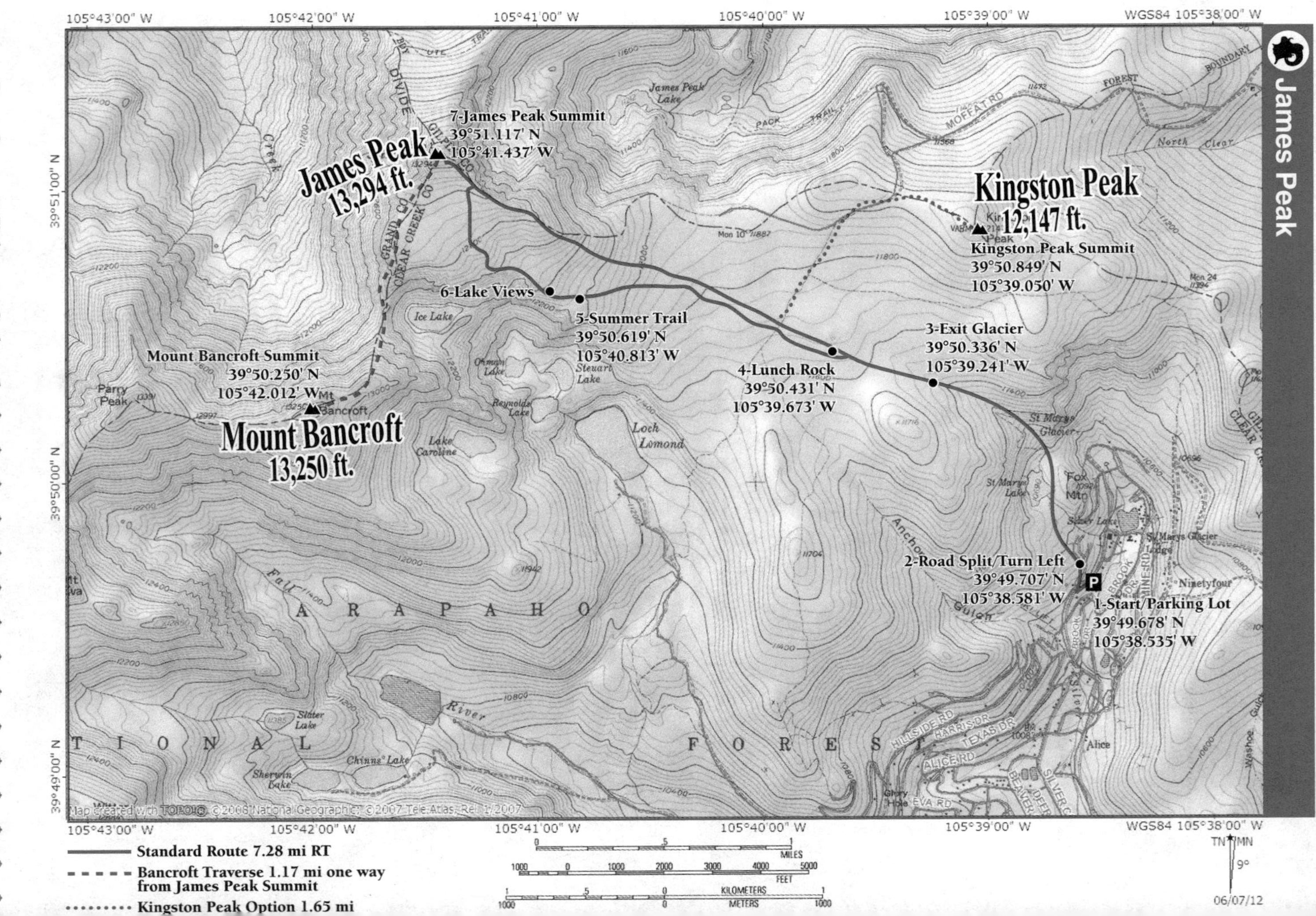

James Peak
7-James Peak Summit
39°51.117' N
105°41.437' W
James Peak
13,294 ft.
Kingston Peak
12,147 ft.
Kingston Peak Summit
39°50.849' N
105°39.050' W
6-Lake Views
5-Summer Trail
39°50.619' N
105°40.813' W
3-Exit Glacier
39°50.336' N
105°39.241' W
4-Lunch Rock
39°50.431' N
105°39.673' W
Mount Bancroft Summit
39°50.250' N
105°42.012' W
Mount Bancroft
13,250 ft.
2-Road Split/Turn Left
39°49.707' N
105°38.581' W
1-Start/Parking Lot
39°49.678' N
105°38.535' W
Ice Lake
Lake Caroline
Loch Lomond
Steuart Lake
Chinns Lake
Parry Peak
St Marys Glacier
St Marys Lake
ARAPAHO NATIONAL FOREST
Standard Route 7.28 mi RT
Bancroft Traverse 1.17 mi one way from James Peak Summit
Kingston Peak Option 1.65 mi

1 James Peak

James Peak offers stunning alpine scenery and glacial goodness. Start your hike on St. Marys Glacier, traverse an alpine meadow, and then ascend an aesthetic dome to the top.

Round-Trip Distance	7.28 miles
Hiking Time	4½–6 hours
Difficulty	4/10
Class	2
Start Elevation	10,300 ft., at St. Marys Glacier Trailhead
Peak Elevation	13,294 ft.
Total Elevation Gain	2,950 ft.
Terrain	Year-round glacier, alpine plains, rocky slopes on the descent ridge
Best Time to Climb	Early June–September
Gear Advisor	Crampons and ice ax in early spring
Crowd Level	Moderate on the peak/High on the glacier

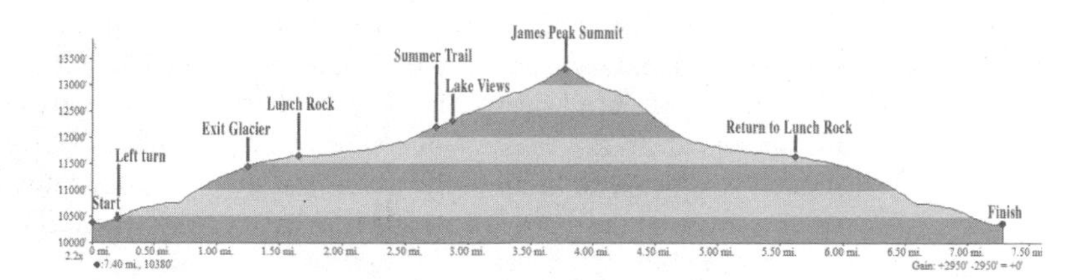

Location Indian Peaks Range in the James Peak Wilderness/Arapaho National Forest near Idaho Springs

Intro James Peak is the centerpiece of the 14,000-acre James Peak Wilderness, a relatively new wilderness area designated in 2002 (prior to that, James Peak was part of the Indian Peaks Wilderness). James stands as the high point of Gilpin County, and its prominent half-dome profile is visible from the east, especially when viewed from the foothills of Boulder County. Relatively speaking, James is one of the easier 13ers to climb, yet it has all the incredible scenery and majestic feel of Colorado's highest mountains.

Why Climb It? James Peak is a year-round attraction, thanks in part to St. Marys Glacier, a permanent ice field that graces the base of the standard ascent route. The glacier offers a great training ground for snow travel and is a short, steep warm-up for the southern slopes that lead to James's summit. Cresting the horizon at the upper terminus of the glacier, James Peak's impressive profile comes into view at the far end of a spacious alpine meadow. The flats leading to the final rise are great places to catch your breath while keeping an eye out for dozens of flowers and the occasional troop of ptarmigans.

Pushing for the summit can be done on a well-maintained, switchbacking trail or by a direct climb of the rolling southeast ridge. Summit views include a unique perspective of the front-side runs at Winter Park and Mary Jane ski areas. Best of all, when James Peak holds snow, it's possible to have some rip-roaring fun glissading down the summit slopes and the glacier.

As a bonus, James Peak's Trailhead is easily accessed from I-70 and is a relatively short drive from Denver, Boulder, or Golden.

Driving James Peak is easily accessible by passenger car. The trail begins off a paved, maintained road.

How to Get There From I-70 (East or West), take the Fall River Road exit (Exit 238, which is also labeled ST. MARY'S/ALICE). In gazetteers, this is listed as 275 RD. If you are westbound on I-70, this exit is roughly 1.5 miles from the town of Idaho Springs. Follow Fall River Road northwest 8.6 miles. Be ready for some steep switchbacks as you get closer to the trailhead. At approximately 8.3 miles, you'll pass the well-hidden town of Alice on your left; a bit farther up you'll see the general store off the main road on your right. You're almost there. Continue to the top of the hill, bypassing a rusted-out ski lift and a parking area blocked off by boulders on the left (this is the old parking area). At the top of the hill, you'll see a fenced-off mining shack and a well-traveled dirt road with a ST. MARY'S GLACIER sign. This is where you start your hike. Drive past the trail approximately 200 yards to a parking area on the left-hand side of the road. Note that this lot gets very crowded on weekends, so arrive early or else you'll have to park farther down the road. Also, please walk up to the main trail you passed; do not scramble up the improvised (and eroded) trails that are cut into the hill directly from the parking lot.

Fees/Camping While there is no fee for entering the James Peak Wilderness, nearby parking areas are privately owned and as of 2012 are charging a $5 fee for using their lots. Don't let the ugly, excessive signage and petty towing threats ruin your day; it's still an incredible hiking area. About a mile in each direction from the trailhead are spots along the road for free parking.

Route Notes None.

Mile/Waypoint **0.0 mi (1)** From the parking lot, walk 200 yards uphill (southwest) on the paved road to reach the wide, well-worn dirt road that leads up to St. Marys Glacier. You'll see a sign pointing out the glacier.

0.2 mi (2) The wide road splits. Head left and uphill. (The road going to the right simply leads to a parking area for people who feel like driving their 4x4s up the 0.1 mile from the road.) Follow the well-worn and rocky path as it winds up to the woods toward St. Marys Lake.

0.5 mi Pass by St. Marys Lake. The enormous, curving profile of St. Marys Glacier will be before you. Cross a small metal bridge and continue to the

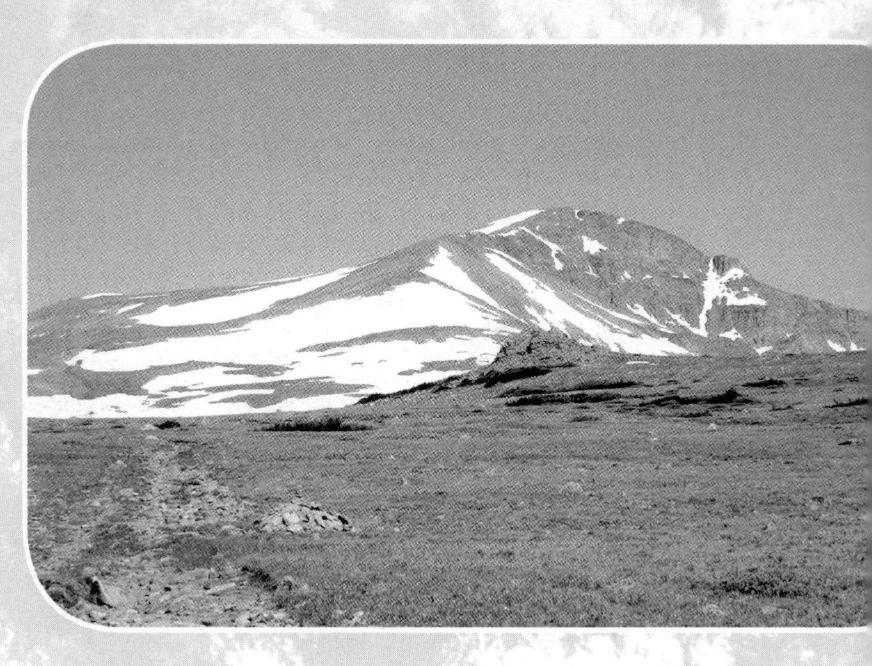

James Peak approach

glacier. It doesn't matter if you take the higher path or the lower path; they both lead to the glacier (though the lower path can be mucky in spring).

0.7 mi Get on the glacier and continue your ascent. Follow the icy snow to the top of glacier. This is a 0.5-mile, steep ascent, with wonderful photo opportunities. The alleyway is notorious for funneling fierce winds, especially in the colder months.

1.2 mi (3) Top out and exit the glacier. Where the snowfield ends depends on the time of the year. A semi-maintained trail fades in on the left (west) side when there is no snow. This is a good waypoint to mark on your GPS; in bad conditions, it's easy to miss the entrance of the glacier. From here, you'll see the expansive flat plains with James Peak dominating the horizon. Continue along the plains to Lunch Rock.

1.7 mi (4) Lunch Rock is a battleship-shaped formation that is the only distinguishing feature on the otherwise flat traverse to the base of James's slopes. There are some small, natural caves and man-made wind shelters in Lunch Rock. This is another good reference point. The faint, "sort of there" trail to the base of James, which is the left fork on the map at waypoint **4**, is the easiest way to make your ascent. From here, continue along the flats, crossing a 4x4 road en route to the south slopes. The trail from the top of the glacier begins to fizzle out, but you can see where you need to go.

2.7 mi (5) Once the snow has melted off, a cairned, switchbacking trail is evident on the southeast slopes. This trail will lead you to the top. Alternatively, you can head directly up the steep hills to James's summit. When there is snow, this is a good option, but be sure to test the snowpack; these slopes are at a prime avalanche angle. Note that when dry, the rocky hill makes for rough climbing (but is a good descent route).

2.9 mi (6) Don't miss the stunning views of the alpine lakes dropping off to the south. Continue to follow the cairns and well-worn trail. There is something of a false summit at 13,000 feet, where you gain James's southeast ridge. A glance north looks down into the impressive couloirs stretching down to James Peak Lake.

3.8 mi (7) Reach the flat summit of James Peak. From here, you can return the way you came or descend directly down the rolling southeast ridge. Following the ridge gives you some new views to the north and is quicker, especially when the snow allows for glissades. When there is no snow, it's a rocky class 2 descent, so if you don't feel like banging up you knees, return via the standard trail.

4.7 mi When you get to the bottom of the southeast slopes and resume the flats, aim for Lunch Rock. You can pass it on either side; on the return, the main trail is to the right of Lunch Rock.

5.7 mi (4) Pass Lunch Rock.

6.1 mi (3) Return to the glacier, and follow it back to St. Marys Lake. Follow the well-worn trail to the road and parking lot. Don't shortcut down the hill to the parking lot just off the top of the trail.

7.28 mi Finish at the parking lot.

Options From the summit of James Peak, Mount Bancroft is a 1.17-mile traverse to the southwest. You may want to bring a rope along for this route: there's a great 80-foot rappel into the saddle between the two peaks. From here, there is some exposed scrambling that is either class 4 or easy class 5 that leads to a class 3+ ridge with plenty of exposure. The route finding is a bit tricky, but for experienced climbers, this is a fine traverse. You can descend class 2 terrain to Three Lakes Basin and head back up to Lunch Rock.

A much more moderate option is to grab 12,147-foot Kingston Peak. From Lunch Rock this is a 1.65-mile class 1 walk up along a jeep road.

Quick Facts James Peak is named for mountaineer, botanist, and historian Edwin James, who served on Stephen Long's Colorado expedition. James's claim to fame was his historic first ascent of Pikes Peak, which initially was dubbed James Peak. Zebulon Pike had surveyed the mountain in 1806 but never climbed it; James and two companions did the trick in 1820. Cartographers used both names—James Peak and Pikes Peak—on early maps, eventually favoring the more phonetically pleasing Pikes Peak for the 14er.

James Peak was officially named in 1866, five years after the death of Edwin James. A fine mountain in its own right, this peak is a respectable consolation for a pioneering Colorado climber.

Contact Info Arapaho National Forest
Boulder Ranger District
2140 Yarmouth Avenue
Boulder, CO 80303
(303) 541-2500

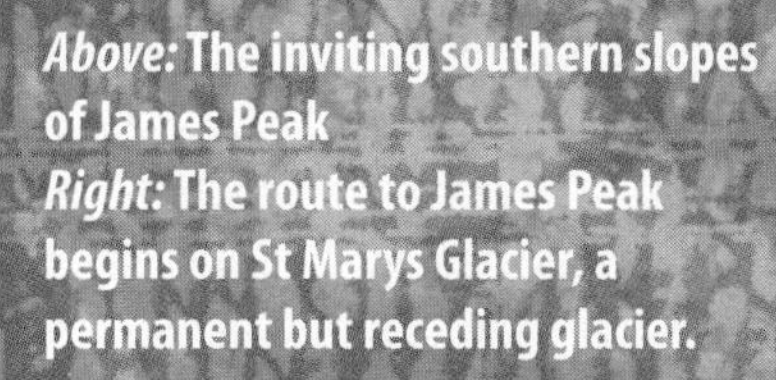

Above: **The inviting southern slopes of James Peak**
Right: **The route to James Peak begins on St Marys Glacier, a permanent but receding glacier.**

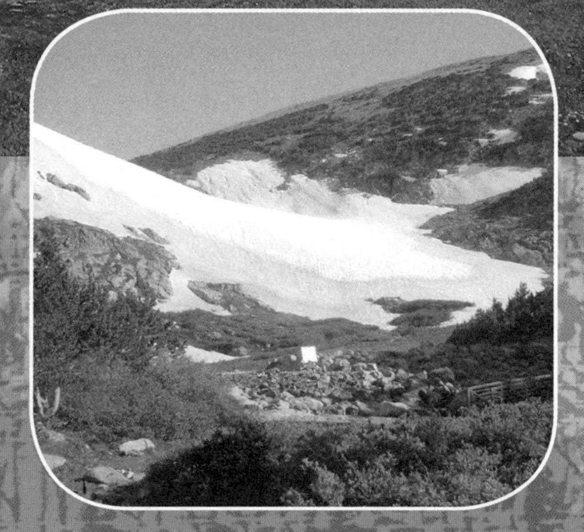

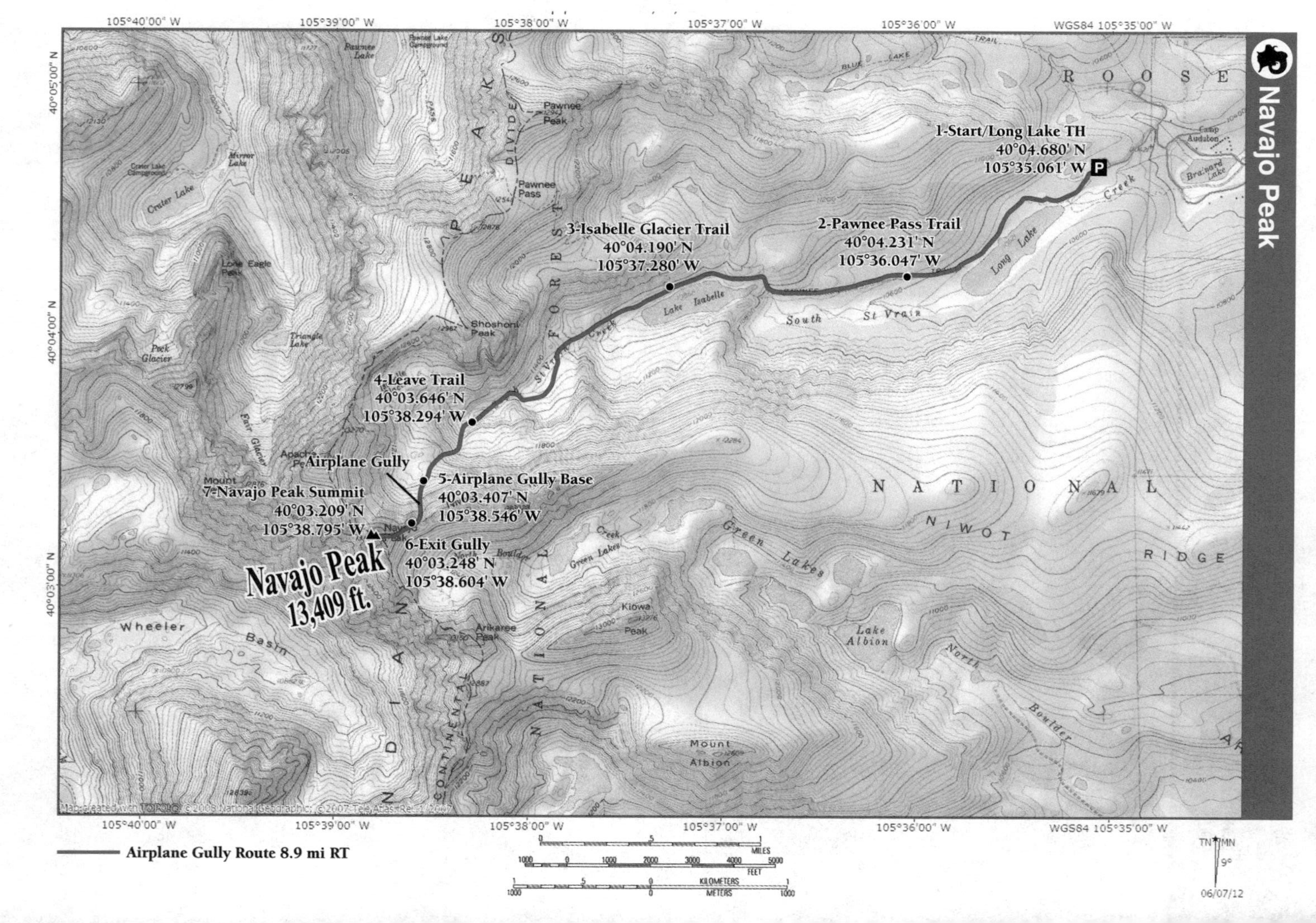
Navajo Peak
1-Start/Long Lake TH
40°04.680' N
105°35.061' W
2-Pawnee Pass Trail
40°04.231' N
105°36.047' W
3-Isabelle Glacier Trail
40°04.190' N
105°37.280' W
4-Leave Trail
40°03.646' N
105°38.294' W
Airplane Gully
5-Airplane Gully Base
40°03.407' N
105°38.546' W
7-Navajo Peak Summit
40°03.209' N
105°38.795' W
6-Exit Gully
40°03.248' N
105°38.604' W
Navajo Peak
13,409 ft.
Long Lake
Lake Isabelle
South St Vrain
Creek
Niwot Ridge
National
Green Lakes
Lake Albion
North Boulder
Kiowa Peak
Mount Albion
Arikaree Peak
Shoshoni Peak
Pawnee Peak
Pawnee Pass
Divide
Fair Glacier
Triangle Lake
Lone Eagle Peak
Mirror Lake
Crater Lake
Peck Glacier
Pawnee Lake
Wheeler Basin
Continental
Camp Audubon
Brainard Lake
105°40'00" W
105°39'00" W
105°38'00" W
105°37'00" W
105°36'00" W
WGS84 105°35'00" W
40°05'00" N
40°04'00" N
40°03'00" N
Airplane Gully Route 8.9 mi RT
MILES
FEET
KILOMETERS
METERS
TN MN
9°
06/07/12

2 Navajo Peak

A trip to the glacial basin below Navajo leads you to the base of Airplane Gully, where ghosts of the past await. A thrilling scramble is the grand finale to Navajo's airy summit.

Round-Trip Distance	8.9 miles
Hiking Time	6½–8 hours
Difficulty	8/10
Class	3
Start Elevation	10,500 ft., at Long Lake Trailhead
Peak Elevation	13,409 ft.
Total Elevation Gain	2,825 ft.
Terrain	Steep, loose gully and airy but solid scrambling on summit block
Best Time to Climb	June–September
Gear Advisor	Gaiters, stiff boots, ice ax in spring, helmet, and GPS
Crowd Level	Low

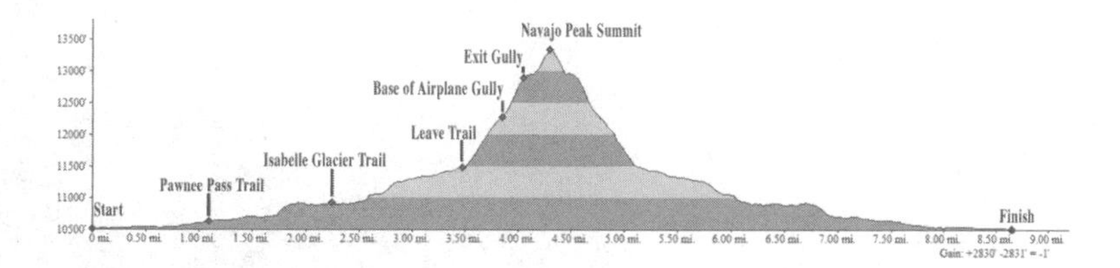

Location Indian Peaks Range in the Indian Peaks Wilderness/Roosevelt National Forest outside the town of Ward

Intro From a distance, the clean, four-sided pyramid block that sits atop Navajo Peak brings to mind ancient Mayan temples. Among the peaks that grace the skyline from Brainard Lake Recreation Area, Navajo offers the most challenging standard route. Half of the hike is off-trail, culminating in a gully climb and an exciting class 3 scramble to the summit. Along the way, you'll have a chance to examine the wreckage of a C-47 aircraft that crashed in January of 1948 en route to Grand Junction. Parts are strewn throughout the gully, and a huge piece of the bulkhead rests near the gully exit.

Why Climb It? Shipwrecks and ghost towns fascinate humankind. We are drawn to relics, the very shells of history, which hold stories of hardship and bravery and are at the same time symbols of mortality. The wreckage on Navajo Peak is half of the appeal of this hike. Debris from the crash is strewn throughout the gully; small, rusty gears are so numerous that they seem like bizarre, metallic sunflowers pushing through the rocks. Besides serving as an archive of aviation history, the scramble to Navajo's summit is exciting itself. Beginning on-trail in the beautiful Long Lake area of Indian Peaks, an easy start leads to an off-trail adventure, where you'll pass two of Colorado's permanent glaciers (Isabelle and Navajo). After a loose scramble up the gully, the remaining ridge climb to the summit concludes with an exposed but very solid scramble 35 feet to the summit block.

Driving Passenger cars can make it to the trailhead with ease: the road is paved all the way.

How to Get There Take Colorado Highway 72 (Peak-to-Peak Highway) to the Brainard Lake Road, which is above the town of Ward. From Nederland, it is 12 miles to this turnoff; from Lyons, it's 10.2 miles from the junction with Colorado Highway 7. If you are approaching from Boulder, it's quicker to take US Highway 36 north out of town approximately 6 miles and take a left onto Left Hand Canyon Drive. Stay on this road 17 miles, all the way through the car graveyard/town of Ward. At the top of the road, take a right on CO 72 and then a quick left to Brainard Lake Road. Follow this road 5 miles

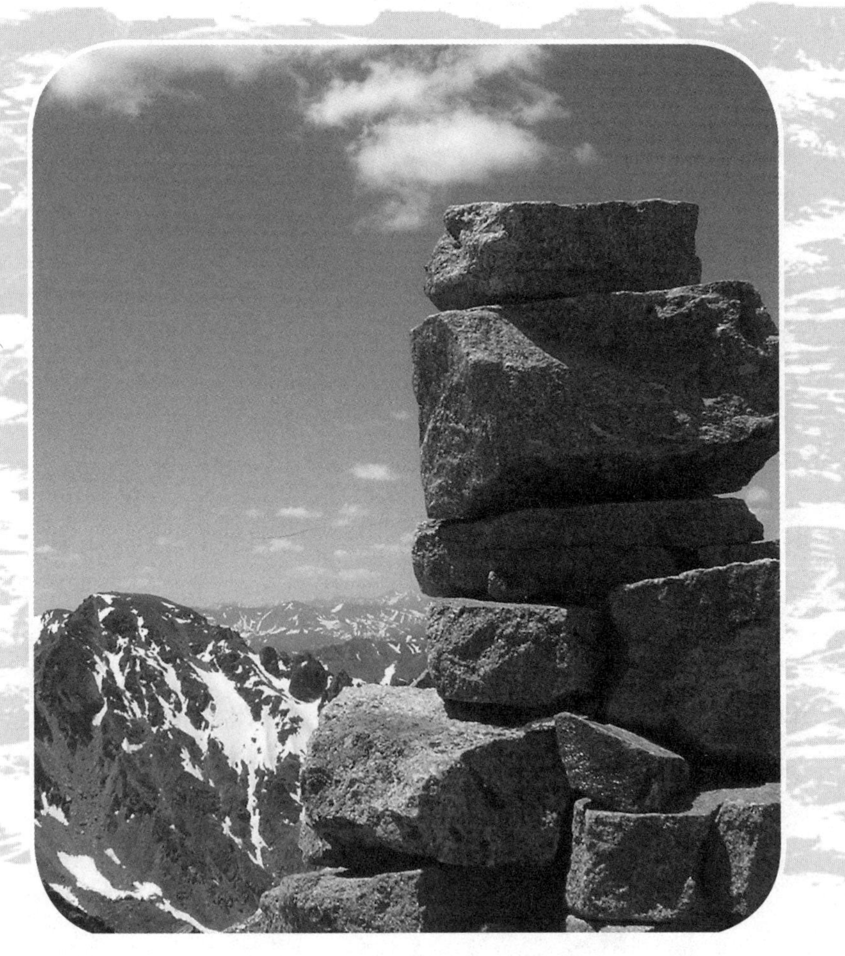

Cairn on the summit of Navajo Peak

(you'll pass a pay station and Brainard Lake), and follow the well-marked signs for 0.5 mile to Long Lake Trailhead.

Fees/Camping As of 2012, the permit for the Brainard Lake Recreation Area is $9 for a three-day pass. You can buy an American Land & Leisure seasonal pass for $45. Pawnee Campground fills up very quickly; if you're able to get a site, it's $12 per night. Backcountry camping requires a permit and a small fee ($5) June 1–September 15. Note that you'll have to go over the west side of Pawnee Pass to reach the designated backcountry camping zones.

Route Notes The off-trail portion of this hike is a little easier in spring, when snow covers the boulders in the basin above Lake Isabelle. Snow in Airplane Gully melts out early, so you shouldn't have to bring crampons after early May. The moves to reach the summit are exposed, but the rock is very solid. The crux of the climb is the short down climb off the summit.

Mile/Waypoint **0.0 mi (1)** Start at the Long Lake Trailhead and go west. Enjoy the flat trail, which is a great warm-up. At the west end of Long Lake, stay right and follow the trail to Pawnee Pass (for the time being).

1.1 mi (2) Pawnee Pass Trail. Continue west to Lake Isabelle.

1.9 mi (3) After hiking up some switchbacks and crossing a cool waterfall, you've arrived at Lake Isabelle and the Isabelle Glacier Trail. Follow the lake on its north side; do *not* go up the trail to Pawnee Pass. Instead stay on the trail to Isabelle Glacier. This trail climbs above Lake Isabelle, eventually coming to a flat, marshy section with a small lake at 11,500 feet.

3.5 mi (4) You will need to get off-trail at the marshy section. However, do *not* follow the steep switchbacked trail to the north going to Isabelle Glacier. Instead, head southwest to the dry basin at the foot of Airplane Gully. It is best to stay on the left (west) slopes instead of dropping down to the flat part of the basin, as the tracks indicate.

3.9 mi (5) This is the base of Airplane Gully (12,280 feet). Finding the right gully can be tricky. Looking up at Navajo Peak, you'll see the Navajo Glacier on the right, the lumpy north face, and a steep gully that ends where the summit pyramid joins the ridge—this is *not* your gully. To the left of this gully is an outcrop of rock; Airplane Gully runs to the left of this rock. There is a minor talus fan of large boulders at the base (as well as a silver wing from the plane, with identification numbers). When you go over to the base of the gully, it will seem very climbable.

There are many loose rocks in Airplane Gully, so be careful if you are scrambling above people. It's steep, but I'd still only rate the gully class 2+. More difficult than its grade is its total of 900 vertical feet. About halfway up (at approximately 12,550 feet), the gully forks. Take the right fork, despite the fact that the straight south route offers a keyhole of blue sky through the rocks topping its exit. The correct fork climbs southwest. At 12,900 feet, just before the exit, lies the largest part of the wreckage. A major section of the bulkhead, motors, gears, and wires are everywhere. Do not touch or take any of the wreckage. It's illegal to take pieces of the plane, as it's a recognized crash site. Furthermore, the heavy metal pieces sit in a loose, unstable gully—they may shift at any time. Above the wreckage, a grassy slope exits onto Navajo's east ridge.

4.2 mi (6) At the gully exit, the final pyramid looms before you. To reach the summit, hike up to the base of the block, favoring the south (left) side of the slope. Head west until you reach about 13,260 feet. There is a perilously balanced rock on the west side known as the Monkey Fist. This is your cue to begin scrambling north on exposed but solid rock. It's a short push, maybe 30–40 feet with several class 3 moves. Note that more experienced climbers can find a way up the face to the right (east face) via several class 3+ and class 4 sections. Novice or inexperienced hikers may find the exposure a bit unsettling.

4.4 mi (7) Navajo Peak's tiny summit has a register tube and a cairn. It can accommodate two people, though there are places for others to sit just below the summit. The down climb back to the east ridge can be tricky. The safest and easiest way is to retrace the way you came, even though it looks like the rocks drop off into oblivion. There are several slightly more direct exits you can take by going down the southeast side; if you take them, you'll have short sections of face-in down climbing, with some fall potential—class 4 stuff.

Once you are safely on the ridge, return via Airplane Gully. The loose rock makes this descent tough; I'd recommend using an ice ax/trekking poles for stability, even when there is no snow. Once you're out of the gully, return to Lake Isabelle, regain the well-worn trail, and enjoy the hike out.

8.9 mi Finish.

Options Hiking Navajo Peak makes for a fairly demanding day, so linking to other routes isn't really an option for a day hike. There are some good views if you explore northeast on Niwot Ridge, which would require a left turn at the top of Airplane Gully (waypoint **6**). Navajo's southeast ridge looks as if it would provide an exciting class 3+ traverse over to nearby 13,150-foot Arikaree Peak, but Arikaree has the unfortunate fate of being in the off-limits Boulder watershed. The impressive stand-alone peak you see from atop Airplane Gully to the east, 13,276-foot Kiowa Peak, is likewise forbidden. Fines are strictly enforced for trespassing in this area.

Quick Facts Ellsworth Bethel advocated naming a series of peaks to honor native peoples; that series is now known as the Indian Peaks. Navajo Peak is one example; others include Apache, Shoshoni, Arapahoe, Pawnee, and Arikaree Peaks, as well as Niwot Ridge. A mountain was named in Bethel's honor also, though not in this range. You can spot Mount Bethel when driving east on I-70 just past the Eisenhower Tunnel, thanks to the snow fences high on its slopes, which are its trademark.

The airplane wreckage is from a crash that occurred on January 21, 1948. Three men were killed when the C-47, en route from Denver to Grand Junction, was caught in bad weather and was pushed into the ridge by strong winds. The crash site was not discovered for several months. There are some who believe that the wreckage should be left alone. It is my opinion that one should not feel guilty or morbid for wanting to see the crash debris. The accident was tragic, but it serves as an example of how man and mountain are intertwined by the threads of fate. Like many scenes that remind us of our mortality, such an experience can also manifest itself as an affirmation of life.

Contact Info

The good news: The Brainard Lake Recreation Area is free from sometime in October–early June. The bad news: The road is closed at the pay station, roughly 2 miles from Brainard Lake. You can park there and bike, ski, or hike in if you want to try an off-season ascent. This area is very popular in the winter for snowshoeing and cross-country skiing.

Grand Country Wilderness Group
(This group helps the US Forest Service manage the Brainard Lake Recreation Area)
P.O. Box 2200
Fraser, CO 80442
(970) 726-4626
Recorded Voice Information Hotline: (303) 541-2519

Arapaho/Roosevelt National Forest
Boulder Ranger District
2140 Yarmouth Avenue
Boulder, CO 80301
(303) 541-2500

Jasper Peak

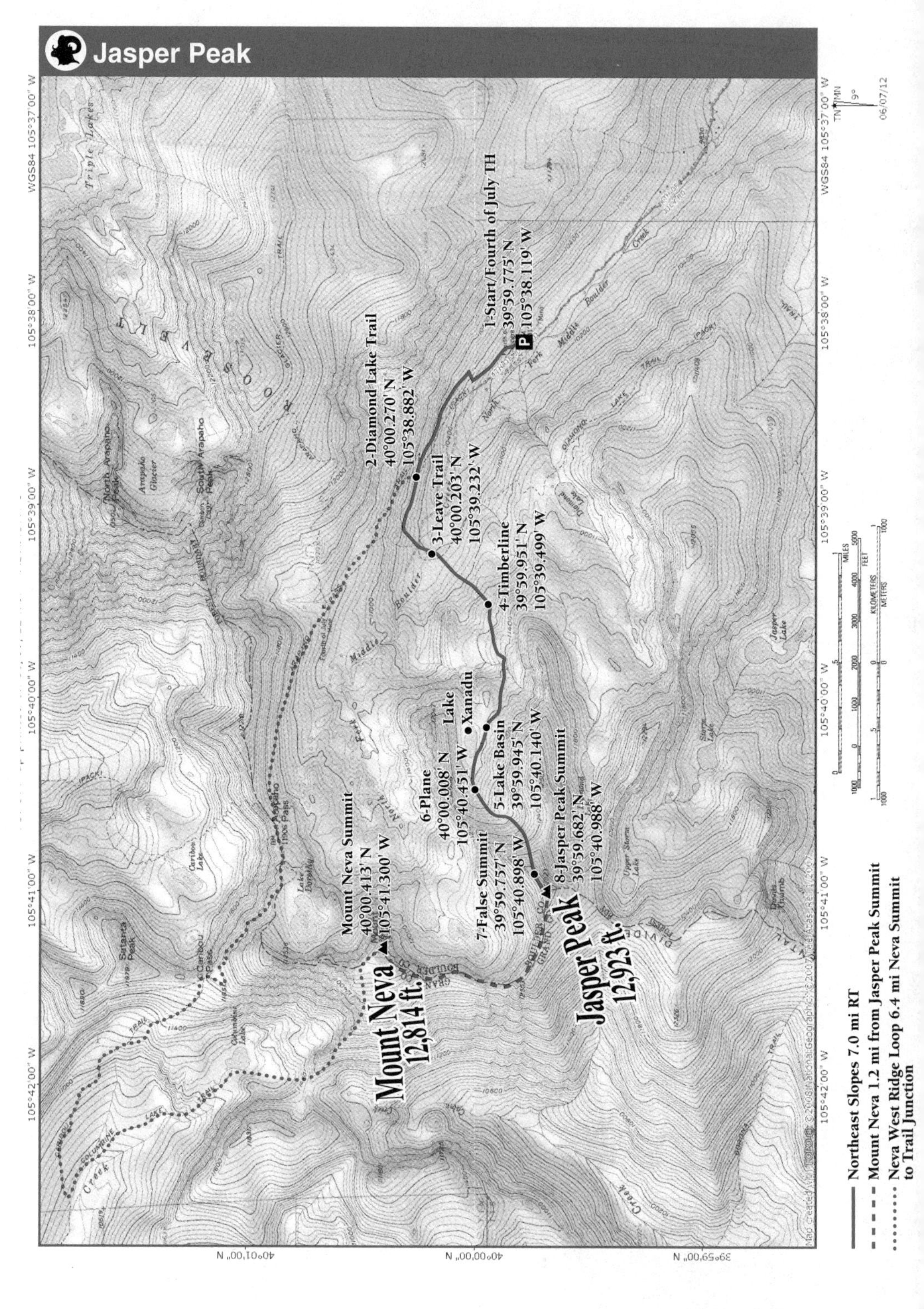

1-Start/Fourth of July TH
39°59.775' N
105°38.119' W
2-Diamond Lake Trail
40°00.270' N
105°38.882' W
3-Leave Trail
40°00.203' N
105°39.232' W
4-Timberline
39°59.951' N
105°39.499' W
5-Lake Basin
39°59.945' N
105°40.140' W
6-Plane
40°00.008' N
105°40.451' W
7-False Summit
39°59.757' N
105°40.898' W
8-Jasper Peak Summit
39°59.682' N
105°40.988' W
Mount Neva Summit
40°00.413' N
105°41.300' W
Mount Neva
12,814 ft.
Jasper Peak
12,923 ft.
Lake Xanadu
North Arapaho Peak
South Arapaho Peak
Arapaho Glacier
Caribou Lake
Satanta Peak
Lake Dorothy
Jasper Lake
Storm Lake
Upper Storm Lake
Diamond Lake
Devils Thumb
Triple Lakes
Columbine Lake
Caribou Pass
Arapaho Pass
Middle Boulder Creek
Northeast Slopes 7.0 mi RT
Mount Neva 1.2 mi from Jasper Peak Summit
Neva West Ridge Loop 6.4 mi Neva Summit to Trail Junction

3 Jasper Peak

Jasper is such a secret that it doesn't even appear on the map. This great climb requires off-trail navigation and passes by the most beautiful unknown basin in Indian Peaks.

Round-Trip Distance	7.0 miles
Hiking Time	5½–7 hours
Difficulty	7/10
Class	2+
Start Elevation	10,170 ft., at Fourth of July Trailhead
Peak Elevation	12,923 ft.
Total Elevation Gain	3,010 ft.
Terrain	Spongy, off-trail forests leading to snowfields and grassy rock slopes
Best Time to Climb	Late May–September
Gear Advisor	GPS, gaiters, ice ax, and crampons in early spring
Crowd Level	Hermit

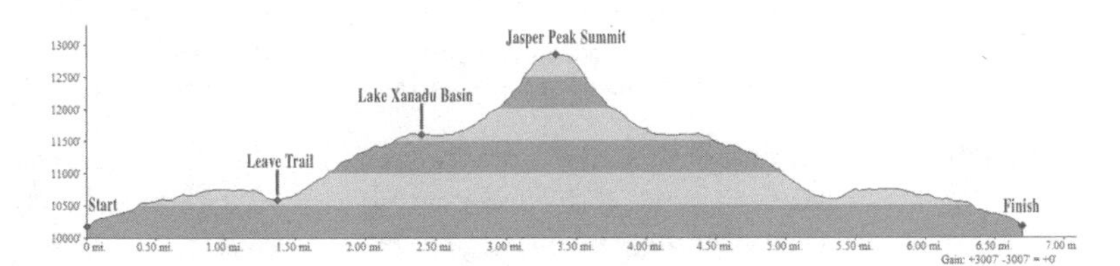

Location Indian Peaks Range in the Indian Peaks Wilderness/Roosevelt National Forest north of Nederland

Intro Jasper Peak (also known as Mount Jasper) has held its name informally for years, despite not appearing on official maps. It is a hard mountain to spot from lower elevations. When the peak becomes visible at higher elevations, it has a very alluring pyramid shape, just begging to be climbed. It takes solid navigational skills to reach Lake Xanadu Basin, a stunning alpine lake tucked away in the folds of the Indian Peaks. Prime hiking time for Jasper is in late May and early June, when snow on the northeast face is stable enough for an ascent and for blazing glissades on the way down.

Why Climb It? It's good that Jasper doesn't appear on the map. The on-trail hikes in this area of the Indian Peaks see a lot of traffic, yet this mountain remains a mystery to most. Once you leave the trail, navigation through the trees is a fun challenge (without severe repercussions if you take a wrong turn). After finding your way through woods and meadows, you'll find yourself in a pristine basin with the small, sparkling Lake Xanadu as the centerpiece. There is also a small plane wreck at the west end of the lake, a curious relic in such a remote area. Climb to a false summit that hides the true apex a short distance beyond. Strong hikers can continue the fun by taking the optional trek over to Mount Neva.

Driving Tough passenger cars can make it to the Fourth of July Trailhead. The road is rocky, with sections of washboards and ruts, but it is passable by cars. I've driven up in my Honda Accord many times, and I've seen other similar cars in the parking lot. Road maintenance is performed every spring, so the road may be in better shape in mid-June.

How to Get There To reach the Fourth of July Trailhead, start in the town of Nederland and go south on Colorado Highway 119 toward Eldora Ski Area. About 0.2 mile out of town, turn right and follow the signs for Eldora Ski Area (Road 130). At 1.4 miles down this road, there is a left turnoff for Eldora Ski Area—do not take this road. Instead, continue straight and at mile 2.9, pass through the small town of Eldora. At the end of town, the road turns to dirt. Continue on for 1.4 miles to a split; stay right (the left road goes to the Hessie Trailhead). The road gets rougher but is still passable in normal conditions. Drive 4.4 miles farther and the Fourth of July Trailhead will be on your right, just past Buckingham Campground. The little access road into the parking lot may be the toughest driving of the whole trip.

Fees/Camping There are no fees to hike in this area. Overnight camping trips in the Indian Peaks require a backcountry permit June–September; the cost is $5. Buckingham Campground is a free, first-come, first-serve site.

Route Notes A majority of this hike is off-trail, and you'll need to perform basic navigational skills to reach Lake Xanadu Basin. (Once you are there, the route is visually clear on good days.)

Mile/Waypoint **0.0 mi (1)** Start at the Fourth of July Trailhead. Get on the well-worn Arapaho Pass Trail and follow it for 1.0 mile to the junction with the Diamond Lake Trail. You'll get a preview of Jasper from viewpoints on this section of the trail.

1.0 mi (2) Bear left onto the Diamond Lake Trail. You will be going downhill and into deeper woods.

1.4 mi (3) Say goodbye to the trail once you reach Middle Boulder Creek. Cross the modest stream, and head southwest through the woods. The ground is spongy, but the trees are well spaced. If the weather is clear, in the clearings you'll have glimpses of where you need to go. The difficult navigation (in trees) is only for about 0.5 mile.

1.8 mi (4) You will reach timberline around 11,060 feet. There will be a large mountain ridge due west and a small bulge south of the mountain. The easiest way to reach Lake Xanadu Basin is to find the gap south of the small bulge (between the small bulge and a ridge to your left, farther south). Find a good route up to the basin from here; it's easier when snow covers the boulders.

2.4 mi (5) Soak in the views at the flat and accommodating Lake Xanadu Basin. The moderate slopes to the southwest become obvious.

Note on Alternate Route: Those who like ridge walks can make the steep scramble directly north of Lake Xanadu and gain Jasper's northeast ridge. Follow it on class 2+ terrain to Jasper's summit.

2.7 mi (6) On the west end of the lake is the wreckage of a small silver-and-red airplane. It's an interesting sight, especially in contrast to the beauty of the area.

Gain the northeast slope and find a good line up to connect with the northeast ridge. In early spring, you may need crampons for the snow. Follow these slopes west and intersect with the northeast ridge.

3.3 mi (7) False summit! At 12,887 feet, you're almost there. The actual summit is just beyond, via an easy scramble heading southwest.

3.5 mi (8) Jasper's summit may surprise you. When the snow is melted, it's a grassy patch with small wildflowers. The Winter Park and Mary Jane ski areas can be seen to the west and Mount Neva is visible to the north. Return the way you came, or continue north on the optional route to Mount Neva.

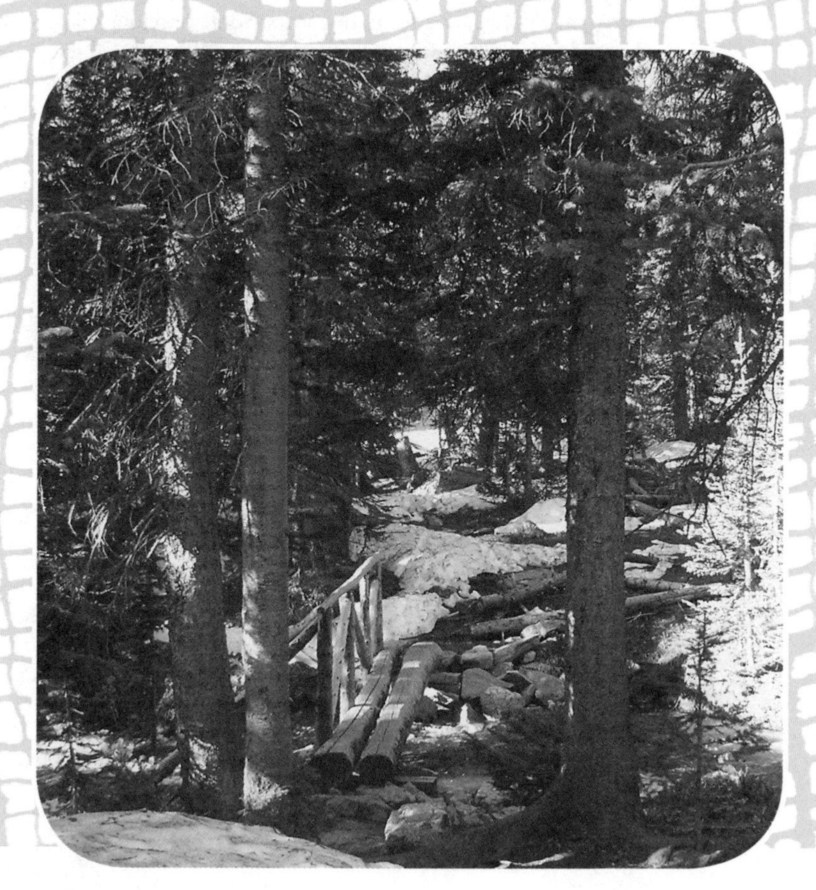

Enjoy your last glimpse of on-trail hiking; from here on out, you'll be off the beaten path.

If returning via the standard route, take care when navigating back to the Diamond Lake Trail (GPS is a huge help at this point).

7.0 mi Finish.

Options Mount Neva is 1.2 miles from the summit along a class 2+ ridge. Head north to reach Neva. Once you are there, it's best to return to Jasper and descend via the standard route—Neva's north ridge to Arapaho Pass is a class 4 route, which may require ropes.

One option that looks like fun (though I have not tried it) is to do a super loop as a two-day endeavor. Camp the first night at Lake Xanadu, and go light because you won't be coming back this way. The next day, climb Jasper and traverse to Neva, and then descend Neva's northwest ridge down to Columbine Lake. Pick up the Columbine Lake Trail and go north to the junction with the Caribou Trail. Return east over Caribou Pass to Arapaho Pass, where you can follow the Arapaho Pass Trail back to your car. From Lake Xanadu, this loop is about 10 miles (12 or 13 total, depending on your navigation skills). It would be difficult to do in a single day, due to afternoon storms, which could catch you high on Caribou Pass or Arapaho Pass.

Quick Facts Jasper is not the official name of the peak (technically, it is unnamed), but it has gone by the name for many years. Some previous maps and guidebooks have identified it as Jasper Peak or Mount Jasper; we'll use Jasper Peak. For that matter, Lake Xanadu is an unofficial name but one that seems to fit the area well. The only landscape feature with an officially recognized name around here, Mount Neva, is named after the brother of Arapaho leader Chief Niwot.

Contact Info Arapaho/Roosevelt National Forest
Boulder Ranger District
2140 Yarmouth Avenue
Boulder, CO 80301
(303) 541-2500

Recorded Indian Peaks Information Hotline: (303) 541-2519

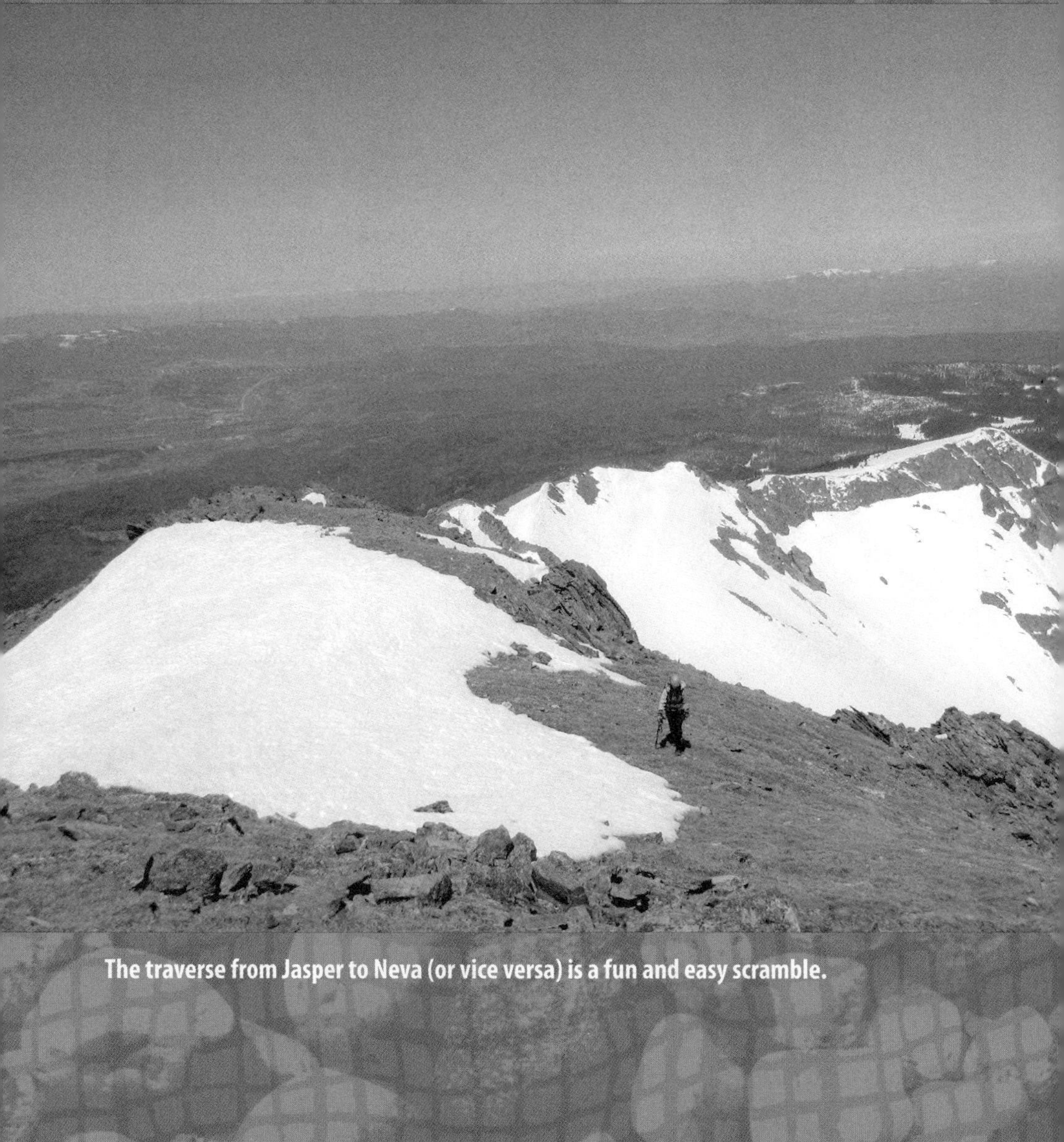

The traverse from Jasper to Neva (or vice versa) is a fun and easy scramble.

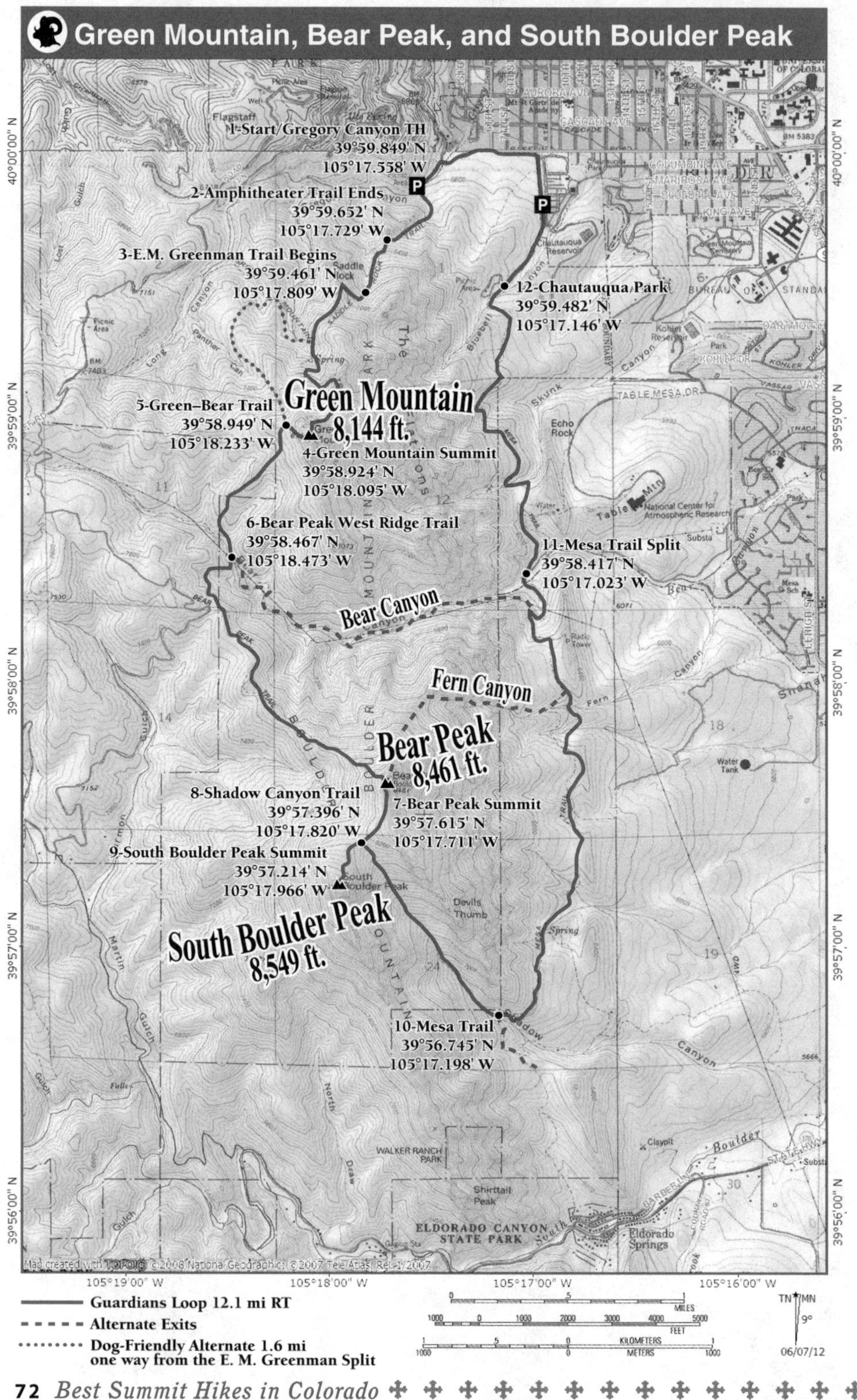
Green Mountain, Bear Peak, and South Boulder Peak
1-Start/Gregory Canyon TH
39°59.849' N
105°17.558' W
2-Amphitheater Trail Ends
39°59.652' N
105°17.729' W
3-E.M. Greenman Trail Begins
39°59.461' N
105°17.809' W
Green Mountain
8,144 ft.
5-Green–Bear Trail
39°58.949' N
105°18.233' W
4-Green Mountain Summit
39°58.924' N
105°18.095' W
6-Bear Peak West Ridge Trail
39°58.467' N
105°18.473' W
Bear Canyon
Fern Canyon
Bear Peak
8,461 ft.
8-Shadow Canyon Trail
39°57.396' N
105°17.820' W
7-Bear Peak Summit
39°57.615' N
105°17.711' W
9-South Boulder Peak Summit
39°57.214' N
105°17.966' W
South Boulder Peak
8,549 ft.
10-Mesa Trail
39°56.745' N
105°17.198' W
11-Mesa Trail Split
39°58.417' N
105°17.023' W
12-Chautauqua Park
39°59.482' N
105°17.146' W
National Center for Atmospheric Research
ELDORADO CANYON STATE PARK
Eldorado Springs
WALKER RANCH PARK
Shirttail Peak
Devils Thumb
Map created with TOPO!© ©2008 National Geographic; ©2007 Tele Atlas, Rel. 1/2007
40°00'00" N
39°59'00" N
39°58'00" N
39°57'00" N
39°56'00" N
105°19'00" W
105°18'00" W
105°17'00" W
105°16'00" W
Guardians Loop 12.1 mi RT
Alternate Exits
Dog-Friendly Alternate 1.6 mi one way from the E. M. Greenman Split
MILES
FEET
KILOMETERS
METERS
TN MN
9°
06/07/12

4 Guardians of the Flatirons: Green Mountain, Bear Peak, and South Boulder Peak

This three-peak traverse is the pride of Boulder, giving you a deluxe tour of the local mountains and the slanted pinnacles of the Flatirons. A big hike that's right in town.

Round-Trip Distance	12.1 miles
Hiking Time	7–10 hours
Difficulty	6.5/10
Class	2
Start Elevation	5,833 ft., at Gregory Canyon Trailhead
Peak Elevations	Green Mountain: 8,144 ft.; Bear Peak: 8,461 ft.; South Boulder Peak: 8,549 ft.
Total Elevation Gain	5,171 ft.
Terrain	On-trail tour of Boulder's Flatirons
Best Time to Climb	Year-round; may be very hot midsummer
Gear Advisor	Normal gear
Crowd Level	Moderate overall; high on Green Mountain and the Mesa Trail

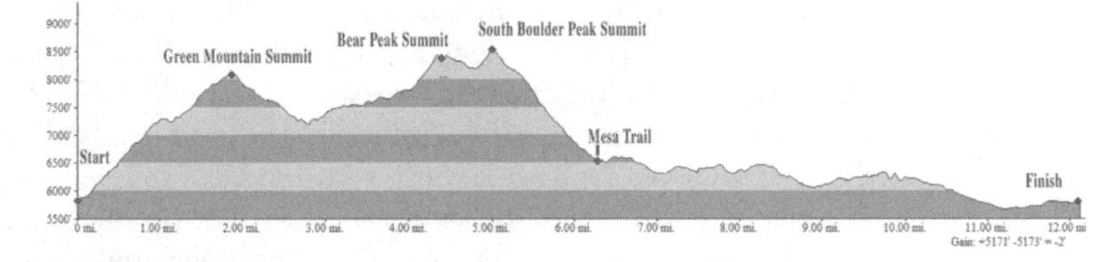

Location Boulder Mountain Park in beautiful Boulder, Colorado

Intro Who says that you need to have your head in the clouds to have an epic day? This three-peak traverse begins in the civilized confines of Boulder. First, wind your way through shady, vanilla-scented pine forests bracketed by towering rock formations to Green Mountain. Descend from Green into a hidden world of alpine flowers and grandiose valleys. It will seem hard to believe that a city of 90,000 people is just on the other side of the ridge as you drop into Bear Canyon. Gradually ascend to the rocky summit of fashionable Bear Peak, and complete the traverse by visiting the less-popular (but slightly higher) South Boulder Peak. Descend via the rocky Shadow Canyon Trail, where the Devil's Thumb will be poised to your left, frozen mid-smite. Complete the loop with a casual return hike below the impressive Flatiron rock formations.

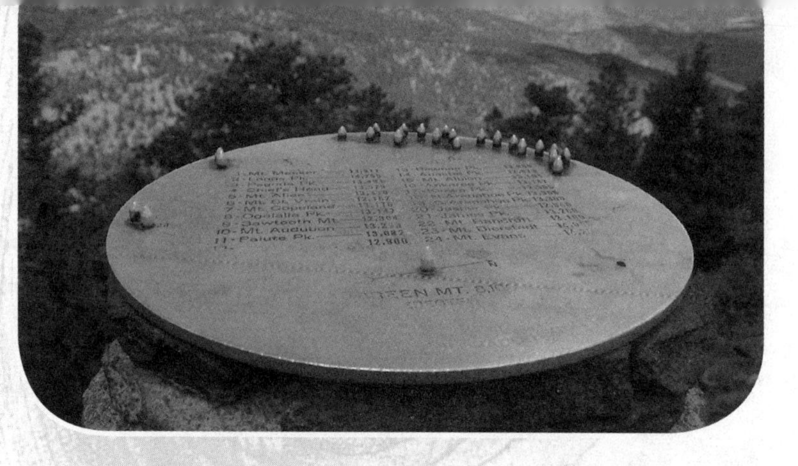

This metal disk atop Green Mountain shows you what mountains are visible on the horizon.

Why Climb It? The Flatirons serve as the mountainous backdrop to Boulder and denote the eastern terminus of the Rocky Mountains. Their abrupt angles and reddish hues make them the perfect ambassadors for the subsequent peaks that rise to the west. This hike gives you an extended tour of the area, offering great views of Boulder and Denver to the east and the Indian Peaks and Front Range to the west. On clear days, you can see from Longs Peak to Pikes Peak. The western side of these mountains is surprisingly wild; standing on the summit of Bear Peak feels as though you're on the dividing line between civilization and wilderness. As the trail drops down to the base of the Flatirons, it bypasses dozens of amazing rock formations. Even though it's in town, the elevation gain and mileage gives you a workout on par with one you'd experience on higher mountains.

Driving Any vehicle can make it to the trailhead; it is paved all the way.

How to Get There From US Highway 36 in Boulder, take the Baseline Road exit, turn west onto Baseline Road, and continue for 1.8 miles. You'll pass Chautauqua Park on your left. Just after the large signs for Boulder Mountain Parks and the fire danger warnings, turn off left as the road bends abruptly uphill to Gregory Canyon Trailhead. If this parking lot is full, you can park on the designated south side of the short access road or simply go 0.1 mile back to Chautauqua's parking lot. On weekends, these parking lots fill up fast.

Fees/Camping There is a $3 parking fee for cars at the Gregory Canyon Trailhead (this fee does not apply to Boulder Country residents). Free parking can be found at Chautauqua Park or along the side roads (such as Ninth Street) to the north of Baseline. As for camping . . . you're in a major city. There's no real legal camping to speak of nearby, but there are plenty of nice hotels in Boulder.

Route Notes There are many trails that intersect this route, especially once you drop down onto the Mesa Trail. Read the description closely so that you don't take a wrong turn along the way. This route is very well marked, with signs at most junctions.

Mile/Waypoint **0.0 mi (1)** Start at Gregory Canyon Trailhead. There are two trails you can take to start your hike; this route favors the Amphitheater Trail (on the east side of the parking area). Get on this trail (staying right at the early intersection with the Bluebell-Baird Trail) and begin hiking upward, quickly reaching a section of steep "stairs." Bypass the Amphitheater Express Trail on your right (which leads to rock climbing routes). You'll know the juncture to avoid when you see a sign previewing the neat formations to come at the Amphitheater.

0.4 mi (2) The Amphitheater Trail ends and joins the Saddle Rock Trail, which comes in from the right (this is the other route that leaves from the parking area). Stay left on the Saddle Rock Trail and continue hiking uphill through the vanilla- and pine-scented forest. Continue to follow the Saddle Rock Trail. Do not turn off at the Saddle Rock climbing access trail on your left, at 0.7 mile.

1.3 mi (3) The Saddle Rock Trail ends and becomes the E. M. Greenman Trail, which comes in from the right. Bear left and continue your ascent on the E. M. Greenman Trail. This trail will lead you to the summit of Green Mountain. Note that there is one slightly tricky part at mile 1.45—the trail takes a turn to the left over some large tree roots. A worn but incorrect path to the right has been blocked off with rocks and sticks. Stay left over the roots and the trail will become obvious again. Follow it to Green Mountain's summit.

2.0 mi (4) Green Mountain summit. There is a register here and a neat metal plaque that identifies the mountains on the horizon to the west. You can see at least four other mountains that this book details hikes for: Mount Alice (Hike 9), Longs Peak (Hike 8), Jasper Peak (Hike 3), and James Peak (Hike 1). Continue south off the summit and down a well-worn, switchbacking trail.

2.1 mi (5) At this four-way intersection, turn left onto the Green-Bear Trail, which goes downhill to the southwest. Keep your eye out for any green bears! The trail feels worlds away from the city din of Boulder. Enjoy the wildflowers. There are also good views of the back sides of Bear Peak and South Boulder Peak.

2.9 mi (6) The Green-Bear Trail ends in Bear Canyon. At the well-marked sign, take a right onto the Bear Peak West Ridge Trail. This well-traveled and well-marked path starts out as a series of gentle switchbacks and then begins climbing more steeply up the rocky slopes of Bear's west ridge.

4.4 mi This trail ends just below the rocks that make up Bear Peak's summit. The scramble up looks tough, but there is an easier way. Traverse a short distance left (north), where you can scramble directly south on a "ramp" to the top. (This is the most difficult scrambling on the hike, and it's only class 2.)

4.5 mi (7) Bear Peak summit! These are the best 360-degree views on the entire hike. To the south is Pikes Peak; to the west, the Indian Peaks; to the north, Longs Peak and Fort Collins; and to the east, the sprawling metropolis of Denver and its suburbs. Exit the summit the way you came up, and return to the west side of the peak below the summit, where the Bear Peak West Ridge Trail ended. Pick up the connector trail, in the rocks, that goes south to South Boulder Peak.

4.9 mi (8) A dip in the ridge between Bear and South Boulder Peaks introduces the Shadow Canyon Trail on your left. Eventually, you will descend on this trail; for the time being, however, stay on the South Boulder Peak trail heading southwest. You can tell from the growth in this area that this peak sees much less traffic than the previous two summits.

5.1 mi (9) South Boulder Peak summit! This is the highest point of your hike, even though it is blocked by trees on the east side. Keep your eyes open for wild raspberry bushes up here. Return to the junction with the Shadow Canyon Trail.

5.4 mi (8) Take the Shadow Canyon Trail southeast and descend via this rocky road. There are a few brief sections where the trail passes over talus fields; follow the cairns to resume the trail after these interludes.

5.9 mi In a slight clearing, look up to your left. The upturned Devil's Thumb gives you its approval.

6.5 mi (10) At the bottom of the rocky trail, you'll enter a small clearing with a few trails intersecting. Turn left (north) onto the marked Mesa Trail and begin the lower tour of the Flatirons. From here on out, you'll be on the class 1 Mesa Trail until you reach Chautauqua Park. You will have many great views of the Flatirons on your left. Several trails intersect with the Mesa Trail along the way. Stay on the Mesa Trail, and continue going north.

9.1 mi (11) This is the only tricky part of the Mesa Trail, though it's still well marked. After passing the Fern Canyon cutoff, you'll pass a small stream on your right. The wide dirt trail you're on continues to the west; make sure that you stay on the Mesa Trail, which cuts off to the left (north) uphill and becomes a single-lane footpath again. Follow it north through a four-way intersection just below the National Center for Atmospheric Research (NCAR) to your right. After this, you'll drop in and out of Skunk Canyon and continue to the boundaries of Chautauqua Park. Several trails continue to come in on both sides of the Mesa Trail.

10.8 mi (12) The Mesa Trail turns into a gravel path as you drop down into Chautauqua. Look west to see the loop you just made over the mountains. To return to Gregory Canyon Trailhead, you can hike west on Baseline Road or take a footpath that parallels the road in the open meadow.

12.1 mi Finish.

Options If you'd like to cut an hour or two off your hike (and still bag the three peaks), bring two cars (or a bike and a car). You can leave a vehicle at the Shadow Canyon/Mesa Trail Trailhead, accessed by taking Colorado Highway 93 (Broadway) out of Boulder and then taking a right onto Colorado Highway 170 at a stoplight (a convenience store is on the right). Follow the road toward Eldorado Springs for 2 miles, and the marked trailhead will be on the right-hand side of the road. At waypoint **10**, instead of turning onto the Mesa Trail after your descent of Shadow Canyon, follow the Shadow Canyon Trail 1.5 miles to this parking lot. You could also park a car at the NCAR lot (no fee), accessed by taking CO 93 and then turning west onto Table Mesa Drive and following it to its terminus. You would end your hike at NCAR by taking the Mesa Trail past Fern Canyon and turning right at the well-marked sign at the top of a small hill (shortly after waypoint **11**); this trail leads to NCAR.

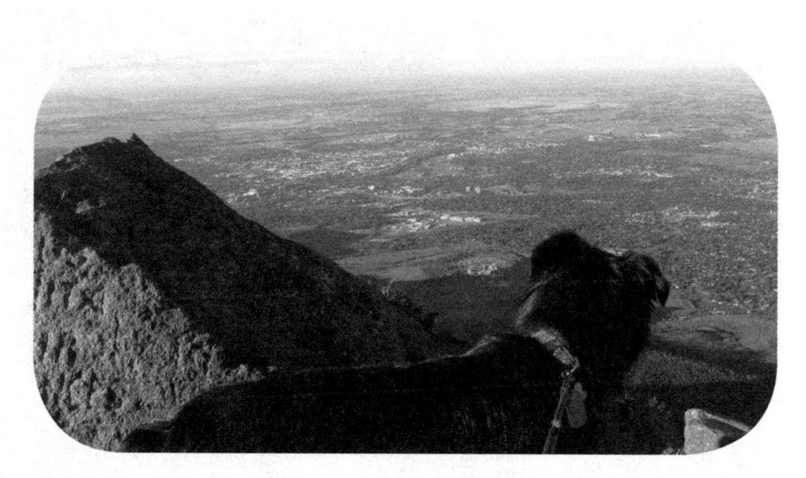

A bird's-eye view of Boulder awaits from the summit of Bear Peak.

If you want an early exit, you can follow the Bear Canyon Trail (at the end of the Green-Bear Trail) or the Fern Canyon Trail (from the summit of Bear Peak) east. Both intersect with the Mesa Trail, shaving time off your hike but still giving you a fun loop.

A dog-friendly detour to the summit of Green goes right (north) to the E. M. Greenman Trail 0.5 mile and then connects with the Ranger Trail. Go left (southwest) on the Ranger Trail 0.9 mile to a flat intersection. Then go left (southeast) to the Green Mountain Summit trail 0.2 mile to the top. The loop is 1.6 miles one-way.

Quick Facts

These three peaks have very common names. Did you know that there are more than 20 Green Mountains in Colorado? One twist on this Green Mountain: It may allude to E. M. Greenman, an early Boulder conservationist. Chautauqua Park was part of an educational movement at the turn of the 19th century that aimed to create communities in which members were encouraged to delve into the arts, sciences, and music as a part of daily life. Touring units of entertainers would visit Chautauqua communities in each state. While the concept was a positive, progressive alternative to mundane living, many of the Chautauqua communities soon became too expensive for normal folks, and the exclusivity stymied the movement, though the practice still exists to some degree in Boulder today.

Contact Info

This hike is especially beautiful on a snowy winter day. If you're hiking in the summer, bring a little extra water, as it can get very toasty in Boulder June–late September. And if you want a good view of fireworks on the Fourth of July, Bear Peak is a fun (and social) place to watch the displays from towns across the Front Range.

Note: This area is undergoing changes as Boulder Mountain Park aims to improve the trail system. Call for more information.

Boulder Mountain Parks
P.O. Box 791
Boulder, CO 80306
(303) 441-3440

Lead Mountain

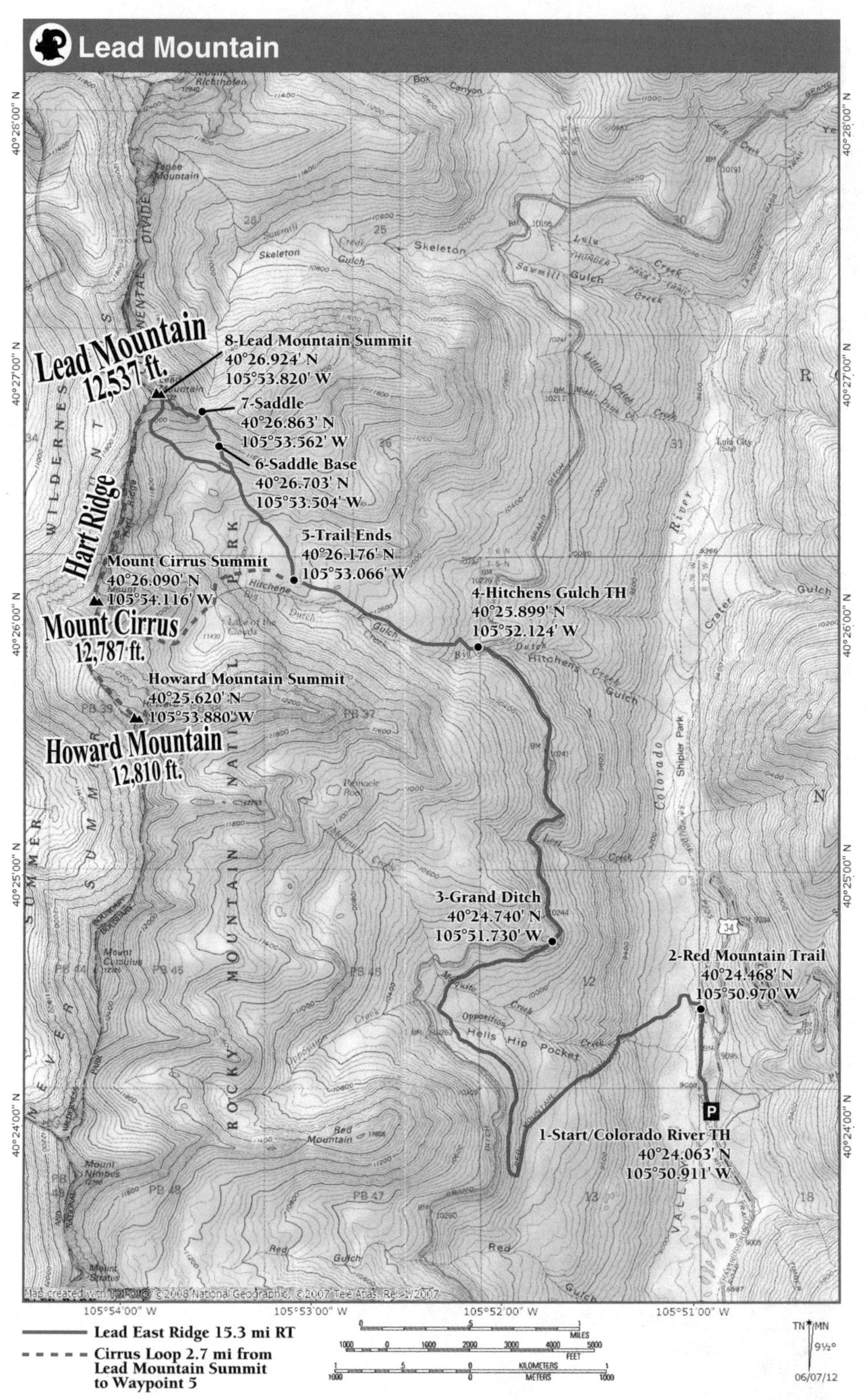
Lead Mountain
12,537 ft.
8-Lead Mountain Summit
40°26.924' N
105°53.820' W
7-Saddle
40°26.863' N
105°53.562' W
6-Saddle Base
40°26.703' N
105°53.504' W
5-Trail Ends
40°26.176' N
105°53.066' W
Hart Ridge
Mount Cirrus Summit
40°26.090' N
105°54.116' W
Mount Cirrus
12,787 ft.
4-Hitchens Gulch TH
40°25.899' N
105°52.124' W
Howard Mountain Summit
40°25.620' N
105°53.880' W
Howard Mountain
12,810 ft.
3-Grand Ditch
40°24.740' N
105°51.730' W
2-Red Mountain Trail
40°24.468' N
105°50.970' W
1-Start/Colorado River TH
40°24.063' N
105°50.911' W
Lead East Ridge 15.3 mi RT
Cirrus Loop 2.7 mi from
Lead Mountain Summit
to Waypoint 5
Map created with TOPO! © 2008 National Geographic; ©2007 Tele Atlas, Rel. 1/2007
06/07/12

5 Lead Mountain

Good Overnight!

This beautiful, airy ridge is a great scramble that will keep you on your toes. The rock is solid, and the views are phenomenal. An optional loop to Mount Cirrus adds to the fun.

Round-Trip Distance	15.3 miles
Hiking Time	9–14 hours
Difficulty	9/10
Class	3/3+
Start Elevation	9,100 ft., at Colorado River Trailhead
Peak Elevation	12,537 ft.
Total Elevation Gain	3,727 ft.
Terrain	Long prelude to exciting class 3 ridge
Best Time to Climb	July–September
Gear Advisor	Helmet and good "grippy" boots
Crowd Level	Hermit

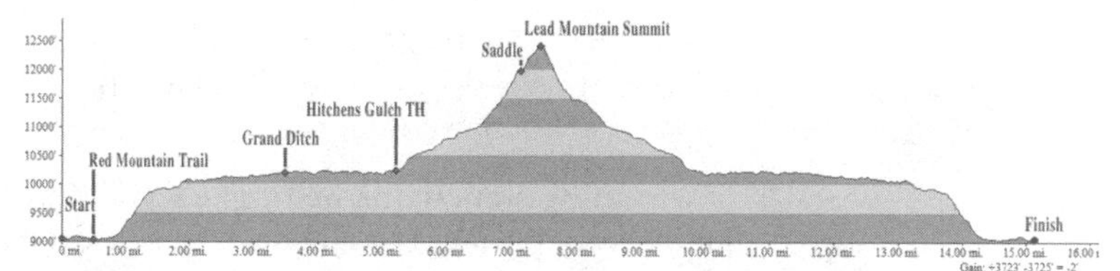

Location Never Summer Range in Rocky Mountain National Park outside of Estes Park

Intro Lead Mountain has one of the premier ridge walks in the state. The exposed, airy, class 3 traverse is short, but it certainly gets your attention. Rock is solid for the most part. Those hikers uncomfortable with hanging out on the spine have the option to drop down slightly to the south side, where terrain is less exposed. The Never Summer Range is a special treat for hikers looking to get away from the crowds. The loop over to Mount Cirrus may be Colorado's best class 3 route that's not in the Grenadiers.

Why Climb It? The mileage looks daunting, but a good deal of this hike is the long and scenic approach. Trails are class 1 from the trailhead, all the way to the end of the Hitchens Gulch Trail, 6.2 miles in. The actual class 3 terrain is only roughly 1.3 miles on the standard route, but every foot is an exciting experience. Lead's east ridge is airy and exhilarating, with sheer drop-offs to the north. Rock is solid, but the exposure will boost your concentration. A few moves may be considered class 4 or 3+ if you stay on the spine of the ridge. The holds are solid and obvious, but if you blow it, you'll be shuffling off this mortal coil with haste. If you aren't used to this kind of exposure, an alternate class 3 route on the south side of the ridge is just as good.

Driving Any vehicle can make it to the trailhead; the entire drive is on paved roads.

How to Get There From the east entrances (Beaver Meadows or Fall River), go about 4 miles (from either) to the intersection of US Highways 34 and 36. Continue on Trail Ridge Road (US 34) 28 miles, up and over the high point near the Alpine visitor center. After the road exits the final hairpin turn downhill, it's about 1.2 miles to the Colorado River Trailhead on the right (west) side of the road. The turnoff is well marked. This trailhead is 11.5 miles north on US 34 from the west entrance at Grand Lake.

Fees/Camping It is $20 for a day pass to Rocky Mountain National Park. There are several drive-in campgrounds in the park that range $10–$14 a night; call for more information. A better option (and one that gives you the time to complete the Hart Ridge traverse to Mount Cirrus) is to camp at backcountry sites at Hitchens Gulch (Hitchens Gulch Campground and Dutch Town Campground—beware of mosquitoes in the summer). It is $20 for a backcountry camping permit but well worth the price for this incredible optional loop.

Route Notes I highly recommend the Mount Cirrus loop, starting with an overnight at Dutch Town and getting an early start to the day. It's a scrambler's delight.

Mile/Waypoint **0.0 mi (1)** Start at the Colorado River Trailhead and head north on the very well-trodden trail (this is the La Poudre Pass Trail). You will be on this smooth section for only a short distance.

0.5 mi (2) Turn left (west) onto the well-signed Red Mountain Trail. The turnoff sign includes mileages to Hitchens Gulch, Grand Ditch, Dutch Town, and Thunder Pass. Stay on this pleasant trail all the way to the Grand Ditch. Along the way, you will pass the rather benign canyon called Hell's Hip Pocket.

3.3 mi (3) After a nice walk in the woods, you come to . . . a road? This is the Grand Ditch. Turn right and hike north on this easygoing road (don't worry that Lead Mountain is directly west; you have to loop around to reach it). Public access to this road is limited to foot traffic, so any vehicle sightings are rare. (And no, you can't drive up here as a shortcut.)

5.2 mi (4) Eventually, you'll come to the Hitchens Gulch Trailhead on your left (west), where the road crosses Dutch Creek. There is a sign here for Hitchens Gulch and Dutch Town. A good trail heads northwest toward Lead's talus-filled basin. Hitchens Gulch Camp area is at mile 5.5; Dutch Town is at mile 5.9. Stay on this trail until it ends abruptly at a post near a mosquito-filled swamp.

6.2 mi (5) Luckily, there is only one small hill to climb after the trail ends (there may still be a faint footpath). Atop this hill, you're out of the trees, and the incredible rock-filled basin is before you. Gradually ascend, first on rocks and then on grassy slopes, northwest to the scree slope that goes to the saddle between Lead and Point 12,438. Some crazy rock formations are

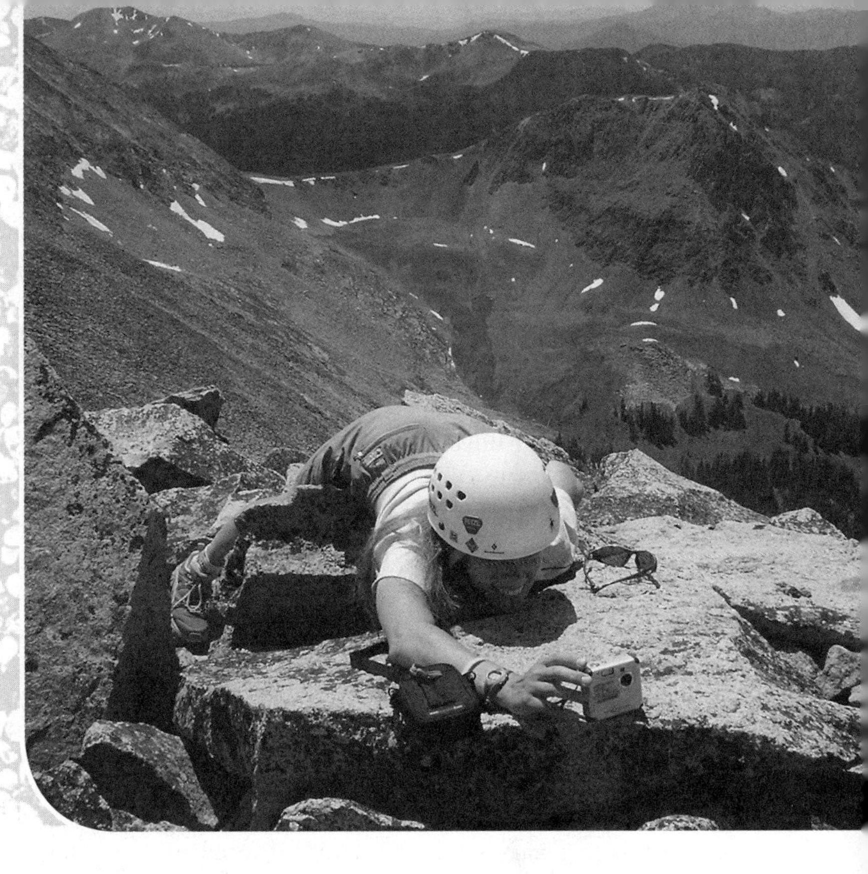

Getting the perfect shot can be tricky on Lead's rocky summit.

on 12,438, and it looks like some large boulders have peeled off the mountain in recent times.

7.0 mi (6) You will come to the base of a loose, red scree gully. The grass on the right side is deceptive; the terrain there is just as loose as the middle of the gully. It's a bit of a knee burner. Make your way to the saddle and get ready to climb.

7.2 mi (7) You are now in the saddle. Don your helmet and get ready to head west on Lead's east ridge. To the north, there is a great view of another mountain featured in this book, Mount Richthofen (Hike 7). You can go a short bit on the north side of the saddle to gain the obvious ramp up to the ridge.

Climbing the east ridge: This ridge is quite short, only about 0.4 mile to the summit, but it will take awhile to get up. As mentioned, the route is all class 3 and 3+ stuff, with the easier sections coming at the lower parts of the ridge. The rock is quite solid but with some big-time exposure. Staying on the ridge all the way up is a thrill, with a few 3+ moves thrown in to keep your heart rate up. Take your time to find and test good holds—they are there. After the initial "connecting ramp" puts you on the east ridge proper, you have the option to drop down to the south side and traverse via rocky ledges just below the ridge. This terrain is still fun class 3, minus the exposure. Scramblers on the ridge will make it directly to the summit, while those on the south side will have a fun, solid rock gully leading to the top. This thrilling little scramble is a great way to wrap up your hike.

7.6 mi (8) Lead Mountain's summit! If you're going for the Hart Ridge Loop, your path awaits. If Lead was your objective (which is probably the case if you're doing this as a day hike), you have two descent options. You can retrace the east ridge, which has some sketchy spots with exposed down climbing but is the fastest way to get back. Experienced scramblers will prefer this route. The other option, which I've outlined on the standard route, goes south via the lower path's ascent gully. Drop down and head right (west) on ledges toward Hart Ridge. Going left onto Lead's face looks more direct, but it cliffs out with difficult and dangerous class 4/5 gullies to down climb. Aim for the ground below the saddle between Lead Mountain and Mount Cirrus: the scrambling is class 3, but it is much safer than other routes. Once you reach the big talus field, head southeast back to where you came up. Return the way you came and bask in the afterglow of this fine summit.

15.3 mi Finish.

Options Hart Ridge runs between Lead Mountain and Mount Cirrus (12,787 feet). This fun class 3 scramble is a great option and may actually provide the safest descent route. It is 1.0 mile between summits. From the top of Lead Mountain, go south along the ridge. It begins with relatively easy terrain; at 0.5 mile, the scrambling becomes similar to stuff on Lead. Again, the holds are solid and the exposure is thrilling. Once you top out on Cirrus, keep going south to the saddle between Cirrus and Howard Mountain at 12,810 feet. (Howard is a quick diversion if you'd like to summit another peak.) Hike/surf down the broad gully of loose scree to Lake of the Clouds at 11,430 feet. From Lake of the Clouds, shuffle down the slopes back into the basin and return via the Hitchens Gulch Trail (waypoint **4**), picking up the route with which you began the hike. This option is approximately 2.7 miles from the top of Lead, over Cirrus, down to Lake of the Clouds, and back to the basin where you hiked up—about 6 miles round-trip from Dutch Town Campground.

Quick Facts Lead Mountain earned its name in 1879. Lead wasn't a particularly coveted ore, and it served more to frustrate miners than to line their pockets.

In 1914, James Grafton Rogers named three sky-high peaks in the Never Summer Range for clouds: Cirrus, Cumulus, and Nimbus. Later, Mount Stratus was added to the mix. Howard Mountain may seem like an atmospheric outcast among these mountains, unless you consider that Luke Howard was the English meteorologist who first named and classified cloud formations. It's a good theory, but according to Rogers's own account, Howard appeared on maps prior to the naming of the cloud mountains. Thus, the true identity of Howard is a mystery. Just for fun, I like to think that it was named after Moe Howard, leader of the Three Stooges. (Harry Moses Horwitz, also known as Moe Howard, was born June 19, 1897, making this theoretically possible, assuming he took his stage name early in life.)

Hart Ridge is named for Lt. Eldon C. Hart, who was killed while flying for the Kansas Air National Guard when his F-100C Super Sabre fighter jet crashed into Mount Cirrus on January 30, 1967. The wreckage is on the west side of the mountain, so you won't be seeing it on this route.

Contact Info

Rocky Mountain National Park
1000 US Highway 36
Estes Park, CO 80517

General Park Information: (970) 586-1206
Visitor Information Recorded Message: (970) 586-1333
Backcountry Information: (970) 586-1242
Campground Reservations: (800) 365-2267

Clark Peak

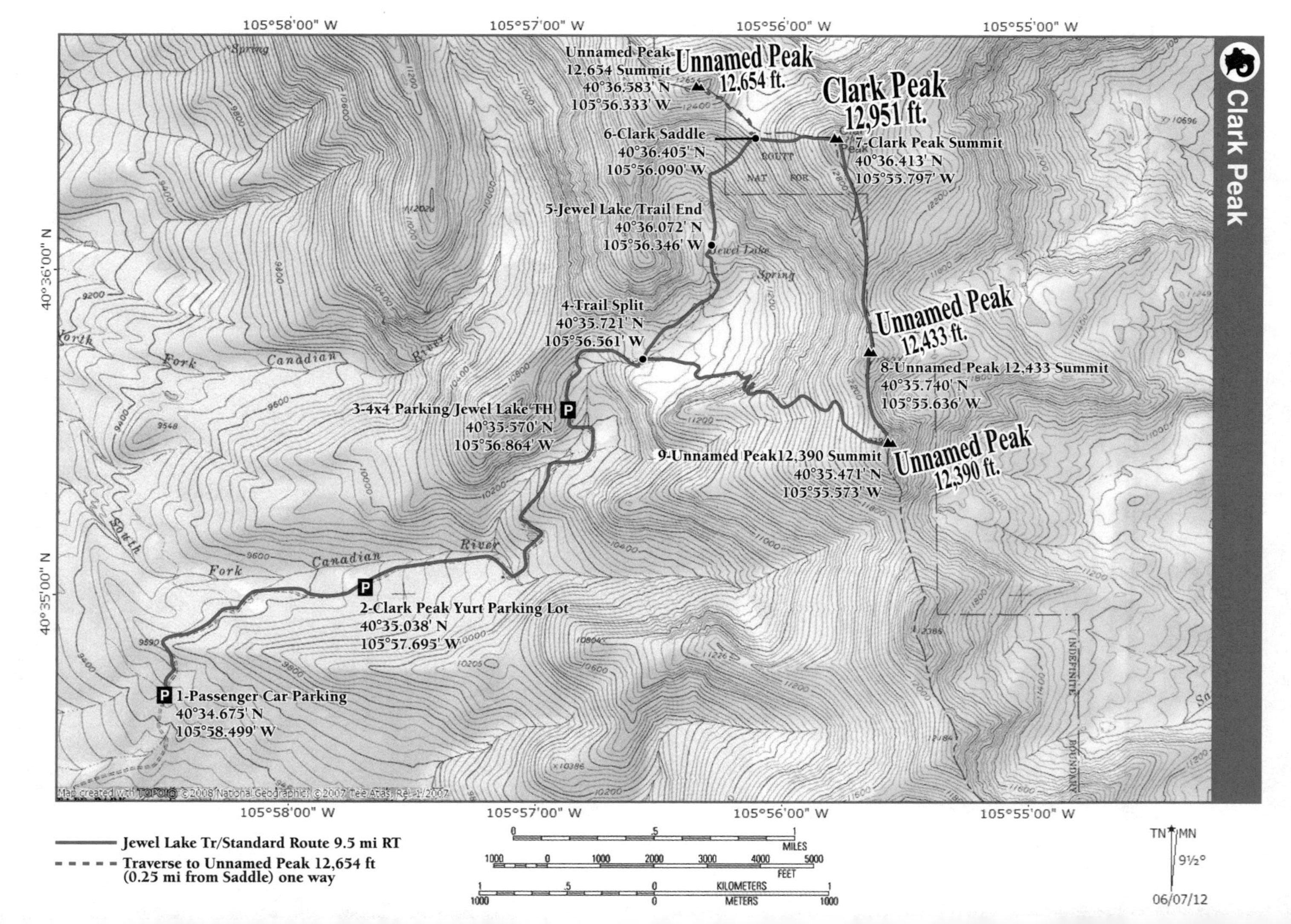

Clark Peak
12,951 ft.
7-Clark Peak Summit
40°36.413' N
105°55.797' W
Unnamed Peak
12,654 ft.
Unnamed Peak
12,654 Summit
40°36.583' N
105°56.333' W
6-Clark Saddle
40°36.405' N
105°56.090' W
5-Jewel Lake/Trail End
40°36.072' N
105°56.346' W
Jewel Lake
Spring
4-Trail Split
40°35.721' N
105°56.561' W
3-4x4 Parking/Jewel Lake TH
40°35.570' N
105°56.864' W
2-Clark Peak Yurt Parking Lot
40°35.038' N
105°57.695' W
1-Passenger Car Parking
40°34.675' N
105°58.499' W
Unnamed Peak
12,433 ft.
8-Unnamed Peak 12,433 Summit
40°35.740' N
105°55.636' W
Unnamed Peak
12,390 ft.
9-Unnamed Peak12,390 Summit
40°35.471' N
105°55.573' W
North Fork Canadian River
South Fork Canadian River
INDEFINITE
BOUNDARY
105°58'00" W
105°57'00" W
105°56'00" W
105°55'00" W
40°36'00" N
40°35'00" N
Map created with TOPO! © 2008 National Geographic; © 2007 Tele Atlas, Rel. 1/2007
Jewel Lake Tr/Standard Route 9.5 mi RT
Traverse to Unnamed Peak 12,654 ft
(0.25 mi from Saddle) one way
MILES
FEET
KILOMETERS
METERS
TN
MN
9½°
06/07/12

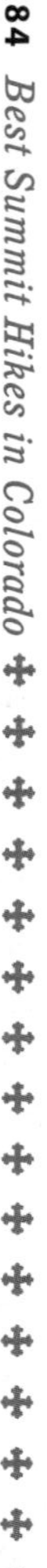

6 Clark Peak

Clark Peak is the high point of the Medicine Bow Mountains, a less-known but beautiful range in the Colorado State Forest. A good hike with a skywalk ridge traverse.

Round-Trip Distance	9.5 miles for cars; 4.2 miles from 4x4 parking
Hiking Time	3–6 hours
Difficulty	5/10
Class	2
Start Elevation	9,470 ft., on Ruby Jewel Road
Peak Elevation	12,951 ft.
Total Elevation Gain	4,087 ft.
Terrain	Nice trail, steep grassy slopes, great flat ridge walk
Best Time to Climb	June–September
Gear Advisor	Trekking poles
Crowd Level	Low

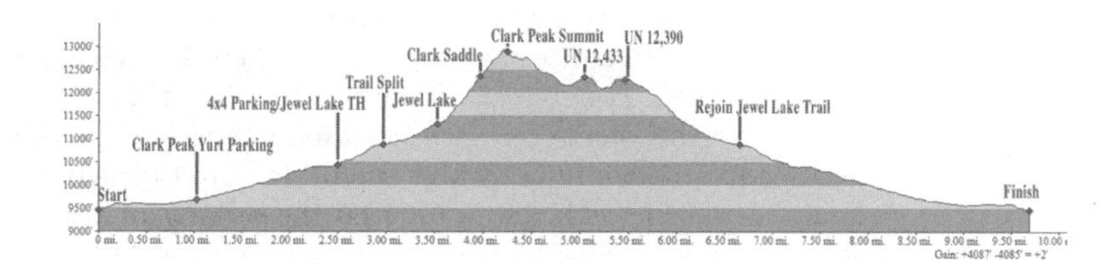

Location Medicine Bow Range in the Colorado State Forest near the small town of Gould

Intro Clark Peak is the high point of the Medicine Bow Range (as well as the high point of Jackson County). Clark's setting in northern Colorado means that you'll be hiking on unique topography, complete with dramatic basins and prolific peaks. Views from the top are awesome, especially the far-off view of the seldom-seen northwest face of Longs Peak. The Colorado State Forest borders the Rawah Wilderness, and both areas offer great backpacking.

Why Climb It? Clark feels very different than most other peaks in Colorado—in a very good way. Those who have hiked in Wyoming's Wind River Range may find the atmosphere in the Medicine Bows familiar. This route goes by Jewel Lake, a dreamy alpine pool at the base of a dramatic basin. The stiff, off-trail hill that goes from Jewel Lake is flooded with flowers of all colors. From Clark's summit (which will be hidden until you actually ascend to the top), the southern skywalk to neighboring unnamed peaks is a transcendent traverse. Many who hike in this area return to backpack and camp (the terrain is similar to the Mount Zirkel Wilderness in Steamboat Springs).

Driving Passenger cars—even tough passenger cars—will be fine on the well-groomed dirt of County Road 41 but can only reach 1.0 mile up Ruby Jewel Road before it gets too rough (read below for more info on the road conditions). High-clearance sport utility vehicles (SUVs) or 4x4s are needed to reach the trailhead; sport utility cars (SUCs) and all-wheel drive (AWD) vehicles can make it most of the way up Ruby Jewel Road but will struggle with the last 1.5 miles. The road is steep and very rocky in sections, with smooth, flat sections between. There is a minor river crossing just before the parking lot.

How to Get There From Fort Collins, turn west onto Colorado Highway 14 (Poudre Canyon) and get ready for a long, twisty ride. You will be on this road for just under 70 miles, but expect the trip to take about two hours, thanks to the curves of the highway. Go up and over Cameron Pass (those cool rock formations you see in front of you are the Nokhu Crags). Drop over the pass, and at mile 69.8, turn right onto CR 41; this turn comes up quickly. The dirt road entrance to CR 41 has info kiosks, self-pay stations, and a campground; it's a gateway to Colorado State Forest. **Note:** There is a ranger station about a mile before this turn on the left side of the road, where you can get additional information.

Stay on CR 41, passing the Michigan Reservoir (and its large concrete sluice) at mile 4.6. At mile 4.9, you'll reach a plateau where Ruby Jewel Road splits off to the right (there are signs). From here, it is 3.5 miles to the Jewel Lake Trailhead. Passenger cars can drive up 1.0 mile and park in a small lot on the right where Francisco Road splits from Ruby Jewel Road. SUCs, SUVs, and 4x4s continue straight uphill (do not turn left onto Francisco Road) on Ruby Jewel Road. At mile 2.0, the parking lot for Clark Peak Yurt appears—this is a good place for lower clearance and AWD vehicles to stop; 4x4s and tougher vehicles can drive 1.5 miles on the rocky, steep road to reach the trailhead. The road is well signed.

Fees/Camping As of 2012, there is a $7 self-pay fee for day use in Colorado State Forest. You will need a permit to backcountry camp, but there is no charge other than the day-use fee. There are several developed campgrounds in the area that range between $10 and $20 per night.

Route Notes You can do this loop either way, though dropping down to Ruby Jewel Lake is rough on the knees. Bring trekking poles.

Mile/Waypoint

0.0 mi (1) This is the passenger car parking lot at the split of Ruby Jewel Road and Francisco Road (1.0 mile from the split with CR 41). There are three to four spots here. Hike, drive, or bike up the road to Jewel Lake Trailhead.

1.0 mi (2) There is a large parking lot for the Clark Peak Yurt.

2.5 mi (3) Reach the fenced-in 4x4 parking lot. The Jewel Lake Trail may not be marked, but it is the obvious footpath that starts north after passing over a footbridge. Stay on the worn path as it crosses a few streams;

you'll eventually come to a clearing and have to follow the path across a talus field.

2.7 mi (4) After the talus field, the trail splits. Stay left for Jewel Lake; you'll return to the main trail later from the right (of course, if you'd like to do the hike in reverse, you can turn right here and loop north instead of south). The Jewel Lake Trail bypasses a lush meadow, which will be on your right. The trail may be overgrown or difficult to find in the mud, especially in early spring. If you get off-trail, remember that Jewel Lake is above you to the north.

3.3 mi (5) Reach Jewel Lake. The trail ends here. Head northeast and pick a line up the steep, grassy slope that heads to the saddle between Clark Peak and Unnamed Peak 12,654. In the spring, this hill is flush with flowers; the route tracked here goes up a shallow gully that I have dubbed Flower Gully. Flower Gully is the path of least resistance. Climb straight up, roughly 1,200 feet, to gain the saddle.

4.0 mi (6) At the saddle, turn directly east and scale your second steep hill to reach Clark's summit (which won't be apparent until you are standing on it).

4.2 mi (7) Clark Peak summit. The huge peak you see to the northwest is South Rawah Peak. You have the option to descend the way you came up, but it is murder on the knees. The more scenic option takes the same amount of time. Leave the summit and traverse the high plains south. This is the beginning of the "skywalk."

5.1 mi (8) Reach Unnamed Peak 12,433. You can drop down here if you like; however, this route carries on to one more unnamed peak.

5.4 mi (9) Reach Unnamed Peak 12,390. Descend the switchbacks to the pack trail below you and follow it to the Jewel Lake Trail (or simply bushwhack back down to the Jewel Lake Trail).

6.8 mi (4) Rejoin the Jewel Lake Trail near the talus field and return to your vehicle.

9.6 mi Finish at the passenger car parking area.

Options From the saddle above Jewel Lake (waypoint 6), it's a short detour (0.25 mile) over to Unnamed Peak 12,654. To get there and back only adds about 0.5 mile to your trip. The back side (north face) of Unnamed Peak 12,654 looks as though it would be a very cool ski descent (though it would drop you into the Rawah Wilderness).

Quick Facts Clark Peak is named for none other than William Clark, of the fabled Lewis and Clark Expedition. There are no mountains to the north in the state of Colorado that are higher than Clark Peak.

Contact Info Colorado State Forest
2746 County Road 41
Walden, CO 80480
(970) 723-8366
parks.state.co.us

Mount Richthofen

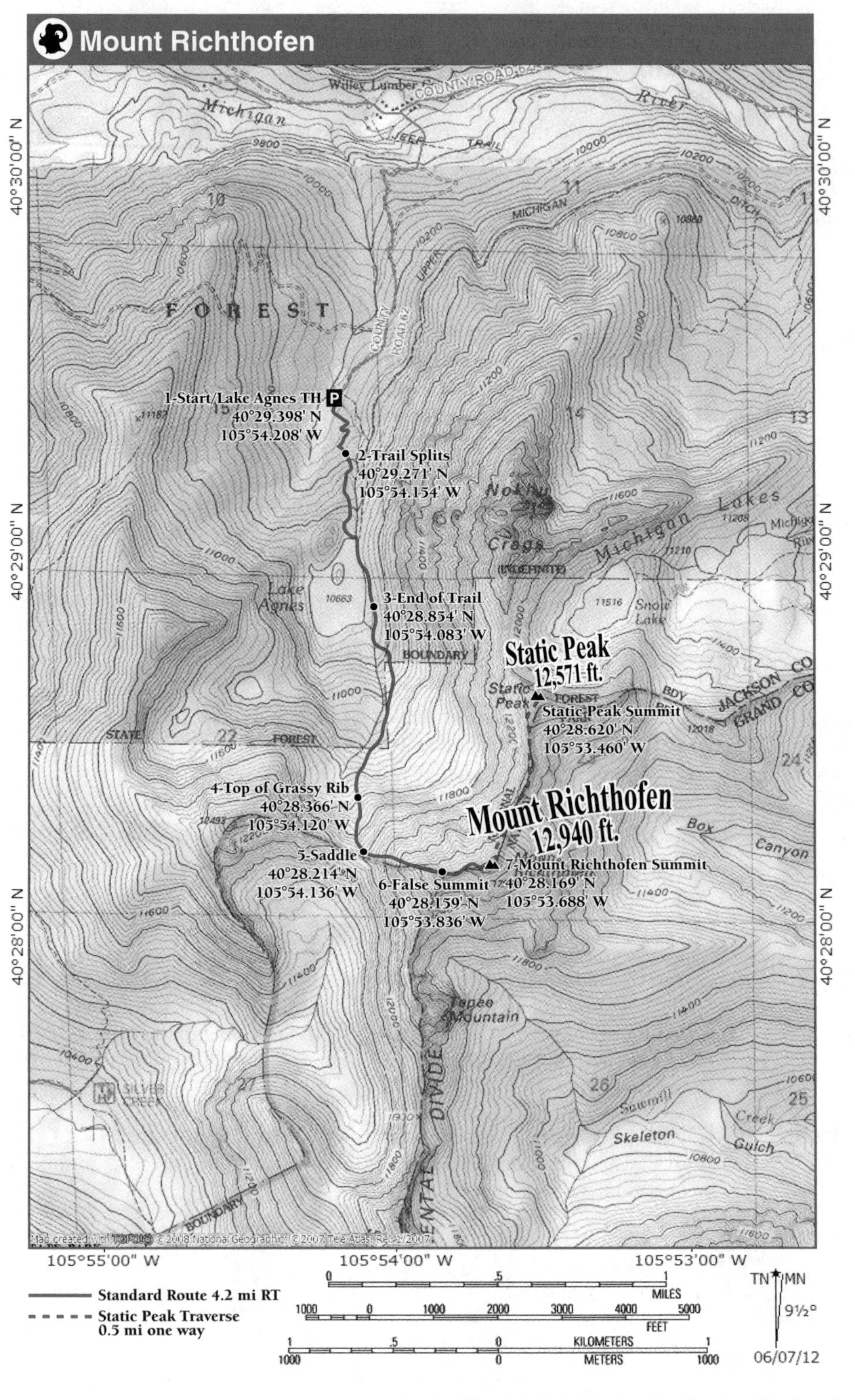
1-Start/Lake Agnes TH
40°29.398' N
105°54.208' W
2-Trail Splits
40°29.271' N
105°54.154' W
3-End of Trail
40°28.854' N
105°54.083' W
Static Peak
12,571 ft.
Static Peak Summit
40°28.620' N
105°53.460' W
4-Top of Grassy Rib
40°28.366' N
105°54.120' W
Mount Richthofen
12,940 ft.
5-Saddle
40°28.214' N
105°54.136' W
6-False Summit
40°28.159' N
105°53.836' W
7-Mount Richthofen Summit
40°28.169' N
105°53.688' W
Nokhu Crags
Lake Agnes
Snow Lake
Michigan Lakes
Tepee Mountain
Skeleton Gulch
Box Canyon
40°30'00" N
40°29'00" N
40°28'00" N
105°55'00" W
105°54'00" W
105°53'00" W
Standard Route 4.2 mi RT
Static Peak Traverse 0.5 mi one way
MILES
FEET
KILOMETERS
METERS
TN MN
9½°
06/07/12

7 Mount Richthofen

Situated in the northern part of the Never Summer Range, Richthofen is a short but sweet scramble with great views. A secret passage grants you access to this impressive summit.

Round-Trip Distance	4.2 miles
Hiking Time	4–6 hours
Difficulty	7.5/10
Class	3
Start Elevation	10,270 ft., at Lake Agnes Trailhead
Peak Elevation	12,940 ft.
Total Elevation Gain	2,627 ft.
Terrain	Rocky scrambling with some loose sections
Best Time to Climb	Mid-June–September
Gear Advisor	Helmets are a good idea if in a group.
Crowd Level	Low

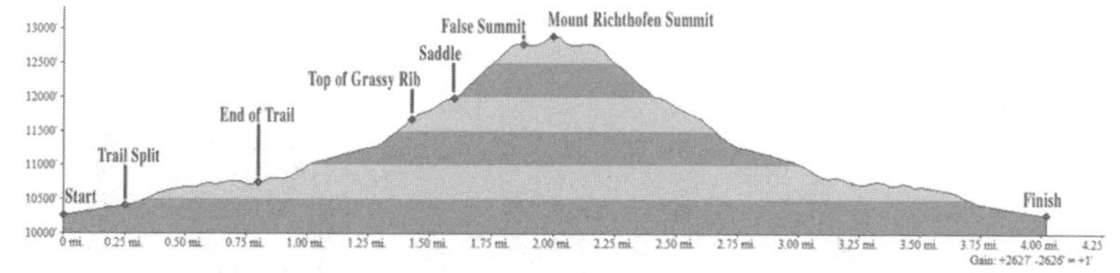

Location Never Summer Range; Richthofen's east and south faces are in Rocky Mountain National Park, while the north and west faces are in the Colorado State Forest. This route approaches from the Colorado State Forest side, just past Cameron Pass.

Intro Good scrambles always appeal to my inner mountain goat. The west ridge on this route starts off a bit loose but becomes increasingly solid as you near the summit block. Richthofen is the highest peak in the burly Never Summer Range, a special range with some of the most rugged mountains in Colorado. Talus is king in the Never Summers, but that doesn't detract from the great hiking and scrambling.

Why Climb It? If you've never been to the Never Summer Range, you owe it to yourself to check out the spectacular terrain that defines the region. Before you even set foot on the trail, you're treated to views of the sinister-looking Nokhu Crags, a collection of crooked spires and crumbling towers that loom west of the access trail. Lake Agnes is a glacial lake surrounded by an amphitheater of boulders. In direct sunlight, the water glows a translucent green hue. As you gain the west ridge, these sights become even more impressive. The final scramble to the top involves a "secret" notch on the north face.

Driving This road to the trail is good for tough passenger cars; you'll probably scrape a low-clearance vehicle here and there, but cars can reach the trailhead without too much trouble. Sport utility cars or vehicles and 4x4s will be fine. The road is a little rocky and narrow, but it never gets too steep or too rocky.

How to Get There From Fort Collins, head west on Colorado Highway 14 for 62 miles (this drive is going to take awhile, thanks to the curvy road). Once you are at Cameron Pass, it is 2.0 miles to the left-hand turn off to County Road 62 (there are signs to Lake Agnes on the road). A self-pay fee station greets you at the turnoff; as of 2012, the day-use fee was $5. At 0.6 mile, the road splits. Stay right and continue to follow the signs to Lake Agnes (you'll be going uphill abruptly after this turn). Continue along this brief road; at mile 1.75 you'll reach the Lake Agnes Trailhead. There are signs that lead you to the trailhead; there are also a few jeep roads that intersect CR 62. Stay on the main road until the parking area, which is home to a weird, football-shaped bathroom.

Fees/Camping It's $7 for a day-use fee at Richthofen. There's really not much in the way of camping near Richthofen, but there are several campgrounds beyond Cameron Pass in Colorado State Forest, where sites are between $10 and $16 per night.

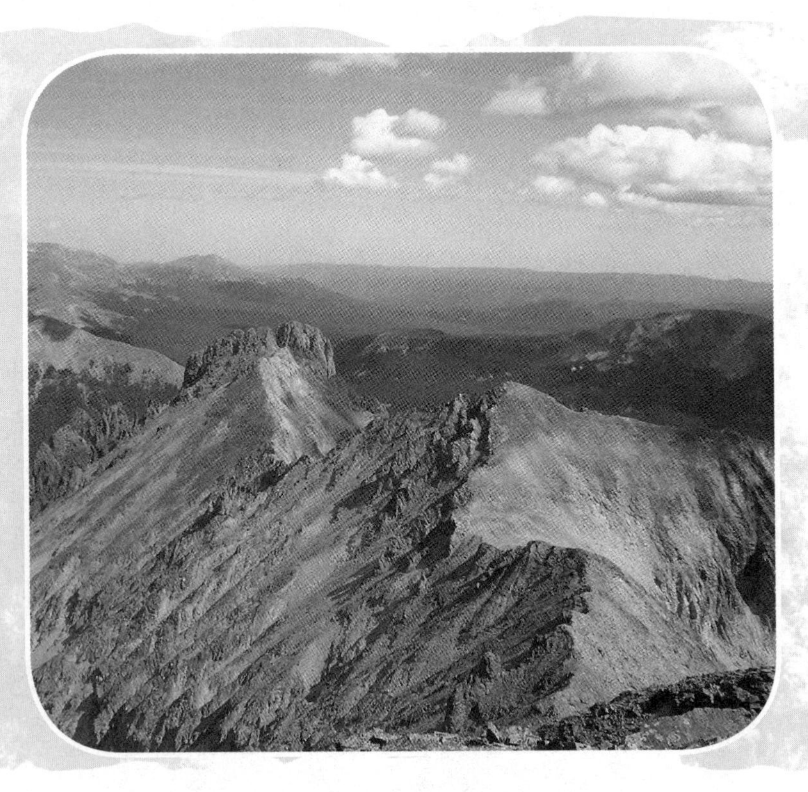

Amazing views of Static Peak and the Nokhu Crags from the summit of Mount Richthofen

Route Notes The mileage here is low, but you'll have to earn every foot of elevation you gain. Your trail ends at the south side of Lake Agnes; from there, you'll need to use some basic navigational skills to reach the saddle between Richthofen and Unnamed Peak 12,942. Most of the hike is out of the trees, so visually following the lines of the mountain is not very difficult.

Mile/Waypoint **0.0 mi (1)** Start at the Lake Agnes Trailhead and take the Lake Agnes Trail. You'll enter the woods and immediately hit a swath of switchbacks.

0.25 mi (2) Stay right (south) on the Lake Agnes Trail at this split. (The left trail goes north and skirts around the Nokhu Crags to the Michigan Lakes.)

0.6 mi Beautiful Lake Agnes, complete with a rocky island, greets you as you come out of the woods. Several trails appear here; you want to stay on the path through the talus on the east side of the lake. Follow it to the southern terminus of the lake. From there, the terrain gets steep: you'll cover 1,250 vertical feet in 1.0 mile to reach the saddle.

0.8 mi (3) The trail ends at the terminus of the lake. Richthofen will be looking down at you, a little bit left of your bearing. Your goal now is to reach the large, obvious saddle to the south. There is a creek (or creek bed in late summer) that can guide you to the easiest path up the saddle. Staying on the grassy sections makes this ascent easier. About halfway up, you can gain a grassy rib that will lead you to the base of the bowl leading up the saddle.

1.5 mi (4) At the top of the grassy rib, you can bear a little to the right and start the push up the saddle. There are some faint trails you can follow, which may help on the loose rock. This is least enjoyable part of the hike, but it isn't very long.

1.7 mi (5) All right—you're at the top of the saddle! The elevation here is just under 12,000 feet. Only 940 vertical feet to go. I hope that your legs are ready because you're going to gain all of that elevation in a mere 0.4 mile. (Now you understand why this low-mileage hike takes so long.) Note that you'll have a good look at Lead Mountain (Hike 5) to the south. Even though it is close to Richthofen, the trailhead for Lead Mountain is a good three hours away, in Rocky Mountain National Park.

As you embark on the west ridge of Mount Richthofen, scramble along the spine. The lower rock is a bit loose but will get more solid as you gain elevation. In the morning, it may be tough to follow the ridge when the sun is breaking just over the top of the mountain (curse these west ridges sometimes!).

2.0 mi (6) There's nothing quite like a false summit. This one isn't too bad; once you're on it, the remaining climb to the summit isn't far. But how *does* one scramble up to the top? That block looks as though it's going to take some tricky scrambling.

When you reach the mini-saddle between the false and true summits, peek around the corner out onto the northwest face of the mountain to find the perfect access gully. This is a short, class 3 scramble that makes topping out on Richthofen a marvelous experience. A wind shelter and a gold U.S. Geological Survey marker await you on the top.

2.1 mi (7) On top of the world, Ma! Mount Richthofen summit! To the south, Tepee Mountain connects Mount Richthofen to Lead Mountain. Orange-tinted peaks of the Never Summer Range twist southwest, where they merge with the Rabbit Ears Range. The Mummy Range and other peaks north of Trail Ridge Road are to the east. Far north, you can see the tips of the Medicine Bow Mountains and the top of Clark Peak, yet another great hike in this book (Hike 6). Return the same way you came up (unless you want to take a quick tour of Static Peak, to the northeast, listed in the "Options" section below).

4.2 mi Finish. That was quite a workout for a 4-mile hike!

Options From the top of Richthofen, it's a clean 0.5-mile traverse to the northeast to reach the top of 12,571-foot Static Peak. This class 2 ridge is a good walk. If the weather (and your legs) allow, check it out. Return back the way you came. The scramble down from the saddle of Static and the Nokhu Crags is loose, dangerous, and prone to rockfall from above. Return back over Richthofen for the safest way home.

Quick Facts Mount Richthofen is named for a famous German but probably not the one of whom you are thinking. Clarence King, director of the Fortieth Parallel Survey, named the mountain after Ferdinand von Richthofen, a globetrotting German geologist. Educated in Berlin, he began his world tour as a geographer and geologist in 1860 by joining a scientific outfit that explored Japan, Taiwan, the Philippines, and Burma. He made his way to the United States in 1862, staying here for six years. He helped discover several gold deposits in California before returning to explore China and other places in Asia. One of his discoveries in China was the dried-up lake bed of Lopnur, a feature visible from space. For his efforts, a mountain range in China is named in his honor.

Oh yes, and Ferdinand von Richthofen was the uncle of Manfred von Richthofen, better known to history as the World War I flying ace "the Red Baron." Manfred's other uncle, Walter von Richthofen, helped found the Denver Chamber of Commerce and is credited with founding the neighborhood of Montclair. He modeled his home in Montclair after the Richthofen family castle in Germany. Admittedly, it seems a little out of the place in the Western frontier.

Contact Info Colorado State Forest
2746 County Road 41
Walden, CO 80480
(970) 723-8366
parks.state.co.us

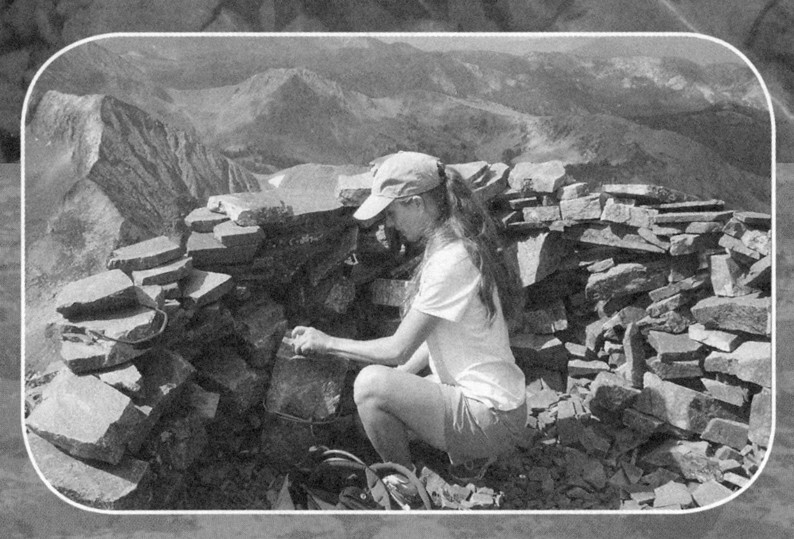

Don't forget to add your name to the list of summiters on Mount Richthofen.

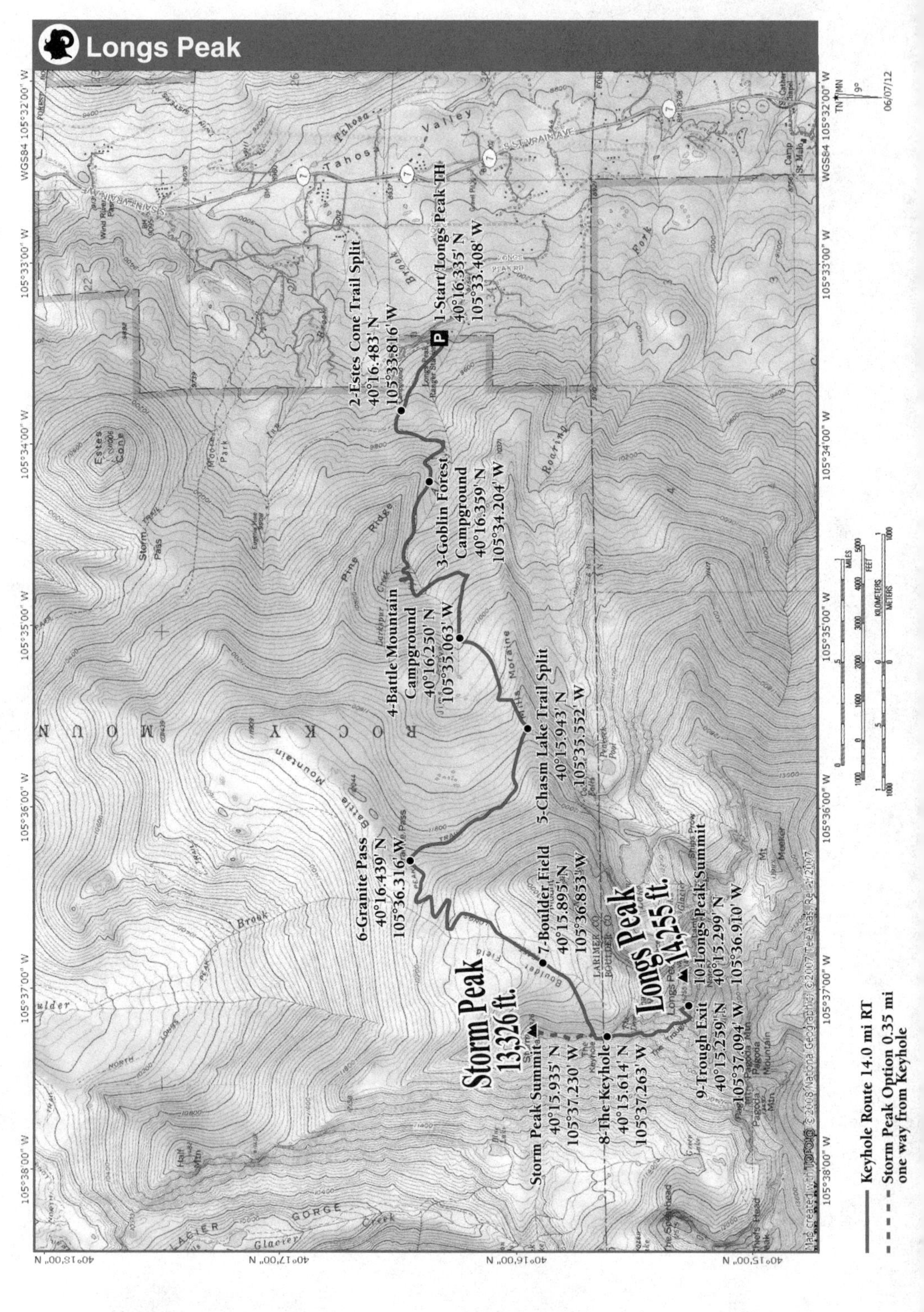
Longs Peak
1-Start/Longs Peak TH
40°16.335' N
105°33.408' W
2-Estes Cone Trail Split
40°16.483' N
105°33.816' W
3-Goblin Forest Campground
40°16.359' N
105°34.204' W
4-Battle Mountain Campground
40°16.250' N
105°35.063' W
5-Chasm Lake Trail Split
40°15.943' N
105°35.552' W
6-Granite Pass
40°16.439' N
105°36.316' W
7-Boulder Field
40°15.895' N
105°36.853' W
8-The Keyhole
40°15.614' N
105°37.263' W
9-Trough Exit
40°15.259' N
105°37.094' W
10-Longs Peak Summit
40°15.299' N
105°36.910' W
Storm Peak Summit
40°15.935' N
105°37.230' W
Storm Peak
13,326 ft.
Longs Peak
14,255 ft.
Estes Cone
Storm Pass
Pine Ridge
Battle Mountain
Tahosa Valley
Keyhole Route 14.0 mi RT
Storm Peak Option 0.35 mi one way from Keyhole
06/07/12

8 Longs Peak

Good Overnight!

Longs is the classic 14er. Despite the fact that it's a strenuous circuit, most people climb the Keyhole route in a single day. The scrambling is among the best in the state.

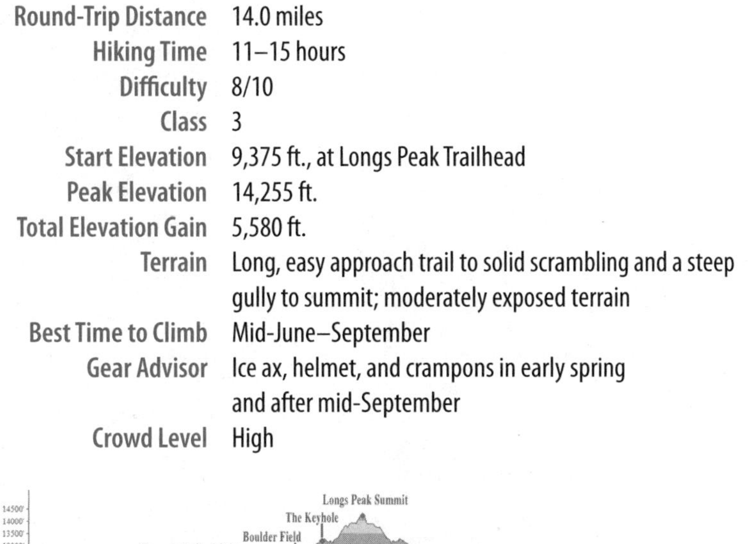

Round-Trip Distance	14.0 miles
Hiking Time	11–15 hours
Difficulty	8/10
Class	3
Start Elevation	9,375 ft., at Longs Peak Trailhead
Peak Elevation	14,255 ft.
Total Elevation Gain	5,580 ft.
Terrain	Long, easy approach trail to solid scrambling and a steep gully to summit; moderately exposed terrain
Best Time to Climb	Mid-June–September
Gear Advisor	Ice ax, helmet, and crampons in early spring and after mid-September
Crowd Level	High

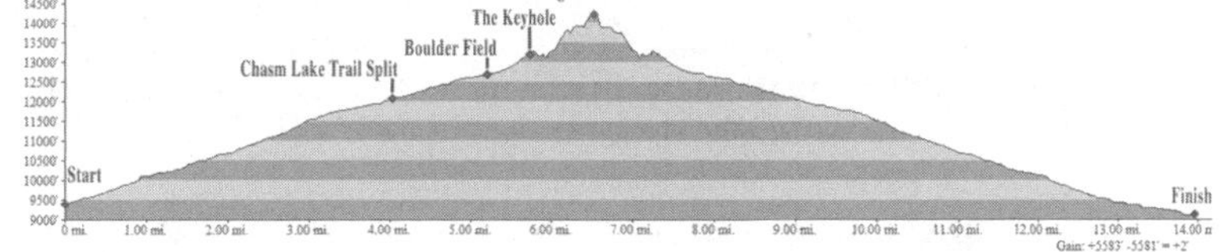

Location Front Range in Rocky Mountain National Park outside of Estes Park

Intro Get ready to make some new friends. Longs Peak is one of the most social summits in the state, even though it's a tough climb. For many, an ascent of Longs Peak is the culmination of their hiking careers. It may be popular, but it's still tough. The classic way to climb the peak is to begin around 3 a.m. (to avoid storms) and summit in the early morning. No other 14er sees more traffic, nor does any other peak bestow everyday glory on the humble hiker more than Longs.

Why Climb It? Yes, you'll be dealing with all kinds of crowds on Longs. In my opinion, this is part of the fun. You'll see it all: families, gutsy weekend warriors, cocky climbers, teenagers, grandparents, guys, girls, the hefty and the slim, all aiming to stand on the flat summit of the mountain whose image is reproduced on the Colorado state quarter. Dreamlike phantom trains of headlamps heading up in the predawn hours are a surreal sight. Passing through the Keyhole is like reaching the next level in a video game. A new world waits on the back side of Longs. Even veteran hikers and scramblers can appreciate the moderately exposed traverses and good class 3 terrain that leads to the summit. Longs is a must-do mountain. I could not in good faith write about the best summits in Colorado and exclude it.

Driving The road to Longs Peak Trailhead is paved and passable by all vehicles.

How to Get There The road to the trailhead is off Colorado Highway 7. From the south, this is 10.4 miles north of the junction of CO 7 and Colorado Highway 72; from the north, it is 9.2 miles from the junction of US Highway 36 and CO 7. Turn west onto the well-marked Longs Peak Road and drive approximately 0.8 mile to the ranger station and Longs Peak Trailhead.

Fees/Camping Longs is in Rocky Mountain National Park, but there is no fee for day hiking the area. Camping requires a permit and a $20 fee. There are three campgrounds along the way: Golbin's Forest, Battle Mountain Group Site, and the Boulderfield. Call for reservations, as these sites fill up quickly in the summer. Longs Peak Campground is just below the trailhead and offers 26 sites for tents only. No overnight camping is allowed in the parking lot.

Route Notes I've noticed that my GPS tracks recorded a slightly shorter round-trip distance than official park publications proclaim (most say either 15 or 16 miles). I stayed on trail where there is a trail; however, I made direct approaches in the boulder field and in the trough, which may have cut my mileage a bit. (I grew up hiking in New England: we don't believe in switchbacks.) As a result, I had a mileage of 6.91 miles to the summit and 6.89 miles on the descent. My elevation profile includes the up and down in the Keyhole, the boulder field, and the slight ups and downs around Chasm Lake. I explain these discrepancies because there is so much literature available providing statistics about Longs.

As mentioned, day hikers should aim to start no later than 3 a.m. (early is better). A considerable amount of this hike is above tree line, with little shelter from the inevitable summer storms. Longs is a serious hike; many people have died on the standard route from falls, lightning, and other accidents. Don't underestimate it just because it is popular.

Note: The Keyhole Route is formally known as the East Longs Peak Trail.

Mile/Waypoint

0.0 mi (1) Start at the Longs Peak Trailhead, gaining the East Longs Peak Trail just behind the ranger station. There's a good chance you'll be hiking in the dark (as you should). The trail is wide, well worn, and easy to follow.

0.4 mi (2) Don't make a rookie mistake in the early morning. At this fork, the Longs Peak Trail goes left, so stay the course. The trail that cuts off to the right goes to Eugenia Mine and Estes Cone. Once you clear this intersection, you have a long approach to the Keyhole. Set a good pace and enjoy the sunrise.

1.1 mi (3) Goblin Forest Campground.

2.4 mi (4) A short distance above timberline, Battle Mountain Campground is off to the right. Stay left on the well-marked trail.

3.1 mi (5) Great views of the Diamond are evident from the flat section that serves as the junction between the Longs Peak Trail and the Chasm Lake Trail (a toilet is here, too). The Diamond on Longs Peak's northeast face is a test piece for advanced rock climbers; practically every line you can see on the sheer face has been scaled. *Do not* descend to Chasm Lake. Continue northwest to Granite Pass and the boulder field.

4.0 mi (6) Granite Pass. Stay left on the trail to the boulder field at the trail junction. In the case of a fast-moving storm, the rocky caves to the north of Granite Pass provide emergency shelters.

5.6 mi (7) This is the heart of the boulder field. There is a toilet here. Gaps in the rock at the west end of the boulder field form the fabled Keyhole. The trail fades out on the rocky slope up to the Keyhole, but your short-term goal is obvious. At the Keyhole is a storm shelter, complete with glass windows. Get ready to climb once you pass this gateway to adventure.

5.8 mi (8) Behold the world beyond the Keyhole! Your route goes left (south) and follows a 0.3-mile trail marked with spray-painted bull's-eye

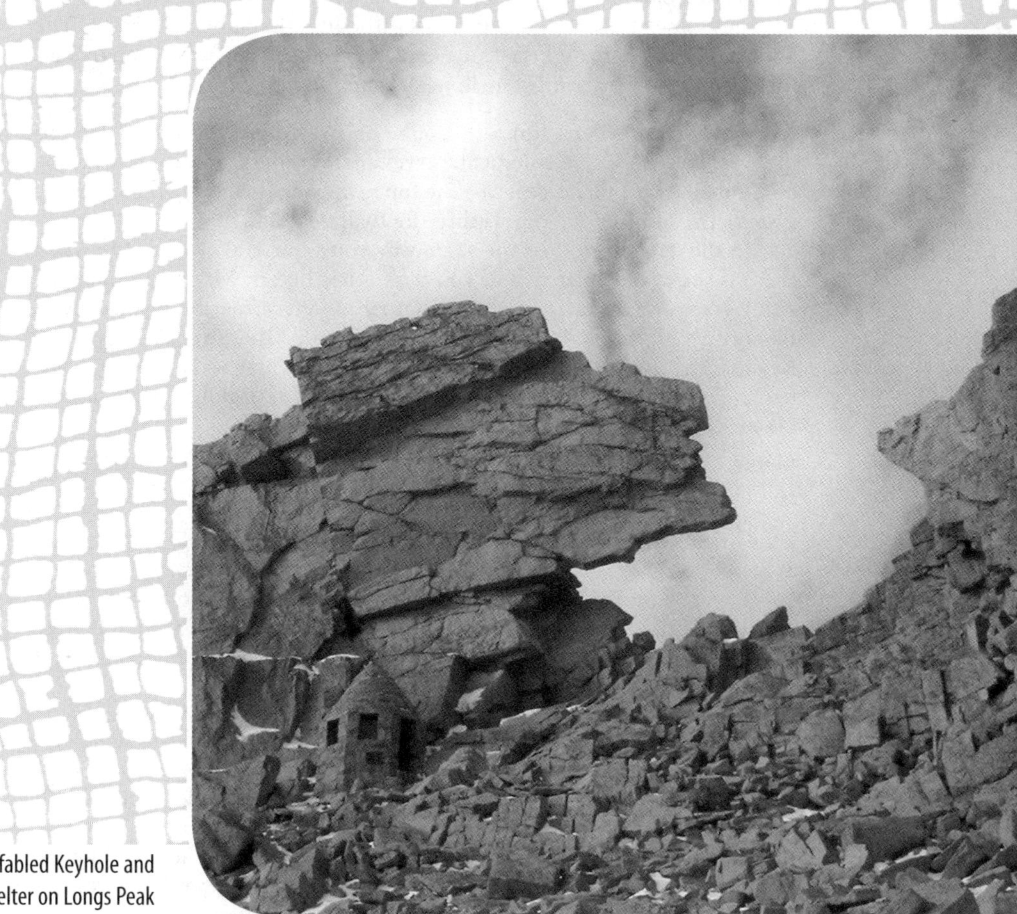

The fabled Keyhole and shelter on Longs Peak

markers. This traverse is slightly exposed and gives you the first real taste of the challenge of Longs.

6.1 mi You are now at the base of a long gully known as the Trough. The base of the Trough is roughly 13,100 feet, so you'll be doing the steepest climbing at dizzying altitude. It's 900 feet to the top of this cardiovascular-pumping chute. Watch out for rocks dislodged by climbers above you, and try not to knock any on the climbers below you.

6.5 mi (9) The Trough tops out just below 14,000 feet. There are great views of another mountain featured in this book, Mount Alice (Hike 9), from this gap. The next short section is known as the Narrows. The exposure may be unsettling for inexperienced hikers. The path is cut into the slope, and there are plenty of good handholds along the way. These sections are short and well marked, so the map of this route will not include them as individual waypoints.

6.7 mi Drop down about 30 feet to 13,980 feet and the beginning of a section known as the Home Stretch. To the southeast, long chimneys of rock are worth looking at while you take a water break.

The Home Stretch entails the most difficult scrambling of the hike. The holds are very good, and the route is marked. Push your way through Victory Gap to the surprisingly mellow, flat summit.

6.9 mi (10) Longs Peak summit! You're halfway done. A rock outcrop to the west has the U.S. Geological Survey marker, the summit log, and the best views. Allow me to describe the top using an all-American measuring system: the summit of Longs is three football fields long.

On the descent, return the same way you came. Take your time when there is snow. Be courteous as you pass other hikers. Many will have the blank stare of exhaustion with a glimmer of determination in their eyes. Be positive! In case of bad weather, remember that there are shelters at the Keyhole and in the rocks at Granite Pass. It's a very long walk down; the last few miles in the trees get tedious. With luck, the afterglow of such a great hike will keep you moving.

14.0 mi Finish the hike and give yourself a pat on the back; you've just completed Colorado's classic 14er.

Options This hike is a big commitment. If doing this as a day hike, you're probably not going to want to add to it. Some people will make the short traverse over to Storm Peak, north of the Keyhole . . . the show-offs! If you really have the legs (or you're camping in the area), the Estes Cone hike is a nice diversion; it's 4.8 miles round-trip (from the trail intersection at waypoint 2) on a good trail.

Quick Facts There is far more history to report about Longs than I can cover in a paragraph. I would suggest reading *Longs Peak: The Story of Colorado's Favorite Fourteener* by Dougald MacDonald, published by Westcliffe Publishers. It is an excellent account of the history of Longs Peak.

The peak is named for Stephen Long, who surveyed the area in 1820 but never climbed the mountain. He didn't formally name the peak after himself. Rather, he described Longs and its 13,911-foot neighbor as the Two Ears, a name given to the peaks by French fur trappers. The sister peak would later be named Mount Meeker, in honor of Nathan Meeker, founder of Greeley.

The first official climb of the peak was recorded in 1868 by a group made up of John Wesley Powell (the famous one-armed Civil War vet), his brother W. H. Powell, William Byers (for whom a mountain was later named), L. W. Keplinger, and three Illinois college students who apparently forgot to sign the register. Upon reaching the summit, they discovered an Arapaho eagle trap, clearly indicating that others had been to the top before them. To his credit, Powell never disputed this fact.

Longs is the highest point in Boulder County and the Front Range. It is also the northernmost 14er. The correct spelling of Longs Peak does not include an apostrophe. Mapmakers agreed long ago that geographical features would not have apostrophes in their official names.

Contact Info

Rocky Mountain National Park
1000 US Highway 36
Estes Park, CO 80517

General Park Information: (970) 586-1206
Visitor Information Recorded Message: (970) 586-1333
Backcountry Information: (970) 586-1242
Campground Reservations: (800) 365-2267

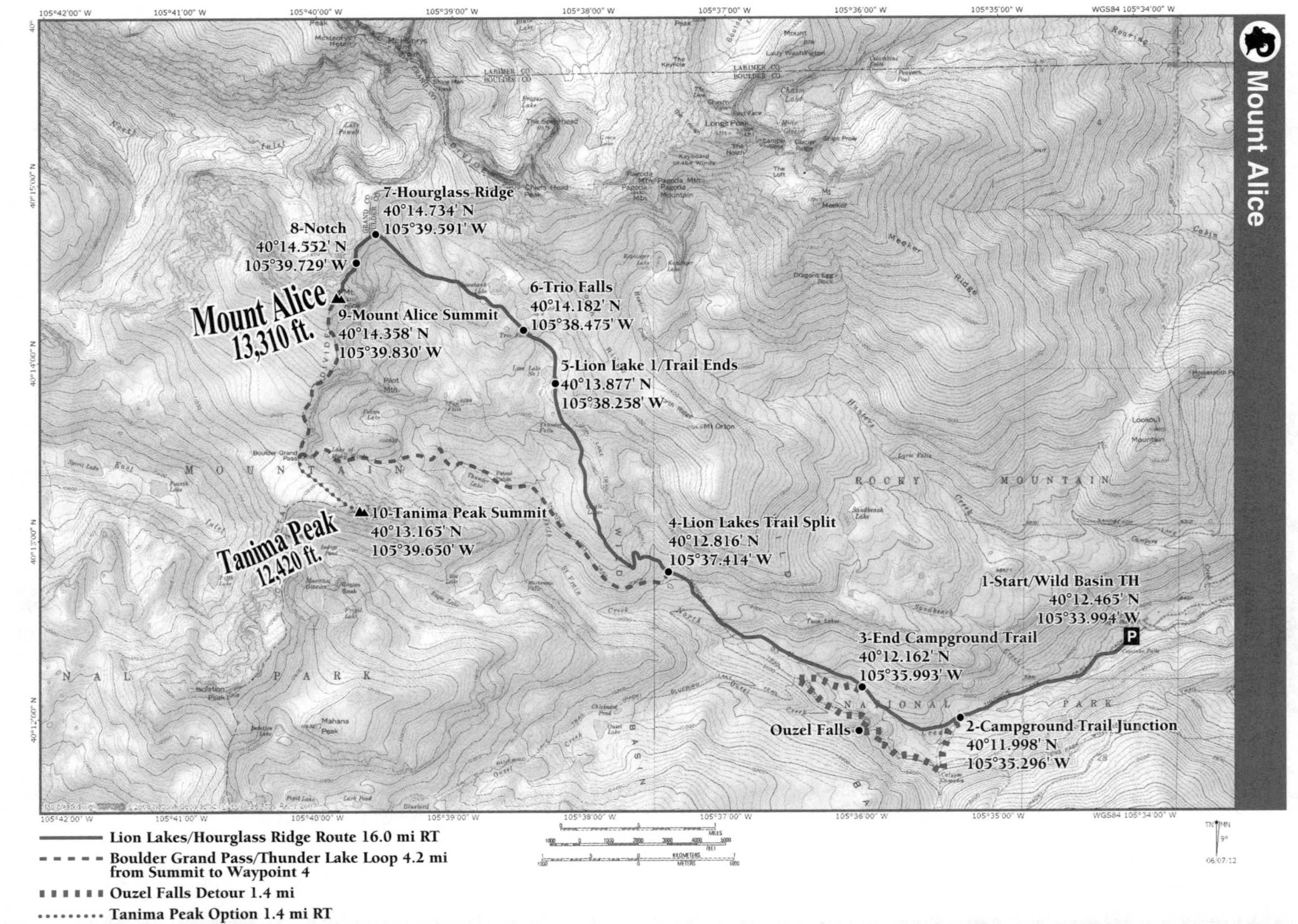

Mount Alice
1-Start/Wild Basin TH
40°12.465' N
105°33.994' W
2-Campground Trail Junction
40°11.998' N
105°35.296' W
3-End Campground Trail
40°12.162' N
105°35.993' W
Ouzel Falls
4-Lion Lakes Trail Split
40°12.816' N
105°37.414' W
5-Lion Lake 1/Trail Ends
40°13.877' N
105°38.258' W
6-Trio Falls
40°14.182' N
105°38.475' W
7-Hourglass Ridge
40°14.734' N
105°39.591' W
8-Notch
40°14.552' N
105°39.729' W
9-Mount Alice Summit
40°14.358' N
105°39.830' W
10-Tanima Peak Summit
40°13.165' N
105°39.650' W
Mount Alice
13,310 ft.
Tanima Peak
12,420 ft.
Lion Lakes/Hourglass Ridge Route 16.0 mi RT
Boulder Grand Pass/Thunder Lake Loop 4.2 mi from Summit to Waypoint 4
Ouzel Falls Detour 1.4 mi
Tanima Peak Option 1.4 mi RT

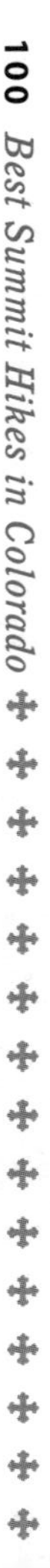

9 Mount Alice

Good Overnight!

Mount Alice is like Longs Peak without the crowds. It even has its own mini-Diamond on the east face. An epic adventure with robust scrambling.

Round-Trip Distance	16.0 miles
Hiking Time	11–15 hours
Difficulty	8/10
Class	3
Start Elevation	8,515 ft., at Wild Basin/Thunder Lake Trailhead
Peak Elevation	13,310 ft.
Total Elevation Gain	4,825 ft.
Terrain	Long, smooth prelude trail to off-trail meadows and rocky summit scramble
Best Time to Climb	July–September
Gear Advisor	Trekking poles and ice ax/crampons in spring and past September
Crowd Level	Low

Location Front Range in Rocky Mountain National Park, Wild Basin Area, outside of Estes Park

Intro Wild Basin is one of the most beautiful areas in Rocky Mountain National Park. Like most places in the park, the crowds thin out the farther in you go. By the time you reach Lion Lakes at the foot of Mount Alice, there's a good chance that you'll be all alone. The beauty of this area is unmatched in the park. Wildflowers and wildlife abound in the lakes area, and all are watched over by the grand matriarch that is Mount Alice.

Why Climb It? The Mount Alice experience is similar to the Longs Peak hike: a long, moderate, on-trail approach leads to a class 3 ascent via an exciting route. Unlike Longs, however, Alice doesn't attract the masses—for most, it's not a "glory peak." The setting is beautiful and remote, a world apart from the rest of the park. Ascending the connecting ridge to Alice's northeast ridge is a wonderful way to start the challenging ascent. Once on the ridge, the class 3 scrambling is steep but solid (it's like an extended version of the scrambling on Pacific Peak, Hike 15 in

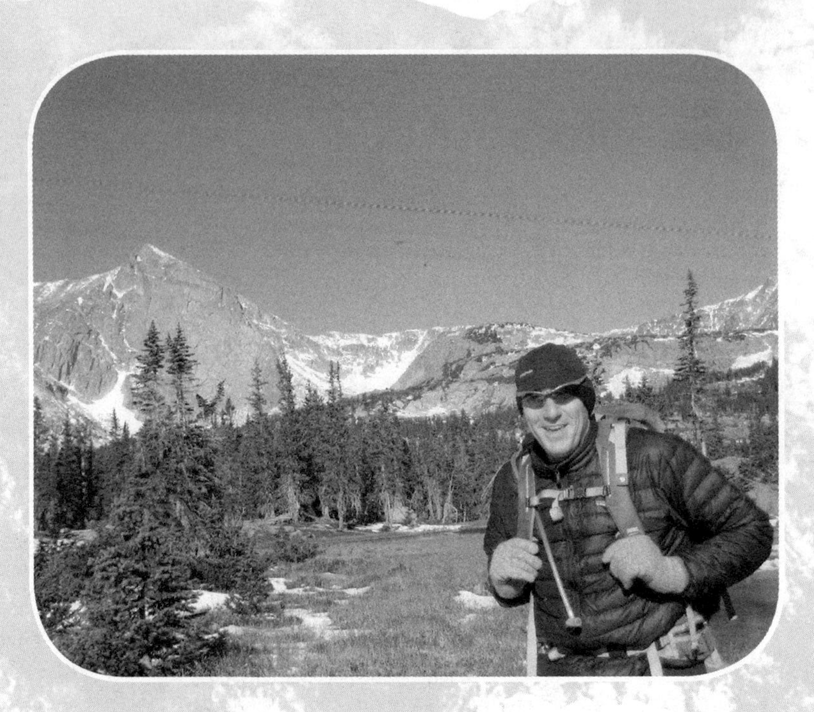

Wild Basin is one of the most beautiful and remote sections of Rocky Mountain National Park.

this book). From the summit, you can return the way you came or make a loop down to Thunder Lake—a nice tour. After the exciting climb, you can further extend your trip by making an easy side trip to Ouzel Falls.

Driving All vehicles can make it to the Wild Basin Trailhead; the dirt road is very well maintained.

How to Get There The road to the trailhead is off Colorado Highway 7. From the south, this is 6.5 miles north of the junction of CO 7 and Colorado Highway 72 after the town of Allenspark; from the north, it is 13 miles from the junction of US Highway 36 and CO 7. Turn west into the well-signed Wild Basin Area and continue along the road 2.6 miles, following the signs to the Wild Basin Ranger Station and the parking area at the end of the road. Try to get there early.

Fees/Camping The day-use fee for Rocky Mountain National Park is $20 for a seven-day pass. Camping at the several sites along the way requires a permit and a $20 fee. Contact rangers before you go to make sure there is site availability. Much like Longs, this hike is feasible as a one-day outing if you get a very early start. The campsites along Campground Trail are good, backcountry sites. There is also camping at Thunder Lake.

Route Notes The route described here uses the Campground Trail to cut a mile off the hike (as well as a bit of elevation gain and loss) by bypassing the Ouzel Falls Trail. This explains the discrepancy between the mileages noted in this section and what you might find in other references (though the accuracy of the GPS plays into that a bit, too). I'd suggest seeing the falls on your descent, which adds a mile to your total trek. If climbing in spring, expect there to be quite a bit of snow on the mountain.

Mile/Waypoint

0.0 mi (1) Start your hike on the Thunder Lakes/Ouzel Falls Trail from the Wild Basin parking area. This is a very easy class 1 trail that serves as a good warm-up. Stay on the main trail when it passes the junction for Copeland Falls.

1.4 mi (2) There is a signpost here pointing to several campgrounds. To save time (and cut about a mile off your hike), take the side Campground Trail to the right instead of taking the tour of Ouzel Falls. This trail is unimproved but still easy to follow, as it goes by four campsites.

2.8 mi (3) The Campground Trail rejoins the main trail at a bridge. The trails then split to Ouzel Falls and Thunder Lake. For now, go north on the trail toward Thunder Lake, which is listed as 3.3 miles away.

3.8 mi (4) At the signed junction, do *not* head toward Thunder Lake. Note that this sign marks the distance to the ranger station as 4.8 miles; this mileage is determined by taking the Ouzel Falls Trail. Stay right (north) on the trail that goes uphill to Lion Lakes. This trail is a bit faded but is still visible as you climb toward the lakes.

5.7 mi (5) After previewing a few small ponds on your left, you'll drop down into the clearing at Lion Lake No. 1. From this point on, consider this an off-trail hike. It's downright beautiful, and the views of Alice are impressive. Pass Lion Lake No. 1 on its right (east) side; a faint trail may or may not be underwater. From here, cairns loosely lead to Trio Falls, a cool waterfall perched on a shelf of rock. If you are unable to follow the cairns, stay close to the stream that leads to the falls.

6.0 mi (6) At Trio Falls, you'll need to do some easy scrambling to get up to the next plateau, where Lion Lake No. 2 awaits. Just left (west) of the falls is a good spot to climb up. From Lion Lake No. 2, you'll be just below the connecting ridge that intersects Hourglass Ridge. Go northwest to the spine of this broad hill and meet up with your goal—Hourglass Ridge.

7.2 mi (7) You've gained Hourglass Ridge, and Alice's imposing north face looks down upon you. It's not as bad as it looks. Go south on the ridge and then downhill just a little to a notch in the ridge.

7.5 mi (8) At the notch (12,520 feet), you'll see your final 0.5-mile scramble as a jumble of blocky boulders. Scramble up, staying closer to the spine on the west side. Too far east, and you'll be on the side of the sheer mini-Diamond (called the Cubic Zirconium by some). This is class 3 territory and is best climbed once the snow and ice have melted off.

8.0 mi (9) Alice's summit. The register here records very few visitors. You have two equally good descent routes from here: return the way you came, or take the optional loop route southwest to Boulder-Grand Pass (read the "Options" section for info on this route). Both are good choices. The first route returns back via Lion Lakes. After scrambling back down the ridge, return exactly the way you came up. However, on the descent, you can take the Campground Trail again or loop over to Ouzel Falls. I recommend the Ouzel Falls Loop if you have the energy.

16.0 mi Finish.

Options Because you're already in for a long day, why not go for the epic loop that traverses over to 12,420-foot Tanima Peak? Tanima is 1.7 miles from the summit of Alice and offers incredible views of Mount Alice to the north and the seldom-seen Moomaw Glacier and Isolation Peak to the south.

To close the loop, you'll need to navigate down Boulder Grand Pass back to Thunder Lake. From the top of the pass to the Thunder Lake Trail (which leads directly pack to the parking lot), it is 1.1 miles of off-trail navigation. The trickiest part is descending from the ridge to the Lake of Many Winds. Look for a dirt couloir on the north side of the pass, which is a steep but nontechnical scramble down. From there, get a bearing to the lake or follow the drainage creek.

For more details and photos on this optional route, check out **tinyurl .com/aliceoption.**

Quick Facts The identity of the Alice for whom this peak was named is unknown. Most signs point to her being a woman of ill repute who earned favor with the survey team. Perhaps a cartographer made a hasty promise to the lady to put her on the map, but when questioned about it later, played dumb in order to save his own bacon (metaphorically speaking). Because there is no known Alice on record, I say that we dedicate this mountain to Alice Cooper, rock-and-roll icon and all-around interesting guy.

Contact Info Rocky Mountain National Park
1000 US Highway 36
Estes Park, CO 80517

General Park Information: (970) 586-1206
Visitor Information Recorded Message: (970) 586-1333
Backcountry Information: (970) 586-1242
Campground Reservations: (800) 365-2267

Boulder Grand Pass leads to a brief off-trail romp to Thunder Lake.

You're already in for a long day. Why not tack on Tanima Peak as a bonus summit?

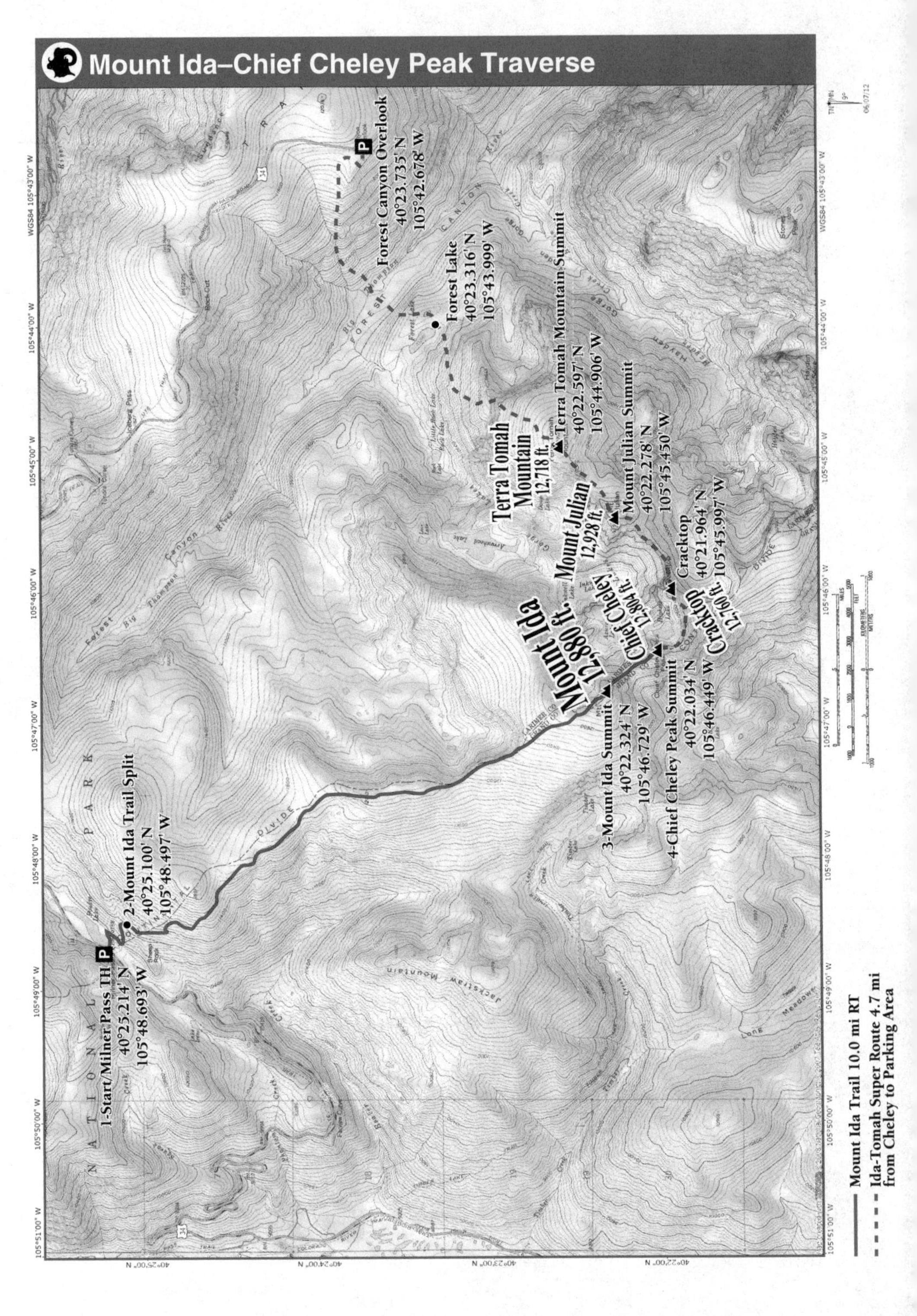
Mount Ida–Chief Cheley Peak Traverse
1-Start/Milner Pass TH
40°25.214' N
105°48.693' W
2-Mount Ida Trail Split
40°25.100' N
105°48.497' W
3-Mount Ida Summit
40°22.324' N
105°46.729' W
4-Chief Cheley Peak Summit
40°22.034' N
105°46.449' W
Mount Ida
12,880 ft.
Chief Cheley
12,804 ft.
Cracktop
12,760 ft.
Cracktop
40°21.964' N
105°45.997' W
Mount Julian
12,928 ft.
Mount Julian Summit
40°22.278' N
105°45.450' W
Terra Tomah Mountain
12,718 ft.
Terra Tomah Mountain Summit
40°22.597' N
105°44.906' W
Forest Lake
40°23.316' N
105°43.999' W
Forest Canyon Overlook
40°23.735' N
105°42.678' W
Mount Ida Trail 10.0 mi RT
Ida-Tomah Super Route 4.7 mi from Cheley to Parking Area

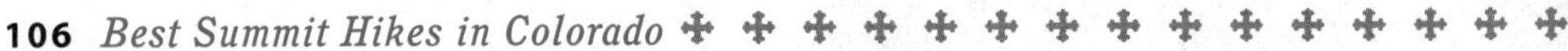

10 Mount Ida–Chief Cheley Peak Traverse

Mount Ida is one of the most beautiful, yet seldom visited, peaks in Rocky Mountain National Park. Cruise the Continental Divide and keep an eye out for the many furry locals.

Round-Trip Distance	10.0 miles
Hiking Time	5–8 hours
Difficulty	6.5/10
Class	2 with long class 1 sections
Start Elevation	10,750 ft., at Milner Pass Trailhead
Peak Elevations	Mount Ida: 12,880 ft.; Chief Cheley Peak: 12,804 ft.
Total Elevation Gain	3,376 ft.
Terrain	Wide-open alpine meadows with class 2 scramble on good rock on Cheley
Best Time to Climb	June–September
Gear Advisor	Normal gear
Crowd Level	Low

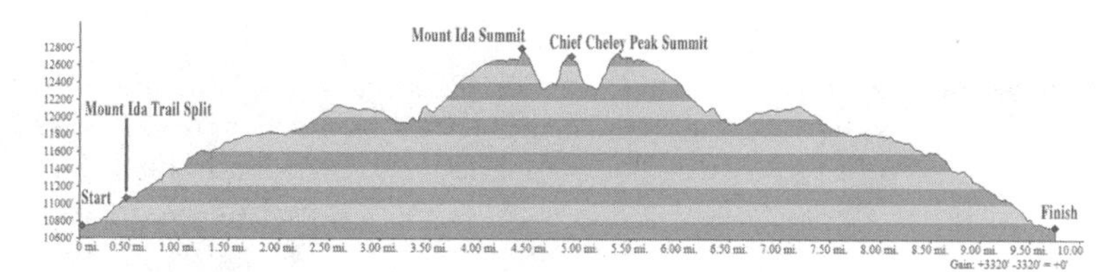

Location Front Range in Rocky Mountain National Park, just below the northernmost point on Trail Ridge Road

Intro With more than 3 million visitors annually to Rocky Mountain National Park (RMNP), it may come as a surprise that Mount Ida is relatively unknown to the masses. The trail to Ida is easy to reach and follows a particularly beautiful line along the Continental Divide. Because it is in the high country of the northern boundaries of RMNP, views of the Never Summer Mountains to the west and the "glory peaks" (such as Longs) to the south are quite impressive.

Why Climb It? As soon as you leave the crowds behind at the parking lot, the walk along the Continental Divide opens up vast tracts of alpine meadows for your enjoyment. Views are spectacular throughout the hike, especially of the pockets of lakes to the east when you near the summits of these two mountains. Wildlife viewing is exceptionally good in RMNP, and this area is no exception. Elk, mule deer, marmots, pikas, ptarmigans, and more mingle in the trees and on the tundra. After you have reached Ida, the solid scramble over to Chief Cheley may inspire you to continue east via the optional route to Cracktop, Mount Julian, and Terra Tomah Mountain.

Driving Passenger cars can make it to Milner Pass Trailhead, which is off the paved Trail Ridge Road. Perhaps the most difficult part of this drive is not getting rattled by the exposure on the thrilling Trail Ridge Road.

How to Get There If you are coming from the east side (Estes Park) of RMNP, enter the park at either Fall River or Beaver Meadows. From both of these points, it is roughly 4 miles to the junction of US Highways 36 and 34. From this junction, follow the always exciting Trail Ridge Road 22 miles, past the Alpine visitor center, over the highest section of road (at 12,183 feet), and descend to the Milner Pass Trailhead, which is on the Continental Divide. You'll see Poudre Lake on your left just before the lot, which has a lot of informative signs.

Fees/Camping The entrance fee to RMNP (which gives you a seven-day permit) is $20 per car (not per person); an annual pass to the park is $35. A backcountry camping permit is $20. There are six drive-in campgrounds in the park; most operate on a first-come, first-serve basis. You can make reservations at Moraine Park and Glacier Basin areas (call [800] 365-2267). Fees are $20 per night, though once the water utilities are shut off in autumn, some sites drop to $14 per night.

Route Notes None.

Mile/Waypoint **0.0 mi (1)** Start at the Milner Pass Trailhead. Your adventure begins on the Ute Trail, which has a sign declaring MOUNT IDA 4.0 as well as distances to other destinations (apparently, everything is 4.0 miles). Hike past the wheezing tourists and up a few modest switchbacks on the very well-worn trail. In the early morning, the reflections on tiny Poudre Lake make for good photographs.

0.5 mi (2) After climbing the switchbacks through the trees, you'll come to a trail intersection. Stay the course to Mount Ida by taking a right (south) and continuing along the well-worn trail as it breaks timberline. Once out of the trees, the trail stretches south as far as the eye can see. Follow it along the Continental Divide, soaking in the awesome views. The orange-tinted Never Summer Mountains to the west contrast with the black, green, and gray Front Range mountains to the south and east. You'll see Ida in the distance; simply continue your southern trajectory on the ridge to reach it. Eventually, the trail fades out (about 3.2 miles in), and you'll have to navigate easy, sparse boulder fields. Staying close to the rim on the western side of the ridge offers great views of the lake-filled basin to the northeast. The navigation here is easy, though the walk to Mount Ida may take a little longer than you think. When the spaces are this wide-open, things are always a little farther away than they appear.

4.5 mi (3) The summit of Mount Ida! Depending on how you navigated the boulder fields, your mileage may be a little more or less than the mileage specified above. Alpine lakes, below to the east, shimmer in the sun and darken to ink black when the clouds move in. To continue to Chief Cheley Peak, drop down 400 feet via the southeast ridge to a saddle between the two mountains. (The scramble is not as hard as it looks from the top of Ida.) A class 2/2+ scramble up to Cheley is done on solid rock. I find it a nice change from the placid pace of the approach.

5.0 mi (4) Huzzah, the summit of Chief Cheley Peak! From here, you can return the way you came, along the Divide, to return to your vehicle. However, I have a sneaking suspicion that you may be tempted to continue east for a few more peaks; read the "Options" section below for more on this route.

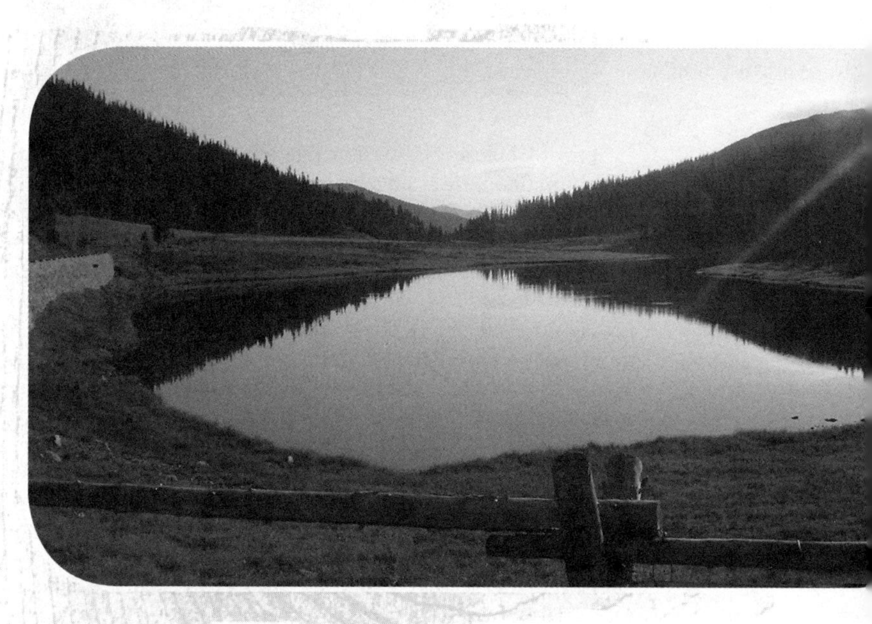

A still morning is reflected in Poudre Lake at the trailhead.

10.0 mi Finish your hike by returning the way you came to the Milner Pass parking lot, which will probably be much more crowded than when you left it in the early morning.

Options The Ida-Tomah Super Route option can be done as an out-and-back or as a two-car endeavor, with one vehicle at Milner Pass and one at the Forest Canyon Overlook parking area. I suggest the two-car option. You'll need to start predawn to get a safe window of weather (getting to RMNP very early has its benefits). The hiking distance to the Forest Canyon Overlook is approximately 4.7 miles from the summit of Cheley and is a class 2/2+ traverse.

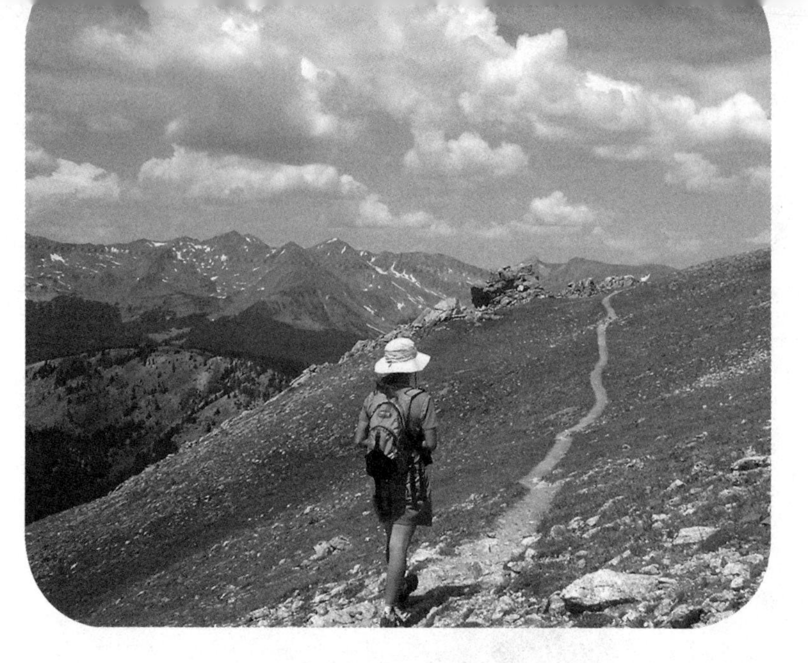

With nearly the entire hike above tree line, you'll have awesome views in all directions.

From Cheley, follow the ridge as it curves east and then northeast to Cracktop (0.6 mile from Cheley), and then to Mount Julian (1.2 miles from Cheley), and then over to the mammoth, glacially carved Terra Tomah Mountain (2.0 miles from Cheley). There are no trails to the Forest Canyon parking area, but the land is very wide-open. From Terra Tomah, head northeast to Forest Lake, and conclude your day with a 1,500-foot push up grassy slopes to the parking area, roughly 4.7 miles from Cheley. This is a good place to use your GPS and compass skills. If you complete the loop, you'll have bagged five of the best summits in the park. You can see all the peaks in this route from the high point on Trail Ridge Road.

Quick Facts If Mount Ida was named after a specific woman, her identity is lost to history. The name Ida was probably transferred from Mount Ida in Crete, Greece. According to ancient Greek mythology, Mount Ida was the birthplace of Zeus, ruler of the gods.

Chief Cheley Peak is named after Frank Cheley, who founded a pre-Outward Bound-style summer camp in the area in 1921, a program that is still active today.

Mount Julian is named after Julian Hayden, a civil engineer who lived in Estes Park.

Terra Tomah's name is a bit of a mistake on the map. In 1914, a hiker named George Barnard was inspired by the sight of a lake near this peak to break out in song, and chanted the Coahuila Native American classic "He northeast Terratoma, northeast Terratoma." Terratoma sounded good, and despite the fact that no one knew what it meant, the word was proposed as a name for the lake and area around it. When James Grafton Rogers, chairman of the Colorado Geographic Board, sent his maps off for approval to Washington, D.C., he was shocked to find that the name had mistakenly been used to identify the mountain. The lake that was to have borne the noble name Terratoma was instead dubbed Doughnut Lake (a name that might entice even Homer Simpson to make this hike!).

So what does Terra Tomah actually mean? The song was allegedly overheard by spying college students in California (and by spying, they probably meant drunk), who heard the song performed at an authentic Coahuila ghost dance in 1892. The students took the melody back to their school, Pomona College, where it became an anthem, even though no one knew what the words meant. As with much of modern pop music, the words didn't make any sense, but the song had a good beat. When questioned, Coahuila natives said they did not know what the words meant. Of course, they may simply have wanted to keep the meaning a secret from white men. Thus, what Terra Tomah means remains a mystery; except, perhaps, to a few Coahuila people who understand the words and keep the meaning to themselves as a century-old inside joke.

Contact Info

Rocky Mountain National Park
1000 US Highway 36
Estes Park, CO 80517

General Park Information: (970) 586-1206
Visitor Information Recorded Message: (970) 586-1333
Backcountry Information: (970) 586-1242
Campground Reservations: (800) 365-2267

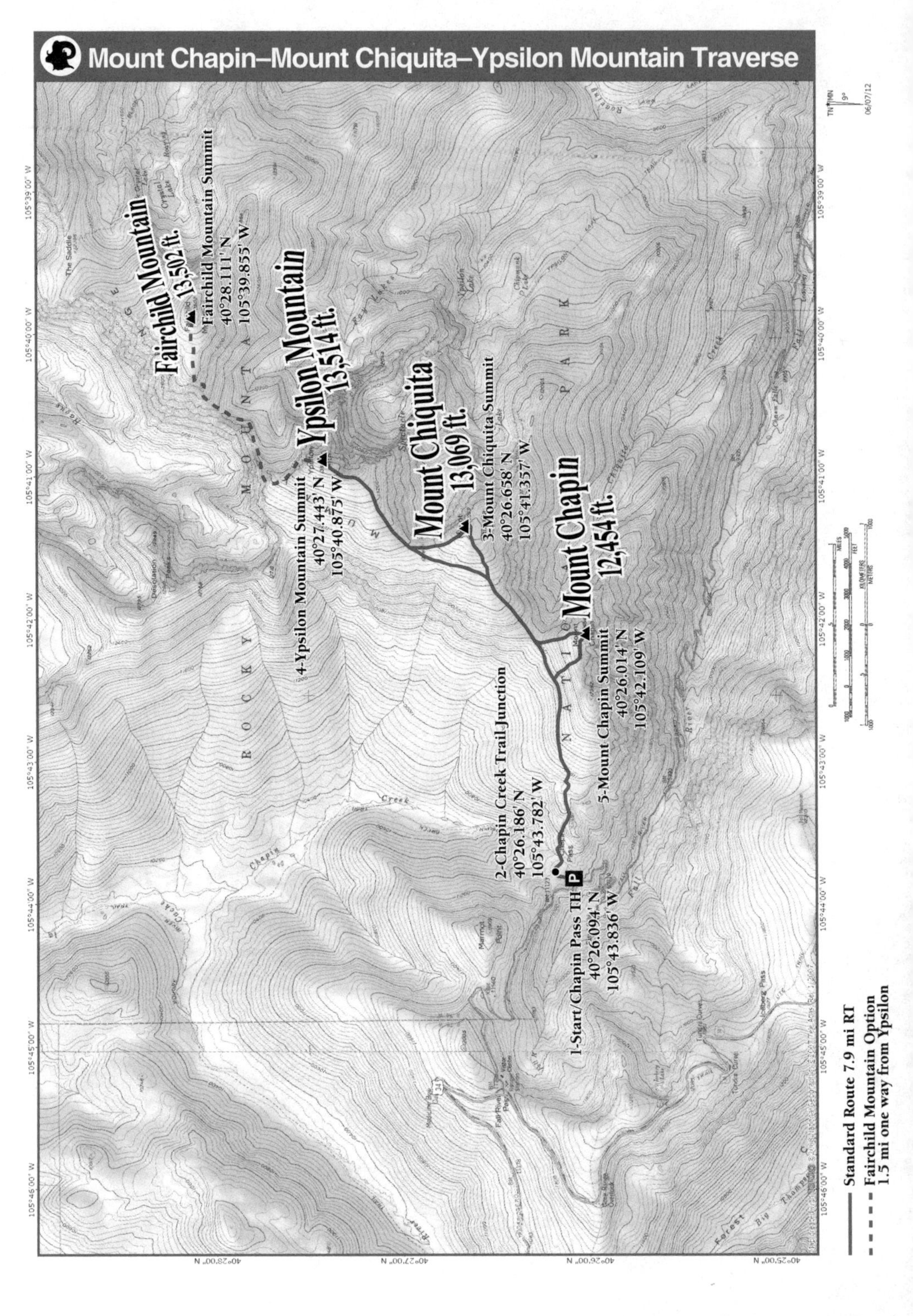
Mount Chapin–Mount Chiquita–Ypsilon Mountain Traverse
Fairchild Mountain
13,502 ft.
Fairchild Mountain Summit
40°28.111' N
105°39.855' W
Ypsilon Mountain
13,514 ft.
4-Ypsilon Mountain Summit
40°27.443' N
105°40.875' W
Mount Chiquita
13,069 ft.
3-Mount Chiquita Summit
40°26.658' N
105°41.357' W
Mount Chapin
12,454 ft.
5-Mount Chapin Summit
40°26.014' N
105°42.109' W
2-Chapin Creek Trail Junction
40°26.186' N
105°43.782' W
1-Start/Chapin Pass TH
40°26.094' N
105°43.836' W
ROCKY MOUNTAIN NATIONAL PARK
Standard Route 7.9 mi RT
Fairchild Mountain Option
1.5 mi one way from Ypsilon

11 Mount Chapin–Mount Chiquita–Ypsilon Mountain Traverse

These peaks are among the farthest north in Rocky Mountain National Park. Views from the high alpine tundra are top-notch on this peaceful, spacious hike.

Round-Trip Distance	7.9 miles
Hiking Time	4–6 hours
Difficulty	4.5/10
Class	2
Start Elevation	11,148 ft., at Chapin Creek Trailhead
Peak Elevations	Mount Chapin: 12,454 ft.; Mount Chiquita: 13,069 ft.; Ypsilon Mountain: 13,514 ft.
Total Elevation Gain	3,373 ft.
Terrain	Good trail to easy alpine tundra
Best Time to Climb	June–September
Gear Advisor	Normal gear
Crowd Level	Moderate

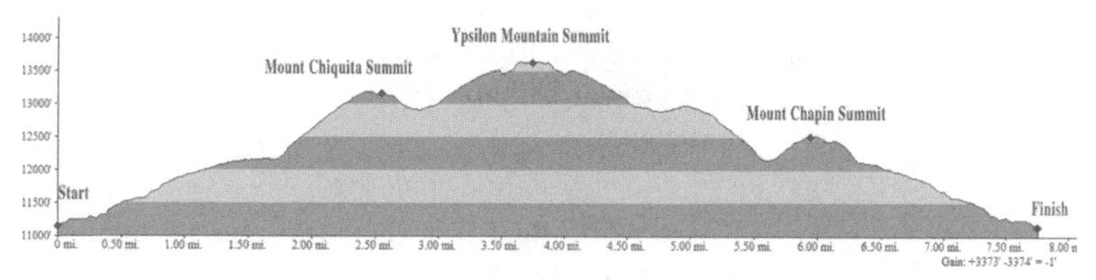

Location Mummy Range in Rocky Mountain National Park, outside of Estes Park

Intro This threesome is very photogenic. Tourists have taken countless pictures of these mountains from the base of Old Fall River Road. Most of the hiking adventure takes place above timberline, offering expansive views of the Front Range, the Never Summer Range, and other Mummy Range peaks to the north. For those hoping to extend the day, there are several options to increase your peak count beyond this trio.

Why Climb It? The chance to bag three scenic peaks is tempting; to do so without heart-busting exertion seals the deal. Moderate alpine terrain brings you to these friendly mountains. The incredible perspective from the top of Ypsilon's southeast couloir down to Spectacle Lakes alone is worth the trip. Every step of the way is chock-full of scenery that elevates your senses. If three summits aren't enough, ambitious hikers can carry on to Fairchild Mountain. A walk along these mountains embodies the freedom of the hills.

Driving Old Fall River Road is a very well-maintained dirt road and is passable by all vehicles.

How to Get There From the Fall River entrance (US Highway 34), it is 2.1 miles to the right-hand turn (west) onto Old Fall River Road at Horseshoe Park. If you are coming from the Beaver Meadows entrance on US Highway 36, go 3.3 miles from the pay station and take the right (northwest) onto US 34. Go downhill 1.8 miles (passing a great photo opportunity of Mount Chapin, Mount Chiquita, and Ypsilon Mountain at a pull-off) and turn left onto Old Fall River Road. Follow the one-way dirt road (which is a novelty in itself) 6.8 miles to Chapin Pass Trailhead, on the right (north) side of the road in the midst of a section of switchbacks. Parking is limited in the area, so try to get in early. Remember when you are done to continue driving up on the one-way road, where you will exit at the Alpine visitor center.

Fees/Camping It is $20 per car to enter Rocky Mountain National Park; annual passes are $35. Backcountry camping is available is designated areas only and requires a permit and $20 fee. There are several pay campgrounds in the park; call ahead to make reservations or to check availability.

Route Notes My route hits the summit of Chapin on the return from Ypsilon and Chiquita; you are more than welcome to summit Chapin first, if you prefer. Both ways are on class 2 terrain.

Mile/Waypoint

0.0 mi (1) Start at the Chapin Pass Trailhead. Get on the trail, and head uphill to a small saddle.

0.1 mi (2) On the quickly reached saddle, turn right at the Chapin Creek Trail junction toward Chapin, Chiquita, and Ypsilon summits. A sign will help point the way.

0.7 mi As you near Chapin, the trail fades a little and goes left of the peak. If you'd like to summit Chapin first, take the optional route to the summit and continue on to Chiquita.

1.8 mi The formal trail disappears as you reach the saddle between Chapin and Chiquita at 12,160 feet. Carry on northeast to Chiquita's summit on good alpine terrain that is a mixture of grass and rocks.

2.6 mi (3) Mount Chiquita's summit has a nice wind shelter and good views. Take a break here, and then continue northeast to Ypsilon.

3.8 mi (4) Ypsilon Mountain's summit looks similar to Chiquita's. As mentioned before, the views down to Spectacle Lakes are astounding. Vistas in every other direction are pretty good, too. For this route, return to the saddle between Chiquita and Chapin, bypassing Chiquita's summit (for the time being).

5.7 mi Back at the saddle, start heading up an intermittent footpath to the summit of Chapin. This climb is only about 400 feet.

6.1 mi (5) Chapin's summit. This is my favorite summit of the three to sit and take in the scenery, which is why I suggest closing your hike with it.

From here, you can descend down the north slopes or take the optional walk down the west ridge back to the trail.

7.9 mi Finish. Remember to drive uphill on the one-way road to exit.

Options So this little sojourn was too easy for ya, huh, tough guy (or girl)? Why not try the traverse over to Fairchild Mountain? Its summit is 1.5 miles from Ypsilon's summit on class 2+/3 terrain. If that's not enough, you can continue on to Hagues Peak. A famous loop can be made by going from Hagues Peak to Mummy Mountain and down to Lawn Lake, where a second car should be parked. (You'll need to pick up additional quad maps if you'd like to give it a shot, as my humble little map doesn't cover these features.)

Quick Facts There are a few theories on which Chapin the mountain is named for. The most plausible is Frederick H. Chapin, another guy from Connecticut who came to Colorado to escape the flatlands and climb some *real* mountains (he was from Hartford). (I, too, hail from the Constitution State, having been born in Waterbury Hospital, elevation: 760 feet above sea level.) Chapin climbed in the state from 1886 to 1888 as a representative of the Appalachian Mountain Club. He also contributed to getting Hallett's Peak named after W. L. Hallett, who had acted as a tour guide for the plucky New Englander.

For some odd reason, Enos Mills (who was responsible for putting names on the map) was smitten by a character in the book *Chiquita, An American Novel: The Romance of a Ute Chief's Daughter.* The story hit a soft spot with old Enos, and the name he gave the mountain stuck.

Spectacle Lakes were named by Roger Toll in 1922 for their resemblance to eyeglasses, though they could just as well have been named for the spectacle they present.

Ypsilon is named after the snow couloirs in its east face that form the letter Y when filled with snow. Because Ypsilon sounds more sophisticated than Y Mountain, that name was applied.

Fairchild Mountain is named after Lucius Fairchild (what a great name!), an accomplished diplomat and three-time governor of Wisconsin. He never climbed the peak, but his admirers did and honored him thus.

One last note: Fall River Road was the first, steep road through the park; it was rendered to second-class duty when Trail Ridge Road was completed in 1932.

Contact Info Rocky Mountain National Park
1000 US Highway 36
Estes Park, CO 80517

General Park Information: (970) 586-1206
Visitor Information Recorded Message: (970) 586-1333
Backcountry Information: (970) 586-1242
Campground Reservations: (800) 365-2267

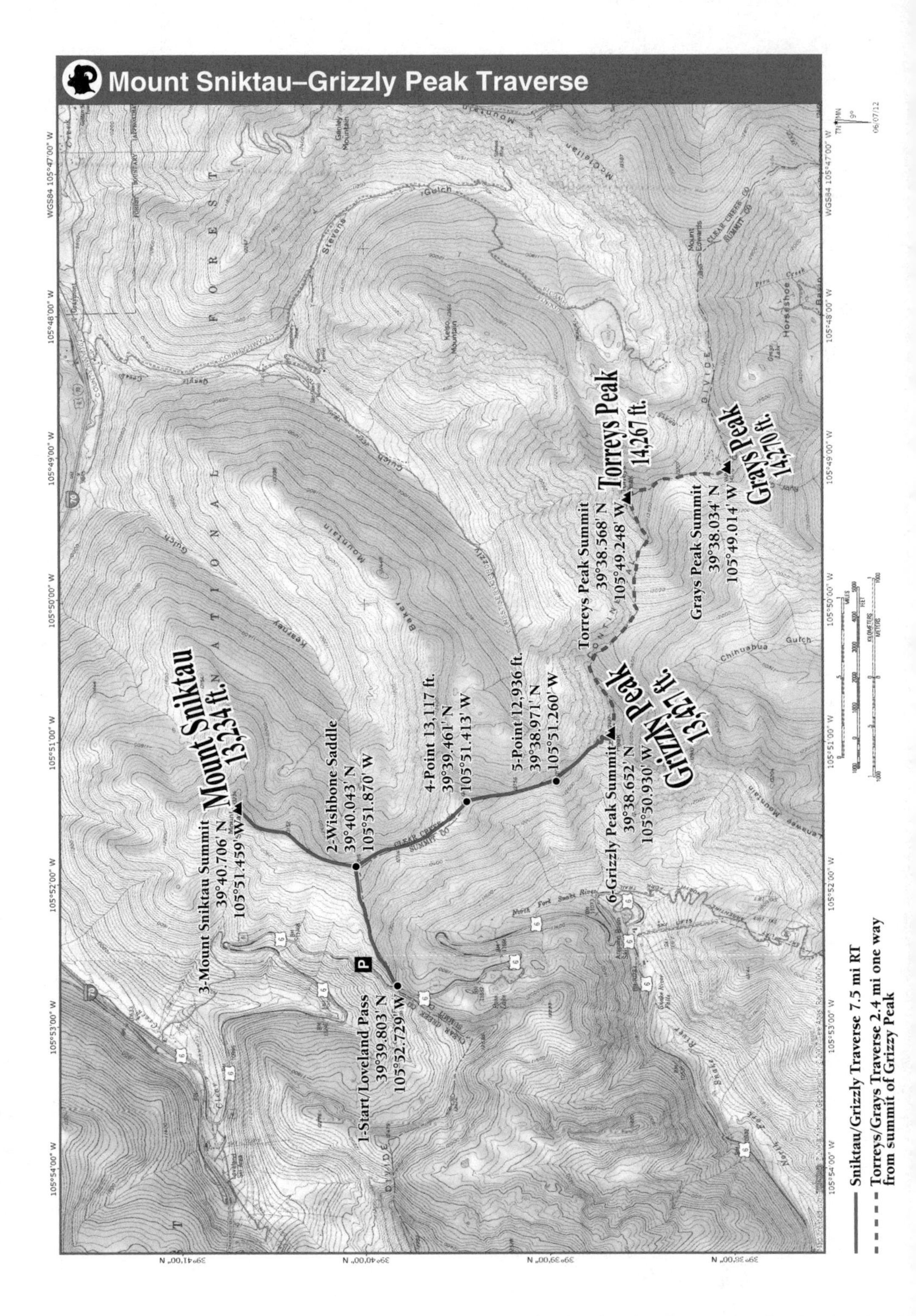

Mount Sniktau–Grizzly Peak Traverse
Mount Sniktau
13,234 ft.
3-Mount Sniktau Summit
39°40.706' N
105°51.459' W
2-Wishbone Saddle
39°40.043' N
105°51.870' W
1-Start/Loveland Pass
39°39.803' N
105°52.729' W
4-Point 13,117 ft.
39°39.461' N
105°51.413' W
5-Point 12,936 ft.
39°38.971' N
105°51.260' W
6-Grizzly Peak Summit
39°38.652' N
105°50.930' W
Grizzly Peak
13,427 ft.
Torreys Peak Summit
39°38.568' N
105°49.248' W
Torreys Peak
14,267 ft.
Grays Peak Summit
39°38.034' N
105°49.014' W
Grays Peak
14,270 ft.
Sniktau/Grizzly Traverse 7.5 mi RT
Torreys/Grays Traverse 2.4 mi one way from summit of Grizzy Peak

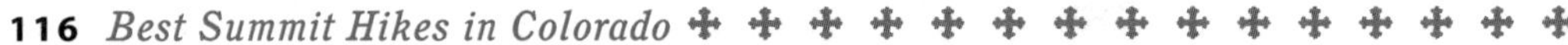

12 Mount Sniktau–Grizzly Peak Traverse

Stay above tree line as you traverse rolling alpine ridges, culminating with a spectacular ascent of Grizzly Peak. Wide-open spaces and views of familiar places await you.

Round-Trip Distance	7.5 miles
Hiking Time	4–6 hours
Difficulty	5/10
Class	2
Start Elevation	11,930 ft., at Loveland Pass summit
Peak Elevations	Mount Sniktau: 13,234 ft.; Grizzly Peak: 13,427 ft.
Total Elevation Gain	4,088 ft.
Terrain	Rolling alpine ridges with good footing
Best Time to Climb	May–October; a good winter hike as well
Gear Advisor	Normal gear
Crowd Level	Moderate

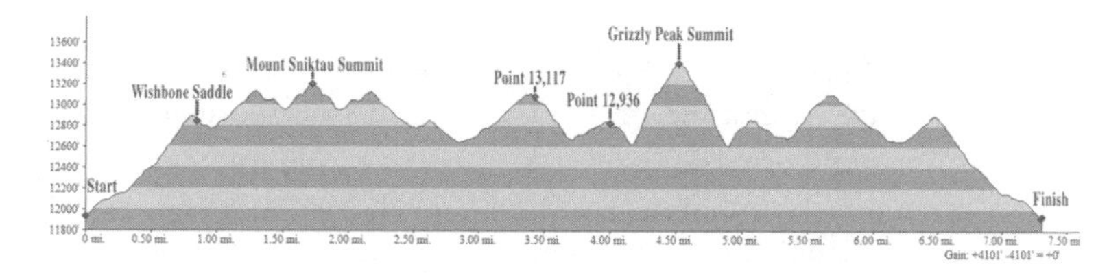

Location Front Range in Arapaho National Forest, just east of Loveland Pass

Intro Mount Sniktau stands out when viewed from I-70 near Loveland Pass; its lower slopes are home to a few runs at Loveland Basin Ski Area. Thanks to a high trailhead located at the summit of Loveland Pass, this entire hike is above the trees. Climbing from the pass to Sniktau is short and sweet; your rewards include amazing views of several mountain ranges and many familiar ski areas: Loveland, Arapahoe Basin, Keystone, and Copper Mountain. Turning south, the trek continues over a rolling ridge of unnamed summits, culminating with an 800-foot push to the top of Grizzly Peak (one of several Grizzly Peaks in the state).

Why Climb It? Sniktau's easy access and familiar confines mean that you'll have a quick drive from the Denver/Boulder/Golden area. An uphill push from the pass grants you access to this scenic ridge, which runs from the valley in I-70 to 14,267-foot Torreys Peak (and beyond). Because the entire hike is above the trees, you'll have grandiose 360-degree views the entire hike. After the moderate climb to Sniktau, roll south on the sky-high ridge to Grizzly Peak. It's a class 2 scramble up the northwest face of the Grizz. From the summit, Grays and Torreys peaks look *enormous*.

Driving Passenger cars can make it up Loveland Pass, which is paved and very well maintained year-round.

How to Get There From I-70, take Exit 216 (Loveland Pass/Loveland Ski Area exit), which is less than 0.5 mile east of the Eisenhower/Johnson tunnel. Exit the highway, and then take a right to proceed up Loveland Pass (US Highway 6), which bypasses the Loveland Ski Area on your right; don't head left (east), or you'll simply end up at the lower part of Loveland. Continue up the steep, exposed pass 4.2 miles to the Loveland Pass summit; parking is on the left. Be warned—it fills up quickly, especially in the winter.

Fees/Camping There are no fees for hiking in this area. Camping is possible, but there are not many water sources. A good place to spend the night is at Herman Gulch, a few miles down I-70 east at Exit 218 (there are no fees there either).

Route Notes None.

Mile/Waypoint

0.0 mi (1) Start at the top of Loveland Pass. There is a large sign with the elevation; the trail uphill starts just behind it. There are no trail signs or markers, but the way up to the saddle is obvious. Follow the spine of the ridge northeast to Wishbone Saddle, 900 vertical feet above.

0.8 mi (2) Wishbone Saddle. Catch your breath and grab a swig of water; the hardest part of your hike is behind you. Turn northeast and continue to follow the ridge.

1.3 mi You'll clear a 13,152-foot false summit en route to Mount Sniktau summit. Between this point and Sniktau, there is often snow, especially on the east side. Continue to stay on the high point of the ridge and make the modest, 400-vertical-foot push up to Sniktau's summit.

1.8 mi (3) That was fast! You're already at the top of Sniktau. Did you bring your snowboard? You can drop directly down to the Loveland Ski Area from here. Wait, you're here to hike! Enjoy the awesome views up here: the Vasquez Mountains are to the north, the Gores to the west, the Front Range to the east, and in the southern distance are the Mosquito Range peaks. Far west, you may be able to see the Sawatch Peaks. Return to Wishbone Saddle.

2.7 mi (2) Back in the saddle again. This time, go south along the footpath that floats over the ridge to the base of Grizzly Peak.

3.5 mi (4) Point 13,117 is a subsummit. From here, you'll need to partake in fun class 2+ scrambling to stay directly on the ridge. Hikers wishing to bypass these outcrops can easily divert left (west). Continue to the base of Grizzly. Note that things get steeper and more rugged from here.

4.0 mi (5) Point 12,936. Grizzly's loose, rocky pyramid looms before you. Climb down to a low point in the ridge, at roughly 12,600 feet. From there, the 800-foot hike/scramble to the top follows a faint climber's trail. Be careful not to kick rocks down as you muscle up to the summit.

4.7 mi (6) Phewwww! Finally, Grizzly Peak's summit. That was quite a push, wasn't it? The incredible views make it all worthwhile, especially panoramic shots to the north of the ridge you just traversed. After you've seen what there is to see, return to the ridge and head north, back to Wishbone Saddle.

5.8 mi (2) Back in the saddle *again!* This time, turn west downhill and back to your vehicle.

7.5 mi Finish.

Options This traverse bags a lot of peaks, but if you really want to push it, continue east from Grizzly Peak to the summit of Torreys Peak. There is a faint trail that follows a scrambly ridge east. It is possible to have an epic day by continuing over to Grays Peak and either making the arduous return the same way you came or looping down the Grays Peak Trail to Bakerville Trailhead (where you should have a second car parked). Torreys is 1.7 miles one way from the top of Grizzly; Grays is 2.4 miles from Grizzly. As an out-and-back, this is 12.4 miles round-trip; as a one-way trek to Bakerville, it's about 11.5 miles.

Quick Facts So what exactly is a Sniktau? A Native American term for "bear nose"? A missing letter of the Greek alphabet? As it turns out, it's neither. Rumor has it that the name was a pseudonym used by pioneer journalist E. Patterson, who borrowed his pen name (with a variant spelling) from fellow journalist W. F. Watkins. Look closely: Watkins spelled backward is "sniktaw." So the peak is named after the nom de plume of a snarky journalist—how'd they slip that one by the cartographers?

There are five Grizzly Peaks in Colorado; all five are 13ers. This Grizzly is the fourth highest of the pack.

Contact Info Arapaho National Forest
Clear Creek Ranger District
101 Chicago Creek Road
P.O. Box 3307
Idaho Springs, CO 80452
(303) 567-3000

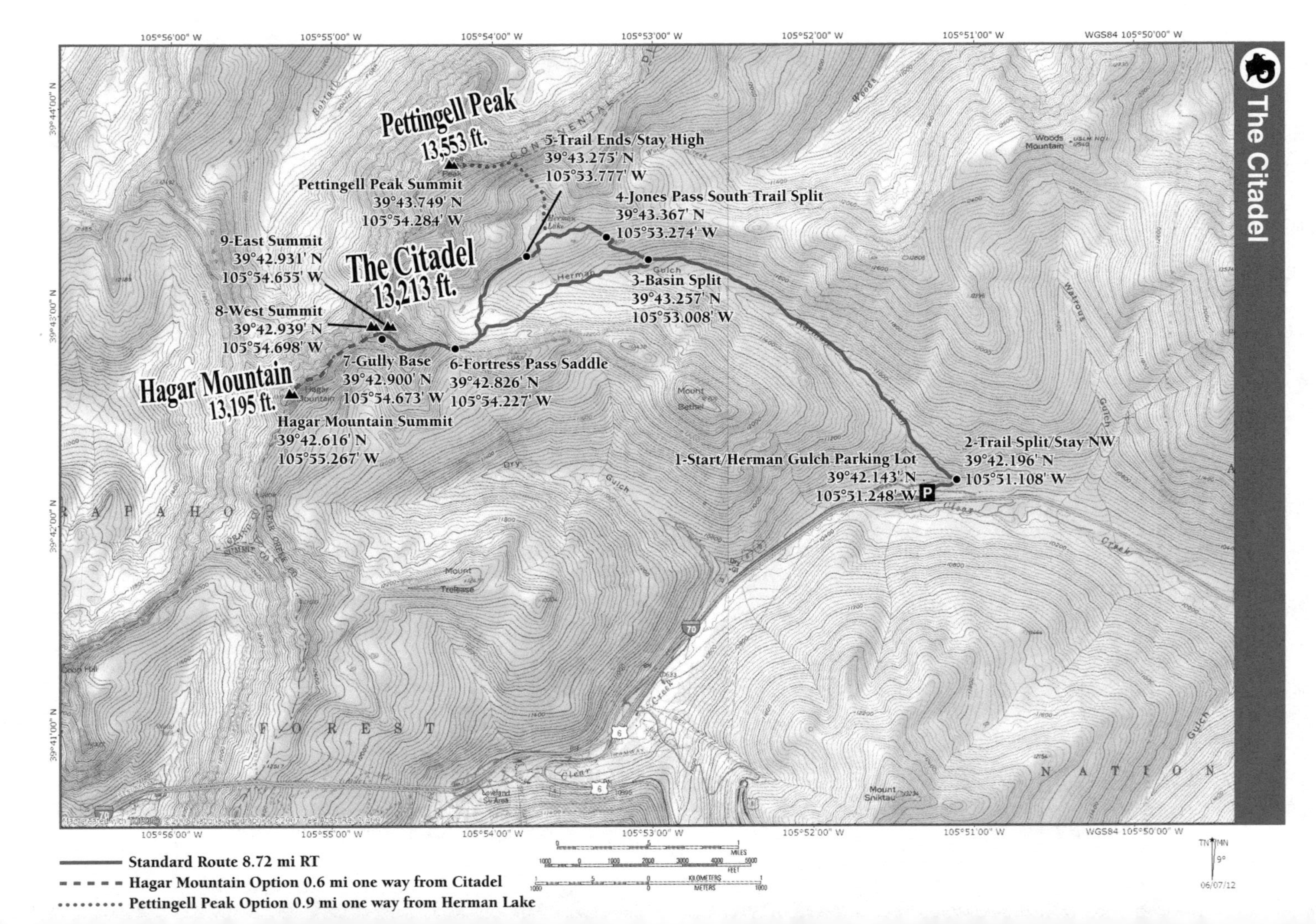
The Citadel
Pettingell Peak
13,553 ft.
5-Trail Ends/Stay High
39°43.275' N
105°53.777' W
Pettingell Peak Summit
39°43.749' N
105°54.284' W
4-Jones Pass South Trail Split
39°43.367' N
105°53.274' W
9-East Summit
39°42.931' N
105°54.655' W
The Citadel
13,213 ft.
3-Basin Split
39°43.257' N
105°53.008' W
8-West Summit
39°42.939' N
105°54.698' W
7-Gully Base
39°42.900' N
105°54.673' W
6-Fortress Pass Saddle
39°42.826' N
105°54.227' W
Hagar Mountain
13,195 ft.
Hagar Mountain Summit
39°42.616' N
105°55.267' W
2-Trail Split/Stay NW
39°42.196' N
105°51.108' W
1-Start/Herman Gulch Parking Lot
39°42.143' N
105°51.248' W
P
Standard Route 8.72 mi RT
Hagar Mountain Option 0.6 mi one way from Citadel
Pettingell Peak Option 0.9 mi one way from Herman Lake

13 The Citadel

The Citadel is a local favorite that you won't find on the map. Fun scrambling and easy trailhead access makes the Citadel a great day hike—a hidden Front Range classic.

Round-Trip Distance	8.72 miles
Hiking Time	5–7 hours
Difficulty	6/10
Class	3
Start Elevation	10,290 ft., at Herman Gulch
Peak Elevation	13,213 ft.
Total Elevation Gain	3,228 ft
Terrain	Mellow class 1 to Herman Lake; Fun, steep hike/scramble to class 3 summit blocks
Best Time to Climb	Late June–September
Gear Advisor	Light hikers or trail runners and helmet
Crowd Level	High to Herman Lake/low from lake to summit

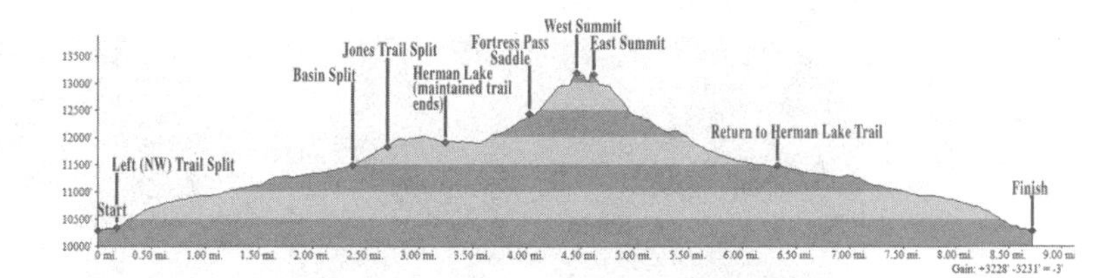

Location Front Range in the Arapaho National Forest near Loveland Pass

Intro You don't want to miss this one. Tucked away just north of I-70, the Citadel is the climber's name for a rock formation that is unnamed on official maps. Citadel's twin summits lie between Pettingell Peak to the north (13,553 feet, the high point of Grand County) and Hagar Mountain (13,195 feet) to the southwest. With very easy access and a surprisingly fun class 3 scramble, these worthy summits are great choices for the Denver/Boulder/Golden crowd who want a great hike with a short drive.

Why Climb It? You'll be surprised that this climb is so close to the familiar stretch of I-70 just before Loveland Pass. An easy, class 1 prelude draws you away from the din of traffic and into a stunning alpine basin. Emerging out of tree line, Herman Gulch opens before you, a beautiful network of streams and small alpine lakes. Imposing views of the Citadel formation contrast with the smooth domes of neighboring mountains. As the trail ends, your trek continues. Cross the basin and head up the steep Fortress Pass. Continue up a burly ridge to the back side of the Citadel's two summits. Reach the tops of both peaks with a good class 3 scramble.

Driving The trailhead for the Citadel is passable for all vehicles and is easy to reach.

How to Get There This one is easy. From either direction on I-70, take the Herman Gulch exit, Exit 218, on the east side of the Eisenhower Tunnel near Loveland Pass. If you exit I-70 westbound, take a right at the end of the exit and then another quick right into the large parking area. If you exit I-70 eastbound, turn left off the exit and proceed to the parking lot. The trail begins at a large sign kiosk.

Fees/Camping There are no fees to climb the Citadel or camp in the area.

Route Notes This is a very avalanche-prone area in winter/early spring.

Mile/Waypoint **0.0 mi (1)** From the parking lot, start your journey on the Herman Gulch Trail (which coincides with a section of the Colorado Trail). The sign lists this as Trail #98. Herman Lake is your first goal.

0.18 mi (2) Early in the hike, the trail divides. Stay left (northwest) on the Herman Gulch Trail at the split. From here, you have an easy-to-follow trail that leads all the way up to Herman Lake. Enjoy the gulch, and be ready for the Citadel's imposing, craggy visage to rise beyond the basin.

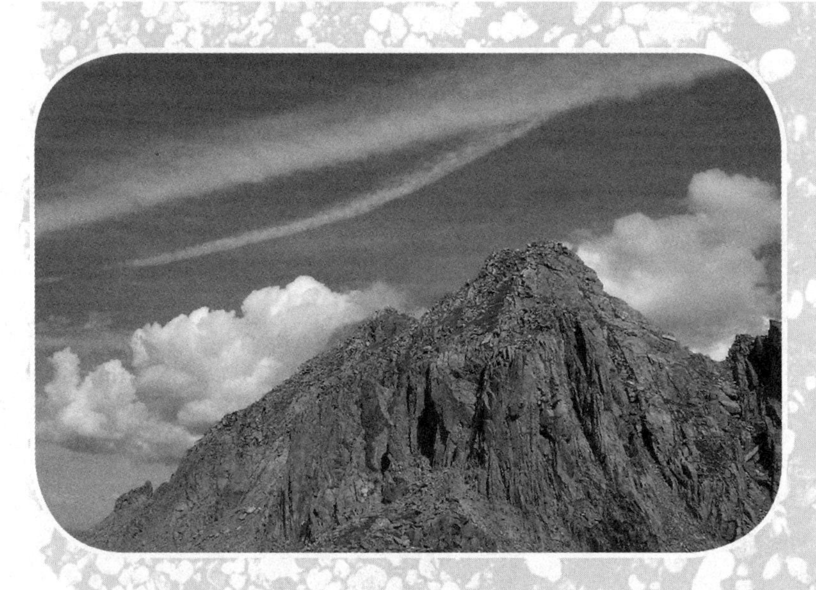

Both the east (forefront) and west summits are accessed by a convenient gully that splits the two.

2.4 mi (3) Where the trail splits in the basin, stay on the main trail and continue uphill. This area is a good place to shortcut through the basin when there is snow; otherwise, stay on the trail. This split is also where you will rejoin the main trail on the way back if you follow the loop detailed in this route description.

2.75 mi (4) The Jones Pass South Trail splits off here; stay on course toward Herman Lake.

3.3 mi (5) Just past Herman Lake, the well-worn trail fades away. You'll need to traverse the basin southwest to Fortress Pass, the saddle between the Citadel and Point 12,674. When the snow is cleared off, you'll see a distinct, switchbacking trail heading up this pass. Stay high in the basin during your traverse, as dropping to the lower section only adds elevation to your climb. Ascend the short, steep trail to the top of the saddle.

4.1 mi (6) From the saddle, head due west up the very steep ridge leading to the Citadel. When you reach the top of this ridge, the east summit of the Citadel will be before you. Do not directly ascend; rather, skirt left (south) on the back side and descend a short distance. You will pass several grayish/black gullies that are very tight; these class 3+/4 paths will lead you to the east summit, but I don't suggest that you attempt them. Pass these gullies and continue 0.1 mile from the ridgetop down to a prominent, wider gully that has dirt and rock (and a small fan of talus) at the bottom.

4.5 mi (7) GPS users might want to note the coordinates of this waypoint, taken at the base of the gully. This class 3 scramble (finally, here it is!) is slightly loose; the rock is fairly solid, but it's easy to kick down smaller, loose rocks. This gully actually terminates directly between the two summits; from here it's a class 3 scramble up to either. My suggestion: Veer left (west) about halfway up the gully, and scramble to the higher west summit.

4.7 mi (8) The west summit of the Citadel, 13,213 feet. Enjoy the views and scramble down to the top of the gully that splits the summits. From here, the scramble up to the east summit (13,203 feet) is a little trickier (perhaps class 3+); there is a great notch to wiggle up directly east of the gully's upper terminus. From here, it's a very short walk to the east summit. (Want a good picture? Take a photo from one summit of your friend on the other.)

4.8 mi (9) From the east summit, descend via the gully (waypoint **7**) you came up (the eastern slopes lead to some sketchy class 3+/4 descents). Return to the ridge, descending back down to Fortress Pass (waypoint **6**).

5.3 mi You can return the same way you came by ascending to Herman Lake, but crossing the basin as you descend is quicker. Follow the streams down (in the spring this may be quite muddy).

6.5 mi (3) As the basin blends in with the pine trees, cut off left (north) to intercept the Herman Gulch Trail. Several faint paths lead from the basin to the main trail; any northward path through the pine trees will eventually connect with the main trail. Follow the trail back to the parking lot.

8.72 mi Finish.

Options Skilled scramblers looking for a good challenge can traverse 0.6 mile one way from the west summit of the Citadel southwest to the summit of Hagar Mountain. This ridge is class 3+ and may require some serious concentration in icy or wet conditions.

County high-pointers can grind up the northeast slopes from Herman Lake to Pettingell's east ridge, and then follow it up to Grand County's highest point, the rounded summit of Pettingell Peak.

The gentle ridge leading over to Mount Bethel (12,705 feet) is another possible climb if you want to scramble over Fortress Pass saddle (waypoint **6**) and continue east along the ridge. While Bethel doesn't look like much more than a nice hill from the saddle, automobiles emerging from the Eisenhower/Johnson tunnel on Loveland Pass will recognize the peak by its prominent snow fences, high upon the southwest face.

Quick Facts

Despite being excluded from maps, the Citadel continues to be a local favorite for Colorado hikers. Climbers bestowed the Citadel's name as a compliment to its fortresslike presence in the Herman Gulch Basin.

Because of its easy accessibility, this area sees a lot of traffic in the winter. It is known for heavy avalanche activity. Skiers and hikers viewing the Citadel from Loveland Ski Area and Loveland Pass have also given it the innocuous title Snoopy's Doghouse because the snow on the twin summits resembles the snoozing beagle of cartoon fame.

Contact Info

Arapaho National Forest
Sulphur Ranger District
9 Tenmile Drive
P.O. Box 10
Granby, CO 80446
(970) 887-4100

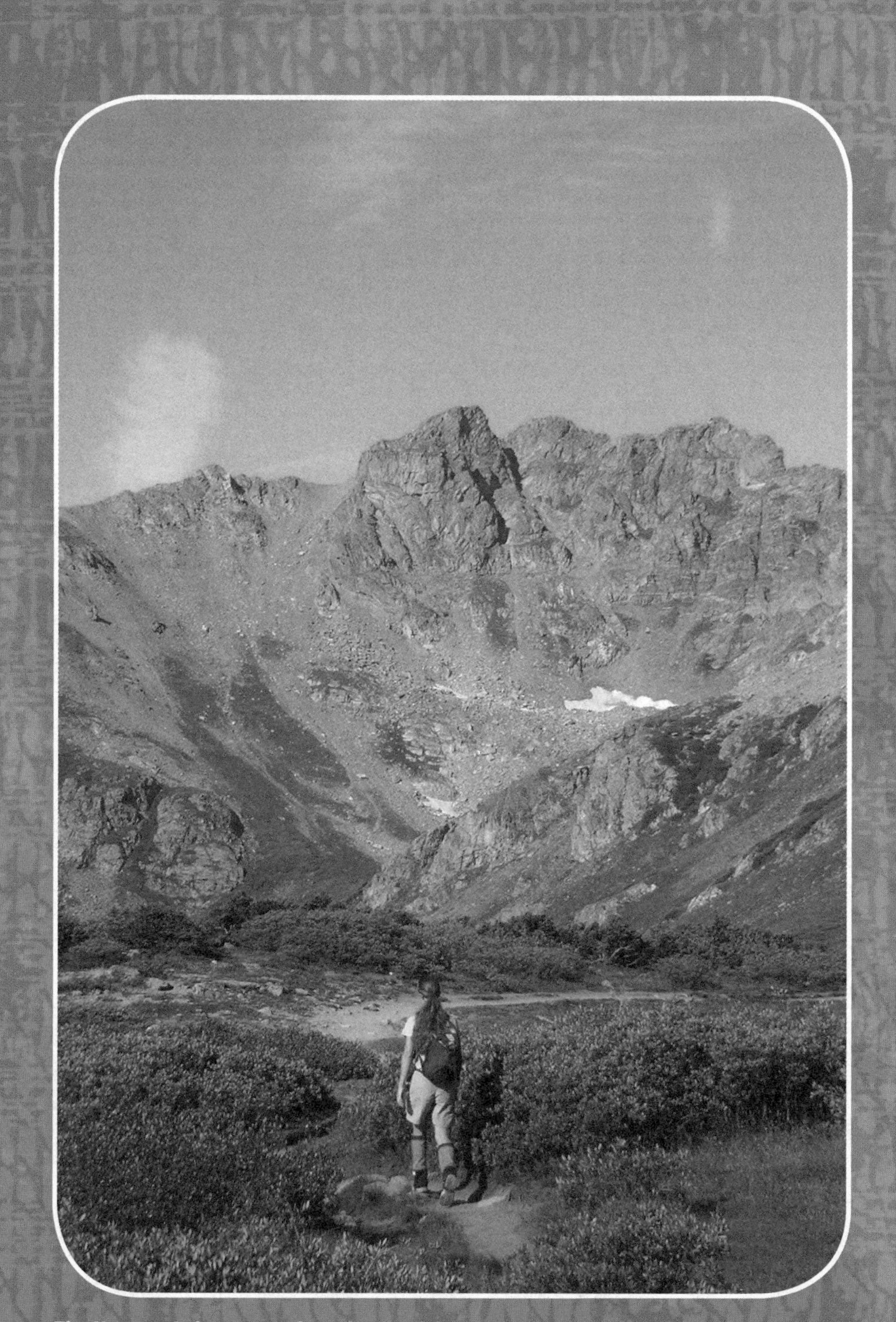

The Herman Lake approach to the Citadel

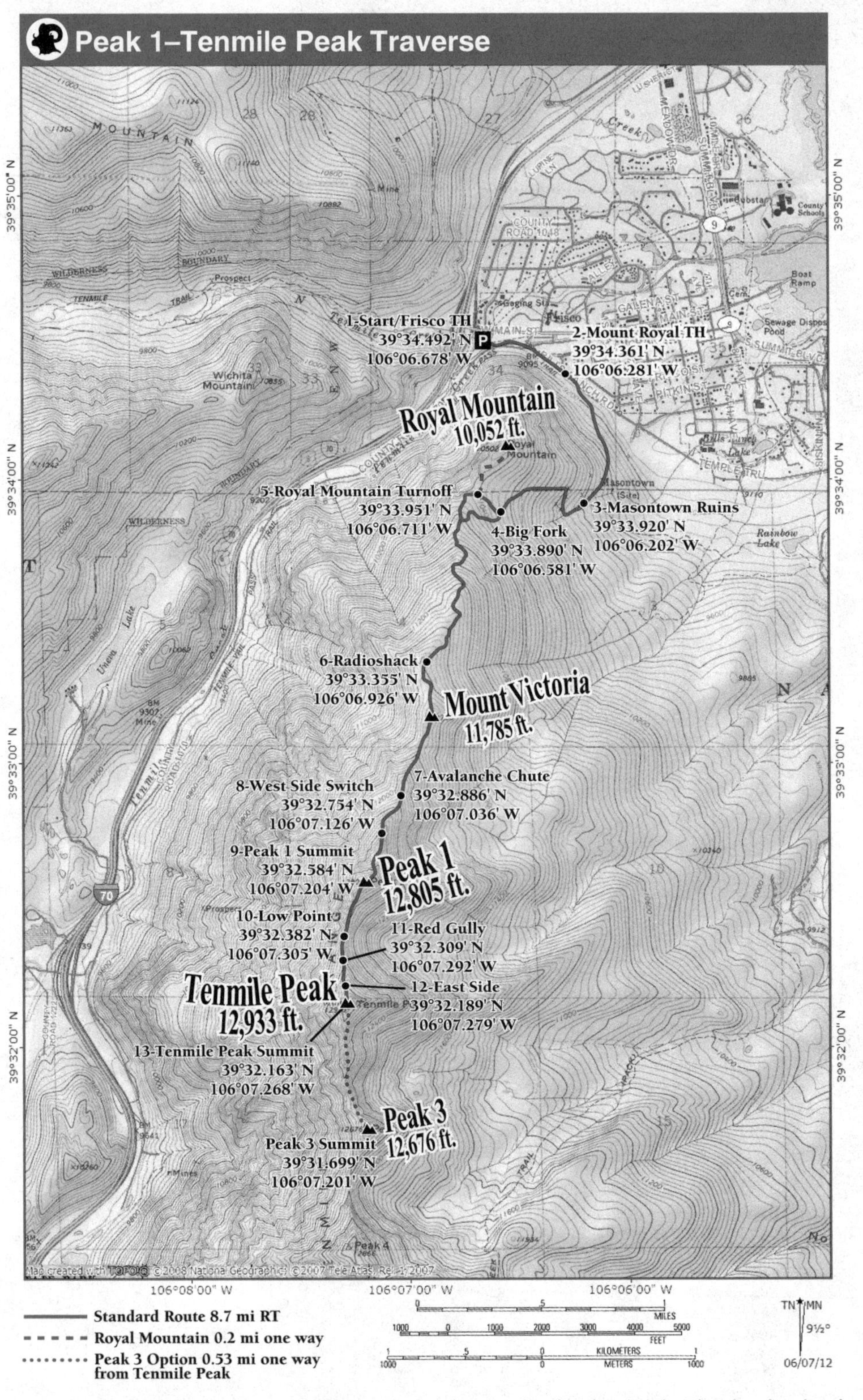
Peak 1–Tenmile Peak Traverse
1-Start/Frisco TH
39°34.492' N
106°06.678' W
2-Mount Royal TH
39°34.361' N
106°06.281' W
Royal Mountain
10,052 ft.
5-Royal Mountain Turnoff
39°33.951' N
106°06.711' W
4-Big Fork
39°33.890' N
106°06.581' W
3-Masontown Ruins
39°33.920' N
106°06.202' W
6-Radioshack
39°33.355' N
106°06.926' W
Mount Victoria
11,785 ft.
7-Avalanche Chute
39°32.886' N
106°07.036' W
8-West Side Switch
39°32.754' N
106°07.126' W
9-Peak 1 Summit
39°32.584' N
106°07.204' W
Peak 1
12,805 ft.
10-Low Point
39°32.382' N
106°07.305' W
11-Red Gully
39°32.309' N
106°07.292' W
12-East Side
39°32.189' N
106°07.279' W
Tenmile Peak
12,933 ft.
13-Tenmile Peak Summit
39°32.163' N
106°07.268' W
Peak 3
12,676 ft.
Peak 3 Summit
39°31.699' N
106°07.201' W
Wichita Mountain
Frisco
Rainbow Lake
Boat Ramp
County Schools
Sewage Disposal Pond
39°35'00" N
39°34'00" N
39°33'00" N
39°32'00" N
106°08'00" W
106°07'00" W
106°06'00" W
Map created with TOPO! © 2008 National Geographic © 2007 Tele Atlas, Rel. 1/2007
Standard Route 8.7 mi RT
Royal Mountain 0.2 mi one way
Peak 3 Option 0.53 mi one way from Tenmile Peak
MILES
FEET
KILOMETERS
METERS
TN MN
9½°
06/07/12

14 Peak 1–Tenmile Peak Traverse

Peak 1 and Tenmile Peak are often admired for their perfect conical shapes, as seen from I-70. The hike over these two is a good challenge; pay attention for seashells on the ridge.

Round-Trip Distance	8.7 miles
Hiking Time	6–8 hours
Difficulty	8/10
Class	3
Start Elevation	9,121 ft., at Frisco Trailhead
Peak Elevations	Peak 1: 12,805 ft.; Tenmile Peak: 12,933 ft.
Total Elevation Gain	4,353 ft.
Terrain	Good trail to rocky ridge traverse
Best Time to Climb	June–September
Gear Advisor	Normal gear
Crowd Level	Moderate to Peak 1; low to Tenmile Peak

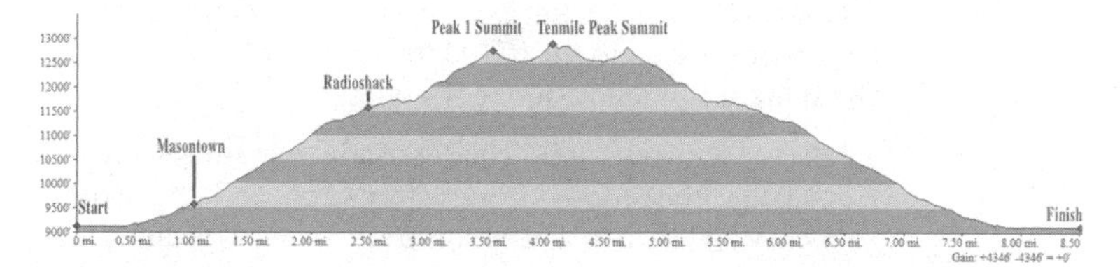

Location Tenmile Range in Arapaho National Forest in the town of Frisco

Intro The pointed summits of these two mountains stand sentry over the town of Frisco. Motorists can't help but be mesmerized by the picture-perfect profiles of the twosome—the view from I-70 westbound is stunning. Even though the trailhead starts in the town of Frisco, these mountains don't see as much traffic as you might think (especially Tenmile Peak). For those who have skied the number peaks in Breckenridge, this route covers the lowest-digit mountains of the Tenmile Range (Tenmile Peak is also known as Peak 2).

Why Climb It? This is the easiest trailhead to reach of any hike in this book; the drive is relatively short from metro areas. I must have passed these mountains a hundred times, every time making a mental note to find out what they were and climb them. My curiosity served me well, as the hike and scramble on these two is a blast. The lower portion of the hike takes you through the ruins of an old mining town that was twice flattened by avalanches. Climbing above tree line offers great views of the city and reservoir below. You also get a sneak peek at hidden lakes and mountains that you can't spot from I-70. The class 3 ridge between the two keeps you on your toes. Much like the nearby Gore Range, the less-traveled parts of these mountains are dotted with fossils and seashells.

Driving Any vehicle can make it to the Frisco Trailhead; it is paved all the way.

How to Get There From I-70, take Exit 201 to Frisco. If you are coming on I-70 westbound, take a left off the exit, pass under the highway bridges, go past the eastbound exit ramp, and take a quick right into a big paved parking area that has restrooms. This area also serves as a launching point for cyclists on the bike path. If you are coming on I-70 eastbound, take Exit 201, and then take a right off the exit and then a quick right into the parking area.

Fees/Camping There are no fees to hike Peak 1 and Tenmile Peak. The campsites around Dillon Reservoir are geared more toward the RV crowd and are a bit expensive. Overnight car camping is allowed in the parking lot.

Route Notes None.

Mile/Waypoint

0.0 mi (1) Start. From the parking lot for the Frisco Trailhead, go left onto the concrete bike path and follow it southeast to Mount Royal Trail on your right.

0.4 mi (2) Turn right (west) onto the marked Mount Royal Trail. This trail sees a lot of local traffic, as it services the Mount Royal viewpoint. A wide trail continues up to the fabled town ruins of Masontown. Don't take any of the side trails that join along the way.

1.0 mi (3) On your right, you'll see a bit of garbage and a few brick foundations from Masontown. The better ruins are a little off-trail on the right side. Stay right when a junction trail comes in around Masontown on your left. It's easy to miss this "town" because there isn't much of it left standing. After the ruins, the trail goes "New England style"—straight up with no switchbacks.

1.5 mi (4) Wow, was that steep! At 1.5 miles, you come to a fairly large fork (I call it Big Fork) with well-worn trails both ways. In 2012 this junction did not have any signs. As the map shows, the right-hand path goes to a neat viewpoint of I-70 and continues over to Royal Mountain **(5)**. Note that there is a very faint wraparound trail that rejoins the main path from here to the left of the viewpoint (I didn't discover this until I was on the way down). This faint trail begins in a sandy area and exits behind an old cabin and then connects with the main trail.

Going left (straight) at the big fork **(4)** is the main trail—straight uphill. A short 0.2 mile up from this point, you'll see the aforementioned cabin on your right. The main trail is obvious from here. It's quite steep up to the next waypoint, which is . . .

2.6 mi (6) . . . the Radioshack, atop the rocky knoll known as "Mount" Victoria. A small radio transmission building and tower announce your exit out of tree line. Pass the shack and level off at a mild saddle between Victoria and Peak 1. The views to the east are really opening up at this juncture.

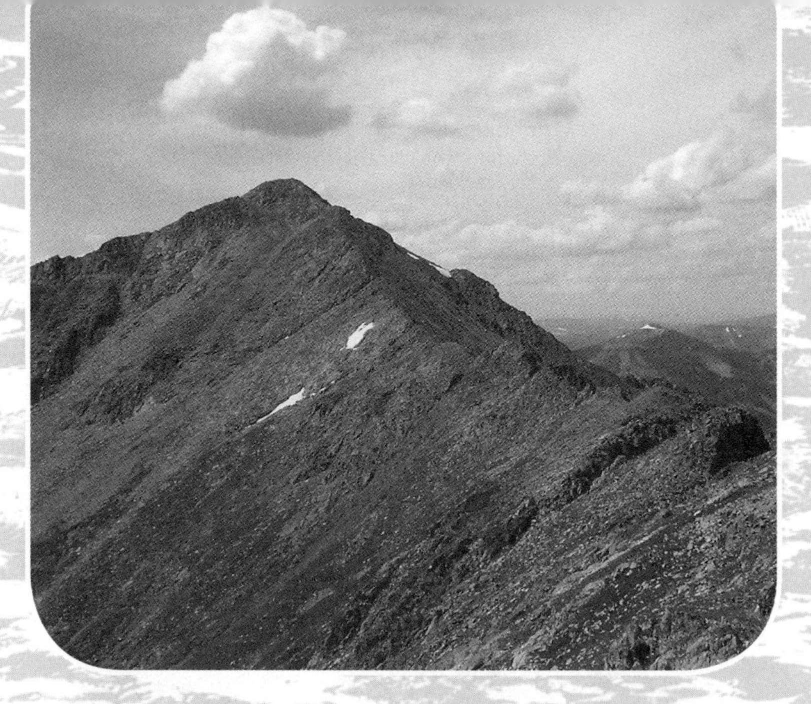

The fun ridge between Peak 1 and Tenmile Peak, as seen from the summit of Peak 1

3.2 mi (7) At the saddle, look down at the swath of aspen trees. This is the path dozens of avalanches have blazed—including the ones that flattened Masontown (twice!). A glance over the west side and down to I-70 reveals a much more rugged side of the mountain. Stay on the trail and continue south.

3.4 mi (8) Get ready to turn to the dark side. Much like the Force in *Star Wars,* this mountain has two sides. The east face is grassy and rounded; the west face is jagged and sharp. If watching movies has taught me anything (which it hasn't, really), it's that humans are always drawn to the dark side. In this case, the west side of the peak offers fun, class 2 scrambling to the upper reaches of the mountain. With all the effort you'll be putting forth, you'll find it hard to believe this isn't even a 13er.

3.7 mi (9) Peak 1's summit! The mileage to here isn't huge, but that was some tough stuff you just came up. The summit is graced with an unusual tripodlike tower.

From the top, keep going south toward the obvious ridge to Tenmile Peak. This is where the class 3 terrain begins. For the most part, you can stay on the ridge or just off to the east side until you reach the low point at waypoint **10**.

3.9 mi (10) At 12,550 feet, you're at the low point of the range. There's a bamboo pole sticking out of the rock just past here, indicating where you should head next. Stay on the ridge or just below it on the east until you reach a sandy, red-colored gully just past the pole.

4.0 mi (11) This is Red Gully. Cross this below the ridge (where it's safest) and quickly get back up on the ridge. This little diversion has a secret: I saw dozens of ancient seashells in the red rock. Please don't take any home, but do take some photos—or else people will think you were hallucinating.

After climbing out of the gully, switch back over to the west side of the mountain, where the scrambling is better.

4.1 mi (12) One more switch. Want more? Get back on the east side and follow the easy, class 2 hill to Tenmile's summit.

4.3 mi (13) Tenmile Peak summit! There's a neat, handmade monument on the spur to the east, perhaps a memorial for a beloved pet. This is a great summit for views. Take your photos, and return the way you came. The return on the ridge has one tricky move, back at Red Gully. Take your time—the route finding is a little tricky, but the scrambling is solid. Go back over Peak 1 and return the way you came.

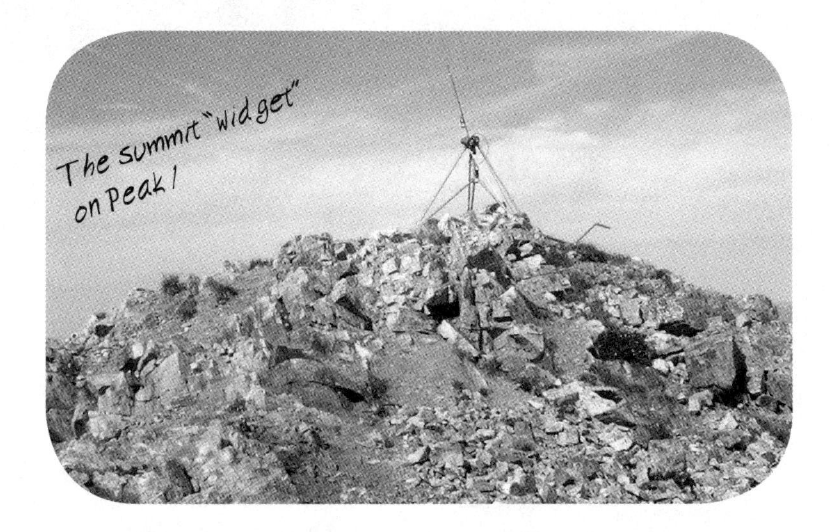

6.8 mi One note on the descent: If you bypassed it the first time, you can take the side trail from the old cabin in the trees down to the Royal Mountain saddle viewpoint (waypoint **5**). Go left on a faint trail (instead of a cairn, there's a bunch of old cans). Follow it down to the viewpoint and then down the wide trail to your right back to Big Fork.

8.7 mi Finish. As with many of these hikes, your mileage may vary slightly, depending on how direct the routes were that you took when off-trail.

Options The only option I've mapped out is the short trek over to Royal Mountain. This 10,502 viewpoint is worth the walk over, and it's only 0.2 mile one way from waypoint **5**.

There are some who get "numbers fever" and continue the traverse (class 3+) south to Peak 3 and over to Peak 4. Friends who have made the trek say the best route is to descend Peak 4 into town, and then take public transportation back to Frisco.

Quick Facts Tenmile Peak takes on the name of the range it's in; it also goes by the alias Peak 2 when it wants to fit in with the guys. The number peaks were labeled by a rather uninspired surveyor.

Masontown was the site of a profitable mill that serviced Victoria Mine. The town lifted its name from a place in Pennsylvania where the company's investors lived. At its peak, there were about 800 residents. The gold and silver from the mine were sent to the Denver mint until operations fizzled, around 1910. The town was demolished by an avalanche in 1912. Bootleggers capitalized on this misfortune and used the damaged town as a center for making moonshine—until they were flattened by an avalanche in 1926. The last structures that still resembled buildings were destroyed—not by ice, but by fire—when the place burned to the ground in 1968.

Contact Info

Arapaho National Forest
Clear Creek Ranger District
101 Chicago Creek Road
P.O. Box 3307
Idaho Springs, CO 80452
(303) 567-3000

Pacific Peak

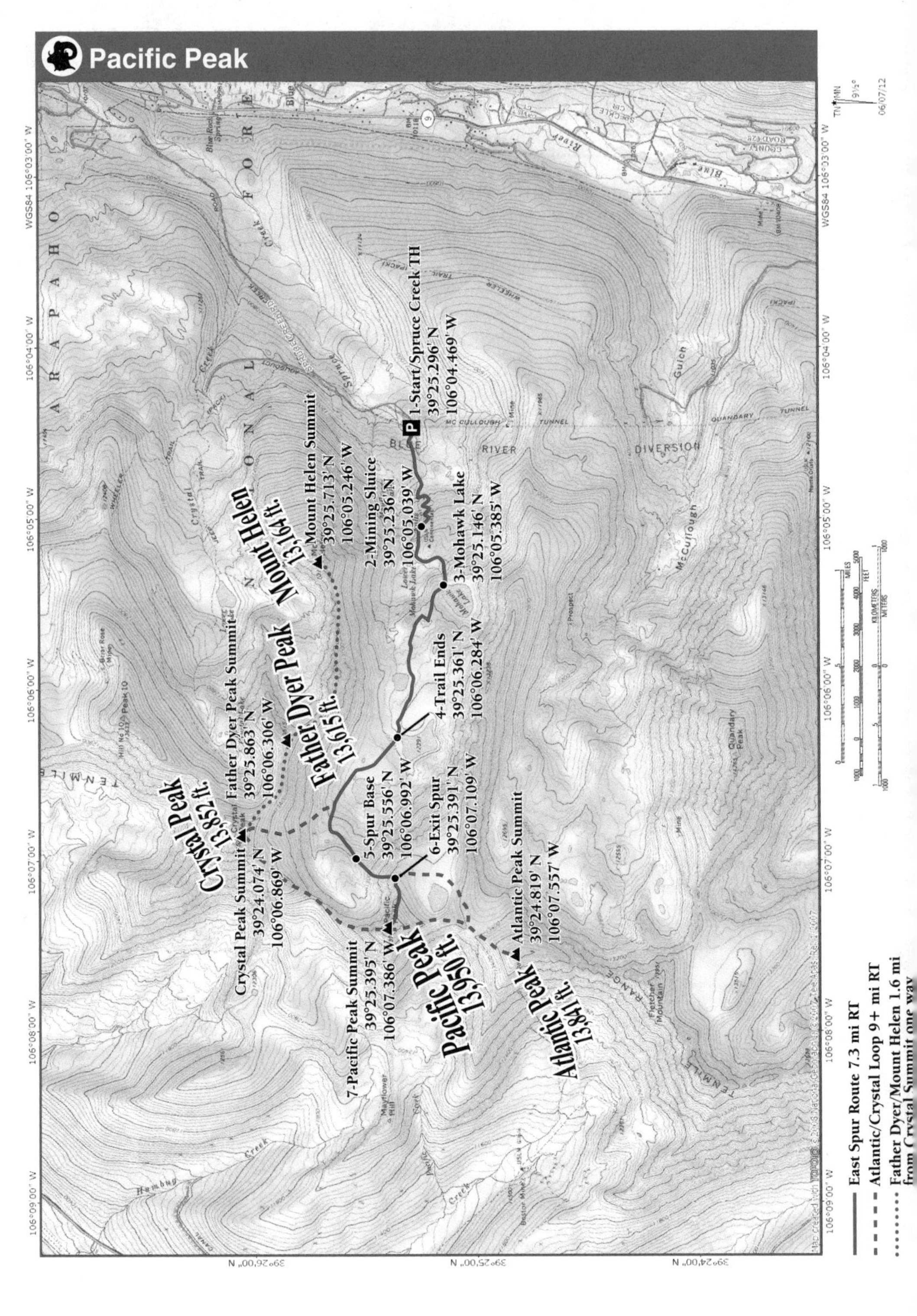

Crystal Peak 13,852 ft.
Crystal Peak Summit 39°24.074' N 106°06.869' W
Father Dyer Peak Summit 39°25.863' N 106°06.306' W
Father Dyer Peak 13,615 ft.
Mount Helen 13,164 ft.
Mount Helen Summit 39°25.713' N 106°05.246' W
2-Mining Sluice 39°25.236' N 106°05.039' W
1-Start/Spruce Creek TH 39°25.296' N 106°04.469' W
3-Mohawk Lake 39°25.146' N 106°05.385' W
4-Trail Ends 39°25.361' N 106°06.284' W
5-Spur Base 39°25.556' N 106°06.992' W
6-Exit Spur 39°25.391' N 106°07.109' W
7-Pacific Peak Summit 39°25.395' N 106°07.386' W
Pacific Peak 13,950 ft.
Atlantic Peak Summit 39°24.819' N 106°07.557' W
Atlantic Peak 13,841 ft.
East Spur Route 7.3 mi RT
Atlantic/Crystal Loop 9+ mi RT
Father Dyer/Mount Helen 1.6 mi from Crystal Summit one way

15 Pacific Peak

Pacific Peak has lots of appeal: mining history, beautiful lakes, and a great scramble. Link up to neighboring summits for extended time in this high-altitude playground.

Round-Trip Distance	7.3 miles
Hiking Time	5–7 hours
Difficulty	7/10
Class	2+/3
Start Elevation	11,095 ft., at Spruce Creek Trailhead
Peak Elevation	13,950 ft.
Total Elevation Gain	2,795 ft.
Terrain	Good trail to rocky scramble to summit
Best Time to Climb	June–September
Gear Advisor	Sturdy boots
Crowd Level	Low

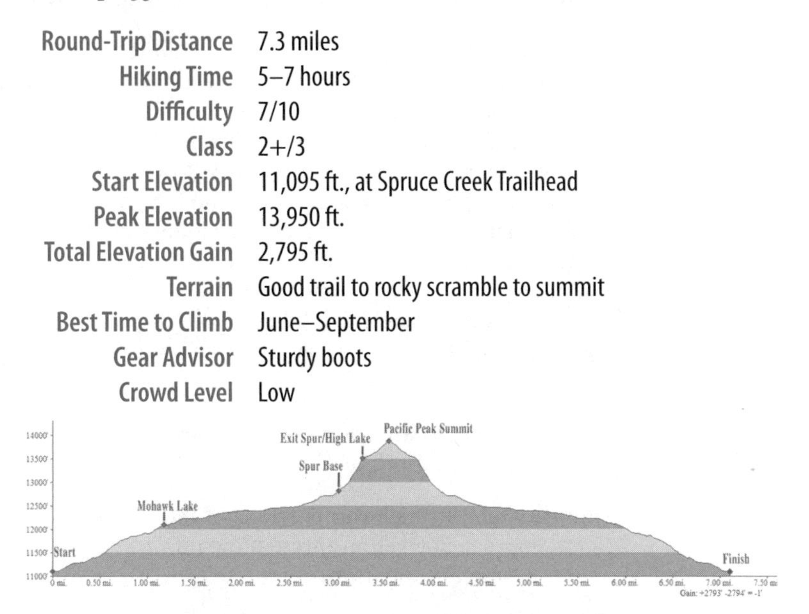

Location Tenmile Range in the Arapaho National Forest outside of Breckenridge

Intro The Tenmile Range possesses riches and stark beauty in abundance. Not only are these mountains perched atop a wealth of minerals (the Colorado Mineral Belt has a strong presence), but these peaks also avoided the heavy glaciations that smoothed out the nearby Sawatch, Mosquito, and Gore Ranges. As a result, the Tenmiles have a jagged and raw appearance. Pacific Peak is in the middle of the range. Its prominent split summit can be seen from miles away.

Why Climb It? Breckenridge was once synonymous with mining, thanks to its hearty gold deposits. The old sluice and cabins at the start of this trail hearken back to the days of the great gold rush. Above the mines, Mohawk Lakes decorate a broad, colorful basin. It's a neat effect to come up to Mohawk Lake and have it appear at eye level, similar to the infinity pools popular at high-end resorts. A solid scramble leads to a very high unnamed alpine lake at 13,420 feet. Finish the climb to the top on a scenic ridge. There are several moderate options available for those who'd like to grab a few more summits.

Driving Driving on Spruce Creek Road pushes tough passenger cars (TPCs) to their limits; I was barely able to make the full length in my Honda Accord. It has all the expected rocks and washboards, but it also has several rutted, water bar–style speed bumps that are difficult for low-clearance vehicles. On the way down, I scraped many, many times, putting numerous dents in my exhaust system. (It wasn't quite as bad as the time I knocked the entire exhaust system off on nearby Kite Lake Road or the subsequent time I again unmoored my exhaust system on a dirt road near Peaceful Valley.) It's passable with a TPC, but you're risking damage from the inevitable bangs and bumps. Sport utility cars or vehicles and 4x4s should have no trouble.

How to Get There Drive south out of Breckenridge on Colorado Highway 9, about 2.5 miles from the edge of town. Just after the town limit sign for Blue River, turn right (west) onto Spruce Creek Road (Forest Service Road 800). There is a small street sign, and the turn comes up quickly. It is 3.0 miles up Spruce Creek Road to the trailhead. Spruce Creek Road begins as a well-maintained dirt road through a housing development; it continues up to a large parking area where several trails (good for mountain biking) intersect. Drive through the parking area and continue on the road, which does not get much rockier. Do not stray onto any of the side roads. After dropping into a low draw, you'll be on the final climb to the parking area, which is the roughest part of the road. The parking area shares space with a small water-treatment facility.

Fees/Camping There are no fees to hike or camp in the area of Pacific Peak. There are a few car camping pull-offs on the way to the trailhead.

Route Notes Volunteers rebuilt the lower portions of the Mohawk Lakes Trail in late 2006 to improve navigation through the mining ruins. The trip up to the lakes is now more straightforward.

Mile/Waypoint **0.0 mi (1)** Start from the Spruce Creek Trailhead and take the trail to Mohawk Lakes/Continental Falls. This trail works its way up through an old mining operation, and you will bypass several cabins and a large sluice within the first mile. Because the mining area has some interesting relics, there are many subpaths that are easy to confuse with the main trail. If you get confused, follow the river up to the large sluice that is anchored with giant wires; the main trail passes by the very top of it.

0.7 mi (2) At the top of the sluice, the trail becomes much easier to follow. Stay on it as it goes by Lower Mohawk Lake and climbs up on the left side of Continental Falls. The cabin ruins along the way add a quaint ambience to this lovely area.

1.2 mi (3) As you reach the basin, the eastern shore of Mohawk Lake will be at eye level. The trail continues up to some higher lakes but begins to fade out as you traverse across the meadow. Pacific Peak's distinct summit looms in the distance.

2.2 mi (4) At this point, north of the unnamed lake at 12,391 feet, the trail is but a whisper, fading away into the grass. Pass the two high lakes in the basin on their north sides. The southern sides of these lakes are a more direct path, but the boulders are big and unstable and will slow you down considerably. Stay north on the grassy slopes and reach the base of the ridge spur (12,825 feet) that intersects with your larger goal, the east ridge.

3.0 mi (5) From the base of the spur, scramble up the slope, picking the line you feel is best. There are a few easy, class 3 moves, especially toward the top.

3.3 mi (6) Exit the spur, taking note of where you do so, so that you will be able to recognize the line down when you descend. Check out the seemingly misplaced lake on a flat tract of land below Pacific's southeast face. Elevation here is roughly 13,500 feet. Follow the obvious east ridge westward to Pacific's summit.

3.6 mi (7) Pacific Peak's summit! From here, you have the option to go south to Atlantic Peak or north to Crystal Peak. Read the "Options" section for more information. Return the way you came.

7.3 mi Finish.

Options

It's a nice walk south to Atlantic Peak. This route is 0.7 mile one way from Pacific's summit on good, class 2 terrain. Note that Atlantic is not named on most maps—it is simply Unnamed Peak 13,841 feet.

The traverse north to Crystal Peak (13,852 feet) is longer and slightly more rugged, at 1.0 mile one way. You can then descend the rocky south slopes (class 2) of Crystal to get back into the lakes basin (rejoining the trail somewhere around waypoint **4**), making this an excellent loop option.

A tour of all three peaks (Atlantic, Pacific, and Crystal) is roughly a 9-mile round-trip. This mileage assumes that you exit the top of the spur (waypoint **6**) and walk past the high lake to Atlantic first, return over to Pacific, traverse to Crystal, and go down Crystal's south slopes. (I highly recommend this route if the weather is good.)

If you want to get yet *more* mountains, Father Dyer Peak (Unnamed Peak 13,615) can be reached via Crystal's east ridge. There is an interesting plaque on the mountain commemorating Father Dyer. From Father Dyer Peak, you can make a class 3 scramble out to Mount Helen (13,164 feet). Father Dyer is 0.6 mile from Crystal's summit, and Mount Helen is 1.0 mile farther to the east, 1.6 miles from Crystal's summit.

Quick Facts

Many men were made wealthy by the riches hidden in these mountains. Gold and silver in particular were found in abundance in this area. Among those who made their fortunes here was Methodist minister John L. Dyer. The "mining minister," Father Dyer met with moderate success at his Warrior's Mark Mine. He built a cabin at the site in 1881; a few years later, he sold the mine for $2,000. A small town sprung up in the area called Dyersville, which died out when the mining ceased.

Contact Info

Arapaho National Forest
Clear Creek Ranger District
101 Chicago Creek Road
P.O. Box 3307
Idaho Springs, CO 80452
(303) 567-3000

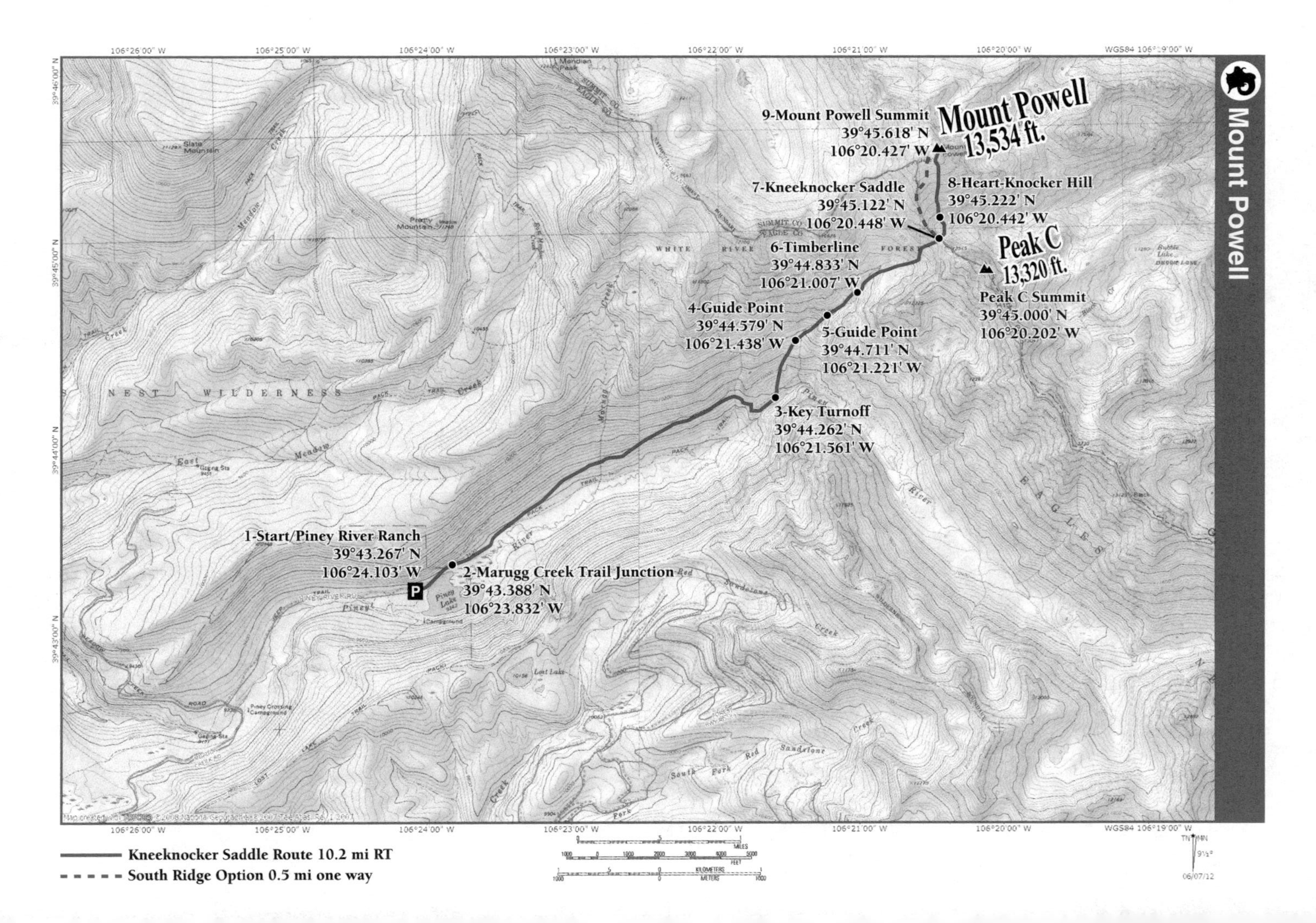

Mount Powell
9-Mount Powell Summit
39°45.618' N
106°20.427' W
Mount Powell
13,534 ft.
7-Kneeknocker Saddle
39°45.122' N
106°20.448' W
8-Heart-Knocker Hill
39°45.222' N
106°20.442' W
Peak C
13,320 ft.
6-Timberline
39°44.833' N
106°21.007' W
Peak C Summit
39°45.000' N
106°20.202' W
4-Guide Point
39°44.579' N
106°21.438' W
5-Guide Point
39°44.711' N
106°21.221' W
3-Key Turnoff
39°44.262' N
106°21.561' W
1-Start/Piney River Ranch
39°43.267' N
106°24.103' W
2-Marugg Creek Trail Junction
39°43.388' N
106°23.832' W
Kneeknocker Saddle Route 10.2 mi RT
South Ridge Option 0.5 mi one way

16 Mount Powell

Isolated in his daunting kingdom, the king of the Gore Range requests your company. Test your legs, lungs, and brains as you find your way to this regal peak.

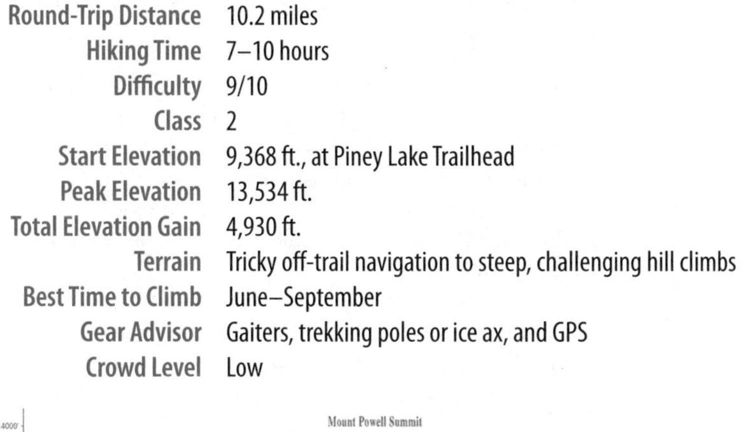

Round-Trip Distance	10.2 miles
Hiking Time	7–10 hours
Difficulty	9/10
Class	2
Start Elevation	9,368 ft., at Piney Lake Trailhead
Peak Elevation	13,534 ft.
Total Elevation Gain	4,930 ft.
Terrain	Tricky off-trail navigation to steep, challenging hill climbs
Best Time to Climb	June–September
Gear Advisor	Gaiters, trekking poles or ice ax, and GPS
Crowd Level	Low

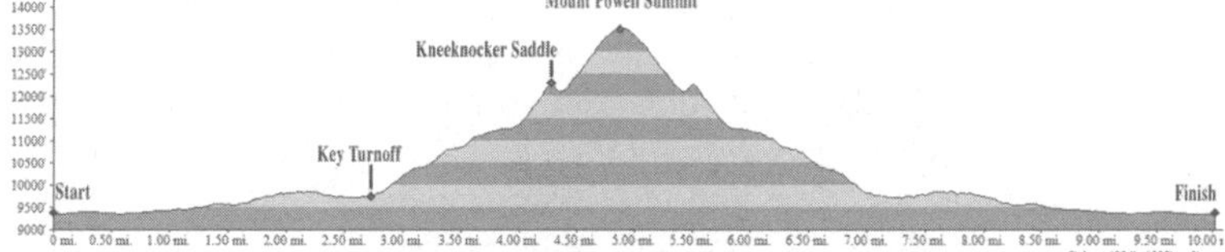

Location Gore Range in the Eagles Nest Wilderness/White River National Forest outside of Vail

Intro Mount Powell is the hidden patriarch of the Gore Range. It takes a bit of backcountry navigation savvy to locate the way up, but once you do, you're in for a heck of a fun day. After a nice approach on class 1 trails through the beautiful Piney Lake area, you will be off-trail for 2.1 miles of rugged terrain. Climb up a foliage-rich slope to a secret alpine basin at 10,800 feet. From here, the route becomes easier to see as you tackle Kneeknocker Saddle and Heart-Knocker Hill. The summit is a special place with incredible views.

Why Climb It? The Gore mountains stand out as some of the most beautiful and geologically significant peaks in Colorado. The Gores were pushed up by fault blocks and further shaped by heavy glaciations. As a result, you have a hybrid range that has jagged peaks and glacial cirques, with terrain that reveals an occasional fossil to the keen-eyed hiker. Powell is the highest of these mountains, yet it has no standard route to its summit—which is part of its appeal. You make the summit in three pushes: a steep climb up a densely overgrown hillside, a steep climb up the basin to Kneeknocker Saddle, and the final summit push up the steep Heart-Knocker Hill. The summit feels like an eagle's nest, with views of wilderness to the north and the Vail Ski Area to the south.

Driving Passenger cars can make it up the dirt road to Piney River Ranch and the start of the trailhead. The road is bumpy at times, but it never gets too rocky or so washed out that you'll need a high-clearance vehicle. Trucks and high-clearance vehicles will fare better and will have no trouble reaching the trailhead.

How to Get There From I-70 westbound, take Exit 176 into Vail. Take a right to enter the roundabout, and then take a left onto North Frontage Road (the sign reads N. FRONTAGE ROAD/WEST VAIL). Stay on this road 1.0 mile and take a right (north) turn onto Red Sandstone Road, which has a sign for Piney Lake. If you are coming from I-70 eastbound, take Exit 173, follow the roundabout to Frontage Road, and continue east for 1.7 miles to reach this same point, Red Sandstone Road.

Follow the paved Red Sandstone Road 0.7 mile uphill, where it turns to a well-maintained dirt road and becomes Forest Service Road 700. Reset your odometer. There will continue to be signs for Piney Lake and Piney River Ranch along the way. At mile 2.6, stay left on FS 700 at a split (at this juncture, you're officially off Red Sandstone Road). Stay on FS 700 as it climbs and drops through an unspoiled part of Vail. You will see several pull-offs for primitive camping along the way; if you plan on camping, wait a few miles for closer (and better) sites. At mile 6.6, stay right on FS 700 at the junction with Forest Service Road 701. Go downhill; eventually you'll be driving next to a river. Be careful of the resident moose that live here. At mile 9.1, turn right where a small sign announces PINEY LAKE 2 MILES. Follow FS 700 to Piney River Ranch at mile 10.6. Park on the left at the end of the road and away from the lots closer to the buildings; the ranch here hosts many functions and needs the spaces for their guests. Please respect the private land around this area, as the ranch owners are the ones who make it possible to hike into the Gore Range.

Fees/Camping There are no fees for hiking or camping in this area. There are great car-camping sites along FS 700, starting around mile 8.9 (once you are near the river). From here to the parking area are several good places to pull off and set up a tent.

Route Notes None.

Mile/Waypoint **0.0 mi (1)** Start at Piney River Ranch, and go west toward Piney Lake. Get on the Upper Piney Trail #1885, and enjoy a morning tour of this misty valley.

0.3 mi (2) At the west end of Piney Lake there is a junction with the Marugg Creek Trail #1899. Stay right on the Upper Piney Trail and follow it as it enters into dark woods, climbs up a hill, and descends back down.

2.8 mi (3) This is the key to your entire hike. Because GPS units are not perfectly precise, expect this turn to come between 2.79 and 2.91 miles on your receiver. You will have gone downhill and will be almost level with the river at roughly 9,750 feet. The barely there trail is usually marked by a few small cairns, which may or may not be there; the uphill trail starts where two skinny pine trees stand in the middle of the footpath. You will need to turn left (north) at this key turnoff and begin climbing. There is a very faint and overgrown trail that you can follow, but if you lose it, don't worry. This climb goes through some dense foliage with the occasional clearing; keep going up with a northeast trajectory.

3.1 mi (4) At this point, the trail is right next to a rocky waterfall/stream and actually crosses over it and continues up. Once you have found this stream, you can use it as a guide to lead you northeast to the basin. Waypoints **5** and **6** are on the map for GPS users to help establish a route.

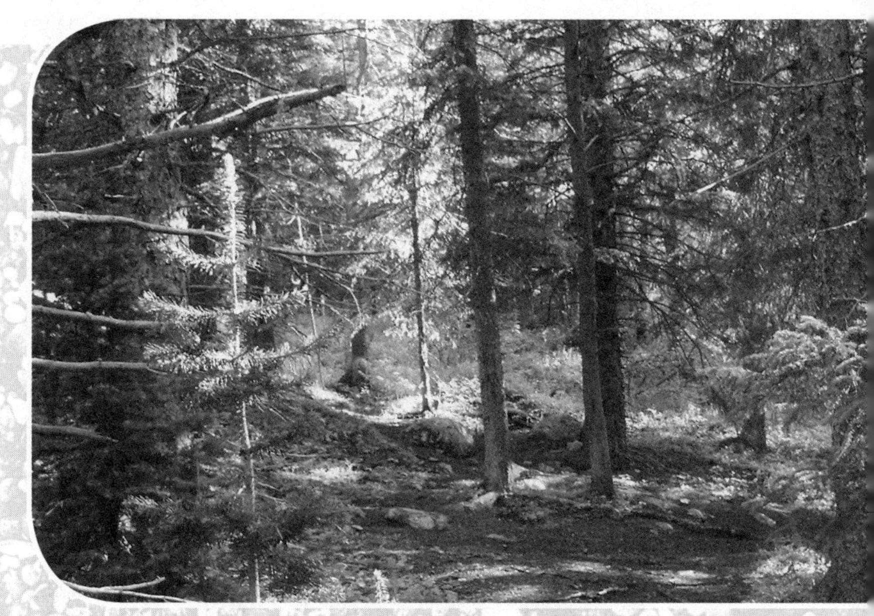

Keep your eyes open for these twin trees—they signal your departure from the main trail onto the barely-there path to Kneeknocker Saddle.

3.7 mi (6) Just above this waypoint, the basin opens up before you at 11,100 feet. It is rocky on the sides but has a nice grassy meadow in the middle. This area holds snow far into the summer. Magically, a hiking trail reappears to guide you to Kneeknocker Saddle. Kneeknocker Saddle is to the northeast, between the shoulder of Powell (you can't see the top from here) on the left and Peak C on the right. Climb more than 1,200 feet directly up to Kneeknocker Saddle, staying on the rockier left side for better footing. The gully in the middle is loose and difficult to ascend, though it makes for good scree-surfing on the descent.

4.4 mi (7) At 12,300 feet, you're in Kneeknocker Saddle, and you'll finally have views of the summit. (A friend related this experience to *The Simpsons* episode in which Homer has to climb Mount Springfield. Each time he thinks that he sees the top of the mountain, a comically larger one appears behind it, much to his chagrin. Same thing here!) There are permanent snowfields on the east side of this pass. To follow the class 2 route, drop down about 100 feet over the east side of the pass to the base of Heart-Knocker Hill to your left (north). Note that when the snowfield is filled in, you may have to descend on snow on the far side of the saddle, to the right, to make your way over to the base of the hill. The direct way to the hill may require you to use kick steps to get down safely (or you can glissade a little, though the terrain may be a bit too steep for some people).

4.5 mi (8) You are now at the base of Heart-Knocker Hill, whose long, grassy, and rocky hill offers the best way up. What are you waiting for? It's only another 1,350-foot climb (in 0.5 mile) to the top. Much like the previous climb, stay to the sides for better footing (in this case, the right side is best). When you get to a flat section at 13,470 feet, atop the gully, you'll need to scramble up a pile of boulders on your right, northeast to the highest point. The rocks are solid, but after all the work to get up here, you may be thinking that you'll never see the summit.

5.1 miles (9) Phew! Finally, Mount Powell's summit! It sure is nice up here. Enjoy the views and let your heart rate slow down. Vail's ski areas are to the south, while there's more Gore goodness to the north.

To return, go back down the basin. (The descent will seem amazingly fast in contrast to your ascent.) The trail through the meadow of the basin is much easier to follow on the way down. You can always follow the stream down (or at least keep it in sight) to return to the main trail. Enjoy your hike out.

10.2 miles Finish.

Options From the top of Kneeknocker Saddle, you can go right onto Powell's south ridge and ascend on class 2+/3 terrain that intercepts Heart-Knocker Hill about three quarters of the way up. It's a nice option for those comfortable with navigating ridges on which you'll need to make a few blind moves.

Quick Facts There are two mountains named after John W. Powell in Colorado; this one and Powell Peak in Rocky Mountain National Park. Powell actually climbed this mountain (with partner Ned Farrell) in the summer of 1868, shortly after his historic "first" ascent of Longs Peak.

To this day, many of the Gore Range peaks lack formal names (such as the letter peaks: C, N, G, and so on).

This is yet another mountain where I found seashells in the dirt.

Contact Info White River National Forest
Eagle Ranger District
125 W. Fifth Street
P.O. Box 720
Eagle, CO 81631
(970) 328-6388

The passes to the summit of Mount Powell are lung busters but worth the grind.

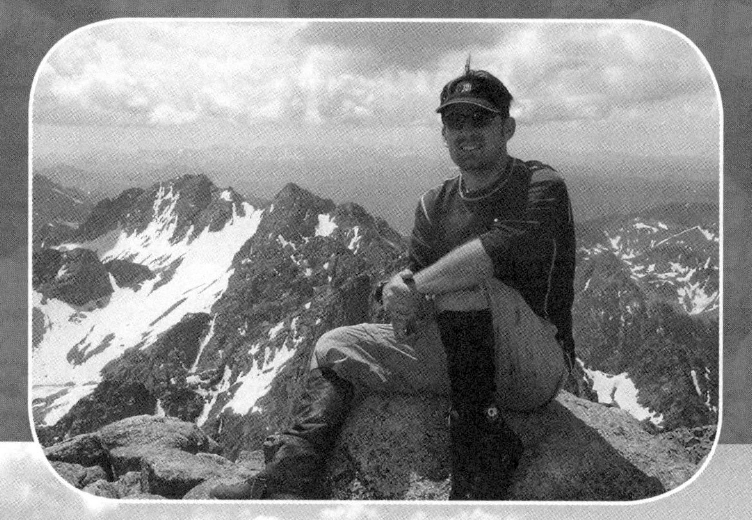

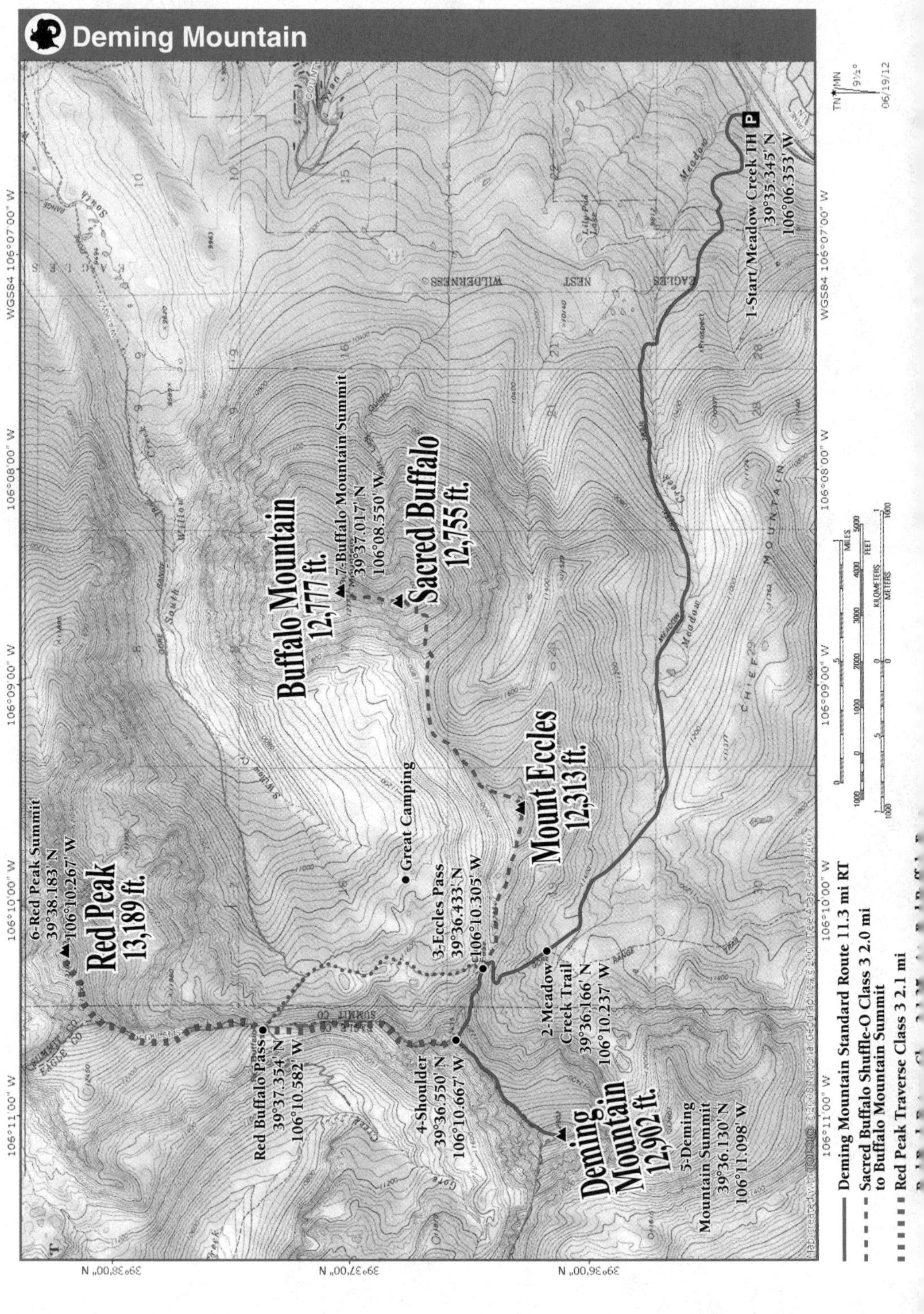

Deming Mountain
Red Peak
13,189 ft.
6-Red Peak Summit
39°38.183' N
106°10.267' W
Buffalo Mountain
12,777 ft.
7-Buffalo Mountain Summit
39°37.017' N
106°08.550' W
Sacred Buffalo
12,755 ft.
Mount Eccles
12,313 ft.
Great Camping
Red Buffalo Pass
39°37.354' N
106°10.582' W
3-Eccles Pass
39°36.433' N
106°10.305' W
4-Shoulder
39°36.550' N
106°10.667' W
2-Meadow Creek Trail
39°36.166' N
106°10.237' W
Deming Mountain
12,902 ft.
5-Deming Mountain Summit
39°36.130' N
106°11.098' W
1-Start/Meadow Creek TH
39°35.345' N
106°06.353' W
Deming Mountain Standard Route 11.3 mi RT
Sacred Buffalo Shuffle-O Class 3 2.0 mi to Buffalo Mountain Summit
Red Peak Traverse Class 3 2.1 mi

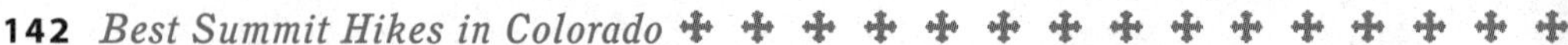

17 Deming Mountain

Good Overnight!

Deming is a truly "Gore-geous" mountain. You have options galore on this overlooked Gore, including a fun class 2+/3 ridge, a class 2 walk up, and an epic loop.

Round-Trip Distance	11.34 miles
Hiking Time	7–10 hours
Difficulty	6/10
Class	2+
Start Elevation	9,153 ft., at Meadow Creek Trailhead
Peak Elevation	12,902 ft.
Total Elevation Gain	3,930 ft.
Terrain	Good trail to open off-trail slopes and ridge to summit
Best Time to Climb	June–October
Gear Advisor	Sturdy boots, hiking poles, and GPS
Crowd Level	Hermit

Deming Mountain Summit
Eccles Pass
Start
Finish

Location Gore Range in the Eagles Nest Wilderness/Arapaho National Forest, outside of Frisco

Intro Deming is a beautiful summit not far from the Denver–Boulder metro area. It offers not only a wonderful day hike but also great camping and several optional summits. There's an excellent class 3 scramble to Red Peak, and the west ridge of Buffalo Mountain is a thrill.

Why Climb It? Poor Deming doesn't see a lot of visitors. Go say hi. The Meadow Creek Trailhead is in the town of Frisco and two minutes off of I-70 (this makes it a nice winter trailhead as well). Meadow Creek and a series of small lakes decorate the landscape en route to Eccles Pass, where incredible views and fantastic camping await. Though there are no established trails to Deming's summit, the off-trail portion is above tree line and easy to navigate. Three other peaks in the area (Eccles, Buffalo, and Red Peak) are equally fun class 2+/3 scrambles. Bears and moose are commonly seen, so keep your bear bells jingling!

Driving All cars can easily make the Meadow Creek Trailhead. From the highway, it is a flat 0.5-mile dirt road to the parking lot.

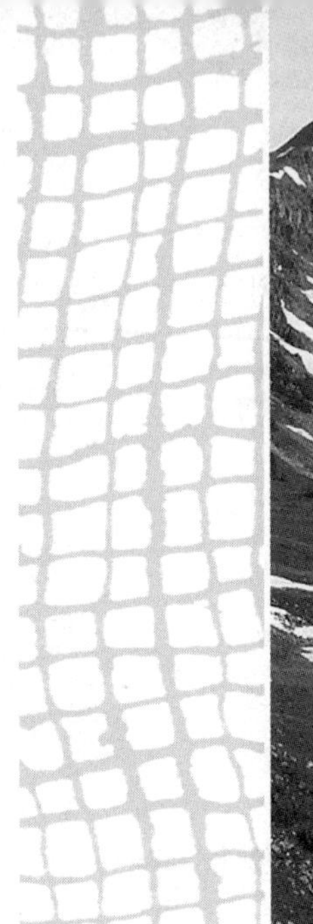

Looking back at Red Peak on the ridge scramble option to Deming

How to Get There Exit I-70 in Frisco at Exit 203. Approaching from the east, simply enter the roundabout at the bottom of the exit ramp and take a right (west) onto County Road 1231 after passing a private road/parking area. From the west, take Exit 203, take a left at the light, and go straight on Summit Boulevard to reach the same roundabout. Follow this dirt road 0.5 mile to the Meadow Creek Trailhead.

Fees/Camping There are no fees to hike or camp in the area. If you do stay overnight, please keep one unfortunate reality in mind: the trailhead is easily accessed and is subject to a bit more crime than backcountry lots.

Route Notes The second edition of *Best Summit Hikes in Colorado* has changed the standard route on Deming from the previous South Willow Creek Route. South Willow Creek is a longer, tougher, and overgrown trail that sees less use every year. Meadow Creek is a much more direct and enjoyable route—and you're less likely to sneak up on an unsuspecting moose.

Mile/Waypoint

0.0 mi (1) Start at the Meadow Creek Trailhead and stay on this well-maintained trail all the way to Eccles Pass. About 0.5 mile in is a split to Lily Pad Lake. Ignore this and stay straight on the trail.

4.2 mi (2) After clearing the aspen groves and pine forests, the trail opens up to a beautiful basin on the south side of Eccles Pass. Technically, this is the end of the Meadow Creek Trail as you now merge with the Gore Range Trail from the south. Continue north up the obvious push to Eccles Pass.

4.7 mi (3) Soak in the views atop Eccles Pass. Red Peak to the north and the fabulous camping basin are especially scenic. It's time to get off trail. Head west along the ridge to Deming's unnamed subpeak.

5.0 mi (4) Reach the 12,435-foot subsummit on the shoulder of Deming's northeast ridge. Turn left (southwest) and follow the ridge to the summit.

5.7 mi (5) Deming's lonely summit features a summit register that has very few names. Add yours to join an exclusive club of Deming summit hikers. From here, simply retrace your path back to the Meadow Creek Trailhead.

11.3 mi Finish.

Options As previously mentioned, the camping on the north side of Eccles Pass is divine. It's worth checking out, especially for a one-night stay, and is a good launching pad for nearby peaks.

Red Peak is an aesthetically pleasing 13,189-foot summit that can be reached via an exciting class 3+ scramble from Deming's shoulder (waypoint **4**) or a more modest class 2+ route that follows the Gore Range Trail over Eccles Pass and then back to Red Buffalo Pass. Both routes bring you to the saddle of Red Buffalo Pass; the class 3 route from waypoint **4** is 0.9 mile to Red Buffalo Pass, while the Gore Range Trail to the same point from Eccles Pass is 1.2 miles. From there it's 1.13 miles one-way along class 2+ ridges to Red Peak's summit.

The locally dubbed Sacred Buffalo Shuffle-O route starts at Eccles Pass (waypoint **3**) and goes east to Buffalo Mountain along Buffalo's seldom-climbed west ridge. Go to 12,313-foot Mount Eccles 0.6 mile from the pass and continue along the ridge. As you get higher, the ridge gets tougher, with several class 3 and 3+ sections. Good route finding helps avoid some sketchy terrain. At 1.9 miles reach Sacred Buffalo, a subsummit of Buffalo. Look for mild terrain on the southeast side of Sacred Buffalo for a cleaner, easier route. After 2.0 miles you're on the 12,777-foot summit of Buffalo Mountain. Return the way you came, or if you want to do a point-to-point hike, leave a car at the Ryan Gulch Parking area 2.3 miles from Buffalo's summit.

To reach the Ryan Gulch parking area, take Exit 205 off I-170 and go north on Colorado Highway 9, and then go west on Wildernest Road. Follow this road 3.5 miles (at 1.0 mile it turns into Ryan Gulch Road). Parking is on the left side of the road, and the trail starts on the right (north) side.

Quick Facts Deming Mountain is named for an old homesteader, John J. Deming, who lived in the Frisco area with his family from 1890 until his death in 1924. It is interesting that the name does not appear on many maps, even though the Bureau of Reclamation has a marker proclaiming DEMING MOUNTAIN on the summit. (The Bureau of Reclamation didn't repossess Deming because the USGS couldn't pay their bills; it's a subgroup of the USGS established in 1902 to deal primarily with environmental water concerns.)

Contact Info Arapaho National Forest
Clear Creek Ranger District
101 Chicago Creek Road
P.O. Box 3307
Idaho Springs, CO 80452
(303) 567-3000

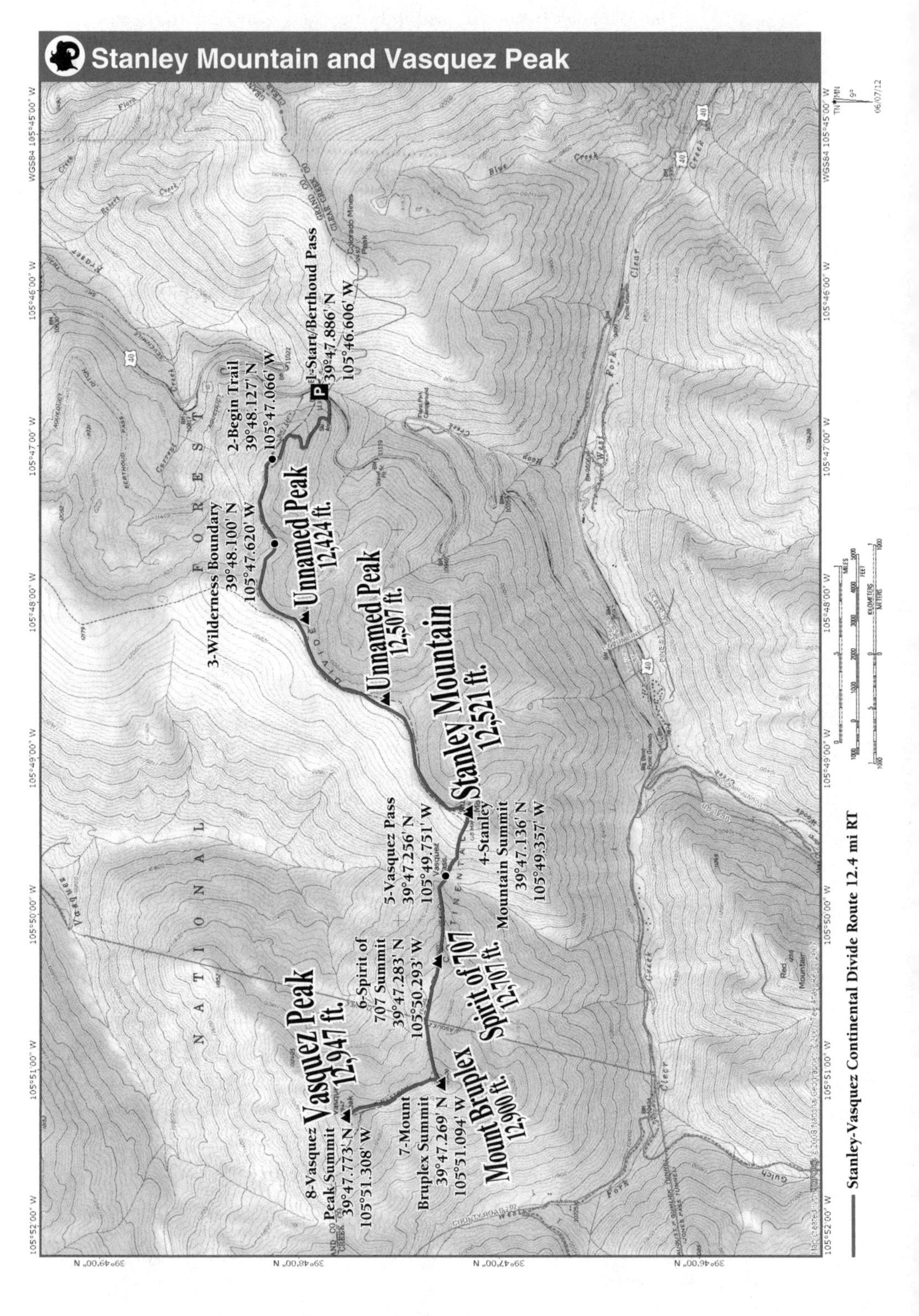
Stanley Mountain and Vasquez Peak
1-Start/Berthoud Pass
39°47.886' N
105°46.606' W
2-Begin Trail
39°48.127' N
105°47.066' W
3-Wilderness Boundary
39°48.100' N
105°47.620' W
Unnamed Peak
12,424 ft.
Unnamed Peak
12,507 ft.
Stanley Mountain
12,521 ft.
4-Stanley
Mountain Summit
39°47.136' N
105°49.357' W
5-Vasquez Pass
39°47.256' N
105°49.751' W
6-Spirit of
707 Summit
39°47.283' N
105°50.293' W
Spirit of 707
12,707 ft.
7-Mount
Bruplex Summit
39°47.269' N
105°51.094' W
Mount Bruplex
12,900 ft.
8-Vasquez
Peak Summit
39°47.773' N
105°51.308' W
Vasquez Peak
12,947 ft.
Stanley-Vasquez Continental Divide Route 12.4 mi RT

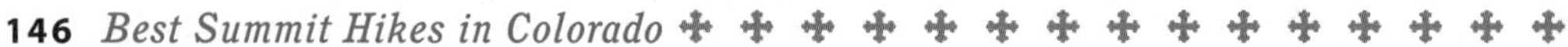

18 Stanley Mountain and Vasquez Peak

BONUS PEAKS: SPIRIT OF 707 AND MOUNT BRUPLEX

Peaks galore are yours for the bagging. Take a walk on the Continental Divide, and discover the charm of the little-known Vasquez Mountains.

Round-Trip Distance	12.4 miles
Hiking Time	6–9 hours
Difficulty	7.5/10
Class	2
Start Elevation	11,304 ft., at Berthoud Pass
Peak Elevations	Stanley Mountain: 12,521 ft.; Vasquez Peak: 12,947 ft.; Spirit of 707: 12,707 ft.; Mount Bruplex: 12,900 ft.
Total Elevation Gain	4,753 ft.
Terrain	Trails and good off-trail alpine tundra
Best Time to Climb	June–September; year-round to Stanley Mountain and back
Gear Advisor	Trekking poles
Crowd Level	Low

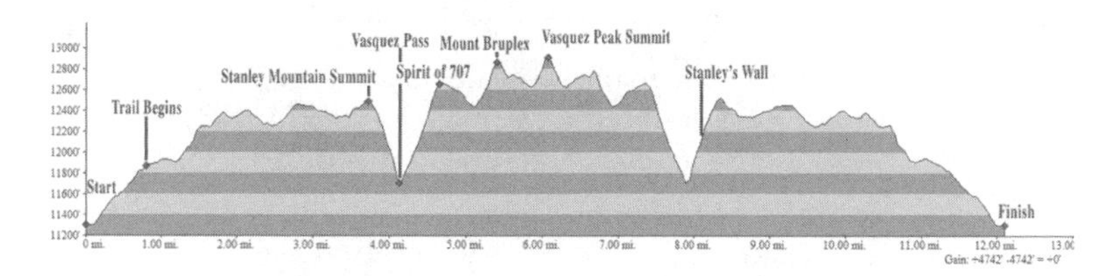

Location Vasquez Mountains in the Vasquez Peak Wilderness/Arapaho National Forest near the top of Berthoud Pass

Intro The Vasquez Peak Wilderness is a relatively unknown area, despite its close proximity to Winter Park and its accessibility from the top of Berthoud Pass. This route begins with a sky-high walk along the Continental Divide to Stanley Peak, a hike that is possible year-round. Dropping down to Vasquez Pass gives you access to three rolling mountains, including the high point of the Vasquez Mountains, Vasquez Peak. The crazy elevation profile shows that this hike is the true-to-life incarnation of that famous old-timer rant: you'll be hiking uphill both ways!

Why Climb It? The Vasquez Mountains make up a small range best known for their northern slopes, where most of the trails for Winter Park and Mary Jane ski areas are cut. This area is popular for backcountry skiers. The beginning of this hike was once within the boundaries of the now-defunct Berthoud Pass Ski Area.

Approximately 95% of this hike is above tree line, giving brilliant views of the Gore and Front Ranges. The first half of the hike follows a mellow trail on high alpine plains to Stanley Mountain. The second half dips down and gives you a chance to test your legs and lungs as you press on to three more mountains. On the west side of Vasquez Pass, the land feels very clean and pure and is punctuated with scarlet grasses and wildflowers. On the way back, get ready to push yourself up the giant grassy feature known as Stanley's Wall.

Driving All vehicles can make it to the top of Berthoud Pass, which is paved and very well maintained. This parking area is open year-round and caters to backcountry skiers, snowboarders, and snowshoers in the winter.

How to Get There From I-70, take Exit 232 (the Winter Park, Empire, Granby exit), and follow US Highway 40 approximately 15 miles to the top of Berthoud Pass. The flat summit of the pass has a large parking area on the right (east) side at the base of a ski hill; you'll see relics of the old Berthoud Pass Ski Area. Park here and cross the street to begin your hike.

Fees/Camping There are no fees to hike or camp in the area. A few pay campgrounds are along Berthoud Pass on both the north and south sides; call the US Forest Service number listed on the opposite page for fee information.

Route Notes None.

Mile/Waypoint

0.0 mi (1) Start at the parking area on the east side of Berthoud Pass. Cross the paved road and begin hiking on the dirt road on the west side. (There will be a gate and a sign for Continental Divide National Scenic Trail; this is also Forest Service Road 786.) As you head up, make sure that you stay on FS 786.

0.8 mi (2) The road ends, and an obvious footpath continues left (northwest). This trail has a cairn at the start. Follow the path to a steep hill, which you'll ascend via several switchbacks.

1.5 mi (3) After climbing the switchbacks, you'll pass the Vasquez Wilderness boundary. You can see your trail stretching far to the west—welcome to the Continental Divide.

1.9 mi The trail intersects with the old Mount Nystrom Trail, which overlaps the ambitious Continental Divide Trail. Stay left (southwest) and hike on the gently rolling hills of the divide, crossing over several small unnamed summits along the way. This is a very peaceful area with great views. Stanley Peak looks far off, but you'll be there sooner than you think.

3.8 mi (4) Stanley Mountain's summit! This is the end of your on-trail hiking (though the barely there Mount Nystrom Trail continues along the route in this description). Drop down Stanley's very steep western slope to the saddle of Vasquez Pass. This grassy hill has good footing but drops very quickly, earning it the nickname Stanley's Wall. Trekking poles will help save your knees at this point.

4.2 mi (5) You're at a low point at Vasquez Pass, 11,700 feet. You may hear the din of machinery from Henderson Mine to the south. From here, a faint path pushes west up to the summit of Spirit of 707 peak. Make up all the elevation you lost, and then some, to reach the top.

4.8 mi (6) The top of Spirit of 707! From here things get much easier—and much prettier. Very few people venture to this section of the Vasquez Mountains. Continue west to Mount Bruplex. A trace of the Mount Nystrom Trail may appear here and there as you hike along the alpine meadows.

5.5 mi (7) After a good class 2 hike/scramble, you're on the summit of Mount Bruplex. The ridgeline between Bruplex and Vasquez is obvious as it heads north. The last brief section before Vasquez's summit has some rocky patches.

6.2 mi (8) You've finally reached the high point of the Vasquez Mountains, Vasquez Peak. Congratulations! On most days, you'll have the summit to yourself, so soak in the solitude and take lots of pictures.

Return the way you came, with the exception of skirting just below the top of Mount Bruplex. It may be tempting to shortcut from the knobby outcrop just north of Bruplex, but the footing is not very good. Continue back up and over 707, and then drop back down to Vasquez Pass.

8.1 mi (5) At this point in most hikes, you'd be done gaining elevation. Not so here—the climb back up to Stanley is a bugger. Again, trekking poles will be a big help. You're going from 11,700 feet to 12,490 feet in less than 0.5 mile. Push, push, push your way back up Stanley's Wall to the summit, and you'll be home free. Enjoy the rest of the walk back to Berthoud Pass.

12.4 mi Finish.

Options If you count the unnamed summits on this hike, you'll be topping seven moderate peaks. What more do you want? The only option that I recommend is hiking to Stanley Mountain in the winter. It's a good adventure on safe terrain. However, going down to Vasquez Pass would be very dangerous (this is prime avalanche terrain) and is not recommended when there is still snow.

Quick Facts Vasquez Peak takes its name from the brothers Vasquez. Louis is known for building a fort at Clear Creek in 1832; Antoine was a member of Zebulon Pike's exploratory expedition. Stanley Mountain honors F. O. Stanley, creator of the Stanley Steamer. Spirit of 707 (an unofficial name) celebrates the long-forgotten events of the year A.D. 707, which included the death of Japanese Emperor Mommu and the Byzantines losing the Balearic Islands to the Moors (the world would never be the same). Mount Bruplex is unnamed on every map save this one, but every good mountain deserves a name. Bruplex happens to be the name of one of my cats.

Contact Info Arapaho National Forest
Clear Creek Ranger District
101 Chicago Creek Road
P.O. Box 3307
Idaho Springs, CO 80452
(303) 567-2901

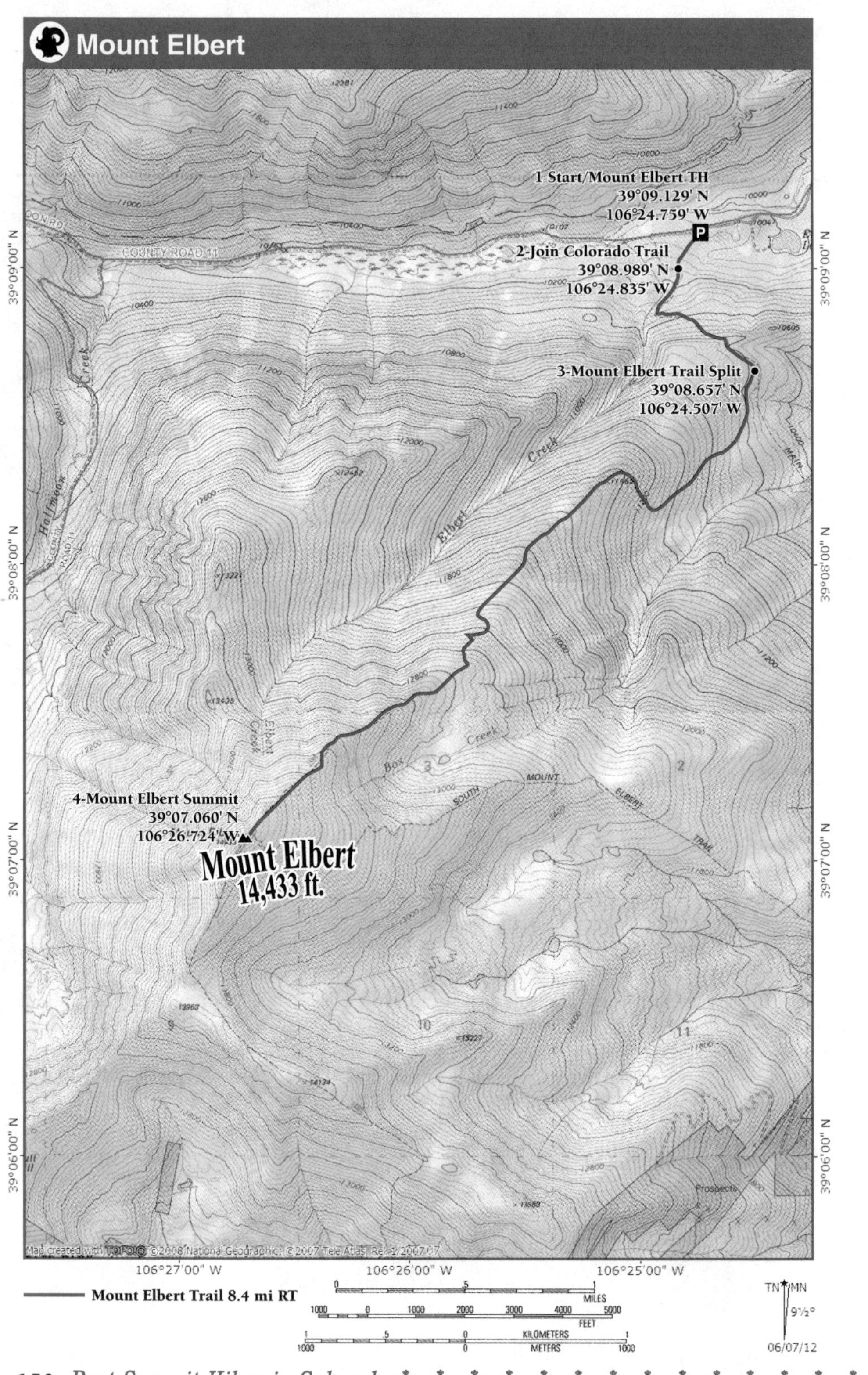
Mount Elbert
1 Start/Mount Elbert TH
39°09.129' N
106°24.759' W
2-Join Colorado Trail
39°08.989' N
106°24.835' W
3-Mount Elbert Trail Split
39°08.657' N
106°24.507' W
4-Mount Elbert Summit
39°07.060' N
106°26.724' W
Mount Elbert
14,433 ft.
COUNTY ROAD 11
Halfmoon Creek
Elbert Creek
Box Creek
SOUTH MOUNT ELBERT TRAIL
Prospects
39°09'00" N
39°08'00" N
39°07'00" N
39°06'00" N
106°27'00" W
106°26'00" W
106°25'00" W
Mount Elbert Trail 8.4 mi RT
MILES
FEET
KILOMETERS
METERS
TN MN
9½°
06/07/12

19 Mount Elbert

Welcome to Colorado's highest mountain. Elbert is a gentle giant whose lofty heights are also tops in all the Rocky Mountains. This king of 14ers is one of Colorado's best hikes.

Round-Trip Distance	8.4 miles
Hiking Time	4½–6½ hours
Difficulty	5/10
Class	2
Start Elevation	10,066 ft., at Mount Elbert Trailhead/Elbert Creek Campground
Peak Elevation	14,433 ft.
Total Elevation Gain	4,643 ft.
Terrain	Well-maintained trail
Best Time to Climb	June–September
Gear Advisor	Light hikers
Crowd Level	Moderate; high on weekends

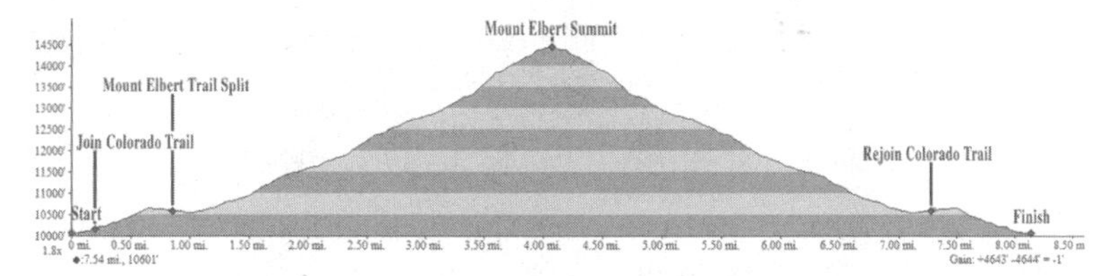

Location Sawatch Range in the Mount Massive Wilderness/San Isabel National Forest near Leadville

Intro Ask folks outside of Colorado what the highest mountain in the state is, and they'll probably guess Pikes Peak or Longs Peak. Humble Mount Elbert has little fanfare outside of the Centennial State, despite being the second-highest mountain in the lower 48 states (and the 21st highest in the entire US, including Alaska). Only Mount Whitney (14,494 feet) in California is higher. Elbert's northeast ridge is a surprisingly moderate hike (roughly 8–9 miles round-trip, and five to seven hours of hiking) and is typical of the rounded, giant Sawatch mountains.

Why Climb It? The obvious draw to Mount Elbert is its height. The gentle northeast ridge that the Mount Elbert Trail follows is a true classic. The lower sections weave through a pristine pine forest and then switchback up to tree line, where Elbert's majesty is revealed. If tree line is reached in the early-morning dawn, the panoramic sunrise looking north to Leadville is stunning, especially when a low blanket of clouds hovers below. Hiking up past the notorious false summits leads to a flat apex with gorgeous 360-degree views. Elbert's moderate difficulty (altitude notwithstanding) makes it a good primer for more arduous hikes.

Driving Elbert Creek and the Mount Elbert Trailhead can be reached by all vehicles. The dirt road is well maintained and easy to drive in normal conditions. Past the trailhead, the road gradually becomes rockier. A tough passenger car can make it far enough past the trailhead to park at some of the better primitive campsites.

How to Get There From downtown Leadville, drive 3.5 miles south on US Highway 24 and turn right (west) onto Colorado Highway 300, which appears just after a service station on the right. Drive 0.7 mile, and then turn left (south) onto County Road 11. Turn right at 1.8 miles (when the road turns to dirt), and follow the signs to Halfmoon Creek Campground. Continue on this good dirt road 6.8 miles (bypassing the Halfmoon Creek Campground) until you reach the Mount Elbert Trailhead on your left; Elbert Creek Campground is across from the trailhead on your right. The Mount Elbert Trailhead is a large lot.

Fees/Camping There are no fees to climb Mount Elbert. If you'd like to camp at Halfmoon Creek or Elbert Creek Campgrounds (which have toilets and maintained sites), the fee is $12 per night, as of 2012. If you prefer to save a few bucks, there are several free primitive campsites past the Mount Elbert Trailhead (and beyond the Mount Massive Trailhead). These sites are between 0.25 and 0.5 mile from the end of the passenger-car-friendly road, though most cars can make it to the first sites.

Route Notes None.

Mile/Waypoint

0.0 mi (1) Start from the Mount Elbert Trailhead and take the Mount Elbert Trail. An informative sign is at the beginning of the trail.

0.2 mi (2) The Colorado Trail joins the Mount Elbert Trail, coming in from the right. Follow the signs for Mount Elbert and bear left (you'll feel silly if you take the wrong turn because it brings you directly back to the road). Get ready to start plugging uphill, passing a few cabin ruins during a level section.

0.9 mi (3) The Mount Elbert Trail splits right (south), while the Colorado Trail goes straight and downhill. Turn right onto the signed Mount Elbert Trail and hike your way up toward tree line. After a straight, steep section, you'll continue to climb to 12,000 feet, where you will emerge from timberline.

2.4 mi Exit tree line (12,000 feet). From here, you'll have a good look at the ridge up to Elbert's summit. Continue on the well-traveled trail.

3.1 mi After a particularly steep section, top out on one of Elbert's false summits. There's one more (sort-of) false summit after this one, before you truly top out.

4.2 mi (4) Mount Elbert summit! You're now the highest thing in Colorado (unless you have a taller hiking companion). Return the way you came up.

7.5 mi (3) It's easy to zone out on the long descent; make sure not to miss the left turn on Mount Elbert Trail when it rejoins the Colorado Trail.

8.4 mi Finish.

Options With so many 14ers and high 13ers nearby, it's easy to pair Elbert up with another Sawatch climb. Some described in this book include Mount Hope (Hike 21), Huron Peak (Hike 22), Mount Ouray (Hike 23), and Carbonate Mountain and Tabeguache Peak (Hike 24). The most logical peak for a weekend excursion with Elbert is Mount Massive (14,421 feet), which is barely Colorado's second-highest mountain (edging out Mount Harvard by a foot). The Mount Massive Trailhead is less than 0.25 mile west from the Mount Elbert Trailhead. Hiking Massive makes for a longer day, but it's still class 2 terrain, with a 13.6-mile round-trip to bag its summit.

Quick Facts Elbert's country-style name comes from former Colorado Governor Samuel Hitt Elbert, who served 1873–74. Elbert, whose term was less than memorable, married the daughter of the next governor, John Evans. Evans had a more notable term in office, but the 14er named in his honor (Mount Evans, 14,264 feet) had a lower elevation. This is another instance in which the mountain is not the measure of the man.

In the 1930s, there was a feud between Mount Elbert supporters and Mount Massive supporters; both argued that their peak was the highest (the actual difference is a mere 12 feet). Massive fan club hikers (who apparently had quite a bit of free time) constructed large cairns on the summit of Massive to boost its height, only to have Elbert supporters tear them down. Ultimately, measurements determined that Elbert is the higher mountain, though it's safe to say that Mount Massive has a more impressive name.

One final bit of interest: In 1949, a Jeep drove to the top of Elbert as part of a survey to gauge the mountain's potential for development of a road or ski area. Several bicyclists have made ascents to the peak as well.

Contact Info Hiking Mount Elbert is a good year-round adventure. During good snow conditions, one can make an enjoyable descent from the peak on skis or a snowboard. Contact the US Forest Service for winter conditions, and remember to bring your avalanche beacon!

San Isabel National Forest
Leadville Ranger District
2015 N. Poplar Street
Leadville, CO 80461
(719) 486-0749

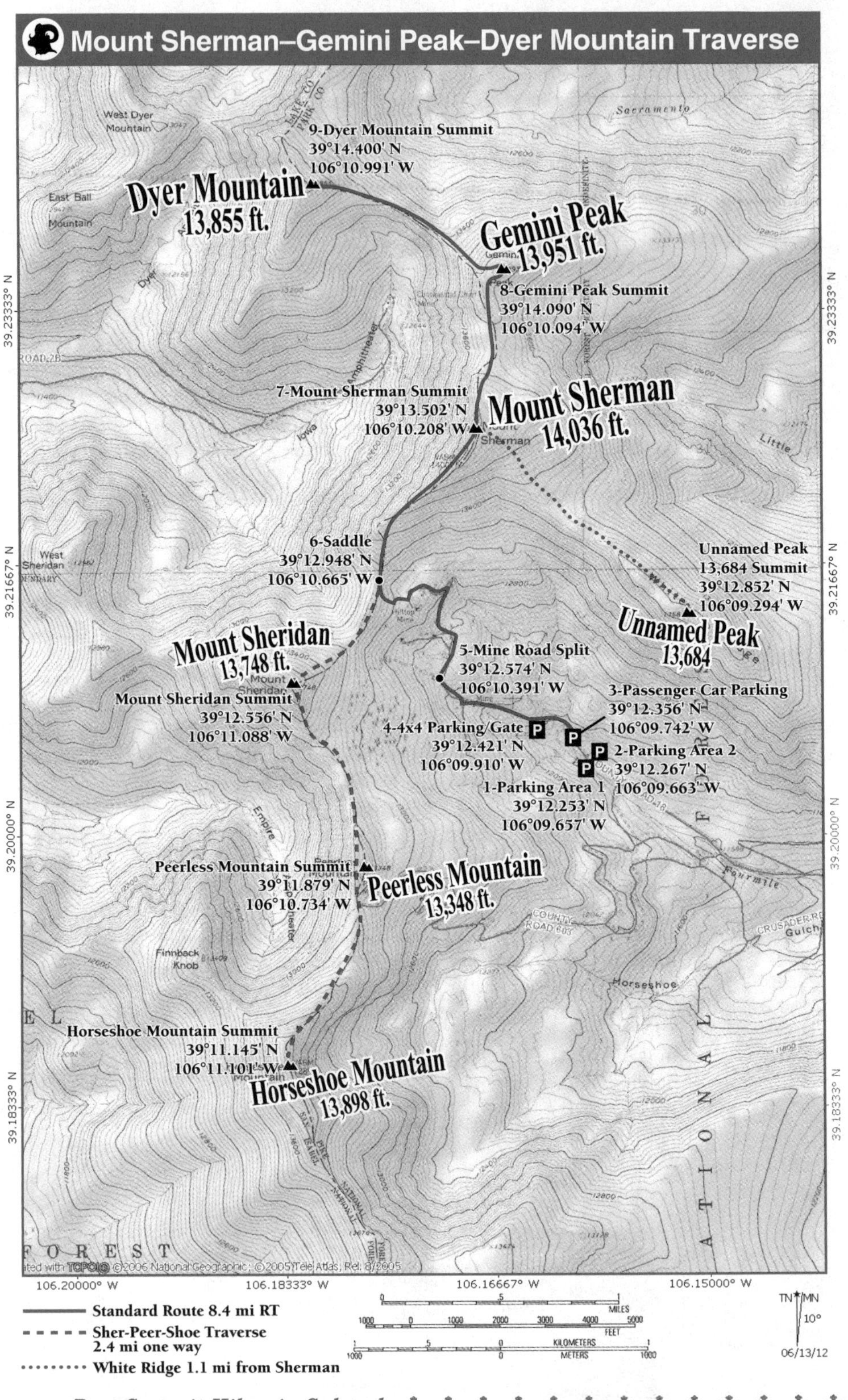
Mount Sherman–Gemini Peak–Dyer Mountain Traverse
9-Dyer Mountain Summit
39°14.400' N
106°10.991' W
Dyer Mountain
13,855 ft.
Gemini Peak
13,951 ft.
8-Gemini Peak Summit
39°14.090' N
106°10.094' W
7-Mount Sherman Summit
39°13.502' N
106°10.208' W
Mount Sherman
14,036 ft.
6-Saddle
39°12.948' N
106°10.665' W
Unnamed Peak
13,684 Summit
39°12.852' N
106°09.294' W
Unnamed Peak
13,684
Mount Sheridan
13,748 ft.
5-Mine Road Split
39°12.574' N
106°10.391' W
Mount Sheridan Summit
39°12.556' N
106°11.088' W
3-Passenger Car Parking
39°12.356' N
106°09.742' W
4-4x4 Parking/Gate
39°12.421' N
106°09.910' W
2-Parking Area 2
39°12.267' N
106°09.663' W
1-Parking Area 1
39°12.253' N
106°09.657' W
Peerless Mountain Summit
39°11.879' N
106°10.734' W
Peerless Mountain
13,348 ft.
Horseshoe Mountain Summit
39°11.145' N
106°11.101' W
Horseshoe Mountain
13,898 ft.
West Dyer Mountain
East Ball Mountain
West Sheridan
Finnback Knob
Sacramento
Fourmile
Horseshoe
39.23333° N
39.21667° N
39.20000° N
39.18333° N
106.20000° W
106.18333° W
106.16667° W
106.15000° W
Standard Route 8.4 mi RT
Sher-Peer-Shoe Traverse
2.4 mi one way
White Ridge 1.1 mi from Sherman
MILES
FEET
KILOMETERS
METERS
TN
MN
10°
06/13/12

20 Mount Sherman–Gemini Peak–Dyer Mountain Traverse

Get ready for great ghost mines, fun scrambles, and hallmark views of Colorado's highest mountains. These mountains are Mosquito Range classics, full of history.

Round-Trip Distance	8.4 miles
Hiking Time	4½–6 hours
Difficulty	5/10
Class	2/2+
Start Elevation	11,885 ft., at County Road 18 parking area
Peak Elevations	Mount Sherman: 14,036 ft.; Gemini Peak: 13,951 ft.; Dyer Mountain: 13,855 ft.
Total Elevation Gain	3,742 ft.
Terrain	Good trail to Sherman; rocky traverse to Gemini and Dyer
Best Time to Climb	June–September
Gear Advisor	Normal gear
Crowd Level	Moderate

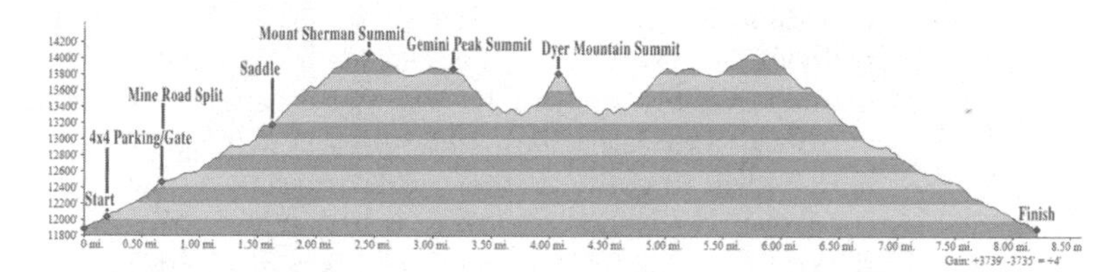

Location Mosquito Range Pike National Forest/Bureau of Land Management land outside of Fairplay

Intro From most perspectives, Mount Sherman's flat summit appears unassuming, perhaps unexciting, as it stands on the horizon. It isn't until you close in on the peak that the allure of this mild 14er becomes apparent. Spooky mining ruins at the base of Sherman, including the enormous mill at the abandoned Leavick townsite, teem with history. The gentle, rolling ridges between several peaks around Sherman make summit-bagging easy. From the central parking area, it's possible to collect six in a single day.

Looking for the ultimate Sherman adventure? Try the 10-peak traverse starting at Weston Pass, listed in the "Options" section of this write-up.

Why Climb It? A trip to Sherman is likely to include more than summiting the 14er. The twisted mine ruins and old Leavick mill site are sure to stir the imaginations of those interested in Colorado's mining history, and the saddle between

Sherman and Sheridan is the perfect place to view Colorado's two highest mountains, Mount Elbert and Mount Massive.

Sherman is generally considered the easiest of the 14ers to climb, making it a good first 14er for the uninitiated. For more experienced hikers, the option to link several mountains is irresistible; the two additional peaks on the main route for this hike go north, while the optional three traverse south.

From the parking area, you can view the amazing glacial cirque on Horseshoe Mountain. The marking is natural, despite its resemblance to a Colorado strip mine.

Driving The dirt road to Sherman is littered with "baby heads"—a cheeky term from the world of mountain biking that refers to dozens of rounded rocks on an otherwise smooth road. In normal conditions, passenger cars will be able to get within 0.2 mile of the closure gate—only a deeply washed-out rut prevents the last portion from being safely passed by low-clearance cars. The last section requires sport utility cars or more rugged vehicles. Note that there are sections of private land en route, so be respectful as you drive through.

How to Get There One mile south of the intersection of US Highway 285 and Colorado Highway 9, just outside of Fairplay, turn west onto Park County Road 18. From here, it is roughly 11.5 miles on PCR 18 to the first of the parking areas, and 12 miles to the final parking area. The road is paved for a short distance; when you reach a four-way intersection, stay straight on PCR 18 as it turns to dirt. Remain on PCR 18 to the end of the road. Be ready for a barrage of small but steady bumps and washboards. You'll go in and out of private land, passing two campgrounds before reaching the enormous Leavick Mill at 10.5 miles. A large parking lot is on the left here, but keep going farther—even passenger cars can make it up the road, and you'll spare yourself a longer walk than is necessary up to the trailhead. Good parking pull-offs begin 1.5 miles after the Leavick Mill on both sides of road. Waypoints **1** and **2** indicate good pull-offs for passenger cars. These lots only add about 0.2 mile max to your already short hike. If you're in a passenger car, pick any of these; sport utility cars or vehicles, as well as trucks, will have no problem making it to the parking area at the closure gate.

Fees/Camping There are no fees to hike Sherman or the surrounding peaks, but please be aware that most of the land is privately owned. There are two campgrounds en route to Sherman: Fourmile Campground (14 sites) and Horseshoe Campground (19 sites). Both sites are $15 per night, as of 2012, and have toilets and water sources.

Route Notes On many maps, there are dozens of trails and subtrails that may confuse the aspiring hiker. It's important to note that the standard trailhead is not officially marked; it's simply a closed gate at the end of the PCR 18. I met several frustrated hikers who had been looking for a sign for Fourmile Creek Trailhead. While you *do* follow Fourmile Creek on the road up,

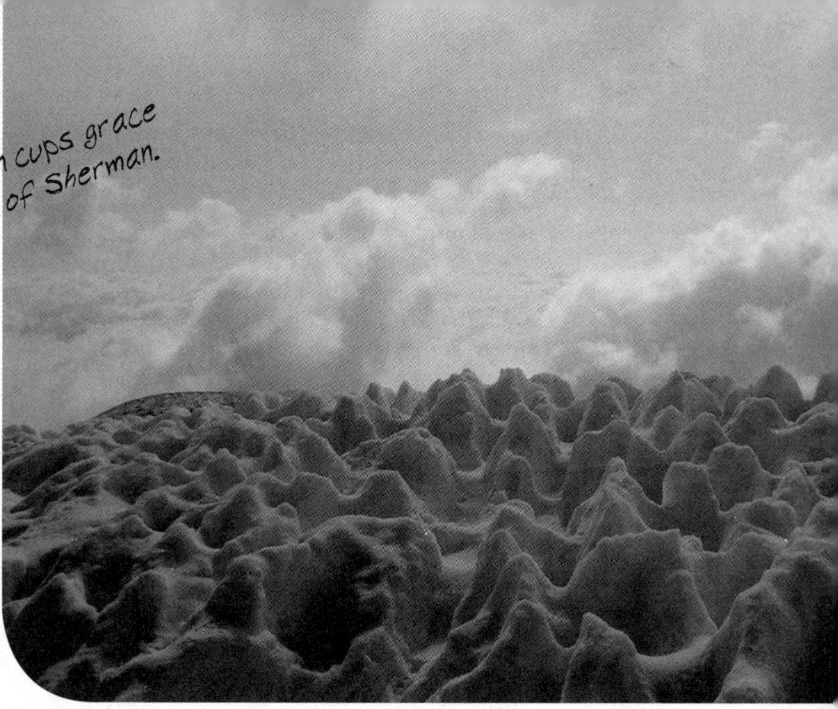

Heavenly sun cups grace the summit of Sherman.

don't frustrate yourself looking for trailhead signage—just get to the end of the road.

Mile/Waypoint

0.0 mi (3) This route starts 0.2 mile east of the final 4x4 parking lot and closure gate. If you park here, walk up the road to the closure gate.

0.2 mi (4) At the gated end of the road, there are about 10 parking spots. You'll see the Dauntless and Hilltop Mines from here. Go through the gate, and continue up the wide dirt road. Check out the mining relics along the way. A tower-supported aerial tramway once ran between the mine and the mill; there are still a few towers between the two (see "Quick Facts" on page 158). Stay straight (due west) on this road until mile 0.7.

0.7 mi (5) Turn right onto the dirt road that switchbacks up to the Hilltop Mine. The saddle between Sheridan and Sherman will be obvious, and you can reach it many ways; this way is the most scenic and easiest to follow. Hike up and past the Hilltop Mine and several abandoned cabins. (This area was actively mined from the late 1800s to the 1960s.) Follow any of the several subtrails behind the cabins to a main trail on the west side of the ruins; eventually, one main trail appears and leads up a small hill to the saddle.

1.6 mi (6) As you gain the saddle, gorgeous views of Mount Massive and Mount Elbert appear on the horizon; you are looking out at the highest peaks in Colorado. Follow a well-worn trail northeast up the gentle, class 2 ridge. This is a pleasant hike with very good views.

2.5 mi (7) Mount Sherman's flat summit! You may be confused as to the actual high point; look for the summit log and U.S. Geological Survey marker. In spring, Sherman is famous for its sun-cupped snowfield, which spikes up on the west side of the summit area. From here, continue north (there will no longer be a trail) to Gemini Peak. This traverse is gentle, dropping only 300 feet before climbing up to Gemini's mini-pyramid block.

3.3 mi (8) Gemini Peak's summit! You can scramble up on the slightly tricky west or south sides (probably class 2+), or find an easier path on the east face to reach the top. Some hikers are content with just these two peaks, which is totally reasonable. The route described here, however, continues on 0.9 mile to Dyer Mountain.

3.8 mi Head northwest 0.5 mile and then 600 feet down Gemini to the saddle between Gemini and Dyer. At 13,300 feet, you'll see huge wire towers. (How the heck did they get those things up here?) Go under the wires, and make the class 2+ scramble up to Dyer Mountain summit (this is like an extended version of the brief scrambling on Gemini).

4.1 mi (9) After a fun scramble, you have attained the summit of Dyer Mountain. Enjoy the views, and note the potential for continuing north for even more summits. Reverse your route back over Gemini and Sherman, returning down Sherman's ridge and back to the parking area.

8.4 mi Finish.

Options You have plenty of options if you want to keep hiking after summiting Mount Sherman. At 1.1 miles southeast of Sherman (waypoint **7**), you can venture out on White Ridge to Unnamed Peak 13,684, which affords some great views of the mining area.

From the saddle between Sherman and Sheridan (waypoint **6**), you can start a 2.4-mile, class 2 traverse that crosses the summits of Mount Sheridan at mile 0.5, Peerless Mountain at mile 1.5, and Horseshoe Mountain at mile 2.4. This southern swing follows the obvious ridgeline that connects all three. Horseshoe Mountain is particularly impressive, with a huge glacial cirque on its east face.

For the ultimate Sherman adventure, try the burly Weston Pass to Sherman and beyond. It's possible to snag 10 official mountains in one day. You'll need two cars, but the mileage isn't impossible (around 12–14 miles total, most of it more than 13,000 feet). For a free map and description of this route, visit **tinyurl.com/westonsherman.**

Quick Facts Mount Sherman was named by the Hayden survey party in 1872 for Civil War General William T. Sherman. Neighboring Mount Sheridan was named at the same time for Civil War General Philip Sheridan. Both were members of the Union Army. It seems just to me that the higher peak is named for Sherman, as Sheridan was involved in a great deal of violence against Native Americans during the US/Native American wars that followed the conclusion of the Civil War.

The mines in this area are evidence of the mineral wealth contained within these mountains. Silver was the draw for Felix Leavick, who bought the Hilltop Mine, following the silver crash of 1893. Along with business partner Brad DuBois, he restored the mining operations, modernizing the process with a railway and aerial tramway.

The prolific Leavick Mill was constructed in the spring of 1897. As in other boomtowns, Leavick's population was briefly sizable enough to warrant a post office. The boom was short-lived, however, as residents began a mass exodus in 1899. Still, mining continued in the area until the 1960s, when most of the valuable veins of ore had been tapped.

Contact Info

Pike National Forest
South Park Ranger District
320 US Highway 285
P.O. Box 219
Fairplay, CO 80440
(719) 836-2031

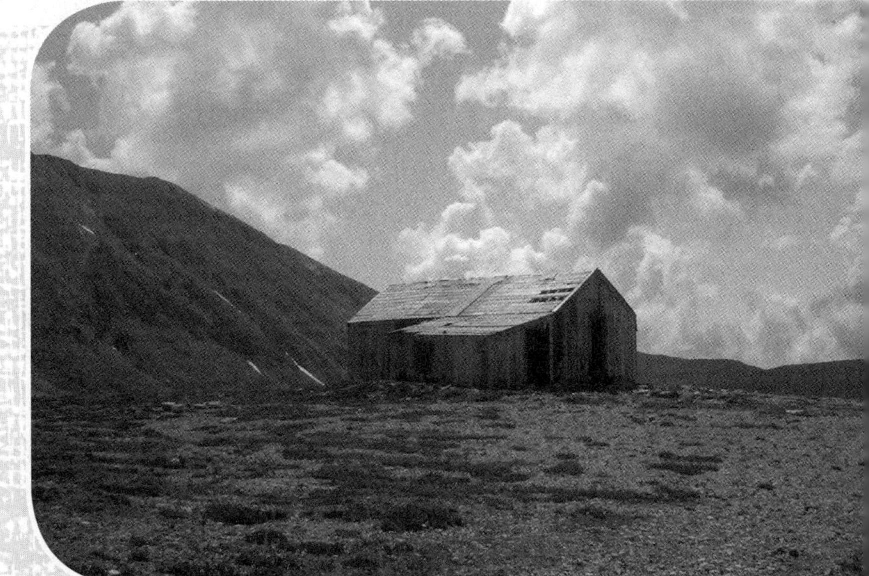

Mount Sherman is a wonderful blend of alpine scenery and mining history.

Mount Hope

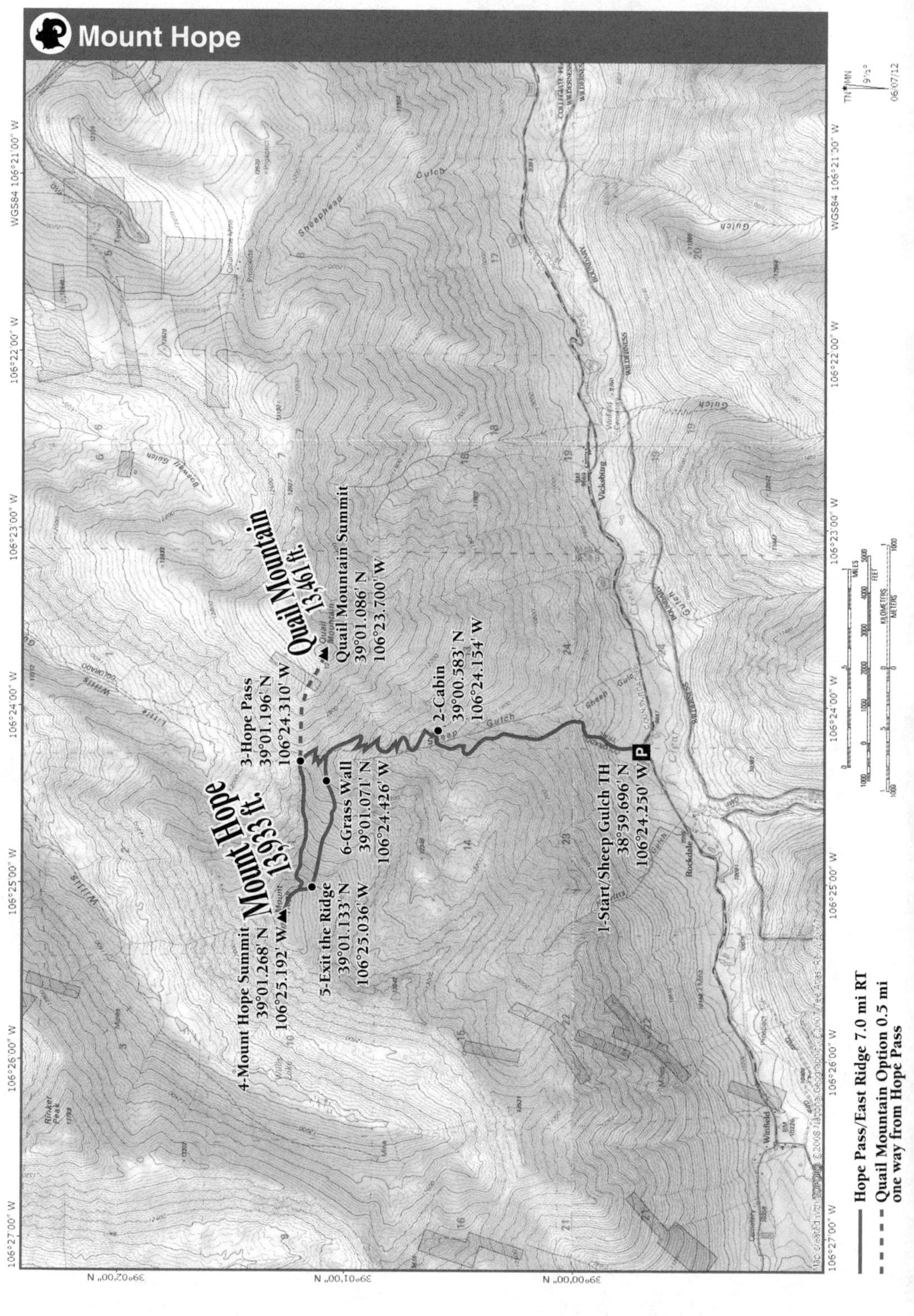

Mount Hope
Mount Hope
13,933 ft.
Quail Mountain
13,461 ft.
4-Mount Hope Summit
39°01.268' N
106°25.192' W
5-Exit the Ridge
39°01.133' N
106°25.036' W
6-Grass Wall
39°01.071' N
106°24.426' W
3-Hope Pass
39°01.196' N
106°24.310' W
Quail Mountain Summit
39°01.086' N
106°23.700' W
2-Cabin
39°00.583' N
106°24.154' W
1-Start/Sheep Gulch TH
38°59.696' N
106°24.250' W
P
Sheep Gulch
Boswell Gulch
Sheephead Gulch
Little Willis Gulch
Willis
Clear Creek
Vicksburg
Rockdale
Winfield
Rinker Peak
106°27'00" W
106°26'00" W
106°25'00" W
106°24'00" W
106°23'00" W
106°22'00" W
WGS84 106°21'00" W
106°21'30" W
39°02'00" N
39°01'00" N
39°00'00" N
Hope Pass/East Ridge 7.0 mi RT
Quail Mountain Option 0.5 mi one way from Hope Pass
06/07/12

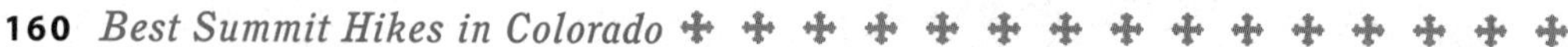

21 Mount Hope

Mount Hope's east ridge is a fun excursion on an overlooked mountain. Scramble on a solid ridge to a flat summit, which may surprise you with a gift of wildflowers.

Round-Trip Distance	7.0 miles
Hiking Time	5–7 hours
Difficulty	7/10
Class	2+/3
Start Elevation	9,875 ft., at Sheep Gulch Trailhead
Peak Elevation	13,933 ft.
Total Elevation Gain	4,070 ft.
Terrain	Good trail to rocky but solid ridge walk
Best Time to Climb	June–September
Gear Advisor	Normal gear
Crowd Level	Low

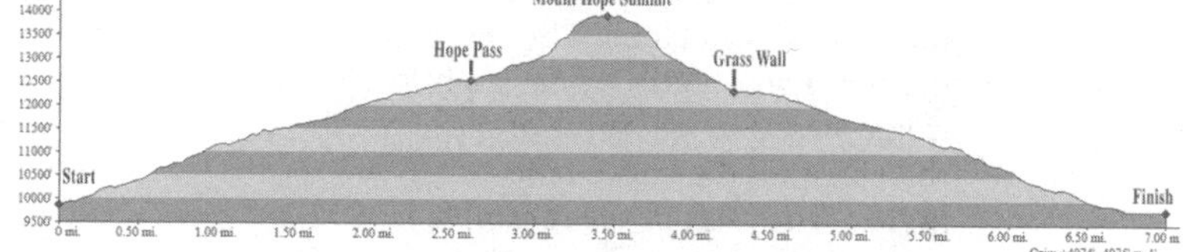

Location Sawatch Range in the Collegiate Peak Wilderness/San Isabel National Forest outside of Leadville

Intro Mount Hope is lost in the shuffle of the Sawatch giants, despite being a mere 67 feet lower than the prized 14ers. Maybe it's for the best because the lack of traffic gives Hope a sense of solitude. The east ridge is a fine way to climb Hope; the scrambling has minimal exposure, which makes it a good first ridge scramble for the uninitiated. The approach to the ridge takes you through aspen forests and emerges from tree line, where stunning views to the south seem to invoke the Rocky Mountain spirit.

Why Climb It? The forest en route to Hope Pass is especially beautiful. Timberline dissipates slowly, with stray bunches of trees guiding you to Hope Pass. Scrambling on the ridge is mostly class 2+ with a few easy class 3 moves thrown in for fun. Daring scramblers can stay on the spine of the ridge and increase the number of class 3 moves. This summit has great views of La Plata Peak and Huron Peak; it is the highest place in which I've ever seen gardens of assorted wildflowers.

Driving Any vehicle can make it to the trailhead. County Road 390 is a very well-maintained dirt road.

How to Get There To reach Sheep Gulch Trailhead, start on US Highway 24 and turn west onto Chaffee County Road 390; this intersection is roughly 20 miles from Leadville and 15 miles from Buena Vista. Follow CR 390 for 9.4 miles, past Clear Creek Reservoir, to Sheep Gulch Trailhead on your right. You can park here or along the road.

Fees/Camping There are no fees to hike or camp in the area. Please note that the town of Winfield, just west of here, is privately owned, so if you're going to camp off the road, find a pull-off before or after that tiny and still functional town.

Route Notes None.

Mile/Waypoint

0.0 mi (1) Start at the Sheep Gulch Trailhead and head north on the Hope Pass Trail, which is also the Colorado Trail. You'll hike by the old parking area as you enter the woods, and then gain an easy-to-follow singletrack trail up to Hope Pass. Enjoy the forest; it's one of my favorites.

1.3 mi (2) On the way up, peek over to the right (east) into the woods. Can you find the cabin hiding in the trees? It must have been a laborious task to build it way up here.

2.7 mi (3) At 12,550 feet you'll arrive at Hope Pass, between Quail Mountain and Mount Hope. The east ridge of Hope looms before you in a series of hills. This entails very straightforward ridge scrambling with the occasional class 3 move. Some of the hike is best done down about 70 feet below the ridge on the south side, where better footing will help you progress higher. The crux of the scramble is at 13,580 feet, where the rocky section to the final summit flats has a few easy class 3 moves that you have to link

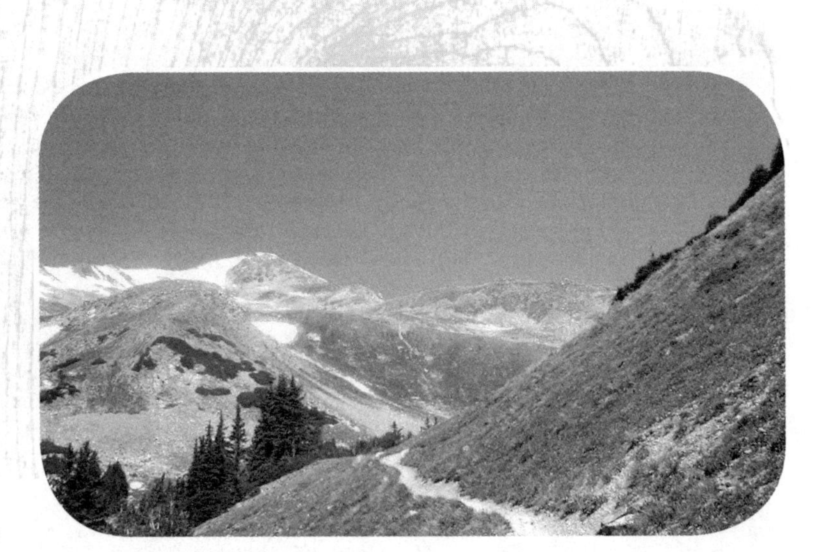

Hope Pass

together. When you emerge on the summit flats, it's a short walk west on gentle terrain to the summit.

3.6 mi (4) Hope's optimistic summit! Views to the west of La Plata Peak are remarkable. To the north, check out Elbert and Massive; to the south are Huron and the Collegiate Peaks. If you like, go back down the east ridge (a good option if you want to climb Quail), but it will be slow going. The route described here is faster. Go south off the summit to the next waypoint.

3.8 mi (5) At 13,670 feet, find a good line down the steep wall, exit the ridge, and make your way into the basin. When there is soft snow, this is a good place to plunge-step with your heels (or glissade). When there's no snow, it's rocky and a bit sketchy. There's no easy way off Hope. The other options are descending the ridge you came up or going down the south ridge—which will give you similar scrambling farther down and present you with a loose talus field to cross to regain the trail in the trees. Better to see where you are going. Stay north in the basin, and find a good high line back to the Hope Pass Trail. There's an easy talus field to cross here, and it is fairly stable.

4.5 mi (6) Just before connecting to the Hope Pass Trail, stay high (north) above the "grass wall." Doing so will give you better footing and reconnect you to the trail more quickly than trying to cut down on steep slopes. Once you are back on the trail, it's a quick hike back down to your vehicle.

7.0 mi Finish.

Options Mount Hope is a stalwart pile of rock that glaciers were forced to flow around. As a result, the only other peak connected to it is Quail Mountain (13,461 feet). From Hope Pass, it's 0.5 mile one way on class 2 slopes to Quail's summit.

Quick Facts Mount Hope is unique in this area of the Sawatch in that it doesn't have a long, gentle slope leading to its summit. The east ridge is arguably the easiest way to reach the top. The south ridge begins as the typical slope but gets broken off before making a smooth connection with the lowlands. This is evidence that the glaciers and rivers that carved the path now followed by Clear Creek were powerful enough to break apart the lower half of the ridge.

The Hopeful Couloir on the north face is a good spring snow climb. Expert skiers can enjoy a run down its thrilling 50-degree slopes.

Contact Info San Isabel National Forest
Leadville Ranger District
2015 N. Poplar Street
Leadville, CO 80461
(719) 486-0752

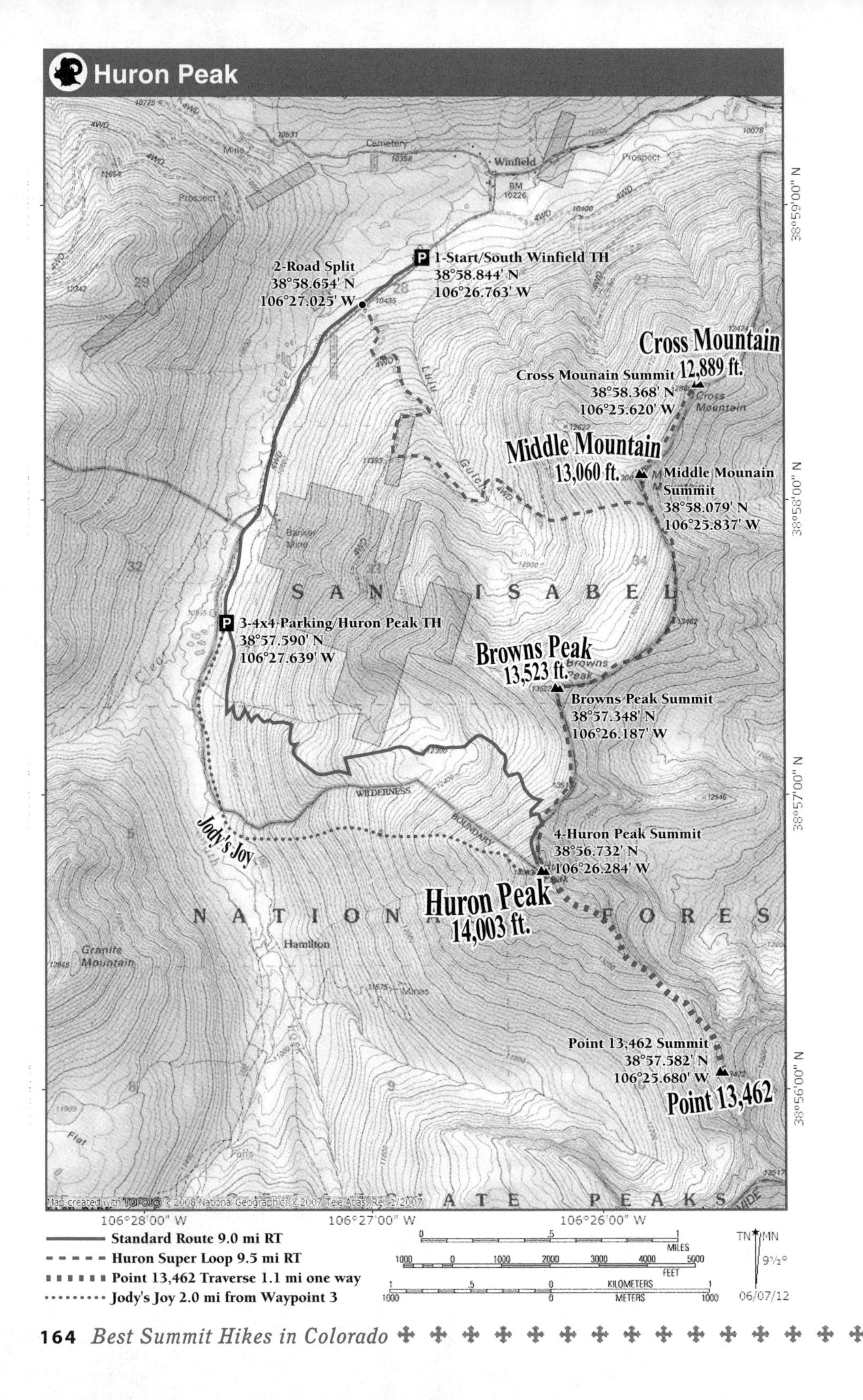
Huron Peak
2-Road Split
38°58.654' N
106°27.025' W
1-Start/South Winfield TH
38°58.844' N
106°26.763' W
Cross Mountain
12,889 ft.
Cross Mounain Summit
38°58.368' N
106°25.620' W
Middle Mountain
13,060 ft.
Middle Mounain Summit
38°58.079' N
106°25.837' W
3-4x4 Parking/Huron Peak TH
38°57.590' N
106°27.639' W
Browns Peak
13,523 ft.
Browns Peak Summit
38°57.348' N
106°26.187' W
4-Huron Peak Summit
38°56.732' N
106°26.284' W
Jody's Joy
Huron Peak
14,003 ft.
Point 13,462 Summit
38°57.582' N
106°25.680' W
Point 13,462
Winfield
Cemetery
SAN ISABEL NATIONAL FOREST
Hamilton
Granite Mountain
Map created with TOPO!® ©2008 National Geographic; ©2007 Tele Atlas, Rel. 1/2007
106°28'00" W
106°27'00" W
106°26'00" W
38°59'00" N
38°58'00" N
38°57'00" N
38°56'00" N
Standard Route 9.0 mi RT
Huron Super Loop 9.5 mi RT
Point 13,462 Traverse 1.1 mi one way
Jody's Joy 2.0 mi from Waypoint 3
MILES
FEET
KILOMETERS
METERS
TN MN
9½°
06/07/12

22 Huron Peak

Huron is a classic climb on a picture-perfect mountain. This 14er may be the most beautiful hike in the Sawatch Range, with excellent views from the summit pyramid.

Round-Trip Distance	9.0 miles/6.5 miles from 4x4 parking
Hiking Time	3–6 hours
Difficulty	4/10
Class	2
Start Elevation	10,286 ft., at South Winfield Trailhead
Peak Elevation	14,003 ft.
Total Elevation Gain	3,576 ft.
Terrain	Good trail; slightly rocky toward summit
Best Time to Climb	June–September
Gear Advisor	Trail runners
Crowd Level	Moderate; high on weekends

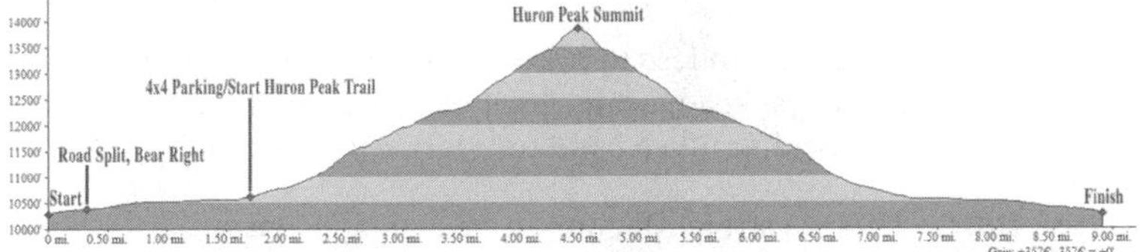

Location Sawatch Range in Collegiate Peaks Wilderness/San Isabel National Forest near Buena Vista and Leadville

Intro Look at that beautiful elevation profile. Huron is a very "clean" mountain with classic contours and a very well-maintained, class 2 trail. It's at the low side for 14ers, with the latest measurement putting its summit at 14,003 feet. Huron Peak has my favorite summit views of any Sawatch mountain, and the hike is a great intro to Colorado's higher peaks.

Why Climb It? Huron's locale in the southern Sawatch makes it the perfect perch for views of Colorado's highest peaks (Elbert, La Plata, and so on) to the north; the amazing views of Ice Mountain and the Three Apostles to the south ain't too shabby, either. The trail is very well maintained, making Huron a very good hike for non-hardcore hikers, dogs, and groups of mixed ability. A direct, on-trail ascent to the summit won't take long for fit climbers. Ambitious peak-baggers looking for more fun are welcome to head north of Huron and summit up to three more peaks, making for a longer day (which is nicely concluded as a loop). Alternately, scramblers can go for a "suicide push" up the steep but stable west ridge, a good off-trail option for those wanting to avoid crowds.

Driving Passenger cars can make it to the South Winfield Trailhead; the dirt road is a little bumpy but passable. Cars will have to park here. The 4x4 road beyond that is good, but it can be very rutted out; sport utility cars, sport utility vehicles, and 4x4s should be able to reach the 4x4 parking in normal conditions (I've seen several Subaru Outbacks and even a Volkswagen Eurovan at the 4x4 trailhead).

How to Get There To reach the South Winfield Trailhead, start on US Highway 24 and turn west onto Chaffee County Road 390; this intersection is roughly 20 miles from Leadville and 15 miles from Buena Vista. CR 390 is a well-maintained dirt road; you'll be on it for just over 12 miles (you can follow the signs to Winfield). After passing the Clear Creek Reservoir on your left, you'll continue down the road until mile 11.8, where you'll see the (revived) ghost town of Winfield, a semi-restored mining town with about 12 active summer cabins. It's worth a visit to Winfield's historic museums and cemetery after your hike. Follow the main road through Winfield (it curves left and then right), and continue 0.3 mile to the passenger car parking area. (The parking area is cleared out a bit; just past it, the road narrows and has a warning sign.) A few camping spots are on the right side here. If you have a 4x4 vehicle, continue 1.7 miles to the end of the road and the Huron Peak Trail. Tons of great camping sites are between the South Winfield Trailhead and the end of the road. Make sure to stay on the main road (see "Mile/Waypoint" section for more info).

Fees/Camping There are no fees to hike Huron Peak or to camp in the wilderness along the access road. Many great camping areas are on the road between South Winfield Trailhead and the Huron Peak Trail.

Route Notes This is a straightforward hike with good views.

Mile/Waypoint **0.0 mi (1)** Passenger cars park here. This is the South Winfield Trailhead. From here, it's a 1.7-mile hike/bike up easy terrain to the Huron Peak Trailhead (you gain only about 300 feet of elevation). Drive on, 4x4s!

0.3 mi (2) Stay straight on the main road. At this intersection, the road forks a bit; bear right (which is pretty much straight ahead). After that, the main road will be easy to follow as it passes a lush meadow on your right. Side roads mostly lead to camping areas.

1.7 mi (3) The Huron Peak Trailhead and 4x4 parking are at the closed US Forest Service gate at the end of the road. Note that the Huron Peak Trail starts left of the sign and gate, not straight ahead (unless you are hoping for an off-trail scramble of the west ridge!). Once you are on the Huron Peak Trail, it's very easy to follow; there are no intersecting trails. Follow the switchbacks up above tree line, and then push up to the ridge between Browns Peak and Huron Peak. Stay right (south) and continue to follow the well-traveled trail to the summit of Huron Peak.

4.5 mi (4) Huron Peak's wonderful summit accommodates quite a few happy hikers. The prominent, powerful-looking mountain to the south is Ice Mountain—you'll have a prime view of the Refrigerator Couloir on Ice, a wildly dangerous snow climb (due to heavy rockfall). The Three Apostles formation is just right (west) of Ice Mountain. Descend the way you came (or check out the "Options" section for more fun).

7.3 mi (3) Return to 4x4 parking lot.

9.0 mi Return to the South Winfield Trailhead.

Options To snag a few more peaks, head north from the summit of Huron Peak along the northern ridge (class 2) to Browns Peak (13,523 feet), 0.7 mile from Huron's top. Traverse northeast over point 13,462, and proceed to Middle Mountain (13,060 feet), which is roughly 1.8 miles from Huron. A full 2.2 miles from Huron will bring you to Cross Mountain (12,889 feet). You can return to the access road by descending the western slopes between Browns and Middle Mountains. There's a jeep trail you can eventually connect with that rejoins the main road (at the fork where you stayed right, 0.3 mile in, at waypoint **2**).

From Huron Peak's summit (waypoint **4**), you can follow the southeast ridge 1.1 miles down to point 13,462.

Finally, for those looking for a fun scramble, try Jody's Joy, a direct climb of the western ridge. Go straight at the forest gate (waypoint **3**) instead of left onto the Huron Peak Trail. Follow this trail 0.8 mile to the wilderness boundary, and then turn left (west) and gain the western ridge. You can stay on the ridge or scramble up the gully just south of the ridge another 1.2 very steep miles (2.0 miles from the 4x4 parking area).

Quick Facts Huron Peak is indirectly named after the Huron Native Americans of Michigan; a mine near the peak was named Huron first, and the moniker was later transferred to the mountain. Because you'll be in the neighborhood, it's worth checking out the revamped ghost town of Winfield. Winfield was formally founded in 1881 after prospectors discovered copper and silver deposits nearby. (The town went through two names, Florence and Lucknow, before the name Winfield stuck.) With a maximum population of 1,500, circa 1890, some of the early residents of Winfield toughed it out until the last mines closed in 1912. Today, the area has a few restored summer cabins and two public museums. The Winfield cemetery is 0.25 mile up the road from the center of town. Vicksburg, a few miles north of Winfield, is another almost-ghost town. (There are a few functional residences in Vicksburg.)

Note that Huron is very close to Sheep Gulch Trailhead, which is the starting point for another hike in this book, Mount Hope (Hike 21). Doing both peaks in a weekend is a grand idea, especially in the early autumn.

Contact Info San Isabel National Forest
Leadville Ranger District
2015 N. Poplar Street
Leadville, CO 80461
(719) 486-0749

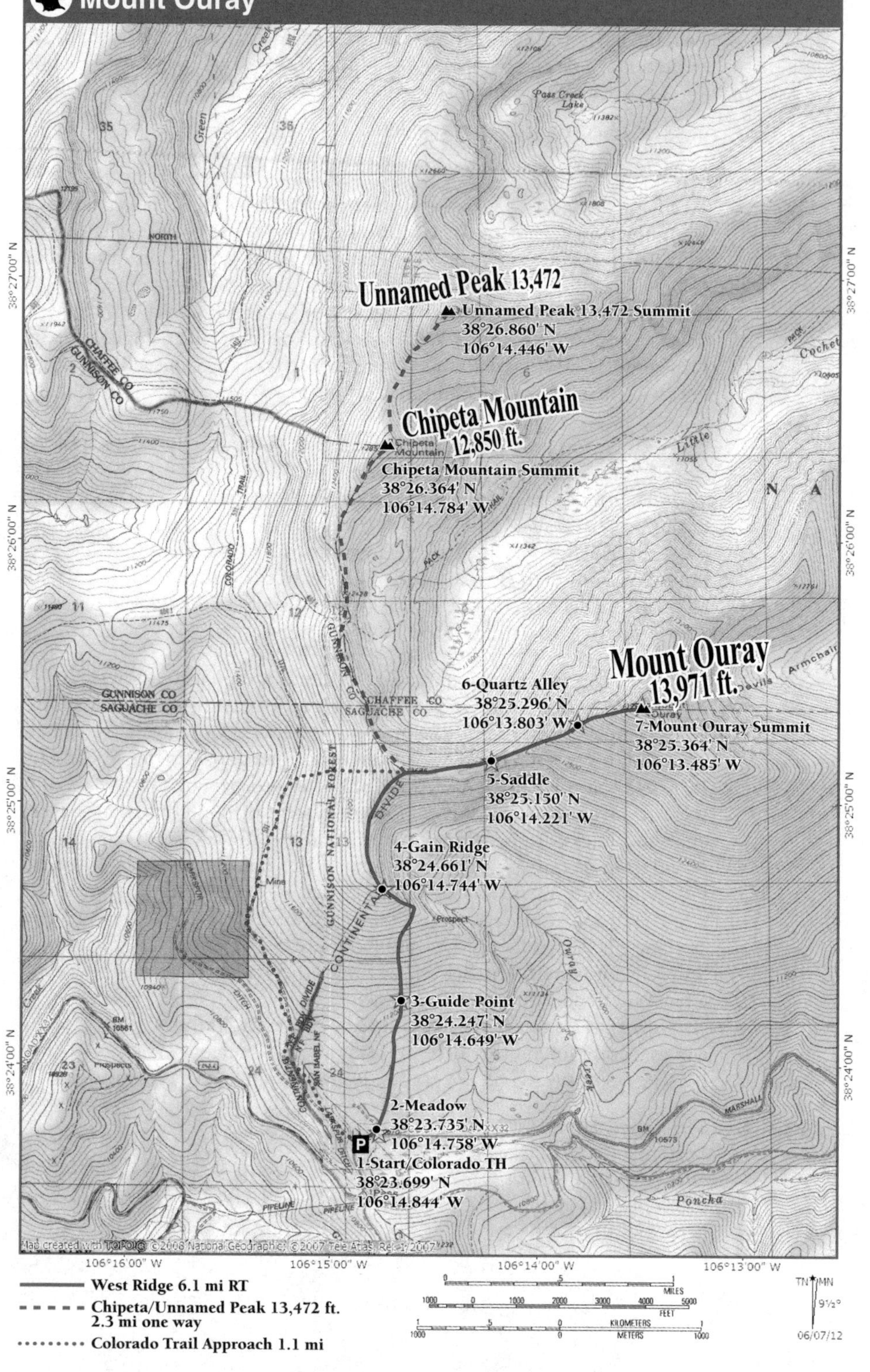
Mount Ouray
Unnamed Peak 13,472
Unnamed Peak 13,472 Summit
38°26.860' N
106°14.446' W
Chipeta Mountain
12,850 ft.
Chipeta Mountain Summit
38°26.364' N
106°14.784' W
Mount Ouray
13,971 ft.
6-Quartz Alley
38°25.296' N
106°13.803' W
7-Mount Ouray Summit
38°25.364' N
106°13.485' W
5-Saddle
38°25.150' N
106°14.221' W
4-Gain Ridge
38°24.661' N
106°14.744' W
3-Guide Point
38°24.247' N
106°14.649' W
2-Meadow
38°23.735' N
106°14.758' W
1-Start/Colorado TH
38°23.699' N
106°14.844' W
GUNNISON CO
SAGUACHE CO
CHAFFEE CO
CONTINENTAL DIVIDE
GUNNISON NATIONAL FOREST
38°27'00" N
38°26'00" N
38°25'00" N
38°24'00" N
106°16'00" W
106°15'00" W
106°14'00" W
106°13'00" W
West Ridge 6.1 mi RT
Chipeta/Unnamed Peak 13,472 ft. 2.3 mi one way
Colorado Trail Approach 1.1 mi
MILES
FEET
KILOMETERS
METERS
TN MN
9½°
06/07/12

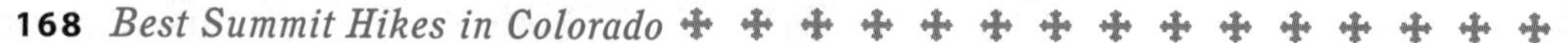

23 Mount Ouray

Ouray's west ridge is an adventure fit for a chief. Named after the great leader of the Utes, this southern Sawatch mountain is a great hike with views to match.

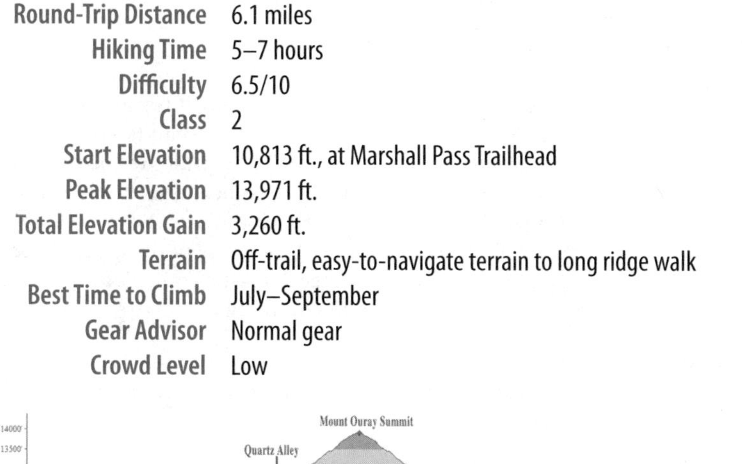

Round-Trip Distance	6.1 miles
Hiking Time	5–7 hours
Difficulty	6.5/10
Class	2
Start Elevation	10,813 ft., at Marshall Pass Trailhead
Peak Elevation	13,971 ft.
Total Elevation Gain	3,260 ft.
Terrain	Off-trail, easy-to-navigate terrain to long ridge walk
Best Time to Climb	July–September
Gear Advisor	Normal gear
Crowd Level	Low

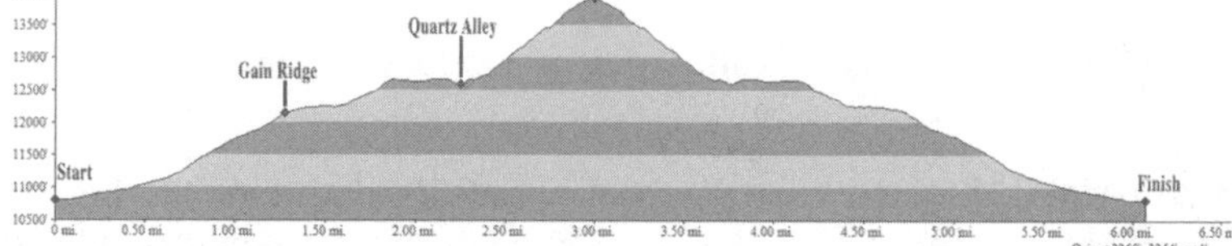

Location Southern Sawatch Range in the San Isabel National Forest outside of Poncha Springs

Intro Viewing it from the south just over Poncha Pass, Mount Ouray looks like a giant, gray, inflatable chair. The rounded contours and large cirque on the east face (another unholy Devil's Armchair) are typical of Sawatch mountains. The long west ridge gives you a catwalk of nearly 2 miles each way, punctuated by views of two major ranges in Colorado: the Sawatch to the north and the Sangre De Cristos to the southeast. (Satan has had quite an influence on Colorado landmarks: Ouray has Devil's Armchair, Lone Cone [Hike 50] is home of the Devil's Chair, and you'll also find Devils Backbone, Devils Cow Camp (for naughty cows?), Devils Elbow, Devils Thumb, Devils Nose, Devils Punchbowl, Devils Kitchen, and Devils Head, to name a few.)

Ouray is one of the southernmost 13ers in the Sawatch Range—though it may actually be a 14er. Several people have noticed GPS readings over 14,000 feet on the top (I had a measurement of 14,005 feet with an error differential of +/- 7 feet.) Perhaps someday it will be admitted into the 14ers club, a fitting honor for Chief Ouray.

Why Climb It? The off-trail approach through flowery meadows is a nice way to start the hike. Navigation is relatively easy, and once you are on the southern curl of the west ridge, you are treated to a long ridge walk to a scenic summit. The scrambling on the ridge is fun class 2 that is sustained the entire way. It's a straightforward Sawatch hike without the tedious switchbacks or gratuitous talus slog, making it a fine bookend to this hiker-friendly range.

Driving Passenger cars can make it to the top of Marshall Pass. The road has a few rocky sections and some potholes but is otherwise well maintained.

How to Get There From the junction of US Highway 50 and US Highway 285 in Poncha Springs, drive 5.1 miles south to the marked turnoff for Marshall Pass. If approaching from the south on US 285, it is roughly 2.4 miles from the top of Poncha Pass. Turn west onto the Marshall Pass Road (County Road 200), which is a dirt road. From here it is 14 miles to the top of the pass. The way up is very well marked. There is a right turn a little past mile 2.0 (it has a sign for Marshall Pass), and from there, the road is easy to follow. The trailhead is just east of Marshall Pass on the left side of the road. There is ample parking and a large sign kiosk for the Colorado Trail. **Note:** If you drive through the cool rock corridor to the top of the pass, you've gone about 0.1 mile too far.

Fees/Camping There are no fees to hike or camp in this area. Campsites abound; there is a small primitive area behind the parking area as well as several similar sites off the summit of Marshall Pass.

Route Notes This hike is quite straightforward; don't be intimidated by the fact that it does not use any trails.

Mile/Waypoint

0.0 mi (1) Start at the Colorado Trailhead lot, just below the top of Marshall Pass. You will not be following trails on this route, though it is possible to take the Colorado Trail north roughly 1 mile and get off-trail east at the base of Ouray's west ridge. The off-trail route is more scenic and easy to follow. Walk east a hundred feet down the road to the open meadows on the north side of the road.

0.1 mi (2) Head into the meadows and aim for the spur of Ouray's west ridge, above tree line. This is easy terrain to navigate; it's mostly open meadows. Get a compass bearing here to the ridge and follow it. A few patches of pine trees are along the way. In a mile, emerge from the intermittent timberline.

0.7 mi (3) This is a guide point for those using GPS.

1.0 mi As you clear the trees, the way to the ridge is obvious. The best footing is found by taking the spur ridge to reach the west ridge.

1.3 mi (4) Gain the spur ridge and follow it as it curves into the west ridge. There are a few ups and downs here. The views of the peak are spectacular from this vantage point.

1.9 mi At 12,670 feet you are now officially on the west ridge. Enjoy the hiking and easy scramble as you head toward the summit.

2.3 mi (5) A windy saddle at 12,600 feet is the low point of the ridge. Keep heading up.

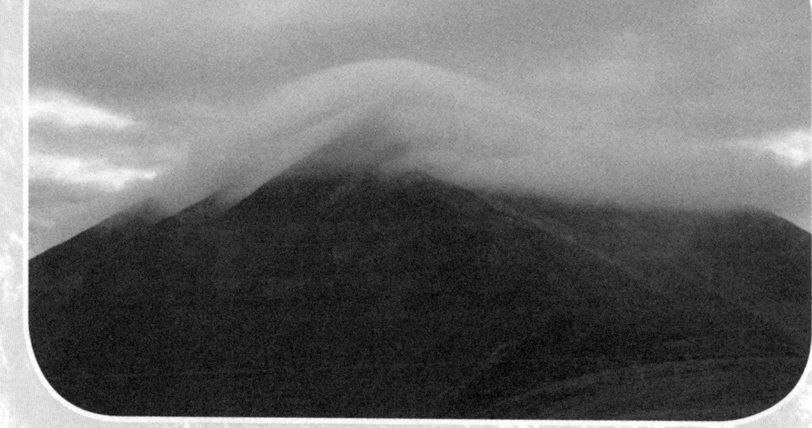

Mystical fog envelops the summit of Mount Ouray.

2.7 mi (6) A band of white quartz is high on the mountain, at 13,350 feet. This quartz alley is the crux of the climb, though you can easily bypass it on the left (west) side. Scrambling up is fun, but the surface is slick when wet. Top the quartz band and continue to the summit.

3.1 mi (7) Mount Ouray's summit! Check your altimeter; you may be on an unrecognized 14er. Return the way you came. The trek through the trees is nothing to worry about. If you get disoriented, just keep heading south and you'll intersect with the Marshall Pass Road.

6.2 mi Finish.

Options Chipeta Mountain (12,850 feet) is an easy walk from the end of Ouray's west ridge (between waypoints **4** and **5**). It is 1.5 miles one way to the north. From here, it is 0.8 mile to a large unnamed peak (UN 13,472). The easy class 2 out-and-back to these two mountains is 4.6 miles round-trip, starting from Ouray's west ridge.

Quick Facts Chief Ouray (pronounced YOO-ray) was a leader of the Tabeguache Utes who tried to negotiate peace between his people and the white men. White leaders appreciated his intellect and willingness to compromise (he met two presidents in his lifetime); Utes respected his leadership and drive. Unfortunately, all his good intentions were in vain—his people were exiled to a Utah reservation in 1880, the year of his death.

Chipeta Mountain honors Ouray's wife, who was exiled to Bitter Creek, Utah, along with the rest of the Utes. She passed away in 1924 and was brought back to Colorado to be buried next to her husband.

Mount Ouray's status as a high 13er or a low 14er has yet to be resolved. Some sources claim that the peak is 29 feet higher than its official height. While it seems apparent that the peak is slightly higher, it may still fall short of being a 14er. Let the controversy rage on!

Contact Info San Isabel National Forest
Salida Ranger District
325 W. Rainbow Boulevard
Salida, CO 81201
(719) 539-3591

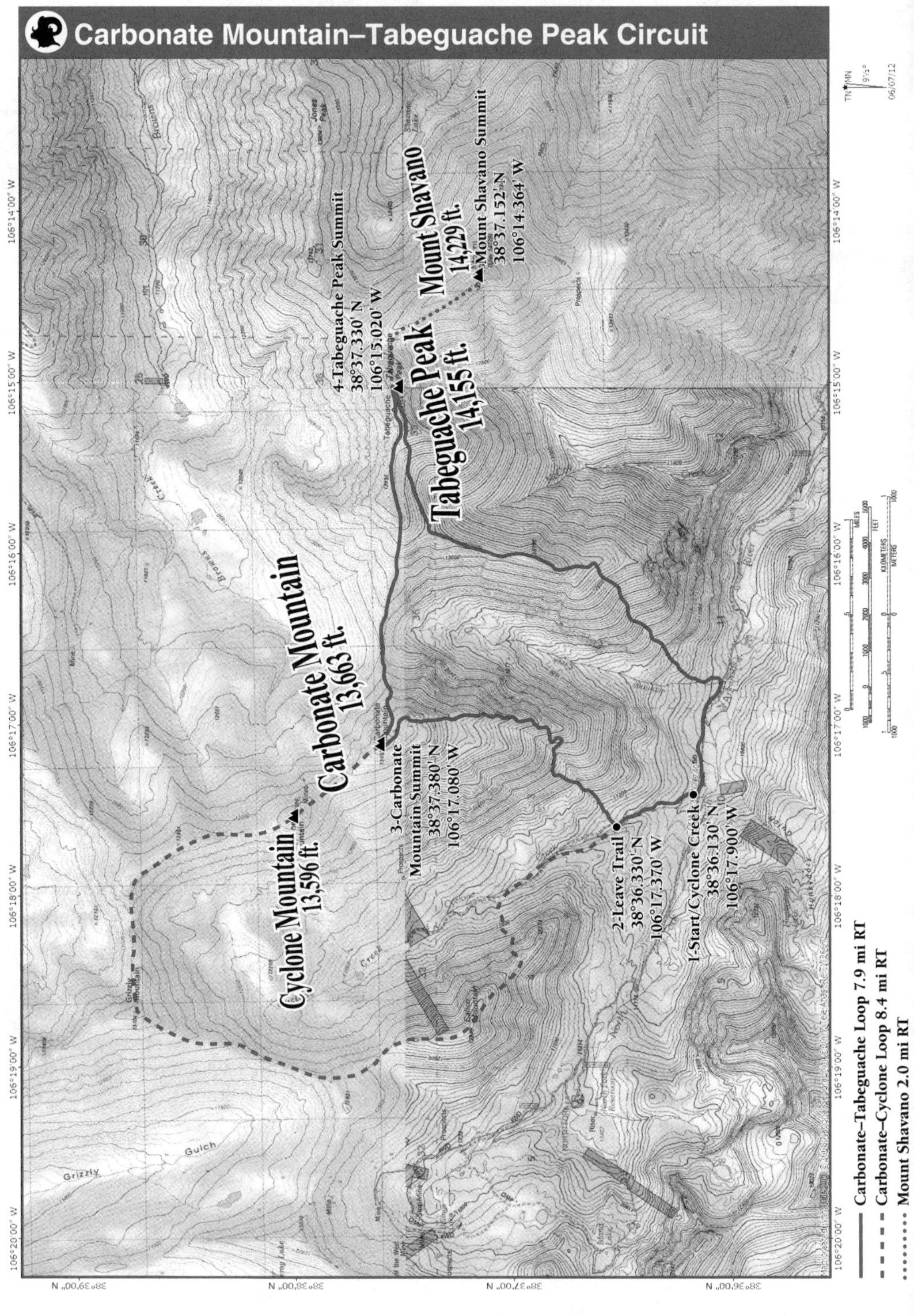

Carbonate Mountain–Tabeguache Peak Circuit
Cyclone Mountain
13,596 ft.
Carbonate Mountain
13,663 ft.
3-Carbonate
Mountain Summit
38°37.380' N
106°17.080' W
Tabeguache Peak
14,155 ft.
4-Tabeguache Peak Summit
38°37.330' N
106°15.020' W
Mount Shavano
14,229 ft.
Mount Shavano Summit
38°37.152' N
106°14.364' W
2-Leave Trail
38°36.330' N
106°17.370' W
1-Start/Cyclone Creek
38°36.130' N
106°17.900' W
Grizzly
Gulch
Browns
Creek
Jones
Peak
106°20'00" W
106°19'00" W
106°18'00" W
106°17'00" W
106°16'00" W
106°15'00" W
106°14'00" W
38°39'00" N
38°38'00" N
38°37'00" N
38°36'00" N
06/07/12
Carbonate–Tabeguache Loop 7.9 mi RT
Carbonate–Cyclone Loop 8.4 mi RT
Mount Shavano 2.0 mi RT

24 Carbonate Mountain–Tabeguache Peak Circuit

A seldom-climbed high 13er is your gateway to amazing ridgeline adventures along Colorado's highest mountain range. Head east to tack on a pair of 14ers, or circle north for the chance to stand atop remote, rugged Sawatch summits.

Round-Trip Distance	7.6 miles
Hiking Time	9–11 hours
Difficulty	8/10
Class	2+/3
Start Elevation	10,765 ft., at Cyclone Creek and County Road 240
Peak Elevations	Carbonate Mountain: 13,663 ft.; Tabeguache Peak: 14,155 ft.
Total Elevation Gain	4,585 ft.
Terrain	Rugged, rocky off-trail with sturdy ridges and semi-loose descents
Best Time to Climb	June–October
Gear Advisor	Sturdy boots, hiking poles, and GPS
Crowd Level	Hermit

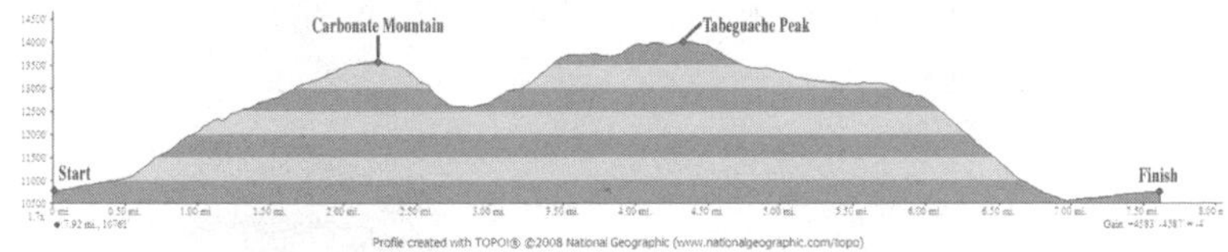

Location Sawatch Range in the Collegiate Peaks Wilderness/San Isabel National Forest near the town of Poncha Springs

Intro Carbonate Mountain is a rarely visited 13er with ridges that connect it to the popular 14er Tabeguache Peak to the east and Cyclone Mountain to the northwest. There's some steep climbing and off-trail navigation, but experienced hikers will have no problem connecting the dots. It's possible to tack on the 14er Mount Shavano as well, a moderate 1-mile traverse from the summit of Tabeguache. This route is drastically less crowded and more enjoyable than the standard Blank Gulch route used for Shavano and Tabeguache.

Why Climb It? The option to run the circuit in either direction means that you can camp at this trailhead and do a new set of peaks each day. Besides avoiding the crowds, the hidden side of the Sawatch Range is a beautiful and magical place, with enticing ridge walks and fun scrambling. Even though this is a fairly remote setting, you're still not far from civilization, and the relics of old ghost mines can be found along Cyclone Creek.

Driving County Road 240 is rocky and steep in sections. A sport utility vehicle or rugged sport utility car, such as a Subaru Outback, will do just fine, and 4x4s with high clearance will have no problem. Cars can get within 4 miles of the trailhead and park at the Angel of Shavano Campground. Because you already have a long day if you start from here, it might be a good idea to hike in and camp if you need to take the road; tacking 8 miles to an already long hike can make for a tough day in the mountains.

How to Get There From the intersection of US Highway 285 and US Highway 50 in Poncha Springs, head west on US 50 for 6.2 miles to the small town of Maysville. Turn right onto CR 240 (there will be signs just before pointing to the Angel of Shavano Campground). This is a paved road that becomes a solid dirt road for the 4 miles to the Angel of Shavano Campground. From here, it is another 4.1 miles along CR 240, high-clearance vehicles only, to the Cyclone Creek Trailhead. Keep an eye on your mileage from the Angel of Shavano Campground as the trailhead for Cyclone Creek is not marked, and there is no real parking lot, just pull-offs on the side of the road. If you reach the old ghost town of Shavano or the North Fork Campground, you've gone a bit too far. There's plenty of great car-camping sites along the way.

Note: Cyclone Creek is one drainage away from Jennings Creek, which was the old standard route up Tabeguache and is closed for restoration. Please make sure that you are starting from the correct place, and avoid disrupting the Jennings Creek Basin.

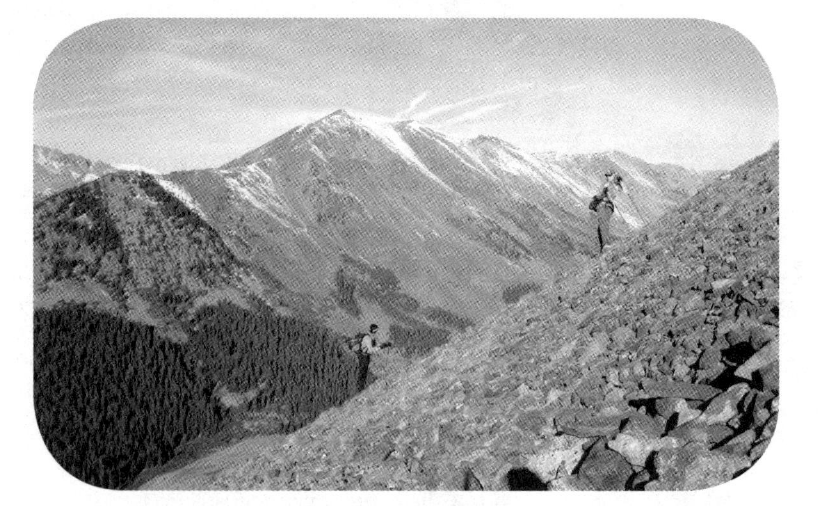

The Cyclone Creek approach to Carbonate Mountain is off-trail and steep—bring poles.

Fees/Camping There are no fees for hiking this area, and there is ample, very good car camping along CR 240. The developed campsites at Angel of Shavano Campground are $15 a night as of 2012.

Route Notes The start of this hike begins at an old, worn-out jeep road that may or may not be easy to find. Check your maps and don't be afraid to freelance a little on the way up. You can always use Cyclone Creek itself as a guide to make sure that you're starting in the right place.

Mile/Waypoint

0.0 mi (1) Start at Cyclone Creek by either following along the creek itself or following the faded jeep road that winds next to it.

0.4 mi (2) At a clearing, look north for the path of least resistance on the south ridge of Carbonate at about 11,036 feet. As you progress, you'll have the option of going east or west of the gully that splits the ridge. Staying on the ridge proper on the right (east) side of the gully may seem tougher at first but ultimately is an easier way to the summit. The slopes to the left of the gully bypass some great old, gnarly trees but present a tougher line.

1.6 mi You will have cleared the tough, steep start and are now ascending Carbonate's moderate southern slopes with a clear and easy shot to the summit.

2.3 mi (3) Way to go—you're on top of Carbonate Mountain! To stay on the standard route, head east and drop down a saddle to go to Tabeguache Peak. If you're taking the optional circuit to Cyclone Mountain and Grizzly Mountain, head northwest here.

4.5 mi (4) After a long and enjoyable scramble along the ridge, you're atop Tabeguache Peak. Mount Shavano's summit is a mile east of here and takes strong hikers 30–40 minutes each way. Return to Tabeguache and get ready to descend. Be careful not to take the direct southern slopes into McCoy Creek. This is a tough, off-trail descent that does eventually hit the road but puts you a few miles out from your start. Instead, aim for the long southern ridge directly south of point 13,936.

5.2 mi This is the ridge below point 13,936. Follow it south, avoiding the temptation to drop down into Jennings Creek to the west. Not only is this basin closed, but it's also a lousy, loose descent.

6.1 mi Follow the ridge to a south-facing gully, which offers the path of least resistance. You can also stay on the ridge proper as both will eventually lead to the road. This is a steep descent, so bring your hiking poles. You may intersect with the old Jennings Creek Trail when you level out about 0.5 mile from the road.

7.2 mi Regain the road and walk west back to you car. If you're really lazy (or happen to have two vehicles), leaving one here can cut out the road finish.

7.9 mi Finish.

Options Options are what this hike is all about. From the standard route, the triple-header of Carbonate, Tabeguache, and Shavano makes for a very satisfying day. Shavano is 1 mile from the summit of Tabeguache, and the hike over is easy class 2 scrambling. A fast hiker can make it over in 30 minutes or so.

Another very fun route is to head north off Carbonate 0.6 mile to the summit of Cyclone Mountain, 13,596 feet. If this is all you want to do, a bailout gully between Carbonate and Cyclone leads back to Cyclone Creek. From Cyclone, it is 1.7 miles to Grizzly Mountain at 13,708 feet (and bypassing point 13,591). Want to keep rolling? Head southwest from Grizzly 1.9 miles to 12,949-foot Calico Mountain, then follow Calico's southeast ridge to a north-facing gully just before point 12,274, and take the gully back to Cyclone Creek and about 1.3 miles back to your car. This super loop is about 8.4 miles round-trip and is ideal for those looking for a wilderness scramble with fun, off-trail mountain navigation. Most of the route is above tree line, so as long as you have line of sight, you'll be able to see Cyclone Creek the entire hike. Bailout lines are plentiful.

Quick Facts

First off, the correct pronunciations of the peaks are "SHAV-uh-no" (with an emphasis like *bungalow*) and "TAB-uh-wahsh." Not Shimano and Tabber Guchie, nor Shamu and Tubberclutch, nor any other odd pronunciation. Taberguache was the white man's spelling of the word the Southern Ute people used for the Northern Utes.

Shavano is a phonetic spelling of the name of a Ute chieftain known as Che-Wa-No. Che-Wa-No was a highly respected, intelligent, and wise leader who received his rank from the greatest Ute of all, Chief Ouray. He did his best to promote peace between Native Americans and whites, acting as a mediator to resolve several major conflicts. He was even taken to Washington and honored by white men for resolving an uprising led by Chief Kaneache. Despite his noble intentions and peaceful demeanor, he and his people were exiled to Utah in 1881.

Mount Ouray, a very high 13er, is climbed less often than Mount Shavano, Chief Ouray's higher rank notwithstanding. Both Ouray and Che-Wa-No were peaceful and strong leaders who were overpowered by the white man's ambitions to control the land.

The famous Angel of Shavano has been compared to the Cross Couloir on the Mount of the Holy Cross for its religious significance, though native people referred to it as the Indian Princess.

Contact Info

San Isabel National Forest
Leadville District
2015 N. Poplar Street
Leadville, CO 80461
(719) 486-0749

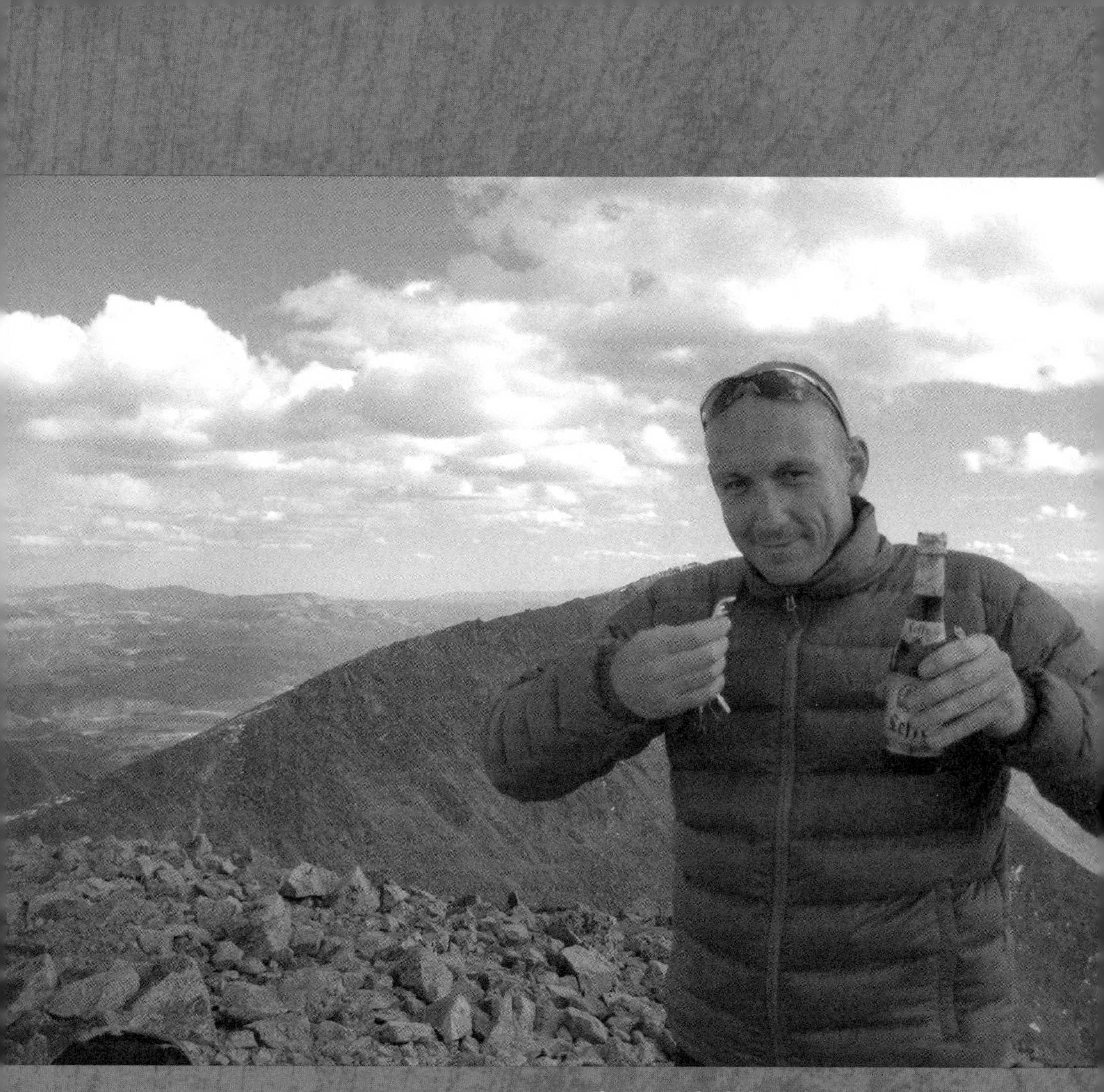

Cheers to the lofty summit of Tabeguache!

Mount Yale

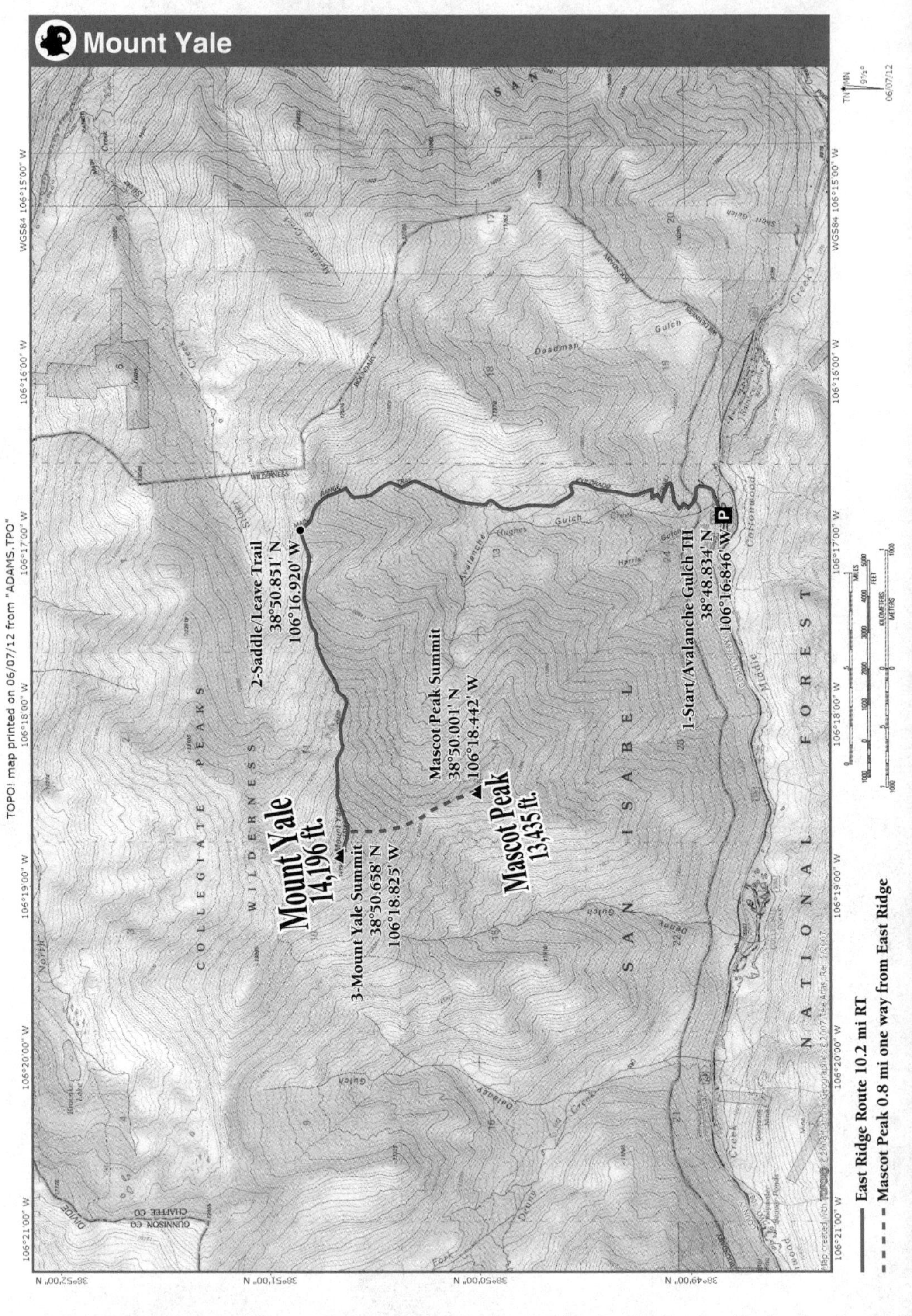

TOPO! map printed on 06/07/12 from "ADAMS.TPO"
Mount Yale
14,196 ft.
3-Mount Yale Summit
38°50.658' N
106°18.825' W
2-Saddle/Leave Trail
38°50.851' N
106°16.920' W
Mascot Peak Summit
38°50.001' N
106°18.442' W
Mascot Peak
13,435 ft.
1-Start/Avalanche Gulch TH
38°48.834' N
106°16.846' W
P
COLLEGIATE PEAKS
WILDERNESS
SAN ISABEL
NATIONAL FOREST
Avalanche
Hughes
Gulch
Harris
Deadman
Gulch
Cottonwood
Middle
Creek
Denny
Gulch
Delaney
Gulch
GUNNISON CO
CHAFFEE CO
DIVIDE
106°21'00" W
106°20'00" W
106°19'00" W
106°18'00" W
106°17'00" W
106°16'00" W
WGS84 106°15'00" W
38°52'00" N
38°51'00" N
38°50'00" N
38°49'00" N
TN
MN
9½°
06/07/12
East Ridge Route 10.2 mi RT
Mascot Peak 0.8 mi one way from East Ridge

25 Mount Yale

Yale's 2-mile east ridge is an exciting scramble that prolongs the fun of hiking on a narrow ridge. Exposure is minimal, but the route is thrilling nonetheless.

Round-Trip Distance	10.2 miles
Hiking Time	6–8 hours
Difficulty	7/10
Class	2+
Start Elevation	9,389 ft., at Avalanche Gulch Trailhead
Peak Elevation	14,196 ft.
Total Elevation Gain	4,950 ft.
Terrain	Good trail to rocky ridge walk
Best Time to Climb	July–September
Gear Advisor	Normal gear
Crowd Level	Low

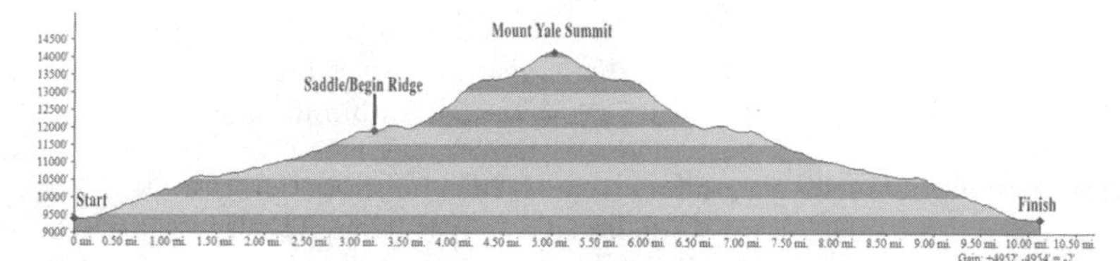

Location Sawatch Range in the Collegiate Peaks Wilderness/San Isabel National Forest outside of Buena Vista

Intro One can only ponder the way our maps would look if this mountain was named after a *different* Connecticut college. We could have been hiking Mount Mattatuck Community College! No matter what you call it, Yale is a prominent 14er cast from the classic, rounded Sawatch mold. The east ridge is not the standard route on Yale, perhaps due to the slightly technical nature of the ascent. At 2.0 miles one way, it's one of the longest ridge walks in Colorado.

Why Climb It? The drawn-out east ridge has good, easy scrambling. It's a fine first ridge walk for those who have only done on-trail hiking. This slight variation on the Sawatch theme means that you won't be grinding up miles of talus. The east ridge is broad and gives the excitement of a narrow walkway without the dangerous exposure. Views from Yale are great, as it is smack in the middle of the Sawatch Range, standing apart from the other Collegiate Peaks.

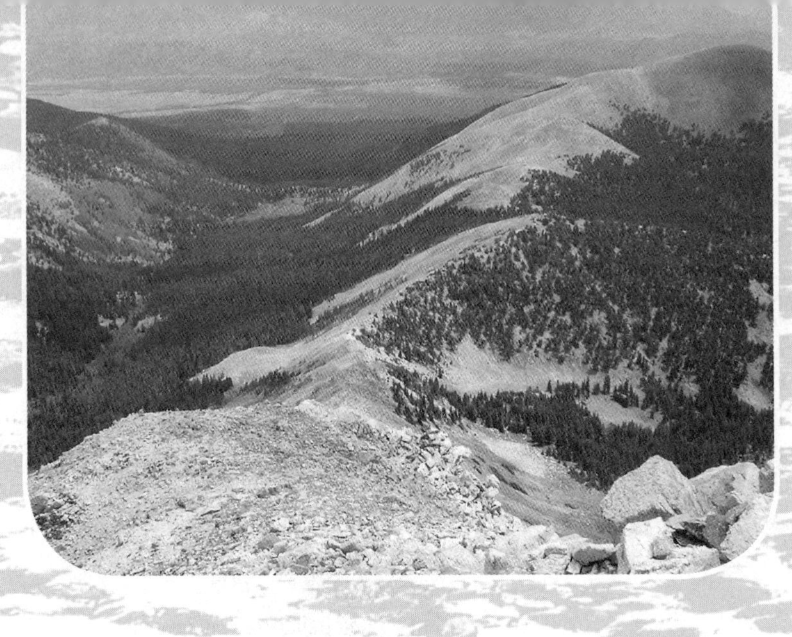
A look back to the saddle from halfway up the east ridge of Mount Yale

Driving Avalanche Gulch Trailhead is off a paved road, and any vehicle can make the trailhead.

How to Get There From downtown Buena Vista on US Highway 24, turn west onto County Road 306 (Cottonwood Pass Road). Follow the road 9.2 miles and turn right (north) into the Avalanche Gulch Trailhead parking lot, which is quite large. The turnoff is just west of Rainbow Lake.

Fees/Camping There are no fees to hike Yale, but note that camping is not allowed at the spacious Avalanche Gulch Trailhead. The large and beautiful Collegiate Peaks Campground is 1.7 miles farther west on CR 306. There are 56 sites available, and the cost is $10 per night. There are some good backcountry campsites 1.4 miles in along this trail.

Route Notes If you got a late start or weather seems to be moving in quickly, you may want to reconsider getting out on the ridge. You'll be walking 4.0 miles (round-trip) on exposed terrain with very little shelter. It's not technical, but you won't be moving as fast as you would on a trail. Start a little extra early on this peak; I've seen some of the most violent and fast-forming storms in Colorado in this area of the Collegiate Peaks.

Mile/Waypoint **0.0 mi (1)** Start at the Avalanche Gulch Trailhead. Get on the Colorado Trail and go north toward the saddle of Yale and point 12,505. From lower elevations, you won't be able to see Yale's summit; the large, rocky peak to your left (west) is Unnamed Peak 13,435, on Yale's south shoulder. Some call this mountain Mascot Peak.

0.2 mi A small connector trail joins from the right; stay left on the Colorado Trail. This should be obvious, and it is just before the trail starts switchbacking up an open hillside. From here, the well-worn Colorado Trail is very easy to follow as it winds through the woods. Enjoy the warm-up.

3.2 mi (2) Your time in the woods comes to an end as you reach the saddle at 11,900 feet. There are a few trees, but the views are mostly open, especially to the north. Here you will leave the trail, turning left (west) onto the east ridge. There are intermittent trails you can follow. Use them as you see fit.

From this point, the hiking is very straightforward. You'll see Mount Yale directly in front of you. The ridge is long and without any major obstacles. A few rock outcrops can be scrambled or skirted, and none of the easier routes exceeds class 2+. Navigation is easy—just stay on the high point of the ridge and head west. At points 13,420 and 13,900 there are some larger outcrops that may be considered false summits (though you'll have views of Yale's true summit the entire time). At 13,600 feet, you'll actually go downhill slightly before the final push to Yale's lofty summit.

5.2 mi (3) Yale's summit! To the north, you'll see many of the Collegiate Peaks, notably Mount Columbia, Mount Harvard, and the Missouri group. To the south, Mount Princeton, Mount Antero, and Tabeguache Peak will stand out. Try to reach the top of this peak no later than 10 a.m. (it's about a four-hour ascent).

On your descent, be aware that it takes quite awhile to get back down the ridge. Return the way you came.

10.2 mi Finish.

Options You can drop off Yale's east ridge just below the final summit hill and take the south ridge 0.8 mile over to 13,435-foot Mascot Peak. While it's feasible to descend Mascot's southeast ridge, going through the woods is rocky, rough, and not much fun. You may be inclined to do so if your navigation skills are adequate (or if the thought of reclimbing 600 feet to the east ridge is not your cup of tea).

Quick Facts Mount Yale was named by Professor Josiah D. Whitney, head of the Harvard Mining School. Did he lose a bet? Why would he name it after Harvard's Ivy League rival? As it turns out, Whitney graduated from Yale and thus honored his alma mater after a surveying trip in 1869. Of course, he named the higher 14,420-foot peak to the north Mount Harvard. Take that, old chap!

Contact Info San Isabel National Forest
Leadville Ranger District
2015 N. Poplar Street
Leadville, CO 80461
(719) 486-0752

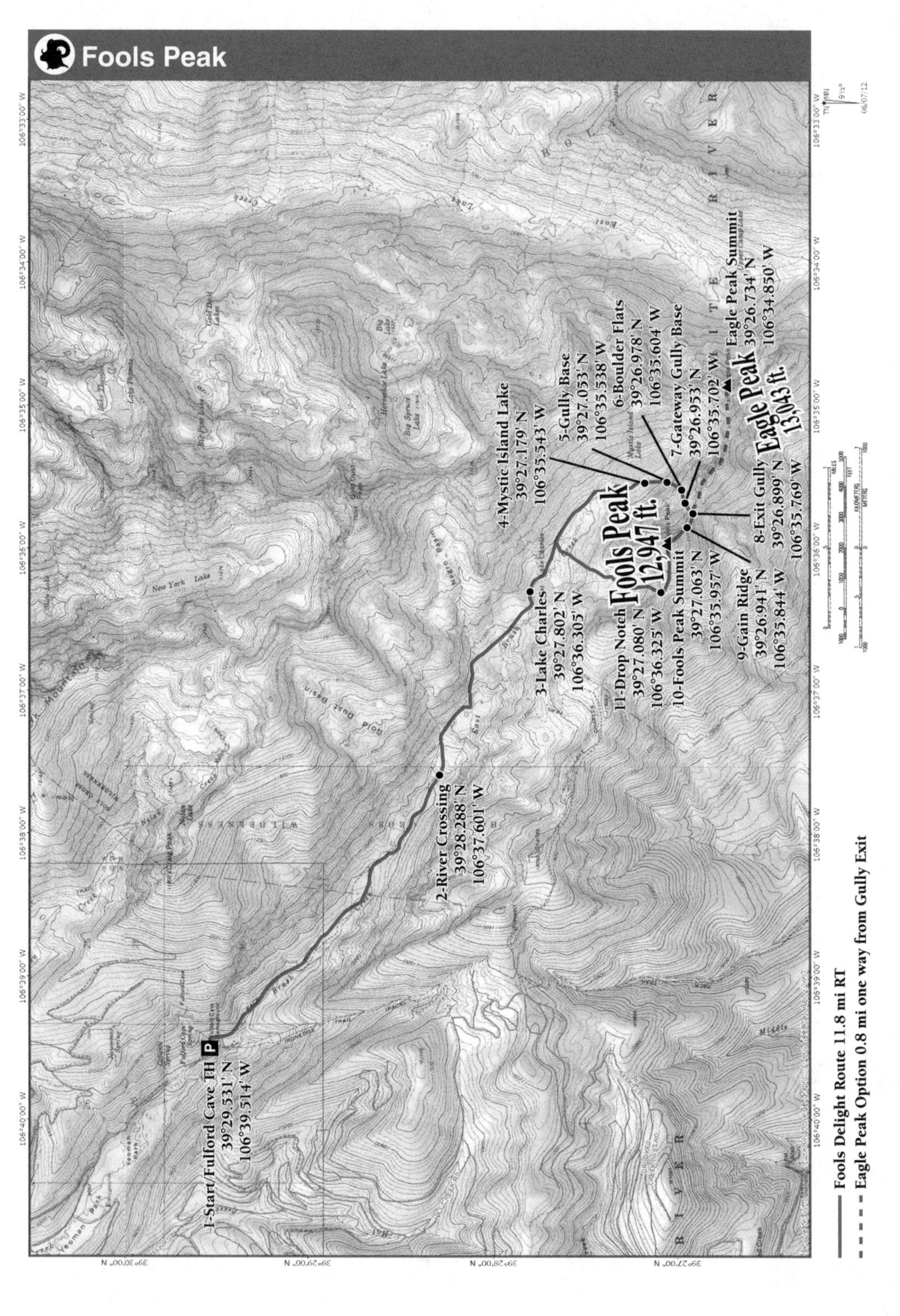
Fools Peak
1-Start/Fulford Cave TH
39°29.531' N
106°39.514' W
2-River Crossing
39°28.288' N
106°37.601' W
3-Lake Charles
39°27.802' N
106°36.305' W
4-Mystic Island Lake
39°27.179' N
106°35.543' W
5-Gully Base
39°27.053' N
106°35.538' W
6-Boulder Flats
39°26.978' N
106°35.604' W
7-Gateway Gully Base
39°26.953' N
106°35.702' W
8-Exit Gully
39°26.899' N
106°35.769' W
9-Gain Ridge
39°26.941' N
106°35.844' W
10-Fools Peak Summit
39°27.063' N
106°35.957' W
11-Drop Notch
39°27.080' N
106°36.325' W
Fools Peak
12,947 ft.
Eagle Peak
13,043 ft.
Eagle Peak Summit
39°26.734' N
106°34.850' W
New York Lake
Fools Delight Route 11.8 mi RT
Eagle Peak Option 0.8 mi one way from Gully Exit

26 Fools Peak

Good Overnight!

You'd be foolish to miss this spectacular peak! A unique gully scramble tops out on a ridge that features exceptional class 3 terrain. This is a great climb with very good camping.

Round-Trip Distance	11.8 miles
Hiking Time	7–10 hours
Difficulty	8/10
Class	3
Start Elevation	9,430 ft., at Charles Lake/Fulford Cave Trailhead
Peak Elevation	12,947 ft.
Total Elevation Gain	3,470 ft.
Terrain	Good trail to interesting, mixed terrain gully; rocky descent
Best Time to Climb	July–September
Gear Advisor	Gaiters, helmet, and solid boots
Crowd Level	Low to lakes; hermit on peak

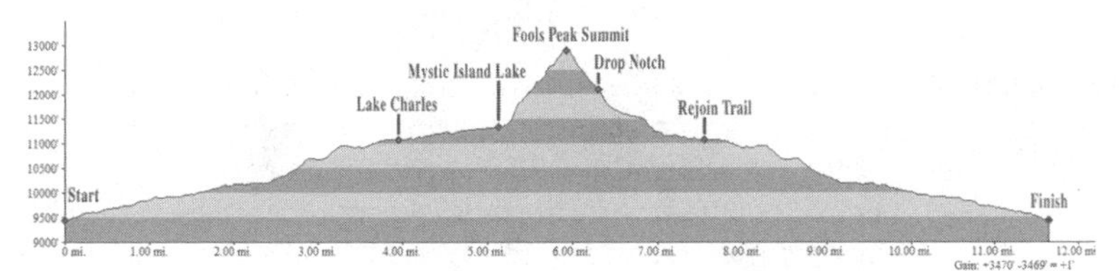

Location Sawatch Range in the Holy Cross Wilderness/White River National Forest outside of Eagle

Intro Mystic Island Lake and Lake Charles are grand destinations for overnight camping. Situated in a brilliant basin, surround by high-rising mountains, this rugged area is unlike any other in the Sawatch Range. Fools Peak is a visually stunning mountain, especially when viewed from the small lakes just east of Lake Charles. If you're ready for an off-trail adventure to one of Colorado's best-kept secrets, this is the hike for you.

Why Climb It? I could rave on and on about the beauty of the lakes below Fools; only the Lion Lakes at Mount Alice rival them for pure splendor. Even though this is a very feasible day hike, I highly recommend camping. Not only does an overnight give you an early jump on the mountain, but it also gives you glorious views of the deep, dark night sky. On clear evenings, stars sparkle in the black canopy, often smeared with the faint glow of the Milky Way. The pure ambience is complemented by a great class 3 gully that scrambles up watery cliffs and steep boulders. A final gully deposits you on Fools's southwest ridge, a short section that features some of the best class 3 scrambling around. A rocky descent lets you loop back down to the lakes.

Driving Passenger cars can make it to the Fulford Cave Trailhead on a well-maintained dirt road. Please note that you are heading toward Fulford Cave, not the ghost town of Fulford.

How to Get There From I-70, take Exit 147 to Eagle. Exit south toward the town of Eagle. At the roundabout, take the first right. From the right at the roundabout, turn left onto Broadway, then left onto Fifth Street, and then right onto Capital. The distances between these turns are only 0.1 to 0.2 mile each, so keep an eye out for signs. Going south on Capital will bring you to a stop sign. Turn left onto Brush Creek Road (note that going straight instead brings you to a nice park—a good place to hang out after the hike). At 0.7 mile after the left at the stop sign, turn right to continue on Brush Creek Road, which is now labeled Forest Road 400. Follow this paved road 9.0 miles to the junction of Brush Creek Road and Forest Road 415 (this split turns to dirt).

Take a left and continue on this road 7.4 miles, following the signs for Fulford Cave Campground/Fulford Cave. Stay on the obvious main road (a few 4x4 road turnoffs are along the way). At mile 6.3, you'll see a sign that reads FULFORD CAVE CAMPGROUND 1 MILE and FULFORD 4 MILES. Do not take the road up to the ghost town of Fulford; stay on the main road to its terminus at 7.4 miles. A small campground, toilets, and some sign kiosks are at the trailhead (there's also a stinky, swampy pond). Don't camp here unless you have to—the bugs are atrocious!

Fees/Camping There are no fees to hike here, though the Holy Cross Wilderness requires you to acquire a permit, which is free. The camping is $7 per night at Fulford Cave Campground; there are only six sites. Only camp here if you have to—the backcountry camping is free. The best campsites are between Charles and Mystic Island Lakes and on the south side of Mystic Island Lake.

Route Notes This scramble requires good route finding in the gully; it's not a good choice for inexperienced scramblers. Because this is a loop, you can feel confident that any tricky sections you ascend won't have to be down climbed.

Mile/Waypoint **0.0 mi (1)** Start at the Fulford Cave Trailhead and head east on the Lake Charles Trail (#1899). Do not take the Ironedge Trail (at the very beginning of the hike), which goes west and downhill. The Lake Charles Trail starts uphill and climbs steadily before following East Brush Creek.

Once you are on the trail, it is well-worn and easy to follow. Two river crossings are accomplished by means of downed trees and rocks in the water—nothing too serious.

2.5 mi (2) At the second river crossing, you'll begin gaining elevation. There are a lot of windblown trees down, so you'll need to take detours where they block the trail. As you get higher, you'll see spectacular black rock walls on both sides of the trail. These are your clues that you are nearing the first of the lower lakes.

4.2 mi (3) The trail emerges into a large meadow; you'll come to a few small lakes before reaching Lake Charles. The hill above Lake Charles is a good place to camp. Not only are the views good, but you will also end the loop portion of the hike in this area. Trails get sort of spotty between here and Mystic Island Lake, but the way up is obvious: just follow the creek.

5.2 mi (4) The trail officially ends at Mystic Island Lake. Continue along the west side of the lake (there's good camping here, too). You'll see several gullies on the right; finding the correct one to continue up can be tricky.

5.3 mi (5) The proper gully to ascend is here at waypoint **5**, at an elevation of 11,480 feet. A dirt patch that looks like a possible trail is at its base; it is the first notch after a large gray rock with black water "stains" and lichen.

It's only 0.15 mile to your next goal, Boulder Flats, but you'll be gaining 450 vertical feet on tricky terrain. This is the hardest scrambling of the hike. The best line stays to the right of the gully, near the solid rock that makes up the right wall. You'll alternate between rocky outcrops and grassy ledges; there are also some mini-waterfalls running down the safest routes. Good scramblers will have no problem finding a good route. Keep climbing. Even when it looks like you may top out, there are always good options—and remember that you don't have to descend what you climb up.

5.5 mi (6) I like to call this semi-flat ledge Boulder Flats. (It would be a very neat place to pitch a tent.) The hardest climbing is behind you, and from here, you can see the good line to the ridge. The dirt-filled Gateway Gully beckons. Hop on the boulders to its base.

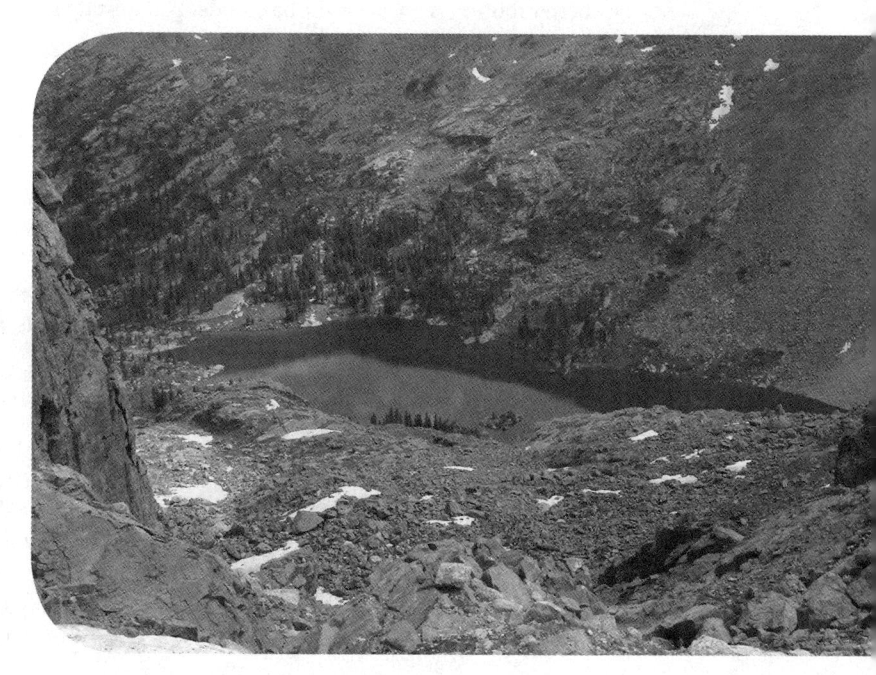

Mystic Island Lake from the gully up Fools Peak

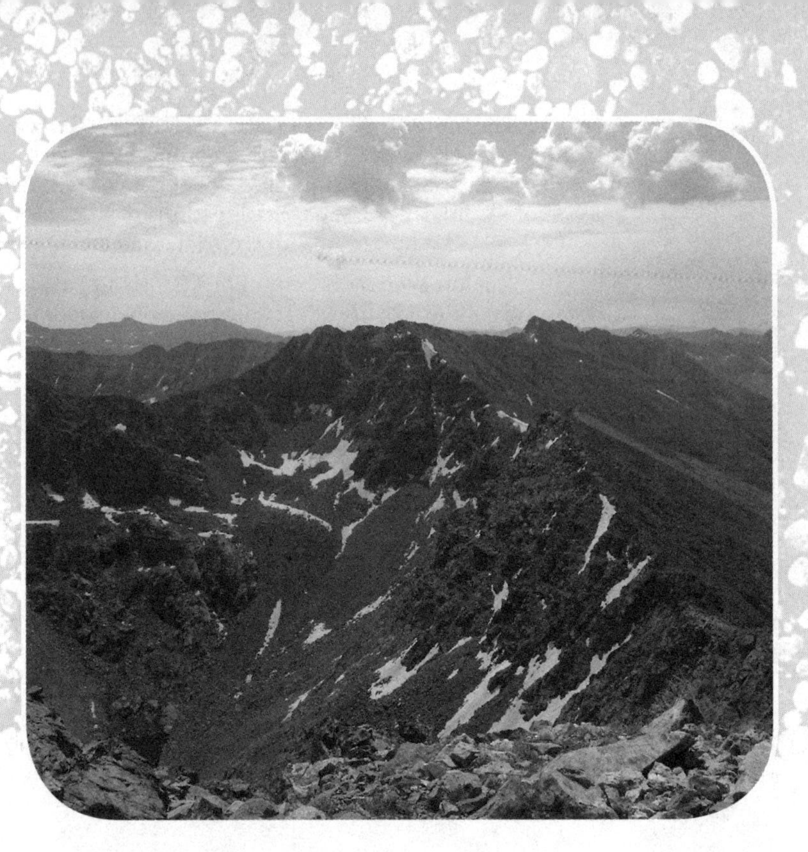

Eagle Peak is one of the more remote 13ers.

5.6 mi (7) This is the base of the gully (a waypoint for those using GPS). The better footing is on the right-hand side. Follow it up to the ridge.

5.7 mi (8) Exit the gully. The optional traverse to Eagle Peak goes to the left (east) from here. If you plan to get it, camp out and get an early start. The way to Fools is to the right (west). There is a steep rock outcrop guarding the ridge, so you'll need to skirt around the south side of the mountain. Go around the outcrop and take the first "lane" up to the ridge that you feel comfortable scrambling. Boulders are set in the grassy slope, and the scrambling is good. Climbing should not exceed class 3; if you feel the route is too tricky, go slightly farther west before ascending north onto the ridge.

5.8 mi (9) Gain the ridge. All the fun scrambling has led to this last hike to the summit, which tops out in dramatic fashion. You'll feel as though you're on top of the world in just a few more steps.

6.0 mi (10) White rock surrounds you on the summit of Fools Peak. The yodeling is quite good up here! The 360-degree views are awesome. Peer over the north edge and wave to hikers down at Mystic Island Lake—they may be shocked to see you up here. Once you've had your fun, continue down the west ridge. Proving it is in fact a Sawatch peak, the slope down to Drop Notch is paved with boulders of all sizes. It's class 2, but step lightly. At the low point of the west ridge, you'll exit north to a high, swampy area.

6.4 mi (11) Get off the ridge and scramble down the steep, talus-filled slopes of Drop Notch. Aim for the ponds at the base of the gully. The rock here is loose and a bit annoying, but it is not exposed. When you finally reach the spongy grass around the lakes, your knees will thank you. Bushwhack north to intercept the trail—the foliage isn't dense, but there are a few areas where you might "cliff out" on small cliffs. I found that staying slightly right (east) gave me the best line. You'll have good sight lines to Charles Lake, so just keep going north, and you'll eventually hit the trail.

7.4 mi Rejoin the trail and return the way you came. Well done!

11.8 mi Finish.

Options The hike to 13,043-foot Eagle Peak is a class 2 traverse covering 0.8 mile from the top of Gateway Gully. If you hike over to it, return back over Fools and follow the standard route down.

Though it's not covered in this book due to its technical nature, a May or June ascent of the April Day Couloir on the north face of the mountain is a great snow climb once the avalanche danger has cleared.

Spelunkers should take a trip up to Fulford Cave, a large labyrinth of stalagmites and stalactites. Please call rangers for more information on exploring this unique cave.

Quick Facts The rangers and historians I consulted were unable to tell me the origin of the name Fools Peak. It was likely named for some joker who probably got into a heap of trouble on the mountain. Mystic Island Lake is so named for the small, enchanting island on the southern side of the chilly lake.

Fulford Cave and the ghost town of Fulford honor the memory Arthur H. Fulford, an affable prospector who perished in an avalanche in 1892.

Contact Info White River National Forest
Eagle District
125 W. Fifth Street
P.O. Box 720
Eagle, CO 81631
(970) 328-6388

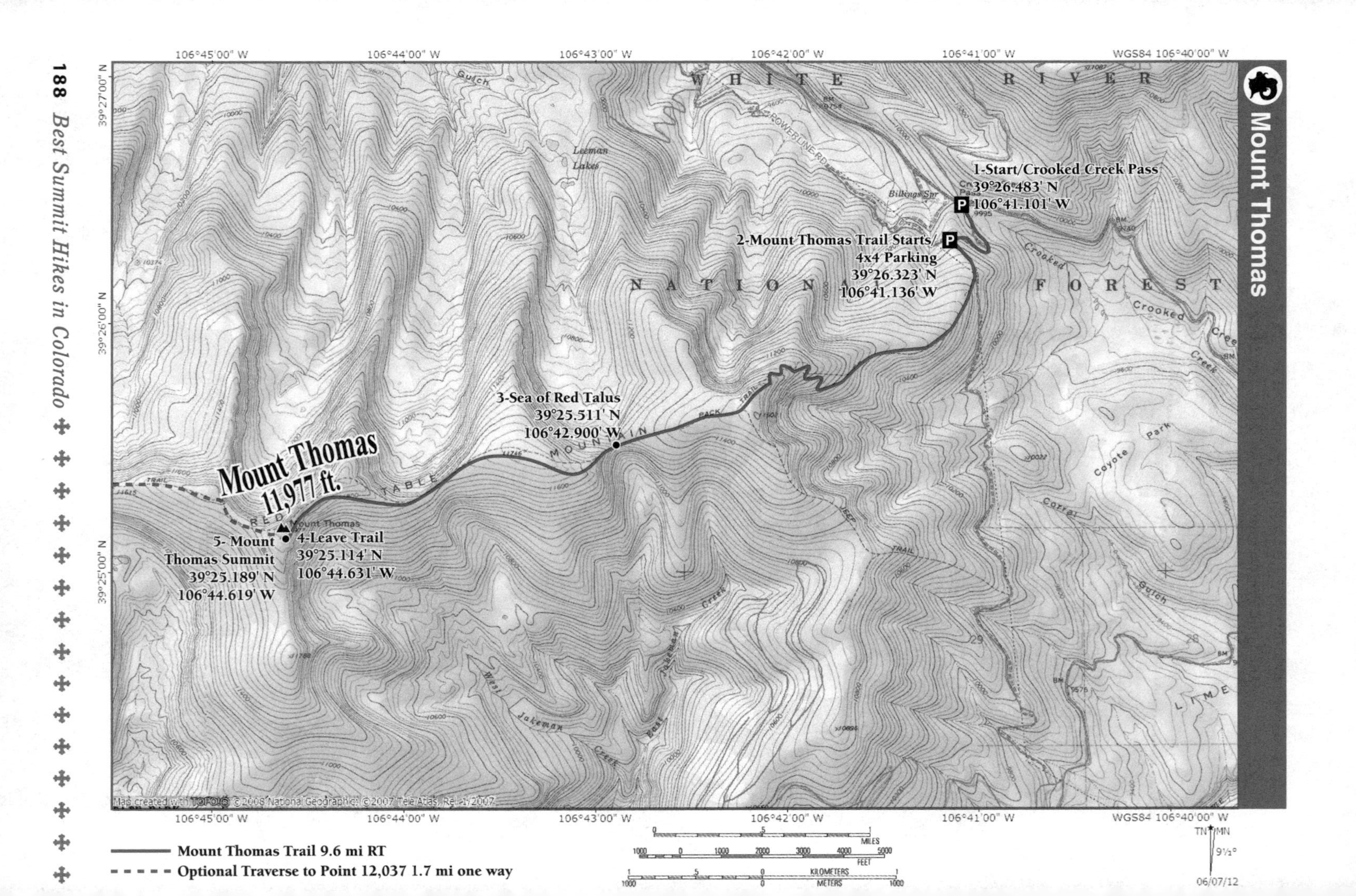

Mount Thomas
1-Start/Crooked Creek Pass
39°26.483' N
106°41.101' W
2-Mount Thomas Trail Starts/
4x4 Parking
39°26.323' N
106°41.136' W
3-Sea of Red Talus
39°25.511' N
106°42.900' W
Mount Thomas
11,977 ft.
5- Mount
Thomas Summit
39°25.189' N
106°44.619' W
4-Leave Trail
39°25.114' N
106°44.631' W
WHITE RIVER NATIONAL FOREST
Mount Thomas Trail 9.6 mi RT
Optional Traverse to Point 12,037 1.7 mi one way
Map created with TOPO! © 2008 National Geographic; © 2007 Tele Atlas, Rel. 1/2007
06/07/12

27 Mount Thomas

Mount Thomas is a relatively easy hike but one filled with many surprises. This wildflower haven features unique geology with great talus rivers and spicy red rocks.

Round-Trip Distance	9.6 miles
Hiking Time	4½–6 hours
Difficulty	2/10
Class	1
Start Elevation	10,007 ft., at Crooked Creek Pass
Peak Elevation	11,977 ft.
Total Elevation Gain	2,850 ft.
Terrain	Easy trail on unique terrain and amid gorgeous scenery
Best Time to Climb	May–October
Gear Advisor	Normal gear
Crowd Level	Low

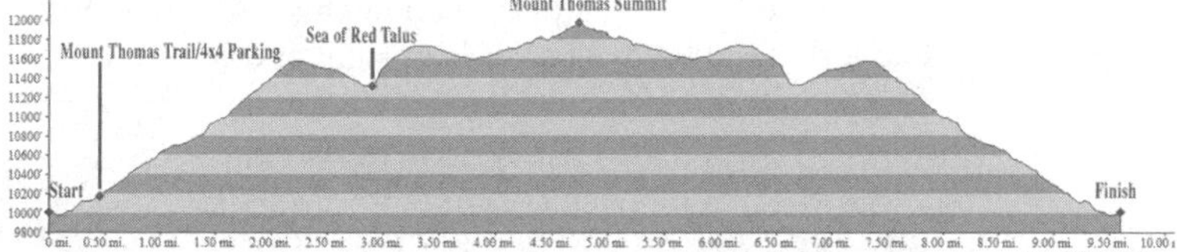

Location Red Table Mountain in the White River National Forest near Eagle and Sylvan Lake

Intro Mount Thomas has a different flavor than other hikes in this book; it's a mellow, peaceful hike with an emphasis on the beauty and unique geology of Red Table Mountain. From a distance, the crimson cliffs resemble the foundation of a giant, unfinished mountain. Because it lacks the glamour and notoriety of other wilderness areas, the chances of seeing pure Colorado alpine scenery are greatly increased. Climbing Mount Thomas affords views into five different wilderness areas, not to mention exceptional views of Pyramid Peak, Mount Sopris (Hike 35), Fools Peak (a class 3 climb, Hike 26), and panoramic vistas of the towns of Aspen and Snowmass Village.

Why Climb It? If the Garden of Eden was to be relocated to an alpine setting, Mount Thomas would be an obvious choice. Wildflowers grow in ponds of swirling colors, complemented by legions of vibrant butterflies patrolling for pollen. After a deceptively modern start under crackling power lines, it soon becomes apparent that mankind has left a softer boot print in these immaculate alpine meadows. Wildlife has taken refuge in the vanilla- and pine-scented forest; mountain lions, black bears, badgers, elk, porcupines, marmots, and even the rare lynx are all acquainted with Red Table Mountain. Half of this hike is above tree line, and the 360-degree views are among the best in the state. At times, the beauty of this area is overwhelming; it will recharge your spirit in the same way that clear, fresh mountain air refreshes your body.

Driving Passenger cars can make it to the top of Crooked Creek Pass, a well-maintained dirt road. The walk from the top of the pass to the formal trailhead is short and pleasant. If you have a Jeep or rugged 4x4, you can try to drive the 0.4 mile on a violently rutted and washed-out road to a small parking area. Sport utility vehicles would probably not make it or would get banged up in the process. When I hiked the peak, I was able to walk up the road faster than a Jeep was able to drive up.

How to Get There From I-70, take Exit 147 to Eagle. Exit south toward the town of Eagle. At the roundabout, take the first right. From the right at the roundabout, turn left onto Broadway, then left onto Fifth Street, and then right onto Capital. The distances between these turns are only 0.1 to 0.2 mile each, so keep an eye out for signs. Going south on Capital will bring you to a stop sign. Turn left onto Brush Creek Road (note that going straight instead brings you to a nice park—a good place to hang out after the hike). At 0.7 mile after the left at the stop sign, turn right to continue on Brush Creek Road, which is now labeled Forest Road 400. Follow this paved road 9.0 miles. Where the road forks (and turns to dirt), bear right and continue to follow the signs to

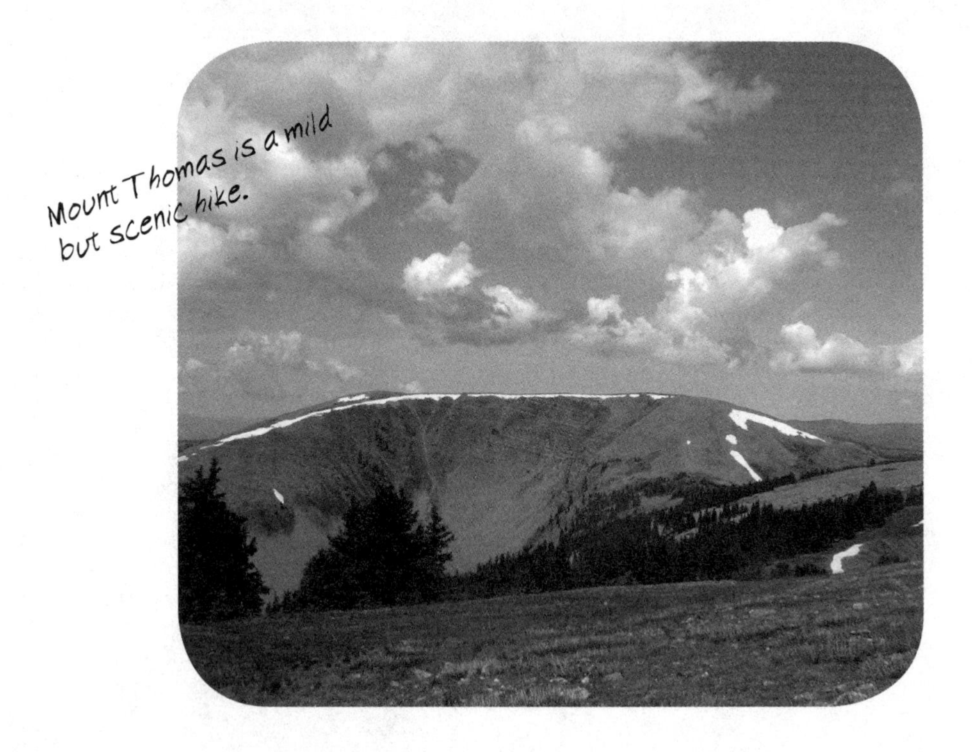

Mount Thomas is a mild but scenic hike.

Sylvan Lake. From the intersection, it is 4.4 miles to Sylvan Lake. Go past the lake and continue up the road toward Crooked Creek Pass. After you pass through an opened gate, this road gets a little narrow but is still in very good condition. Continue 5.3 miles (you'll cross a cattle gate) to the top of Crooked Creek Pass, where a sign reads EAGLE 20/THOMASVILLE 12. You can park here on the right. Your hike will begin by going right on the dirt road that drops down off the top of the pass. (Do *not* start on the trail marked RED TABLE MOUNTAIN 8). Those driving 4x4s can try the road to the trailhead if they feel so inclined.

Note: Even passenger cars can drive a short distance down this road and park in a bumpy lot on the left at the bottom of the hill. There are some nice, big pine trees here to keep your vehicle in the shade while you hike.

Fees/Camping

There are no fees to hike or camp in the Mount Thomas area. There are some primitive camping sites at the top of Crooked Creek Pass and several fee sites below at Sylvan Lake.

Route Notes

None.

Mile/Waypoint

0.0 mi (1) Start at the top of Crooked Creek Pass. After the cattle gate, start by walking (or driving if you have a 4x4) right (south) down a shady 4x4 road. Stay on this road to the Mount Thomas Trailhead. Note that there is one split in the road; stay left (you'll see a sign for Forest Service Road 431), and hike up the steep hill. As you continue up the road, you'll see and hear crackling power line towers above you.

0.5 mi (2) Look for a worn parking lot off to the right, near the top of a hill. You'll be hiking directly under the power lines just before reaching the right turnoff (it can fit about three Jeeps). Cross under the power lines, and to your surprise, you'll see a nice sign for the Mount Thomas Trail (#1870). The hardest part of your hike is over. Once you're on this trail, you can turn on cruise control and take in the sights, smells, and sounds of untainted nature.

0.7 mi The trail is easy to follow and diverts from the intrusive power lines. Head southwest and continue a steady climb. I don't want to ruin any surprises, but get ready for some stunning wildflower meadows. You'll climb in and out of aspen and pine trees, with views opening up the higher you get. There isn't much signage, but the trail is very well worn. Continue west on this fine trail.

2.6 mi Though this hike never truly breaks tree line, you'll come to an open mountaintop area where the trees will be spaced out in sporadic pockets. The views just keep getting better.

2.9 mi (3) Continue on the trail as it crosses the sea of red talus, a giant slide of red boulders that looks like a stone river cascading down the mountainside. Stay the course on the trail (which you'll note is slightly south of the mapped trail, as it doesn't quite follow the ridgetops—though you are welcome to do so if you wish).

4.7 mi (4) At mile 4.7, you'll be just below the summit of Mount Thomas. Get off the trail for a short distance to make your way up.

4.8 mi (5) Mount Thomas's summit! Enjoy the incredible views, especially of the continuing chain of peaks on Red Table Mountain, to the west. Check out the "Options" section for a bonus trek over to the highest peak on Red Table Mountain. Regardless of which option you take, simply follow the trail back to your car.

9.7 mi Finish.

Options As you can see from the top of Mount Thomas, the pack trail continues west over to the high point of Red Table Mountain, the unnamed point at 12,037 feet. The traverse from Thomas's summit covers 1.7 miles, one way. It's a nice peak, but you won't be seeing too much more than you do from Thomas (though you get a nice view of Mount Thomas from point 12,037).

Quick Facts Red Table Mountain has remained unspoiled by humans throughout history. Outside of a few grazing pastures and short-lived sawmills, the area has remained relatively untouched. Geologically, Thomas is made of the same metamorphic sedimentary mudstone that makes up the Maroon Bells. This hardened mud gives both Red Table Mountain and the Maroon Bells their ruddy hue. Mount Thomas is one of the areas that was on the bottom of the ancient inland sea that covered Colorado some 70 million years ago.

Contact Info White River National Forest
Eagle Ranger District
125 W. Fifth Street
P.O. Box 720
Eagle, CO 81631
(970) 328-6388

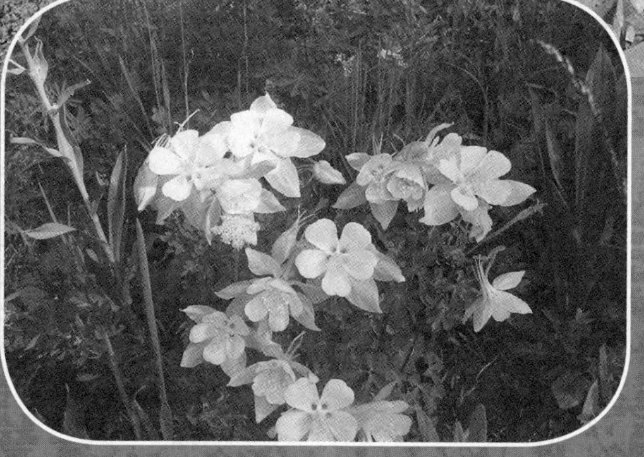

The geology of Mount Thomas is unlike any other in the state of Colorado. Red rocks, talus rivers, and a great variety of wildflowers await.

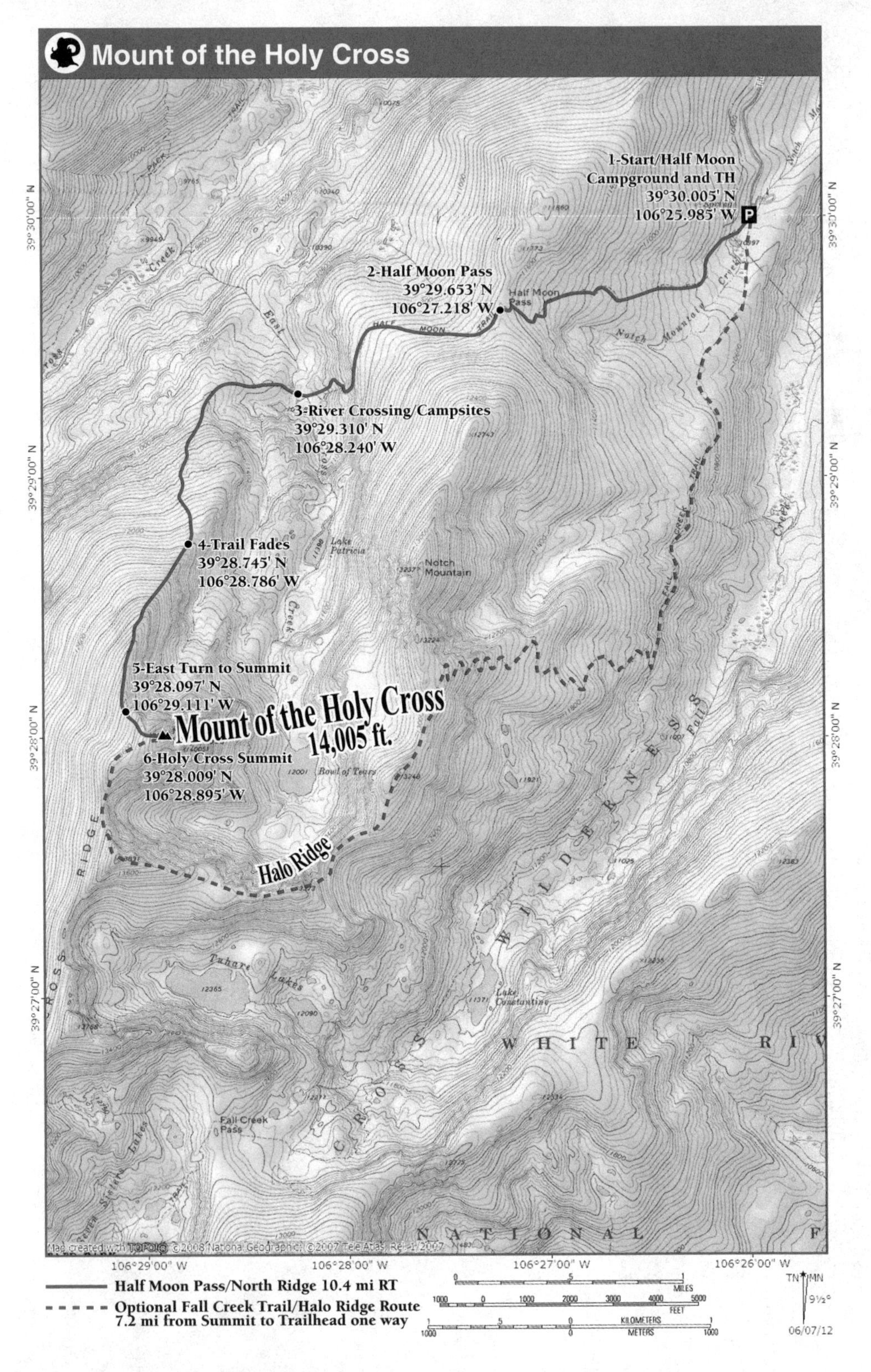
Mount of the Holy Cross
1-Start/Half Moon Campground and TH
39°30.005' N
106°25.985' W
2-Half Moon Pass
39°29.653' N
106°27.218' W
3-River Crossing/Campsites
39°29.310' N
106°28.240' W
4-Trail Fades
39°28.745' N
106°28.786' W
5-East Turn to Summit
39°28.097' N
106°29.111' W
Mount of the Holy Cross
14,005 ft.
6-Holy Cross Summit
39°28.009' N
106°28.895' W
Halo Ridge
Half Moon Pass
Notch Mountain
Lake Patricia
Bowl of Tears
Tuhare Lakes
Lake Constantine
Fall Creek Pass
HOLY CROSS WILDERNESS
WHITE RIV
NATIONAL F
CROSS RIDGE
Map created with TOPO!® ©2008 National Geographic; ©2007 Tele Atlas, Rel. 1/2007
Half Moon Pass/North Ridge 10.4 mi RT
Optional Fall Creek Trail/Halo Ridge Route 7.2 mi from Summit to Trailhead one way
MILES
FEET
KILOMETERS
METERS
TN MN
9½°
06/07/12

28 Mount of the Holy Cross

Good Overnight!

Holy Cross, Batman! This sturdy 14er is a favorite for hikers of all denominations, thanks to some heavenly routes that utilize the mountain's long, stable ridgelines.

Round-Trip Distance	10.4 miles
Hiking Time	7½–10 hours
Difficulty	7.5/10
Class	2
Start Elevation	10,315 ft., at Half Moon Campground and Trailhead
Peak Elevation	14,005 ft.
Total Elevation Gain	5,627 ft.
Terrain	Good trail leads to big, stable boulders to summit
Best Time to Climb	June–September
Gear Advisor	Normal gear
Crowd Level	Moderate

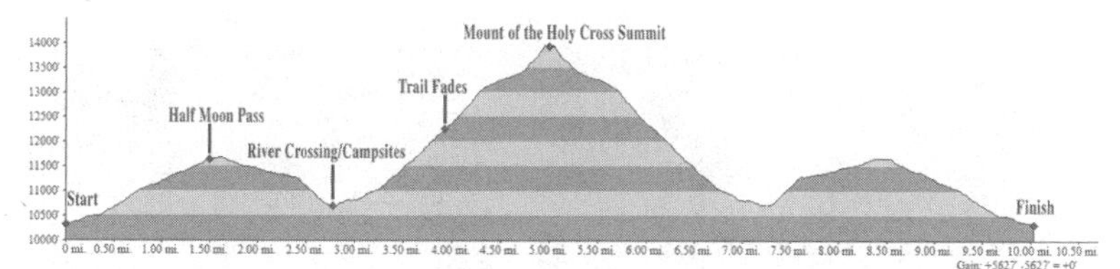

Location Sawatch Range in the Holy Cross Wilderness/White River National Forest near the town of Minturn

Intro Mount of the Holy Cross is named for the enormous, crumbling cross of couloirs and crevasses that dominate its east face. The cruciform has drawn hundreds of pious pilgrims of many faiths; those who believe in the power of a good hike won't be disappointed. Once considered a national monument, Holy Cross was demoted to a plain ol' mountain in 1954. In classic Sawatch style, Holy Cross has several drawn-out ridges that are perfect for class 2 ascents. Alpinists can take a shot at the fabled Cross Couloir or the more subtle Angelica Couloir on the northeast face.

Why Climb It? Does Holy Cross have divine healing powers, as professed by dozens of visitors? It could be, though any visions you receive might be due to a lack of oxygen. As with other Sawatch peaks, the standard routes to the summit are solid, gradual ascents. One difference is the summit massif, which is mildly steep and will require some easy scrambling. While the Cross Couloir is an impressive site, the enormous north face is equally as beautiful. The hiking is very good on Holy Cross, and you'll have many opportunities to peer down the steep northeast features from the safety of the north ridge. Those looking for an epic day can tour the mountain via the optional 13-plus-mile loop.

Driving Passenger cars can make it to the trailhead, though they will encounter some bumps and bangs; if you have a tough passenger car, no problem. Tigiwon Road is a rutted dirt road. I made the trailhead unscathed with my Honda Accord. Cars will have to drive slowly to avoid legions of potholes; the entire road looks as though it has sustained a mortar attack. Sport utility cars, sport utility vehicles, and 4x4s will have no problem. Tigiwon Road is open seasonally and is closed once the snow piles up.

How to Get There Take Exit 171 (Minturn) off I-70; this exit is approximately 5 miles west of downtown Vail. Go south on US Highway 24 (east) for 2.0 miles to the charming town of Minturn. Roughly 3 miles after the end of town, turn right onto Tigiwon Road (Forest Service Road 707; there's a National Forest Access sign). Tigiwon is a dirt road that goes under a trestle before climbing into the woods. It is a slowgoing 8.5 miles to the Half Moon Campground and Trailhead. Along the way, you'll pass the Tigiwon Community House at mile 6.0 and Tigiwon Campground at mile 6.2. Reach the trailhead at mile 8.5.

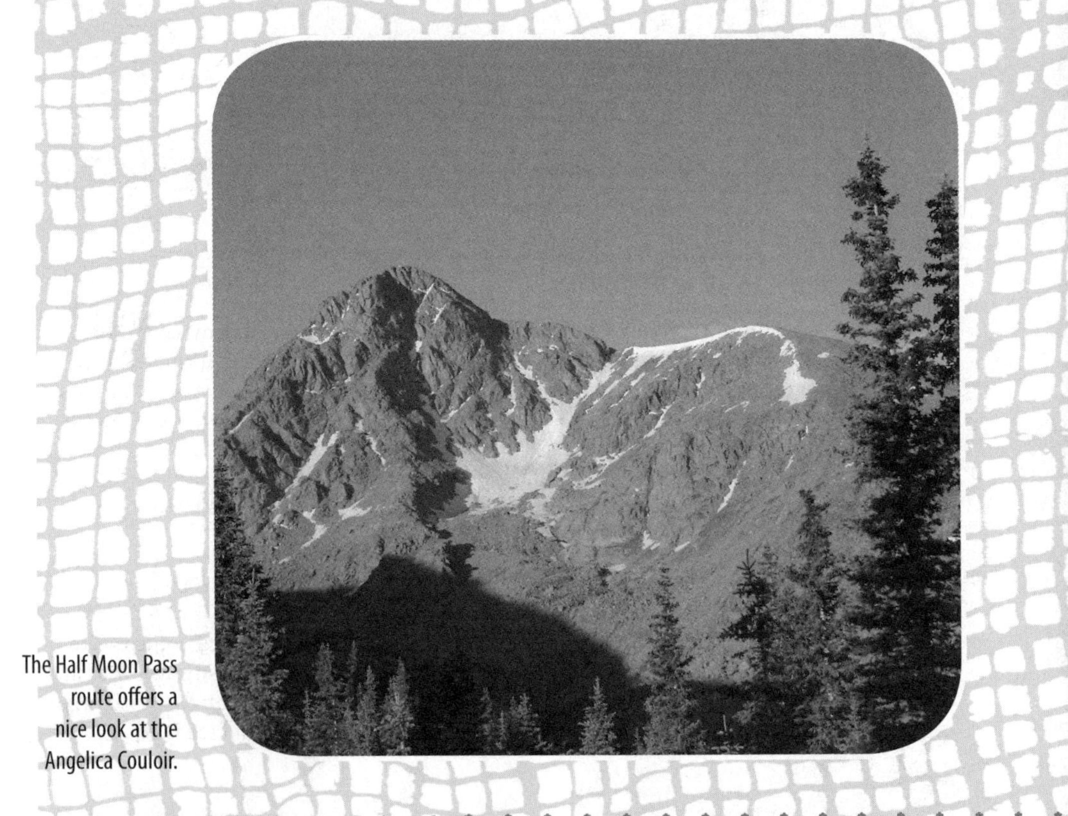

The Half Moon Pass route offers a nice look at the Angelica Couloir.

Fees/Camping There is no fee to day hike the peak or to backcountry camp, though you need to fill out a free user permit. Great backcountry spots to pitch a tent are near the River Crossing waypoint; if you don't mind a short hike, there are also good areas near Patricia Lake. If you'd like to camp at Half Moon Campground, be warned: the few spaces fill up quickly, though you can always retreat to Tigiwon Campground 2.5 miles down the road. As of 2012, sites were $11 a night.

Route Notes Many hikers are intimidated by the elevation gain presented by this hike. While you need to be in good shape to climb Holy Cross, the climb isn't as strenuous as the raw measurements make it seem (unless you do the entire Halo Ridge Loop). On the standard route, you climb to Half Moon Pass and then descend roughly 1,000 feet to the riverbed below. There are dozens of great, free campsites here for backpackers (and it's only 2.8 miles in).

The out-and-back mileage on the standard route is 10.4 miles, which makes this a better day hike than some people suppose—though the dread of hiking 1,000 feet back up to Half Moon Pass after descending the summit is intimidating. I had the good fortune to double-check the distance with a park ranger using an advanced Trimble GPS system, as the distances published in various other guides were different than those I had recorded

Note: The standard route does not offer a view of the Cross Couloir; you can see it by making the full Halo Ridge Loop or by hiking up the Fall Creek Trail to the south saddle of Notch Mountain.

One more thing: Many people have become disoriented above tree line on Holy Cross. Bringing a compass and GPS will increase your margin of safety.

Mile/Waypoint **0.0 mi (1)** Start your hike out of the Half Moon Campground and Trailhead. Note that there are two major trails here: the Half Moon Trail, which is the start of the standard route and goes uphill; the other is the Fall Creek Trail, which descends initially and leads to Notch Mountain and the Halo Ridge route. For the route detailed here, take the well-traveled Half Moon Trail.

1.5 mi (2) In a brief 1.5 miles, you'll have climbed 1,350 feet to the top of Half Moon Pass. From the top, you'll see a phalanx of mountains in the distance. Which one is Holy Cross? Continue down the trail a few hundred yards, past the obstructive shoulder of Unnamed Peak 12,743. Look to your left and prepare to have your jaw drop. Follow the switchbacking trail downhill to the riverbed.

2.8 mi (3) At the bottom of the hill, there's an easy river crossing. Make sure to stay on the correct trail after the crossing; the Holy Cross Trail goes west and uphill. Avoid the trail that follows the river south to Lake Patricia. Dozens of great campsites are along this stretch of trail; the last good sites are about 0.25 mile west of the river.

3.5 mi Hike uphill through a rocky forest and pop out of tree line at 11,600 feet. A confusing series of cairns denoting a few different routes will appear. I prefer to stay close to the spine of the ridge, though it is steeper and lacks knee-preserving switchbacks. The terrain gets steep and rocky for a while.

4.0 mi (4) For all intents and purposes, the main trail has disappeared by mile 4.0. Continue south on the ridge; as long as visibility is good, the way up will be obvious.

4.5 mi Finally, a reprieve from the steep climbing. The ridgeline gets less sharply inclined and more defined. A trail reappears on the spine of the ridge, leading to the base of the final summit pyramid.

4.9 mi (5) This is the base of the final summit pyramid. Glance down to the left to see one of the exits of the Angelica Couloir. The push to the summit has the same multicairned confusion as you encountered on the lower section of the mountain. Pick a good line and head east to the top.

5.2 mi (6) Mount of the Holy Cross summit. Return the way you came up; this is often easier said than done. The perspective on the descent can be momentarily confusing. Take your time and regain the north ridge. Once you pass the Angelica Couloir, it gets easier.

6.3 mi (4) About here, regain the original trail and follow it back into tree line. If visibility is bad, remember that you can head east-northeast to reach the river basin and follow it north to the trail. From the river crossing, slog back up to Half Moon Pass.

8.8 (2) Revisit Half Moon Pass. Good news: It's all downhill from here!

10.4 mi Finish.

Options As noted on the map, ambitious folks can make a monster loop of this hike by continuing on from the summit of Holy Cross (waypoint **6**) and following Halo Ridge, a class 2+ traverse that circles the Bowl of Tears Lake and rejoins a well-worn trail at a shelter house on the south saddle of Notch Mountain. This vantage point is ideal for photos of the Cross Couloir. From the saddle, a trail zigzags down to a juncture with the Fall Creek Trail; follow it north to return to the Half Moon Trailhead. You can also reverse the route by starting at the Fall Creek Trail instead of Half Moon Pass Trail, which is a less strenuous option because the north ridge descent is easy to follow, and you can go on autopilot once you find the trail in tree line.

The Halo Ridge option is 7.2 miles from the summit of Holy Cross to Half Moon Trailhead (a full loop is between 12.5 and 13.3 miles, depending on how well you navigate and how many switchbacks you take).

Quick Facts Mount of the Holy Cross was a hidden treasure for many years. Many doubted that it even existed until it was officially surveyed in 1873. William H. Jackson took the first famous photo of the cross that captured the imagination of the public. In 1874, Thomas Moran (famous for his Yellowstone paintings) made an ethereal painting of the cross hanging in mist, which added to the mountain's mystique. Images of the peak inspired Henry Wadsworth Longfellow (who never saw Holy Cross in person) to write "The Cross of Snow," a depressing poem that uses the obscure word *benedight* (which means "blessed").

From the 1920s on, religious pilgrimages made up a large portion of the tourism in the area. Mount of the Holy Cross was made a national monument in 1950, only to lose its status in 1954 due to a lack of visitors. For a

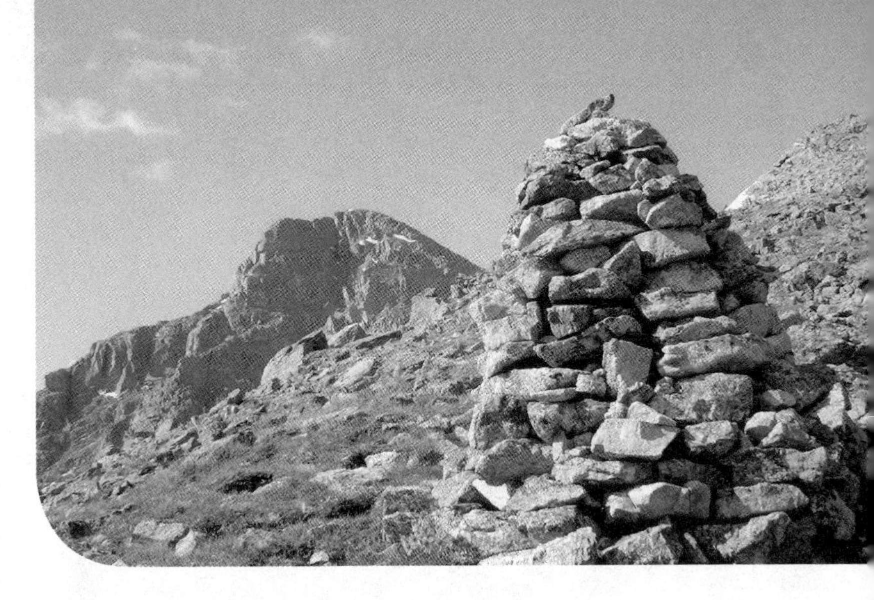

Cairns mark the initial part of the trail above tree line but slowly fade out. Stay close to the ridge and you'll be fine.

long time, Holy Cross was very difficult to reach. It did not receive official 14er status until 1964. It wasn't until the establishment of a good road that traffic finally increased (for better or for worse). Observant historians have noticed that the right side of the cross's horizontal bar is rapidly eroding, which may eventually cause the name of the peak to be changed to Mount of the Holy T-Square.

One more fact: Tigiwon Community House has served as the launching point for religious retreats since 1927. Tigiwon is the phonetic English interpretation of the Ute word for "friend."

Contact Info

White River National Forest
Holy Cross Ranger District
24747 US Highway 24
Minturn, CO 81645
(970) 827-5715

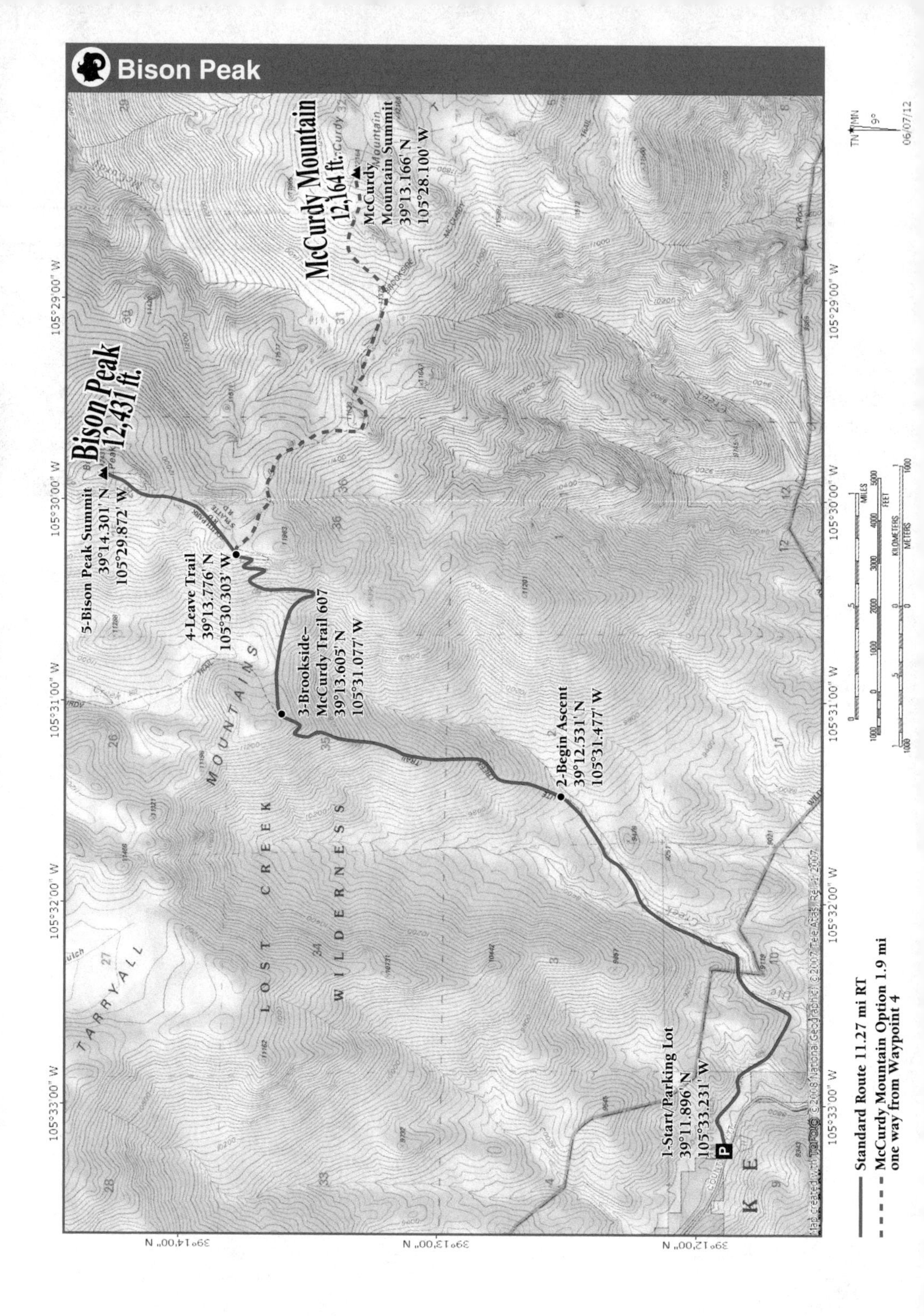

Bison Peak
Bison Peak 12,431 ft.
McCurdy Mountain 12,164 ft.
5-Bison Peak Summit 39°14.301' N 105°29.872' W
4-Leave Trail 39°13.776' N 105°30.303' W
3-Brookside–McCurdy Trail 607 39°13.605' N 105°31.077' W
2-Begin Ascent 39°12.531' N 105°31.477' W
1-Start/Parking Lot 39°11.896' N 105°33.231' W
McCurdy Mountain Summit 39°13.166' N 105°28.100' W
LOST CREEK WILDERNESS
TARRYALL MOUNTAINS
Standard Route 11.27 mi RT
McCurdy Mountain Option 1.9 mi one way from Waypoint 4

29 Bison Peak

Welcome to another planet! Bison Peak's incredible rock formations must be seen to be believed. This all natural super-Stonehenge is a unique Colorado experience.

Round-Trip Distance	11.27 miles
Hiking Time	6–8 hours
Difficulty	3/10
Class	1
Start Elevation	8,719 ft., at Ute Creek Trailhead
Peak Elevation	12,431 ft.
Total Elevation Gain	4,315 ft.
Terrain	Well-maintained trail/grassy meadows
Best Time to Climb	May–October; this is a year-round option due to low grade
Gear Advisor	Trail runners and trekking poles
Crowd Level	Low

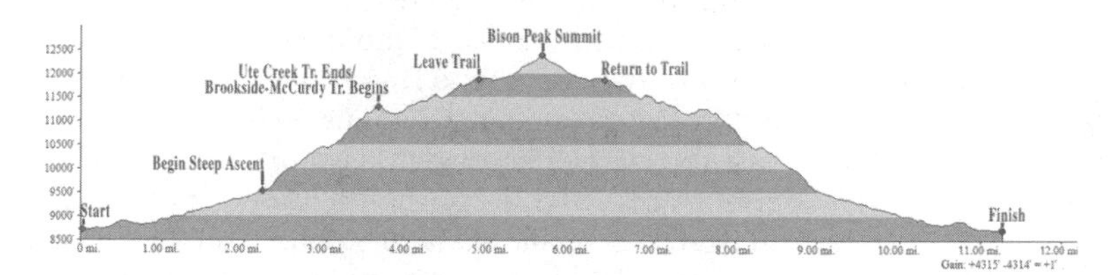

Location Tarryall Mountains in the Lost Creek Wilderness/Pike National Forest outside the town of Jefferson

Intro Bison Peak is unlike any other mountain in Colorado. Don't be intimidated by the mileage and elevation gain. This entire hike is class 1 on a well-maintained trail. After a pleasant walk through the woods, pop out of tree line into another world. Bison's enormous stone monoliths grace the summit in wild and wonderful formations. Rounded rocks sit impossibly atop one another, and there are dozens of fun climbs, caves, and scrambles to enjoy.

Why Climb It? Magical rock formations atop the peak are incredible to behold. The hike in is long but peaceful; anyone in decent shape will be able to handle the class 1 trail. Besides the impressive rock gardens, Bison's place as the high point of the Tarryall Mountains offers beautiful panoramas of Pike National Forest and several Mosquito Range peaks. The isolation and grandeur of this peak bring to mind images of the fabled Elysian Fields of Greek mythology. Blur your vision, and watch the monoliths turn into a herd of giant bison.

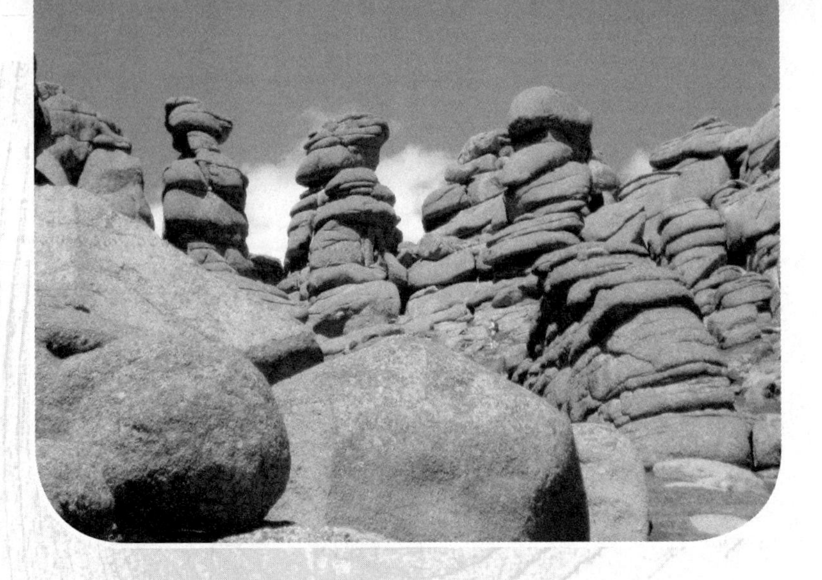

To appreciate the sheer scale of Bison Peak's towers, see if you can find the hiker in this photo.

Driving The Ute Creek Trailhead is reached on paved roads, passable by all vehicles.

How to Get There From US Highway 285, find your way to the tiny town of Jefferson. If you are coming from the Denver area, you'll have to go over Kenosha Pass. From Jefferson, turn southeast onto Park County Road 77, also known as Tarryall Road. An easy way to find PCR 77: The junction is at Jefferson's general store and gas station. Continue on patchy paved road. At mile 17.0, you'll pass the Tarryall Reservoir on your right. At the end of the reservoir, it's approximately 3.4 miles to the Ute Creek Trailhead on the left side of the road (you'll pass some old barn buildings on the left). This parking area has a Lost Creek Wilderness sign, and a bridge spanning Tarryall Creek is visible from the road and parking lot.

Fees/Camping There are no fees to hike Bison Peak. As of 2012, there are no fees to camp in the Lost Creek Wilderness. (Call phone numbers in "Contact Info" section for more up-to-date information.)

Route Notes None.

Mile/Waypoint **0.0 mi (1)** Start your hike from the Ute Creek Trailhead parking lot. Head north, cross the bridge, and begin hiking on Ute Creek Trail #629. You will cross into the Lost Creek Wilderness. This trail is well maintained and easy to follow—assuming there is no snow on the ground. You'll be cruising through beautiful stands of aspens and evergreens as you ascend.

2.2 mi (2) After a nice warm-up, the trail begins to climb in earnest. As you ascend, you'll begin to see the southern rock formations through the trees. It's easy to mistake point 11,963 for Bison Peak at this point.

3.7 mi (3) The Ute Creek Trail ends and the Brookside-McCurdy Trail #607 begins. This trail heads north and east; you'll want to turn right (east) and climb up to tree line.

4.9 mi (4) After you've climbed some switchbacks to this high point, more formations will be visible to the north. Leave the trail (which fades out a bit in the upper meadows) and proceed northeast to Bison's summit. Follow the high, flat ridge until the truly amazing formations appear. You'll descend a short 150 feet, and then climb up to the largest rock formation, where Bison's summit awaits. Don't worry: the summit is an easy scramble and doesn't require any technical or scary moves.

5.6 mi (5) Bison's summit is marked with a U.S. Geological Survey (USGS) marker and summit register (there are actually a few USGS markers up there). There are a few weathered wooden structures and some other debris, including dozens of long metal nails driven into the stone, around. Return the same way you came, regaining the Brookside-McCurdy Trail where you left it.

11.27 mi Finish.

Options Exploring the rock formations and scrambling on them can keep you busy for hours. A southwest traverse over the open meadows leads to McCurdy Mountain (12,165 feet). Even though it may look close, it's about 2 miles one way from Bison to McCurdy, so be prepared to add about 4 miles to an already long hike (which in turn makes for a really long day) if you decide to check it out.

Quick Facts The Lost Creek Wilderness (designated in 1980) is an amazing place of gravity-defying rocks, mostly rounded granite blocks piled in assorted fashions. No other wilderness area boasts such unique terrain, especially in alpine tundra areas above tree line. Bison Peak was named for the similarity the huge monoliths on its summit bear to the tawny brown ungulates.

Contact Info Pike and San Isabel National Forests
South Park Ranger District
320 US Highway 285
Fairplay, CO 80440
(719) 836-2031

Mount Zirkel

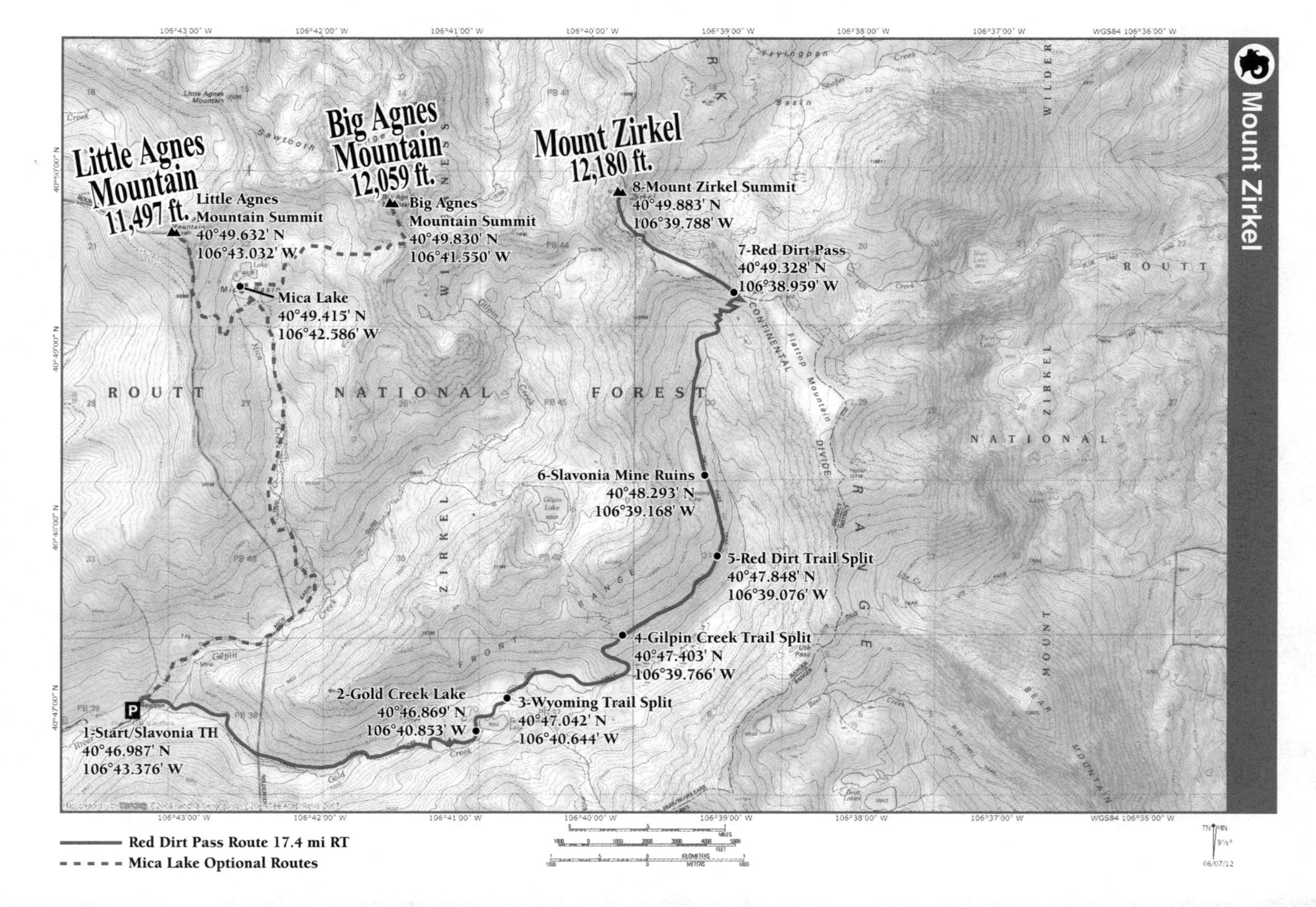
Little Agnes Mountain 11,497 ft.
Little Agnes Mountain Summit
40°49.632' N
106°43.032' W
Big Agnes Mountain 12,059 ft.
Big Agnes Mountain Summit
40°49.830' N
106°41.550' W
Mount Zirkel 12,180 ft.
8-Mount Zirkel Summit
40°49.883' N
106°39.788' W
7-Red Dirt Pass
40°49.328' N
106°38.959' W
Mica Lake
40°49.415' N
106°42.586' W
ROUTT NATIONAL FOREST
6-Slavonia Mine Ruins
40°48.293' N
106°39.168' W
5-Red Dirt Trail Split
40°47.848' N
106°39.076' W
4-Gilpin Creek Trail Split
40°47.403' N
106°39.766' W
2-Gold Creek Lake
40°46.869' N
106°40.853' W
3-Wyoming Trail Split
40°47.042' N
106°40.644' W
1-Start/Slavonia TH
40°46.987' N
106°43.376' W
CONTINENTAL DIVIDE
Flattop Mountain
ZIRKEL FRONT RANGE
PARK RANGE
BEAR MOUNTAIN
Red Dirt Pass Route 17.4 mi RT
Mica Lake Optional Routes

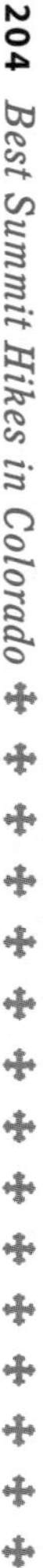

30 Mount Zirkel

Good Overnight!

A northern setting and a low-elevation peak make Mount Zirkel a haven for color. Wildflowers, grasses, red dirt, and snowy summits all decorate this pristine sanctuary.

Round-Trip Distance	17.4 miles
Hiking Time	8–12 hours
Difficulty	7/10
Class	2
Start Elevation	8,388 ft., at Slavonia Trailhead
Peak Elevation	12,180 ft.
Total Elevation Gain	4000 ft.
Terrain	Good trail to good off-trail alpine plateau
Best Time to Climb	June–September
Gear Advisor	Gaiters, trekking poles, and sandals for river crossing
Crowd Level	Low

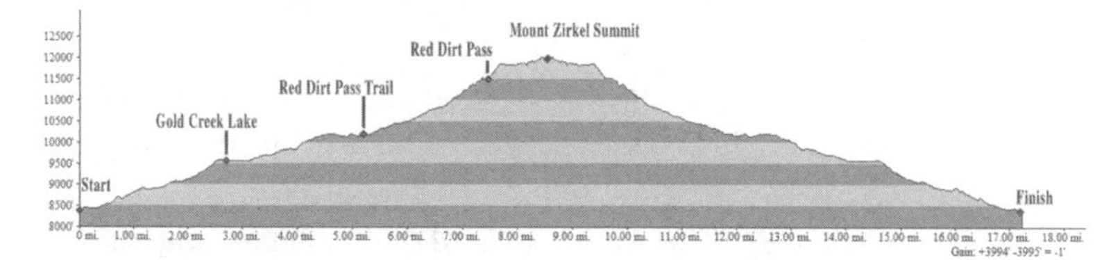

Location Park Range in the Mount Zirkel Wilderness/Routt National Forest outside of Steamboat Springs

Intro Mount Zirkel is the showpiece of the Mount Zirkel Wilderness. The mountains here hold more water than other areas, giving rise to great splashes of color. Hike early in spring to see white snow, green grass, and blue sky. Summer brings wildflowers, and autumn changes aspen leaves bright yellow. There is a calming and refreshing atmosphere in this peaceful and immaculate realm. The abundance of water, wide-open spaces, and nontechnical terrain make this the perfect hike for your canine pals.

Why Climb It? You can climb Zirkel in a day; despite the long mileage, strong hikers will move quickly on the trail up to Red Dirt Pass. Better still, take your time and spend a night out in the alpine basin. The trail up to Zirkel is rich and teeming with flora and fauna. Diverging from the pass, you'll climb up to a secret plateau carpeted by thousands of wildflowers. An easy scramble leads up to an amazing summit. When I last did this hike and topped out, I wasn't alone. Two deer were lounging on the rocks, enjoying themselves on the lofty apex.

Driving The road to Slavonia Trailhead is a very well-maintained dirt road. All vehicles will be able to make it to the trailhead.

How to Get There From Steamboat Springs, start out on US Highway 40, west of town, and turn north onto County Road 129 toward Hahns Peak/Clark. Follow the road 17 miles to the town of Clark; from here, drive another 0.8 mile to the right (east) turnoff on Forest Service Road 400/County Road 64 (Seedhouse Road). Follow this road 11.8 miles to the eastern terminus at the Slavonia Trailhead; the first 5.9 miles are paved, and then it becomes a dirt road.

Fees/Camping There are no fees to hike in the area or to backcountry camp. There are several primitive campsites along FS 400 and two pay campgrounds with facilities: Seedhouse and Hinman. Both places are $12 per night. Fantastic camping is along the trail starting at mile 5.8, the Slavonia Mine ruins.

Route Notes None.

Mile/Waypoint

0.0 mi (1) Start at Slavonia Trailhead and head west on the Gold Creek Trail. This is a good class 1 trail that is easy to follow. Take it to Gold Creek Lake.

2.7 mi (2) Arrive at the lovely Gold Creek Lake. Stay on the north side of the lake; there's a river crossing here that may run high in the spring. Cross it and return to the trail, heading westward.

3.0 mi (3) The Wyoming Trail splits off here on the right. Stay on the Gold Creek Trail toward Red Dirt Pass.

4.4 mi (4) The Gilpin Creek Trail splits off here to the left. Again, stay straight on the Gold Creek Trail, which is turning into the Red Dirt Pass Trail.

5.2 mi (5) An anemic trail sign here designates a split in the trail. Stay left on the Red Dirt Trail that heads north, higher into the basin. The wrong-way Ute Pass Trail heads left and downhill. Do not take it.

5.8 mi (6) As the basin opens up, there is great camping. The Slavonia Mine is just left (west) of the trail and has some interesting ruins to explore. Near the mine is a small pond with some funky water in it; I would advise that you don't drink it for obvious reasons. Note that there is a small, grassy, wet section where the trail disappears. Just keep heading north, and you can pick it back up when it reappears. You'll also get your first look at Red Dirt Pass from here. Drop down into the basin, cross a low-flowing river, and take the switchbacks up to the top of Red Dirt Pass.

7.5 mi (7) Red Dirt Pass. At 11,500 feet, you've reached the top of the saddle. Leave the trail and head up the grassy/rocky slope to your left (northwest). Climb this slope to 11,870 feet, where a broad plateau will reveal your first glimpse of the craggy summit of Mount Zirkel. Walk across the beautiful meadow and make a class 2 scramble on solid rock to Zirkel's prized summit. Note that when you first see it, you may not be able to tell which lump is the top. Luckily, the summit isn't the peak on the far right—it's the blocky piece left of that point, on the other side of the U-shaped saddle.

8.3 mi (8) Mount Zirkel's summit. You have exceptional views from the top, especially of Big Agnes Peak to the west. The optional traverse over

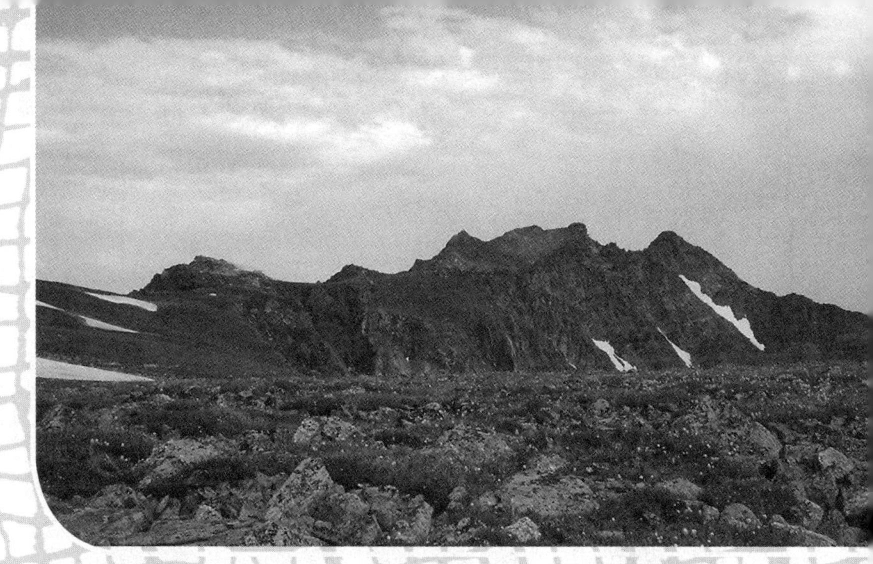

The final approach to Zirkel's summit

to Zirkel's lower north summit is an exposed, class 3 thrill. Be careful; the rock is a little rotten on the way over. Once you have had your fill, drop back down to Red Dirt Pass and return the way you came.

17.4 mi Finish.

Options

From Red Dirt Pass (waypoint 7), you could go right (east) instead of west to check out the rolling mesa of the appropriately named Flattop Mountain. Amazingly, the huge, photogenic mountain you see to the northeast—from the top of Red Dirt Pass—is unnamed; maps list it as Unnamed Peak 11,931. It makes a good second peak to climb if you are camping in the area.

If you want to extend your adventure—or simply do an alternate peak in the Zirkel Wilderness—Mica Lake is a beautiful area to set up camp and explore the surrounding peaks. Little Agnes Peak to the west of the lake is a steep class 2 scramble, while Big Agnes Mountain to the east is a fantastic class 2+/3 scramble. This area may be the most beautiful in all of Colorado for autumn backpacking.

Quick Facts

Mount Zirkel is named for Ferdinand Zirkel, a German petrologist who was a big help to survey parties, despite having a name that sounds like it belongs to a Muppet. I wonder what kind of woman Big Agnes was? Is it a compliment or an insult to have such a mountain named after you if you're a woman? My guess is that she wasn't a delicate flower of femininity but could probably cook some mean flapjacks and pull the family plow if the ox needed a day off.

Slavonia Mine had solid yields of zinc in its prime. If you had to work a mine, this was a beautiful place to do it. There is a bit more information on Slavonia at the trailhead.

Contact Info

Routt National Forest
Hahns Peak/Bears Ears Ranger District
925 Weiss Drive
Steamboat Springs, CO 80487
(970) 879-1870

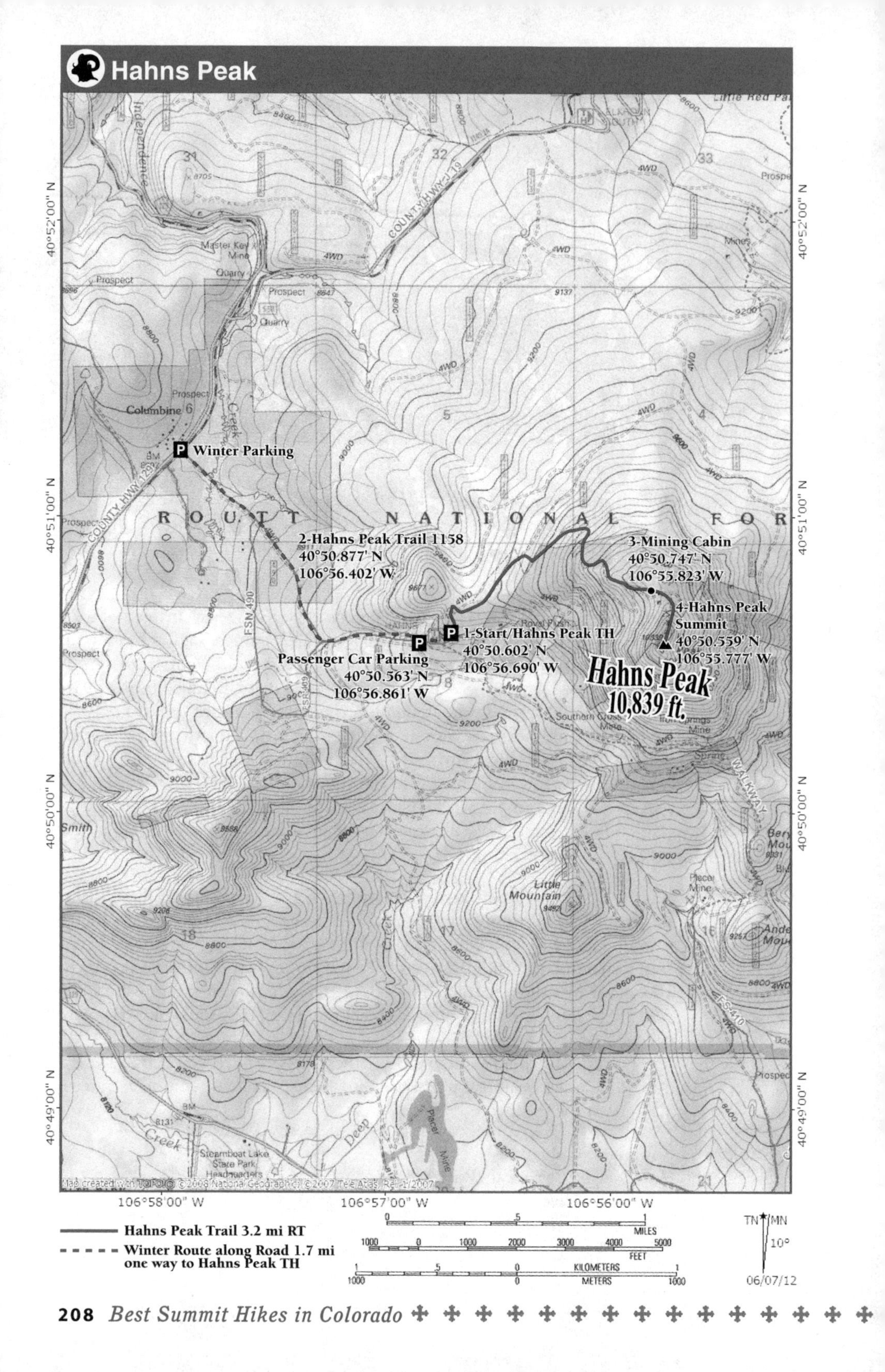

Hahns Peak
Winter Parking
Columbine
ROUTT NATIONAL FOR
2-Hahns Peak Trail 1158
40°50.877' N
106°56.402' W
3-Mining Cabin
40°50.747' N
106°55.823' W
4-Hahns Peak Summit
40°50.559' N
106°55.777' W
1-Start/Hahns Peak TH
40°50.602' N
106°56.690' W
Passenger Car Parking
40°50.563' N
106°56.861' W
Hahns Peak
10,839 ft.
Little Mountain
COUNTY HWY 129
COUNTY HWY J 19
FSN 490
WALKWAY
40°52'00" N
40°51'00" N
40°50'00" N
40°49'00" N
106°58'00" W
106°57'00" W
106°56'00" W
Map created with TOPO!® ©2008 National Geographic (©2007 Tele Atlas, Rel. 1/2007)
Hahns Peak Trail 3.2 mi RT
Winter Route along Road 1.7 mi one way to Hahns Peak TH
MILES
FEET
KILOMETERS
METERS
TN
MN
10°
06/07/12

31 Hahns Peak

Miles of bright aspen trees and crystal clear lakes unfold before you from Hahns Peak's summit. This easy hike is the perfect complement to any trip to the Steamboat area.

Round-Trip Distance	3.2 miles
Hiking Time	2–4 hours
Difficulty	1/10
Class	1; 2 for the last 0.5 mile
Start Elevation	9,407 ft., at Hahns Peak Trailhead
Peak Elevation	10,839 ft.
Total Elevation Gain	1,316 ft.
Terrain	Well-maintained trail with a slightly rocky hike to the top
Best Time to Climb	Year-round
Gear Advisor	Normal seasonal gear
Crowd Level	Moderate

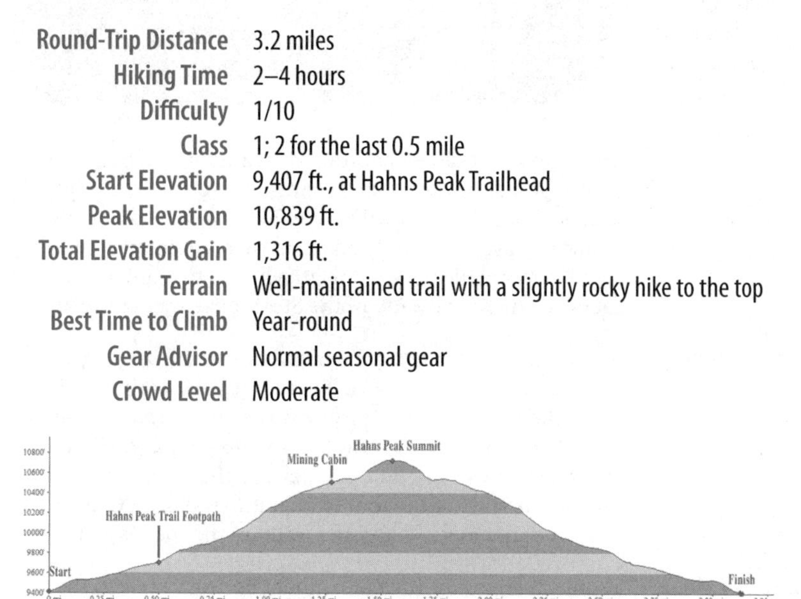

Location Elkhead Mountains in the Routt National Forest outside of Steamboat Springs

Intro Hahns Peak overlooks the aspen forests of Steamboat like a benevolent guardian. From the Steamboat Lake area, the perfectly conical mountain appears much higher than 10,839 feet; this may be due, in part, to the mountain's low timberline. The northern locale of the mountain presents a lush and gentle landscape. In the autumn, expansive acres of aspens turn bright yellow, and the crisp scent of fallen leaves may leave you feeling sentimental for another time and place.

Why Climb It? Hahns Peak is by far the easiest hike in this book. Taken just by the numbers, this mountain may seem too mellow to mention. So why put such a simple trek alongside such brawny adventures as Lead Mountain (Hike 5), Storm King Peak (Hike 45), and Mount Powell (Hike 16)? My rationale for including Hahns is simple. First of all, it's a fun hike that offers the best views I've seen of the beautiful Steamboat Springs and Steamboat Lake areas. The old mining ruins are intriguing, and the fire tower on the summit is a nice touch. But my main incentive to include Hahns is that it's a great complementary adventure to any visit to Steamboat Springs. Chances

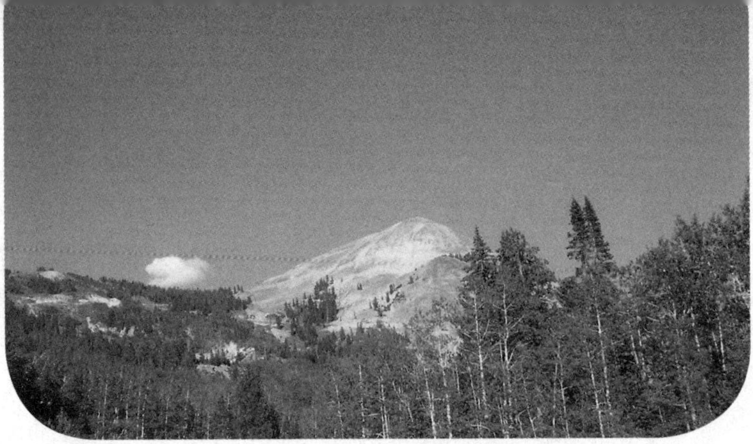

The old fire lookout affords incredible views of the Steamboat Springs area.

are that you would be coming to Steamboat Springs to mountain bike, ski, camp, or just be outdoors. Hahns takes only a half day to climb, meaning that you can mix it in with other activities. In the winter, climbing Hahns from the paved road only adds another 3.0 miles, round-trip, to the adventure. Its low angle makes it relatively safe to climb in snow. Hahns brings to focus the distinct beauty of the Steamboat area year-round.

Driving The road is a bit rocky and rough, but tough passenger cars can make it to the Hahns Peak Trailhead. There is a good bailout point for cars 0.2 mile from the trailhead. Because this is a short hike, it may be a good idea to stop there if you don't want to bang up your car. High-clearance 4x4s and Jeeps have the option to drive beyond the trailhead to a very small parking area at the start of the foot trail, but I recommend that you don't. There is only one spot to park, and the walk up the road is actually quite nice.

How to Get There From US Highway 40 in Steamboat Springs, drive to the north end of town. Turn right (north) onto County Road 129, which has a sign for the town of Clark, the airport, and Hahns Peak. Stay on this scenic road for 29.0 miles, passing the towns of Clark and Hahns Peak. You'll also pass Steamboat Lake and State Park, which will be on your left. At mile 29.0, you'll need to turn right onto Forest Service Road 490 (this is directly across from the Columbine General Store). If you're hiking in the winter, you'll have to park at the store and hoof it or ski in. Follow FS 490 for 1.4 miles on a progressively rockier road; at this point, the road splits. If you like, you can park your passenger car here—the roughest part of the road is the next short section. Stay left on Forest Service Road 418 (there will be signs for Hahns Peak Trail #1158 to guide you) for slightly less than 0.2 mile and arrive at the large, well-marked trailhead. From here, the trail follows a true 4x4 road west and north 0.5 mile to the Hahns Peak Trail. As mentioned above, you can crash your 4x4 up the road, but the parking is limited at the footpath (plus it's very easy to miss if you're not paying attention). My advice is to park in the main lot.

Note: There has been a lot of construction on private land on the first mile of FS 490. There may be turnoffs for driveways and other new dirt roads; stay on FS 490 until the junction with FS 418. Don't camp on the land before the trailhead.

Fees/Camping There's no fee to hike or camp in the Hahns Peak area, which is in the Routt National Forest. Please be aware of the private land. Several pay campsites are at Steamboat Lake and nearby Pearl Lake State Park.

Route Notes None.

Mile/Waypoint

0.0 mi (1) Start at the Hahns Peak Trailhead parking lot. Head north on the 4x4 road (at the very beginning, avoid the downhill road to the left, after the fences). This is a surprisingly nice hike in the trees, with views opening up to the west as you get higher.

0.5 mi (2) Turn right (east) onto the marked Hahns Peak Trail #1158. If you've taken your 4x4 up this road, you'll need to park in the small spot on the left-hand side of the road. This is a well-traveled, class 1 trail. Follow it up through the woods.

1.3 mi (3) As you clear out of timberline (a relatively low 10,330 feet), an old mining cabin is on your right. Shortly thereafter, you'll come to a crisscross of old mining roads that overtake your humble footpath. Getting up to Hahns Peak from here won't be hard: the fire tower is in clear sight, and a trampled path in the rocks goes east and then cuts south to the summit. The rock on this final push is like a giant pile of broken ceramic plates, making audible clangs as you ascend.

1.6 mi (4) That was quick! You've reached the lookout station on the summit. In the autumn, the views are particularly good. To make sure that you are on the right trail when descending, hike down the rock pile, and make sure that you pass the old mining cabin. Return the way you came.

3.2 mi Finish.

Options The options for this hike are a bit different than others in this book. First off, I'd like to suggest this as a winter trip. You'll have to park at the Columbine General Store off CR 129, and it's a great adventure. If you are hiking in the summer, complement your trip with some great mountain biking on Emerald Mountain or a paddle on Steamboat Lake. This is also a good place to bring friends who aren't rabid hikers but still enjoy a good day out. It may be a short and easy summit, but it's too good not to mention.

Quick Facts Hahns Peak is named after prospector Joseph Henn (or Henne); the English version of this German name takes the phonetic spelling Hahn. Ol' Joseph did pretty well getting himself on the map, having both a mountain and a town named in his honor. As with the names of many other Colorado mountains, Hahns Peak lacks an apostrophe, in accordance with a rule instituted by the U.S. Board of Geographic Names that eliminates apostrophes from almost all geographical names.

Contact Info Routt National Forest
Hahns Peak/Bear Ears Road Ranger District
925 Weiss Drive
Steamboat Springs, CO 80487
(970) 879-1870

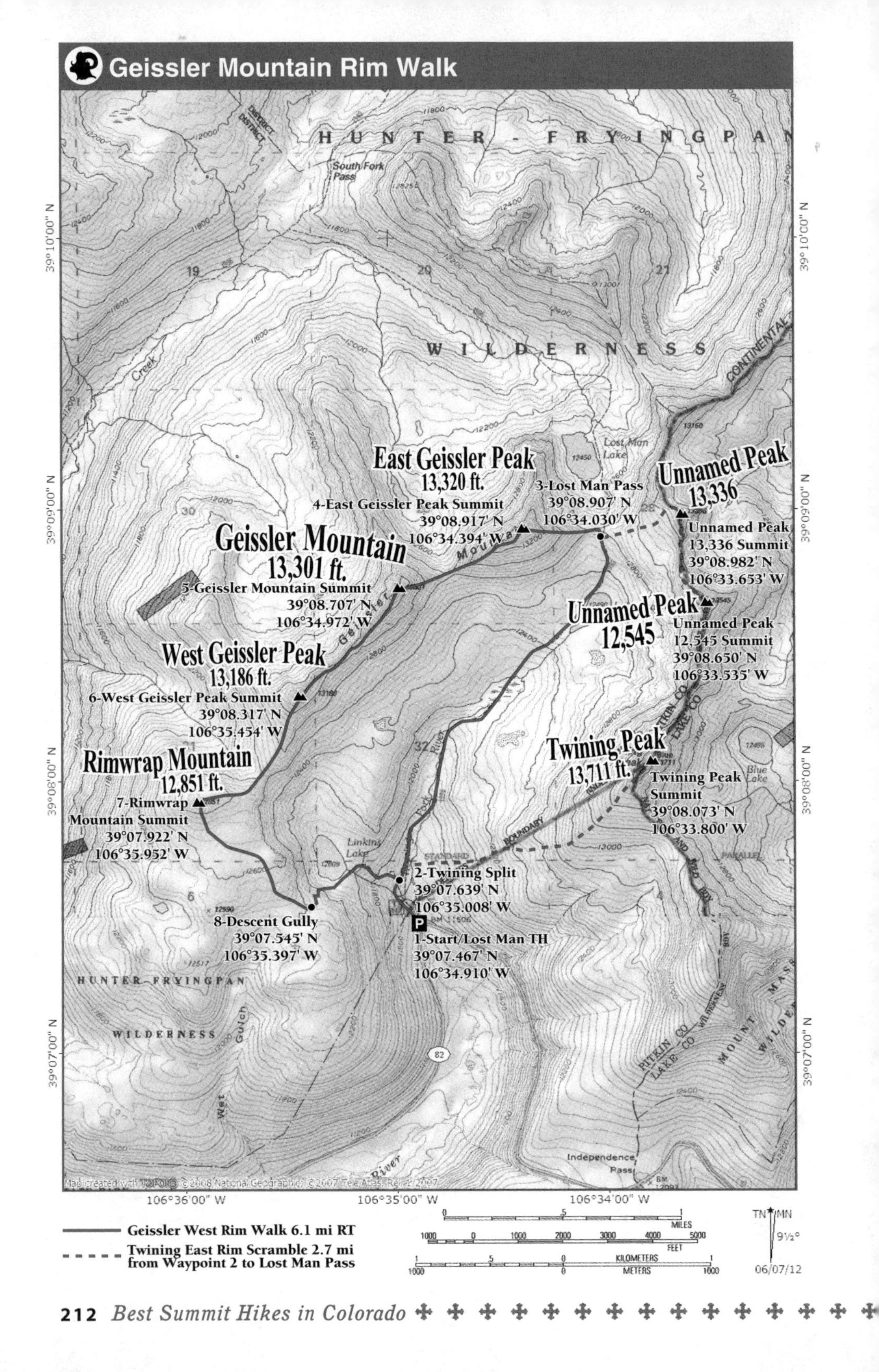
Geissler Mountain Rim Walk
HUNTER - FRYINGPAN
WILDERNESS
South Fork Pass
Lost Man Lake
Creek
East Geissler Peak
13,320 ft.
4-East Geissler Peak Summit
39°08.917' N
106°34.394' W
3-Lost Man Pass
39°08.907' N
106°34.030' W
Unnamed Peak
13,336
Unnamed Peak 13,336 Summit
39°08.982' N
106°33.653' W
Geissler Mountain
13,301 ft.
5-Geissler Mountain Summit
39°08.707' N
106°34.972' W
Unnamed Peak
12,545
Unnamed Peak 12,545 Summit
39°08.650' N
106°33.535' W
West Geissler Peak
13,186 ft.
6-West Geissler Peak Summit
39°08.317' N
106°35.454' W
Twining Peak
13,711 ft.
Twining Peak Summit
39°08.073' N
106°33.800' W
Rimwrap Mountain
12,851 ft.
7-Rimwrap Mountain Summit
39°07.922' N
106°35.952' W
Linkins Lake
2-Twining Split
39°07.639' N
106°35.008' W
8-Descent Gully
39°07.545' N
106°35.397' W
1-Start/Lost Man TH
39°07.467' N
106°34.910' W
Blue Lake
CONTINENTAL
PITKIN CO
LAKE CO
HUNTER-FRYINGPAN
WILDERNESS
Wet Gulch
MOUNT MASSIVE WILDERNESS
82
River
Independence Pass
39°10'00" N
39°09'00" N
39°08'00" N
39°07'00" N
106°36'00" W
106°35'00" W
106°34'00" W
Map created with TOPO! © 2008 National Geographic; ©2007 Tele Atlas, Rel. 1/2007
Geissler West Rim Walk 6.1 mi RT
Twining East Rim Scramble 2.7 mi from Waypoint 2 to Lost Man Pass
MILES
FEET
KILOMETERS
METERS
TN MN
9½°
06/07/12

32 Geissler Mountain Rim Walk

Geissler Mountain is actually a collection of peaks that frame a beautiful, rugged alpine basin. The standard route collects four summits in a single day, while the optional route bags seven.

Round-Trip Distance	6.1 miles
Hiking Time	4–6 hours
Difficulty	5/10
Class	2
Start Elevation	11,535 ft., at Lost Man Pass Trailhead
Peak Elevation	13,301 ft.
Total Elevation Gain	2,615 ft.
Terrain	Good trail to semi-rocky ridge traverse
Best Time to Climb	June–September
Gear Advisor	Normal gear and helmet for the optional loop on Twining
Crowd Level	Moderate

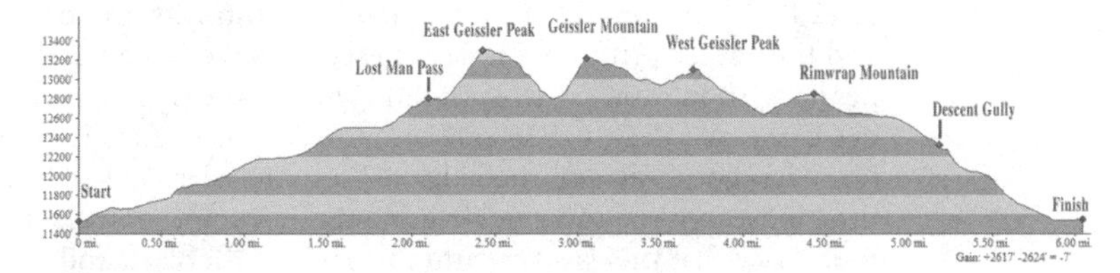

Location Sawatch Range in the Hunter-Fryingpan Wilderness/White River National Forest just past the top of Independence Pass

Intro Even though the Geissler Mountains are easily accessed, not many people know about them. Located just off Independence Pass, the multiple summits on the western rim of Independence Lake Basin make a great day hike that gets to the good stuff right away. The access trail begins a mere 0.3 mile from the middle of the basin. For those who like scrambling and want to tour the whole rim, a thrilling 3+ traverse of Twining Peak and a pair of burly unnamed mountains await.

Why Climb It? If you've ever driven over Independence Pass, you've no doubt looked up at the big peaks in the area and wondered what their names are and how to reach them. The Geissler Mountain may well be among those that have piqued your curiosity. The mountain of many peaks is very easy to access, and you have a ton of options once you are in the area. The Geissler summits (four in all) present a fun, class 2 ridge traverse that opens up incredible views from Aspen to Leadville. For those who love scrambling and want a longer, more challenging day, the Twining-Geissler Loop hits the whole rim—an exciting and novel experience!

Driving Any vehicle can make it to the trailhead; the road is paved the entire way. Note that Independence Pass is closed from mid-autumn to mid-spring.

How to Get There The Lost Man Trailhead is 1.9 miles from the summit of Independence Pass on the Aspen (west) side of the pass. If you are coming from the east, from the junction of US Highway 24 and Colorado Highway 82 (Independence Pass), drive 25.6 miles west on CO 82, up and over the pass, and down 1.9 miles to the trailhead parking area. It is on the north side of the road, off a tight, switchbacking turn. There are signs and a small information kiosk.

Fees/Camping There is no fee to hike or camp in the area; nearby Lost Man Campground (a few miles west of this trailhead on CO 82) provides drive-in camping spots for $13 per night.

Route Notes None.

Mile/Waypoint **0.0 mi (1)** Start at the Lost Man Trailhead. Get on the trail and head north. In almost no time, you're in the basin. How's that for service?

0.2 mi (2) This waypoint is here to show the split (east/northeast) for the Twining-Geissler Loop. Stay on the Lost Man Trail as it passes the inky Independence Lake and continues up to Lost Man Pass.

2.1 mi (3) Two miles of easy hiking have brought you to Lost Man Pass at 12,800 feet. Geissler and its attendant summits are to your left (west), and the western rim walk is easy to see. If you'd like to grab a couple more peaks without doing the optional route, you can go east here and check out Unnamed Peak 13,336 and Unnamed Peak 12,545. The standard route, however, goes west, up the ridge to East Geissler Peak. The rock here is a little loose, but the route never gets more difficult than class 2. Views from here show that this is a very unique basin, with black and gray rock covering everything in sight.

2.5 mi (4) East Geissler Peak is the first of your summits at 13,320 feet. Take in the great views, and then continue southwest along the ridge to a saddle and up to the middle summit.

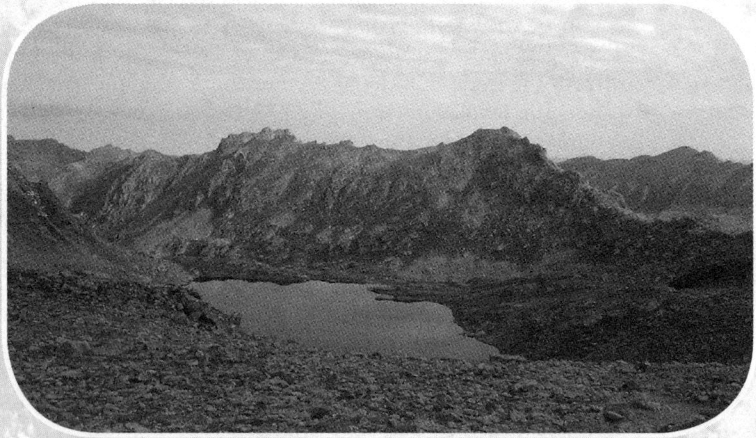

The Hunter-Fryingpan Wilderness is easily accessed from Independence Pass.

3.1 mi (5) The center peak is the official Geissler Mountain summit, despite being lower than the east peak. This 13,301-foot peak has good views of Twining Peak and the eastern rim. Drop down again and head over to your third summit, West Geissler Peak.

3.8 mi (6) West Geissler Peak! This summit is more craggy and rugged than the previous two. At 13,186 feet, it's the wee Geissler of the family. (As of 2012, there was a broomstick poking out of the highest point. Add this to the ravens I saw circling around and the eerie Gothic color scheme, and I might as well have been standing on Halloween Peak!) Continue on southwest to your next summit.

4.5 mi (7) Rimwrap Mountain wraps up the rim walk at 12,851 feet. From West Geissler, it looks impressive, but from down below it doesn't even resemble a mountain. From here, walk on the broad plateau southeast to the top of a trail that drops down to Linkins Lake.

5.3 mi (8) The Descent Gully is more of a slope. A faint trail is here, but you can get down the slope whatever way is easiest. Once you get on the level with Linkins Lake, a cairned trail goes back to the parking area.

6.1 mi Finish.

Options The optional Twining-Geissler full rim hike is an exciting scramble. Bring your helmet for this one—you'll be on loose rock that gets up to class 3+ (maybe even class 4) in difficulty. You shouldn't need ropes in normal conditions, but there are some committing moves. At waypoint **2**, go up the slope to Twining Peak; this is an easy class 2 hump up to 13,711 feet. Twining is the highest mountain in the rim. From here, you'll have a challenging ridge traverse over and around a few tricky rock pillars. You'll need good route-finding skills and a boost of courage to stay on the ridge. You'll eventually get to Unnamed Peak 12,545, a rugged peak that is officially unnamed despite its prominent profile. From here, continue north toward UN 13,336 on some more challenging terrain. There continues to be loose rock and some tough, short sections that require class 3 maneuvers. Once you reach the summit of UN 13,336, the hard stuff is over. Drop down to Lost Man Pass (waypoint **3**), and pick up the Geissler Loop on the west rim from here.

Quick Facts The Hunter-Fryingpan Wilderness is so named because the area serves as the headwaters of the Hunter and Fryingpan Rivers. It is somewhat unique in that the area is easy to access yet sees little traffic. It was designated in 1978 and expanded in 1993, making it a relatively new wilderness region.

The mountain you see directly in front of you (north) when you get into Lost Man Pass is Unnamed Peak 13,001, the lowest officially ranked Colorado 13er (number 637 of 637).

Contact Info White River National Forest
Aspen Ranger District
806 W. Hallam Street
Aspen, CO 81611
(970) 925-3445

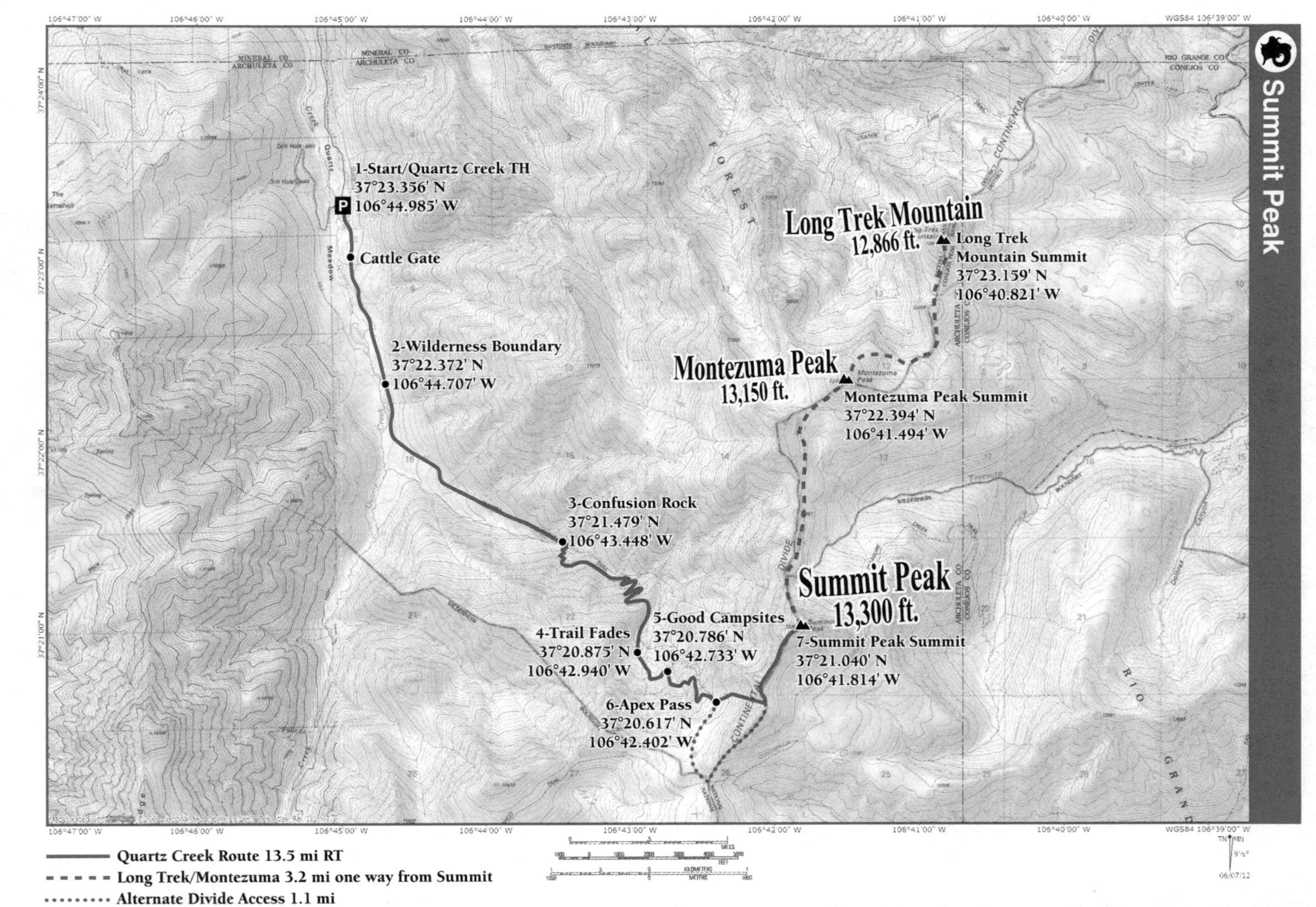

Summit Peak
1-Start/Quartz Creek TH
37°23.356' N
106°44.985' W
Cattle Gate
2-Wilderness Boundary
37°22.372' N
106°44.707' W
3-Confusion Rock
37°21.479' N
106°43.448' W
4-Trail Fades
37°20.875' N
106°42.940' W
5-Good Campsites
37°20.786' N
106°42.733' W
6-Apex Pass
37°20.617' N
106°42.402' W
Long Trek Mountain
12,866 ft.
Long Trek
Mountain Summit
37°23.159' N
106°40.821' W
Montezuma Peak
13,150 ft.
Montezuma Peak Summit
37°22.394' N
106°41.494' W
Summit Peak
13,300 ft.
7-Summit Peak Summit
37°21.040' N
106°41.814' W
Quartz Creek Route 13.5 mi RT
Long Trek/Montezuma 3.2 mi one way from Summit
Alternate Divide Access 1.1 mi

33 Summit Peak

Good Overnight!

Isolation and peace are the themes for this seldom-visited route to Summit Peak. If you are looking for a beautiful escape and a great walk on the Continental Divide, read on.

Round-Trip Distance	13.5 miles
Hiking Time	7½–10 hours
Difficulty	5/10
Class	2
Start Elevation	8,917 ft., at Quartz Creek Trailhead
Peak Elevation	13,300 ft.
Total Elevation Gain	4,460 ft.
Terrain	Good trail leading to pristine wilderness area
Best Time to Climb	July–September
Gear Advisor	Gaiters, trekking poles, GPS, and sandals for river crossing
Crowd Level	Low

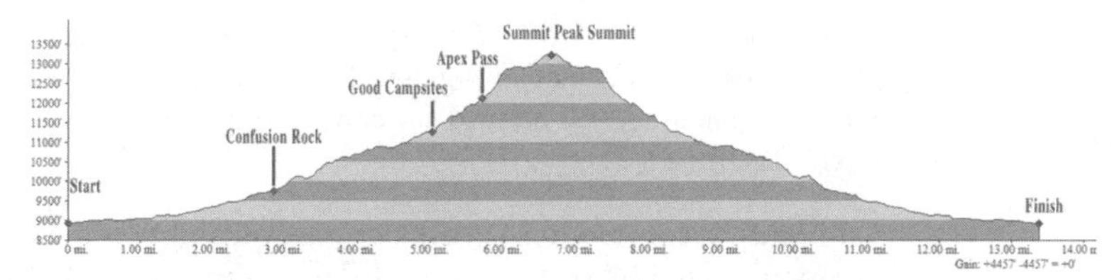

Location San Juan Mountains in the San Juan Wilderness/San Juan National Forest outside of Pagosa Springs

Intro Sometimes you just want to get away. Summit Peak and its attendant trail take you deep into the wilderness, where no signs of civilization are in sight. This hike is a catalog of natural wonders: thundering waterfalls, spacious alpine meadows, soulful forests, elaborate rock formations, dark woods, and grassy plateaus. This serene setting is ideal for a relaxing overnight journey, complemented by a good trek up to Summit Peak. Add the optional Montezuma Peak and Long Trek Mountain into the mix, and you have a trio of summits sure to rejuvenate your soul.

Why Climb It? This is not a hike for adrenaline junkies. That's not to say that there are not challenges; you'll need to navigate an overgrown basin and push up steep slopes to reach the Continental Divide. The raw natural splendor will have you reaching for your camera at every turn. Quartz Creek is especially fetching, as the cold mountain water runs clear over a bed of white and light gray rocks. Once you are on the divide, Summit Peak opens up a wonderful world of gentle ridges and glorious vistas.

Driving Tough passenger cars can make the trailhead, but if there has been a lot of rainfall (which is common in the San Juans), there may be trouble. When East Fork Road drops down next to the river around mile 7.0, there are several runoffs and mud puddles that bisect the road. Heavy rain can make these puddles traps for two-wheel drive vehicles. On Forest Service Road 684, there is a wide river crossing where the water normally flows about a foot and a half deep. If you can clear this, you're home free to the trailhead. Sport utility cars and vehicles and 4x4s will be fine.

How to Get There From the intersection of US Highway 84 and US Highway 160, east of Pagosa Springs, travel 9.7 miles north on US 160 to the East Fork Road turnoff on your right (east). If you are approaching from the north, this turn is roughly 10 miles from the top of Wolf Creek Pass. Turn onto East Fork Road (Forest Service Road 667) and follow it for 9.2 miles. Turn right onto FS 684 (Quartz Meadow Road). At mile 0.1, there is a river crossing that is often too deep for passenger cars, which will have to park here if the water is too high. One plus to this crossing is that the bottom is lined with rocks, not mud. Continue up the road, where a large cattle gate may be closed depending on the time of the year; it's not locked, but you'll have to get out of your vehicle to open and close it. Turn left at mile 2.8 and park at the obvious trailhead near a large meadow. Make sure not to drive into the woods past the trailhead.

Fees/Camping There are no fees to hike or camp in this area. Drive-in camping is available at East Fork Creek Campground's 25 sites at $8 per night, but there are plenty of places to pull off and car camp along the way, including at Quartz Creek Trailhead.

Route Notes I'd highly recommend this hike as an overnight; you can set up a high camp protected by trees at several flat sections around 11,270 feet in the high basin. These spots are mentioned in the route description.

Mile/Waypoint **0.0 mi (1)** Start at the Quartz Creek Trailhead. Get on the Quartz Creek Trail and head south through the open meadow. Don't bother the cows that may be grazing in the area. (Seriously, these are not your normal cows. Alpine cows are a tough breed. They've come to chew cud and kick butt . . . and they're all out of cud.) Pass through a cattle gate and enjoy this trail. For the most part, it is easy to follow, though there are some sections that seem to be washed out, where runoff from the east intersects the trail. If there is a washout, continue south, and eventually you'll regain the well-worn tail.

1.2 mi (2) Wilderness boundary sign. From here, you begin to go away from the creek and enter a pine forest draped with hanging moss. The trail is still easy to follow and gradually gains altitude.

2.8 mi (3) Welcome to Confusion Rock. Confused? The trail you have been following goes down a little hill to the creek. There are faint trails on your side of the river, and they all apparently dead-end. When you are standing at this point, you'll see a giant rock that looks like a big, gray potato. You need to cross the river and get on the right side of this rock, where the trail

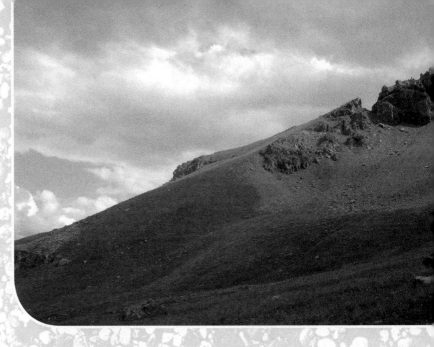

The grassy ridgelines of Summit Peak are seldom visited, so don't expect trails.

resumes in a series of steep switchbacks. This means that you'll need to go downstream a little to get across to the rocky, steep hill. It's a bear to lug a backpack up that section, but once you are up, the trail magically reappears and the going is easy again. When you hike to the top of Confusion Rock, look to the east. You'll see a secret waterfall running in the notched entrance of a cave.

The next section of the trail is easy to follow. The switchbacks are well-designed as they climb higher. With luck, you won't scare any camouflaged pheasants, who will in turn scare the tar out of you with their loud, flapping wings.

4.7 mi (4) As you enter the big, sloped basin, the trail gets overgrown. You need to start heading southeast. If the trail is visible, take it. If not (which was the case when I was last there), find a good route through the foliage. There are several ways to gain the Continental Divide here, but stay on route.

5.0 mi (5) In many of the pockets of pine trees, you can find level ground. These sites are great for camping. They are sheltered, close to water, and have great views. This is a good place to pitch a tent and call it a night. Day hikers will want to continue up toward the grassy slopes below Apex Pass.

5.8 mi (6) This is the base of Apex Pass (12,100 feet), a smooth, loose, scree slope that grants access to the Continental Divide. Starting at the grassy slopes above timberline, march to the base of the pass and push up to the divide—a gain of 700 feet. Those looking for an easier (but longer) way to gain the divide can go south and get on the ridge via mild slopes (this is the way the trail should go, but it's faded out).

6.2 mi Once you are on the divide, the way to Summit is obvious. Walk northeast on the gentle grassy ramp to Summit's highest point.

6.8 mi (7) Summit's summit! You'll feel like the king of your own private empire up here. Continue on the optional route or return the way you came. A GPS is helpful for retracing your tracks. Once you're on the trail on the west side of the basin, it's easy going back down the Quartz Creek Trail.

13.5 mi Finish your hike.

Options If you overnight at the camp spot (waypoint 5), you set yourself up for a great day of peak-bagging. Gain the ridge via Apex Pass and begin a long, easy, class 2 stroll north. The Continental Divide Trail runs along the peaks here. Montezuma Peak (13,150 feet) is 1.8 miles from Summit. The hermit's haven of Long Trek Mountain (12,866 feet) is 3.2 miles from Summit. From high camp, the round-trip mileage to Long Trek and back is 10 miles—a very full day. On the divide, it's easy to hike quickly, so you can do this out-and-back in about four to six hours. Start early (at sunrise) and get back to camp to avoid summer storms. All three summits as a day hike from Quartz Creek Trailhead? You're looking at 20 miles. Fit trail runners may be able to do it, but it would be tough. Break it up and you have two full days of great hiking.

Quick Facts At least Summit Peak's bland name is accurate: it's the high point of Archuleta County. This fact brings a few county high point peak-baggers to Summit every year.

Montezuma is named for the ancient deity who had significance to both the Aztec and Pueblo people. It is also incorrectly cited as the name of two flesh-and-blood emperors of the Aztec empire. Their names were actually Monteczuma I and Monteczuma II: Esta Vez Esto Es Personal. (Every sequel needs a tagline: "This Time It's Personal" seems to work for most!)

Contact Info San Juan National Forest
Pagosa Ranger District
180 Second Street
P.O. Box 310
Pagosa Springs, CO 81147
(970) 264-2268

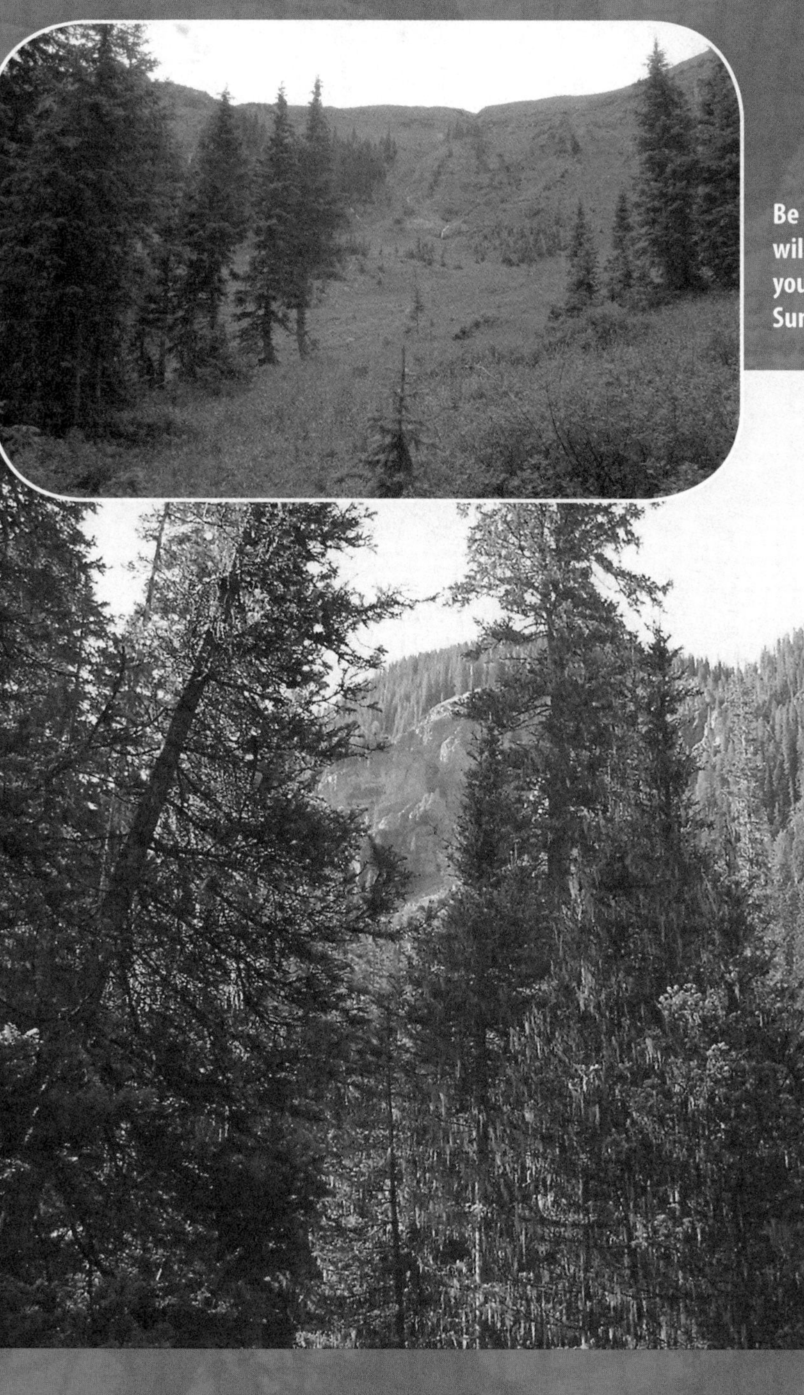

Be ready for a remote wilderness experience on your adventure to Summit Peak.

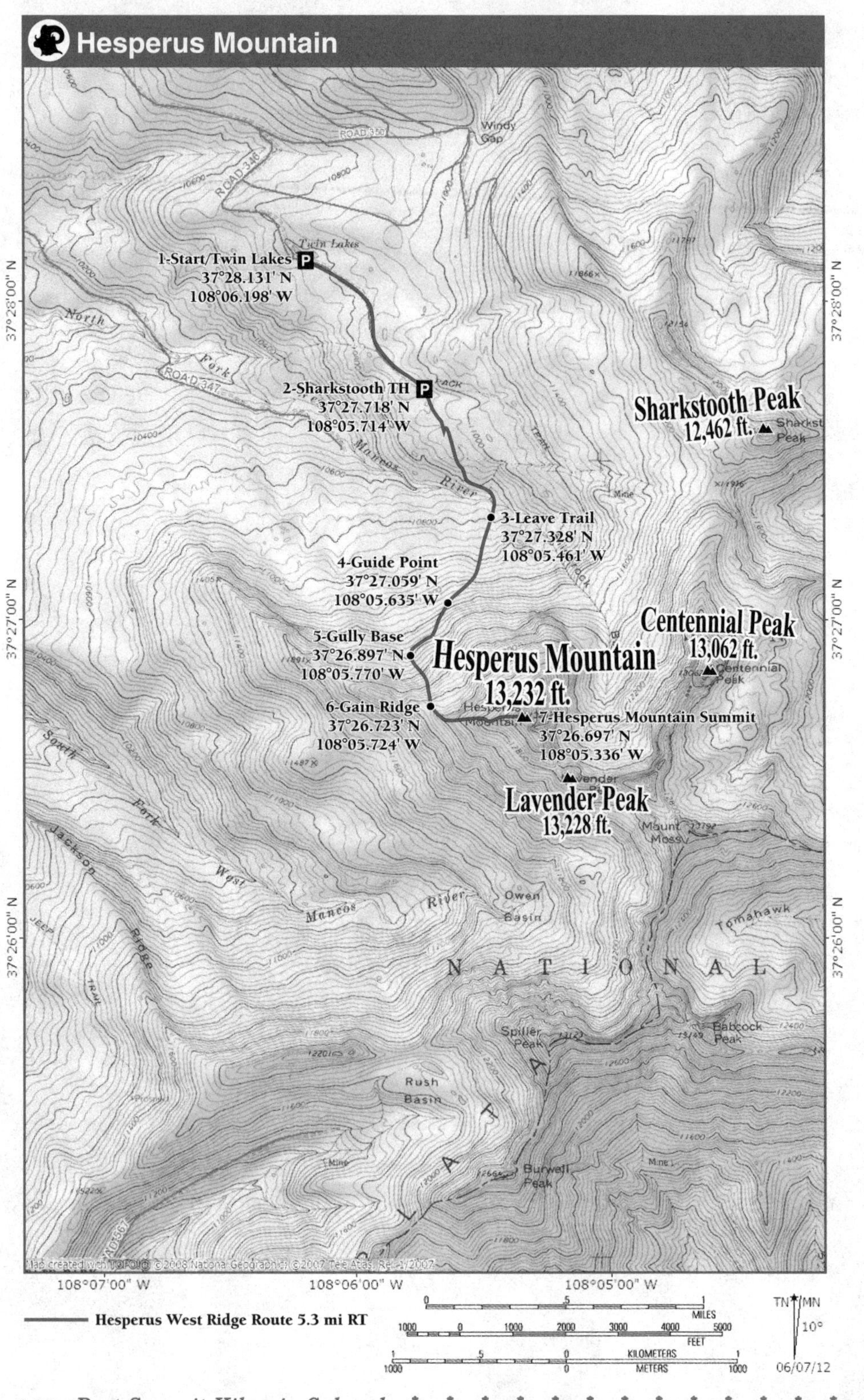
Hesperus Mountain
1-Start/Twin Lakes
37°28.131' N
108°06.198' W
2-Sharkstooth TH
37°27.718' N
108°05.714' W
3-Leave Trail
37°27.328' N
108°05.461' W
4-Guide Point
37°27.059' N
108°05.635' W
5-Gully Base
37°26.897' N
108°05.770' W
6-Gain Ridge
37°26.723' N
108°05.724' W
7-Hesperus Mountain Summit
37°26.697' N
108°05.336' W
Hesperus Mountain
13,232 ft.
Sharkstooth Peak
12,462 ft.
Centennial Peak
13,062 ft.
Lavender Peak
13,228 ft.
Windy Gap
ROAD 350
ROAD 346
ROAD 347
Twin Lakes
North Fork
Mancos River
South Fork
West Mancos River
Jackson Ridge
Owen Basin
Mount Moss
Tomahawk
NATIONAL
Spiller Peak
Babcock Peak
Rush Basin
Burwell Peak
37°28'00" N
37°27'00" N
37°26'00" N
108°07'00" W
108°06'00" W
108°05'00" W
Hesperus West Ridge Route 5.3 mi RT
MILES
FEET
KILOMETERS
METERS
TN MN
10°
06/07/12

34 Hesperus Mountain

Red and white stripes decorate the face of Hesperus; it's a truly unique Colorado color scheme. Go off-trail and make your way to the top of this most sacred mountain.

Round-Trip Distance	5.3 miles
Hiking Time	5–7 hours
Difficulty	7/10
Class	2+
Start Elevation	10,780 ft., at Sharkstooth Trailhead
Peak Elevation	13,232 ft.
Total Elevation Gain	2,840 ft.
Terrain	Short but good trail leads to rocky, rugged gullies and ridge walk
Best Time to Climb	June–September
Gear Advisor	GPS and trekking poles
Crowd Level	Low

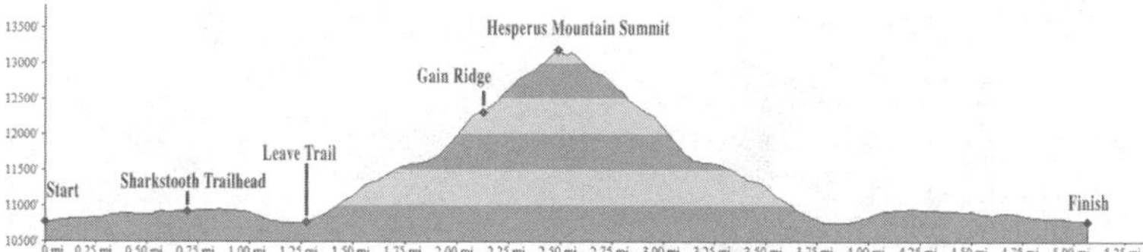

Location La Plata Mountains in the San Juan National Forest outside the town of Mancos

Intro It's easy to see why the Navajo people consider this sacred mountain a special place on Earth. They call it Dibé Nitsaa, which translates to "big mountain sheep." Each of the four sacred mountains was assigned a color that related to its spiritual significance; Hesperus was noted not for the red and white stripes but for the black, powdery obsidian found on its ridges. Obsidian was an important rock to the Navajo because it could be shaped into tools and arrowheads. Dibé Nitsaa is the sacred mountain of the north (find out more about the other peaks in the "Quick Facts" section on page 227).

The Navajo believe that these mountains are vital to their existence; not only do they designate the boundaries of the land given to the Navajo by the Great Spirit, but they also are places where the people can connect with all living things, renew the spirit, and gaze with wonder upon the same lands as their ancestors.

Why Climb It? I would be lying if I said that I didn't feel a spiritual pull to Dibé Nitsaa. The striking profile and coloration of the peak stands out from miles away. Views from the top are incredible, mimicking an eagle's perspective of the land below. Sharkstooth Peak rises from an ocean of talus to the north, and the craggy, broken face of Lavender Peak shares a busted ridge to the west. The hiking is tough at times, but once you have gained the west ridge, you're in business. What begins as a steep ridge on broken plates of rock gives way to better scrambling the higher you climb. It's short mileage-wise, but it's a challenging hike that will take some time and route finding.

Driving Tough passenger cars can make it most of the way; the route described here starts at the car parking area at Twin Lakes. Sport utility cars (SUCs), sport utility vehicles (SUVs), and 4x4s can push on the final 0.7 mile to Sharkstooth Trailhead. The dirt road is rocky and washed out in places; large mud puddles are the main obstacles for two-wheel drive vehicles.

How to Get There From the charming town of Mancos, on US Highway 160, find the intersection of US 160 and Colorado Highway 184. Turn north onto CO 184 for 0.3 mile and turn right onto County Road 42 (there will be signs for Mancos State Park/West Mancos Road/Jackson Lake). This is also known as Forest Service Road 561. It begins as a paved road and turns to dirt at 1.2 miles.

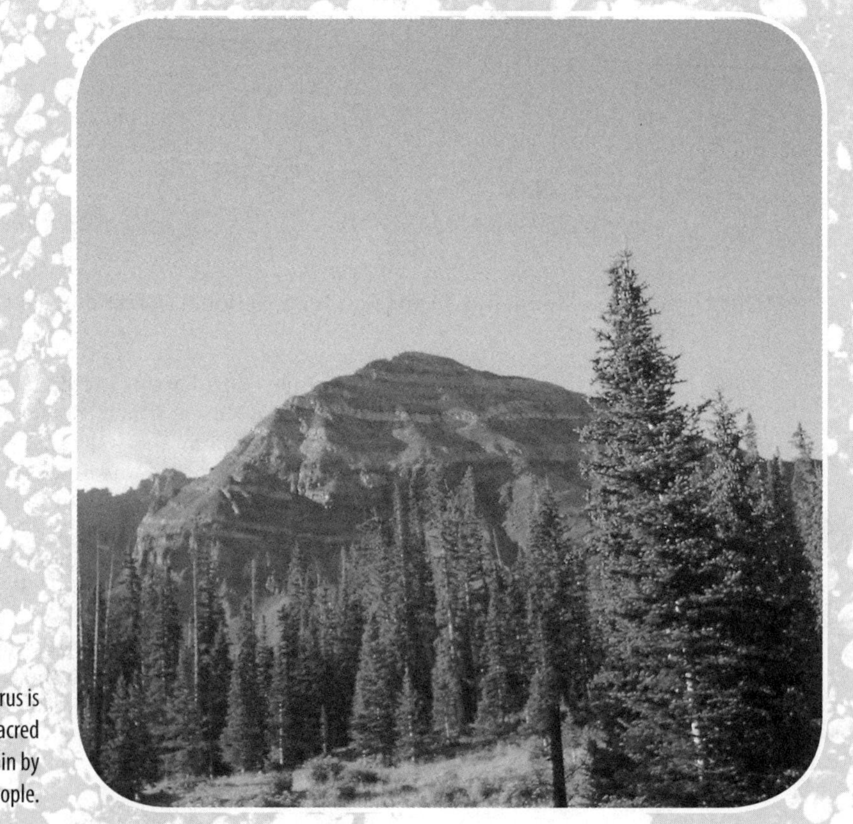

Hesperus is considered a sacred mountain by native people.

Follow this road past the Transfer Campground and Aspen Guard Station, and at mile 12.0, take a right onto Forest Service Road 350 (Spruce Mill Road). There will be signs for the Sharkstooth Trailhead (mile 7.5) here. Stay on this semi-rocky road 6.0 miles (there are nice camping options the last mile), and then turn right and downhill onto Forest Service Road 346. The turn isn't well marked; there are signs for the Aspen Loop ATV Trail, a Mancos 17 sign, and eventually a sign for Twin Lakes and Sharkstooth Trailhead. The road gets significantly rougher here. Cars can make it to within 1.0 mile of Twin Lakes and park on the right; the route described here starts at this point. SUCs, SUVs, and 4x4s can brave some big mud puddles and deeply rutted chunks of road to travel the remaining 0.7 mile to the Sharkstooth Trailhead at the end of the road.

Fees/Camping There are no fees for hiking or camping in this area. The closest pay sites with facilities can be found at the Transfer Campground, where sites are $10 per night. The backcountry car camping is quite good the last 2.0 miles of FS 350.

Route Notes This route is off-trail most of the way. A GPS and trekking poles will help.

Mile/Waypoint

0.0 mi (1) Start the hike at Twin Lakes parking area. Hike or drive up the remaining 0.7 mile to the formal Sharkstooth Trailhead.

0.7 mi (2) This is the official trailhead at 10,925 feet. A few trails start here. You want to go south on the West Mancos Trail #621. This trail doesn't see a ton of traffic, so it's a little faded. It's an easy start—you go downhill! Stay on trail as you drop down to the river. A sign that reads NORTH FORK OF THE WEST MANCOS is visible. Cross the river and stay on trail, due southwest.

1.3 mi (3) From the trail, you'll see a grassy clearing to your left (south). It's time to get off-trail, but take a good look first. A teardrop of talus is in the middle of the slope; to the right of that are some weeds and bushes, and to the right of them is a row of pine trees. Aim to climb on the left fringe of the pine trees, up a grassy slope and right, to the top of the talus pile. From there, you will begin to go right and line up a good path to gain the ridge.

1.6 mi (4) Use this waypoint to stay on course. Under the giant north face, continue to skirt up and right (southwest) toward a grassy slope west of the rocky face. Stay above the patches of willows. I've seen some people trying to get a more direct route up these rocky ledges, and they struggled mightily. The line may be more direct, but it's also on bad rock—rotten, broken, and steep. Keep going right (southwest) through a few pine trees and gullies. Stay low on the flatter parts of the slope while you traverse over.

1.9 mi (5) At 11,646 feet, you will be at the base of a gully with a moderate grade (it's the second big gully after the rocky shoulder of the ridge). The gully is defined by a plethora of scree and a coating of obsidian powder at the top. GPS users should check the waypoint. If it still looks too steep, you can continue to traverse westward and connect with the ridge farther down.

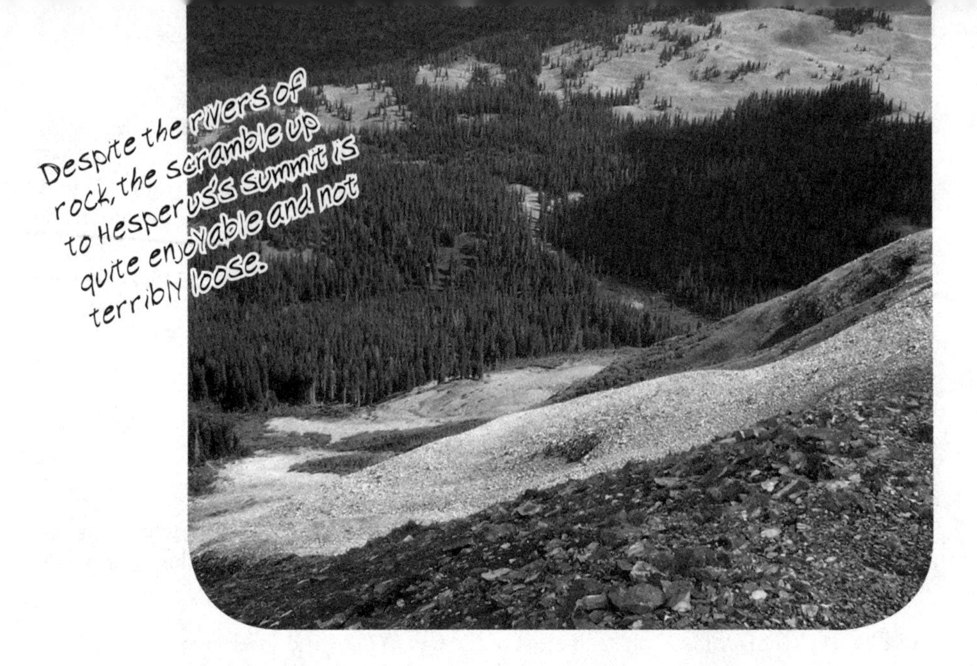
Despite the rivers of
rock, the scramble up
to Hesperus's summit is
quite enjoyable and not
terribly loose.

2.2 mi (6) After a tough push, you've gained the west ridge. From here, all you need to do is head east and get up the ridge. Most of the terrain on the ridge is class 2+, perhaps easy class 3. Staying on the spine of the ridge makes travel easier; the frosted flakes of rocks in the beginning aren't good for your knees. There are some nice notches and gullies to scramble up, just make sure that you don't go onto the north face. There is always a class 2 option to your right (south) if the terrain gets too tricky for you. Continue up, past bands of white rock, and work to the highest point on the horizon (which may be blinded out by the east-rising sun). Eventually, you'll top out; hike about 60 feet north, and you'll be at the summit.

2.6 mi (7) Hesperus Mountain summit! You are standing on the white top of the sacred mountain. There is a summit register here maintained by a very dedicated individual. The views up here rival that of any 14er. As you gaze out upon the homelands of the Navajo, consider this quote:

> We, the five-fingered beings, are related to the four-legged, the winged beings, the spiritual beings, Father Sky, Mother Earth, and nature. We are all relatives. We cannot leave our relatives behind.
>
> —*Betty Tso, Navajo*

Give your thanks to the Great Spirit of your choice and return down the way you ascended. A GPS will help you retrace your tracks back to the trailhead.

5.3 mi Finish.

Options From Hesperus, ridges to other points are fraught with peril. The southeast ridge to Lavender Peak looks to be a tough ticket; I have not tried it, but it appears to be at least class 3+/4. If you're an enterprising scrambler, it may be a fun way to reach Lavender and Centennial Peaks. Oh, and if you're the kind of freak who loves knee-twisting, ankle-wrenching talus fields, you can go up to Sharkstooth Peak from the Sharkstooth Trailhead. Your orthopedic surgeon thanks you in advance.

Quick Facts

Hesperus gets its name from the Hesperus Mine that spawned a boomtown of the same name in 1882, founded by John Porter. The name transferred to the mountain; in Latin it means "the evening star," which referred to the planet Venus.

The four sacred mountains of the Navajo delimit the land of their ancestors. The mountains are:

Mount Blanca (*Tsisnaasjini'*—Dawn or White Shell Mountain)
Sacred Mountain of the East

Mount Taylor (*Tsoodzil*—Blue Bead or Turquoise Mountain)
Sacred Mountain of the South

San Francisco Peak (*Doko'oosliid*—Abalone Shell Mountain)
Sacred Mountain of the West

Mount Hesperus (*Dibé Nitsaa*—Big Mountain Sheep—Obsidian Mountain) Sacred Mountain of the North

Thanks to **lapahie.com,** a Navajo Web page, for this information.

Contact Info

San Juan National Forest
Dolores Ranger District
100 N. Sixth Street
P.O. Box 210
Dolores, CO 81323
(970) 882-6841

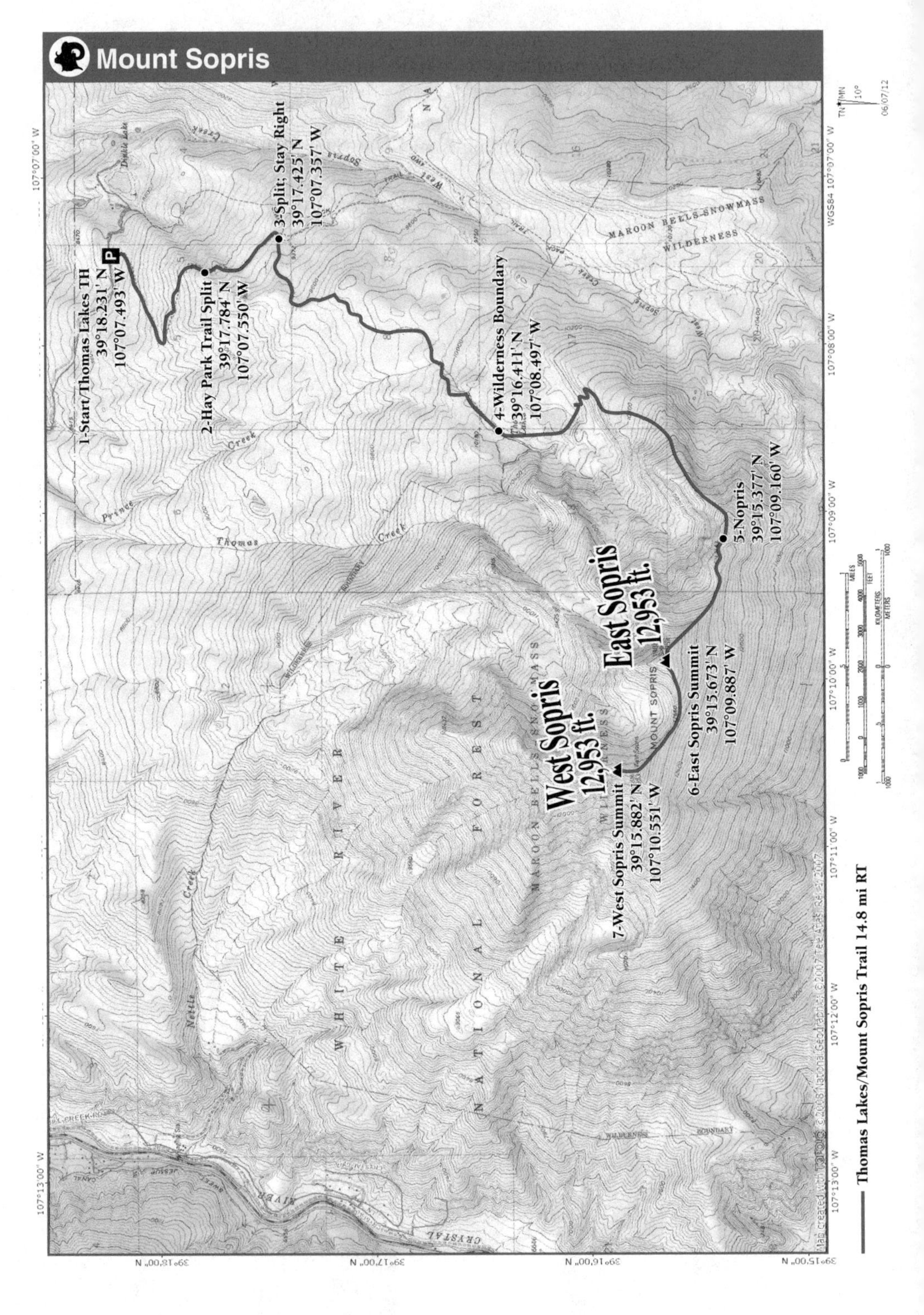
Mount Sopris
1-Start/Thomas Lakes TH
39°18.231' N
107°07.493' W
2-Hay Park Trail Split
39°17.784' N
107°07.550' W
3-Split; Stay Right
39°17.425' N
107°07.357' W
4-Wilderness Boundary
39°16.411' N
107°08.497' W
5-Nopris
39°15.377' N
107°09.160' W
6-East Sopris Summit
39°15.673' N
107°09.887' W
7-West Sopris Summit
39°15.882' N
107°10.551' W
East Sopris
12,953 ft.
West Sopris
12,953 ft.
MOUNT SOPRIS
WHITE RIVER
NATIONAL FOREST
MAROON BELLS-SNOWMASS WILDERNESS
Thomas
Prince Creek
Nettle Creek
Dinkle Lake
West Sopris Creek
CRYSTAL RIVER
Thomas Lakes/Mount Sopris Trail 14.8 mi RT

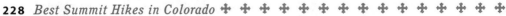

35 Mount Sopris

Sopris is perhaps the most impressive stand-alone mountain in Colorado, especially when viewed from Carbondale. Both east and west summits boast the exact same official elevation; I got the same results with my GPS.

Round-Trip Distance	14.8 miles
Hiking Time	7½–10 hours
Difficulty	6.5/10
Class	2
Start Elevation	8,635 ft., at Thomas Lake/Sopris Trailhead
Peak Elevation	12,953 ft.
Total Elevation Gain	5,072 ft.
Terrain	Good trails to good ridge traverse
Best Time to Climb	June–September
Gear Advisor	Normal gear
Crowd Level	Moderate

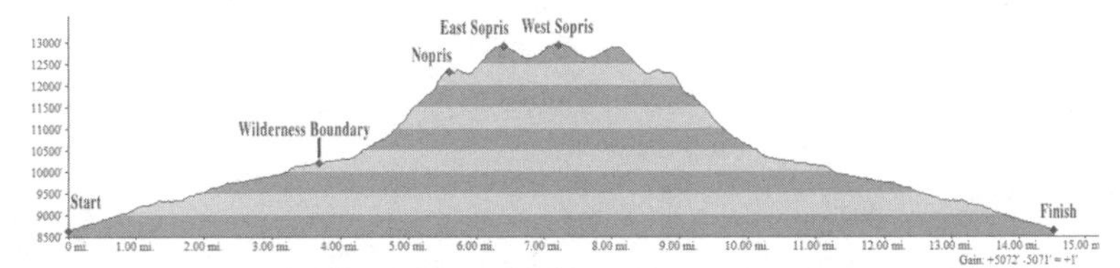

Location Elk Range in the Maroon Bells-Snowmass Wilderness/White River National Forest outside of Carbondale

Intro By all accounts, 12,953-foot Mount Sopris *looks* like the biggest mountain in Colorado when viewed from the north. The twin summits rise more than 6,500 feet from the nearby town of Carbondale. That would be like having a 13er smack-dab in downtown Denver. In comparison, the mountains behind Boulder rise to only 8,500 feet. Not only is this a great-looking mountain, but it's also a great hike. What seems like an arduous task to ascend both summits turns out to be an easy, 1.0-mile saddle traverse between the two. Don't let the high mileage discourage you—this is a very viable day hike. The approach to Thomas Lakes goes by quickly on class 1 trails.

Why Climb It? Sopris is yet another peak that begs to be climbed. The long trail to Thomas Lakes is quite scenic and travels through open meadows and friendly forests. Once you reach Thomas Lakes you'll tour the twin summits via the east ridge. This is one of my favorite ridge walks in all of Colorado. After an initial push on rocky talus to the top of Nopris, you are granted access to the rolling ridge to the east summit. Views of the river of gray talus that flows down the north face are stunning; there are even ripples and contours that make it look like a molten lava flow (or a giant river of cake batter). Gaining the two summits will leave you scratching your head and wondering which is truly higher.

Driving Passenger cars can make it to the Thomas Lakes Trailhead. The dirt road is well maintained and poses no difficult sections.

How to Get There From Carbondale, go south on Colorado Highway 133. From the south end of town, go 0.92 mile from the intersection of CO 133 and the last major road, Snowmass Drive. Pay attention. You want to take a left onto Prince Creek Road, which is very easy to miss. It has an irregularly small blue sign, and it comes up just after passing the high school on your left. If you pass a fish hatchery on the right, you've gone too far.

Stay on the road as it passes through Bureau of Land Management lands. There will be signs for Dinkle Lake along the way. At mile 6.0, you'll come to a somewhat confusing junction. You want to bear right onto County Road 6A, which is marked with signs for Dinkle Lake; essentially this is your second right. The first right is a private road with a gate (which may or may not be open)—do not take it. Staying left on West Sopris Road is also a mistake. Get on County Road 6A and stay the course as it climbs through aspen groves. At 1.85 miles, there is a parking area atop a hill (this comes up before Dinkle Lake). The parking area (on the left) has a large, fenced-off area for horse trailers, as well as a restroom. The Thomas Lakes Trail starts on the right (south) side of the road through a grassy meadow.

Fees/Camping There are no fees to hike or camp in the area. There are backcountry campsites at Thomas Lakes.

Route Notes None.

Mile/Waypoint

0.0 mi (1) Get on the marked Thomas Lakes Trail on the south side of the road. This trail starts as a singletrack through a grassy meadow and then joins a wider dirt "road" as it enters the woods. Note that the road is not used by automobiles—it's a snowmobile path. Stay on this trail as it climbs through the woods.

1.1 mi (2) The Hay Park Trail splits to the left here; stay on the Thomas Lakes Trail.

1.7 mi (3) There is another trail split; again stay right on the Thomas Lakes Trail as it goes up a hill to a grassy meadow. There are very good views of Carbondale from here.

3.7 mi (4) After a pleasant walk through the forest, you arrive at the Maroon Bells-Snowmass Wilderness boundary. Just past this sign are the Thomas Lakes. Stay on the main trail that runs between the two of them. There is a signed trail for Mount Sopris in this area. Note that any side trails simply lead to backcountry campsites.

After passing the east lake, the trail begins to climb steadily on switchbacks to timberline.

4.9 mi At 11,060 feet, you clear tree line and have a good look at the ridge before you (as well as amazing views of the lakes and landscape to the north).

The hardest section of hiking is coming up—a steep trail cut into the talus slopes en route to Nopris. It's a lung burner, even for veteran hikers.

5.7 mi (5) The strong push up the ridge leads to Mount Nopris, officially an unnamed 12,463-foot subpeak of the Sopris massif. You can skirt this summit to the left or scramble up to the top. From here, the east summit looks huge. The little saddle between Nopris and the east summit is one of my favorites. Continue along the ridge westward to the broad East Sopris summit.

6.5 mi (6) East Sopris summit! This is the more spacious of the two tops, with room to stretch out and enjoy lunch. A register and a wind shelter are located here. When you are ready, continue west along the ridge to West Sopris summit. This stretch is 0.9 mile one way on similar terrain, though the very end, near the west summit, is a bit rockier. Some interesting homemade memorials are just off the east summit on the west side: perhaps the ashes of a relative or a pet?

7.4 mi (7) West Sopris summit! A skinny, 7-foot cairn seems to force the issue of which mountain is truly higher. Cheaters never win, West Sopris. Enjoy the views and return the way you came, bypassing the south side of East Sopris to save a little time. For a relatively long walk back, it does not get as tedious as other descents.

14.8 mi Finish.

Options There are no other routes to speak of on this hike; you're climbing on most of everything that is available. You can try some alternate ridges on the north face if you'd like a new way up. Good luck with the talus!

Quick Facts I once had an interesting encounter on Sopris. On my way down, I met a woman from Utah (her name slips my mind) who is a direct descendant of the man for whom the peak is named, Captain Richard Sopris. Captain Sopris surveyed the area in 1860 (he never climbed the peak) and went on to prominence as the mayor of Denver. His present-day relative had driven from Salt Lake City to see the mountain named after her great-great-great-grandfather. As afternoon storm clouds moved in, she realized that she wouldn't make the summit. That's OK because neither did her great-great-great-grandpa!

Nearby Carbondale takes its name from Carbondale, Pennsylvania. It was coincidence that coal mining later helped the economy flourish. Carbondale was originally a "feeder" town, providing potatoes and other foods to nourish the hungry miners working in the nearby silver mines of Aspen. Potato Days celebration in October is still a big event for the town.

Contact Info White River National Forest, Sopris Ranger District
620 Main Street
P.O. Box 309
Carbondale, CO 81623
(970) 963-2266

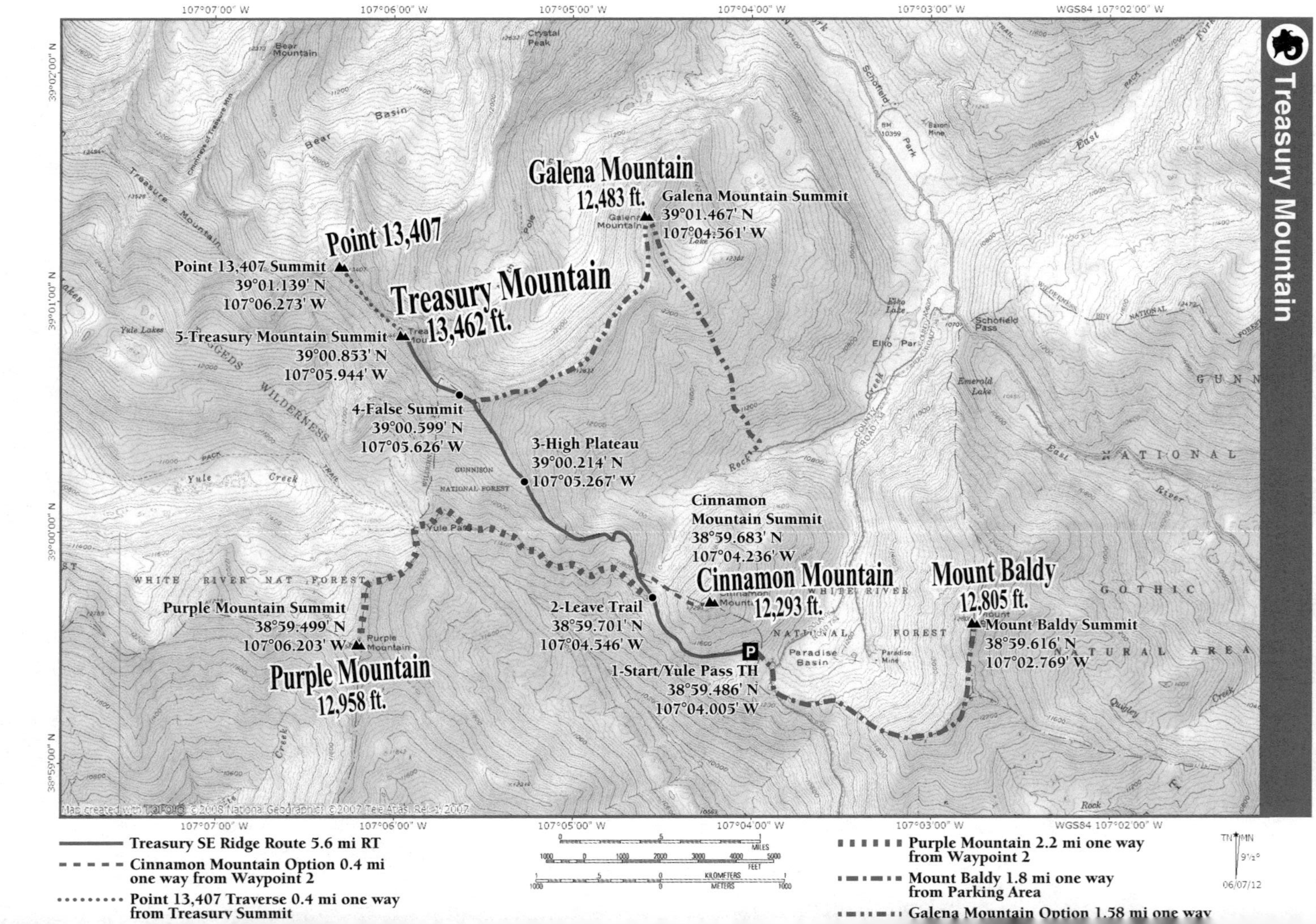

Treasury Mountain
Point 13,407
Treasury Mountain 13,462 ft.
Galena Mountain 12,483 ft.
Cinnamon Mountain 12,293 ft.
Mount Baldy 12,805 ft.
Purple Mountain 12,958 ft.
Point 13,407 Summit 39°01.139' N 107°06.273' W
5-Treasury Mountain Summit 39°00.853' N 107°05.944' W
4-False Summit 39°00.599' N 107°05.626' W
3-High Plateau 39°00.214' N 107°05.267' W
2-Leave Trail 38°59.701' N 107°04.546' W
1-Start/Yule Pass TH 38°59.486' N 107°04.005' W
Galena Mountain Summit 39°01.467' N 107°04.561' W
Cinnamon Mountain Summit 38°59.683' N 107°04.236' W
Mount Baldy Summit 38°59.616' N 107°02.769' W
Purple Mountain Summit 38°59.499' N 107°06.203' W
Schofield Pass
Emerold Lake
Paradise Basin
Yule Pass
Treasury SE Ridge Route 5.6 mi RT
Cinnamon Mountain Option 0.4 mi one way from Waypoint 2
Point 13,407 Traverse 0.4 mi one way from Treasury Summit
Purple Mountain 2.2 mi one way from Waypoint 2
Mount Baldy 1.8 mi one way from Parking Area
Galena Mountain Option 1.58 mi one way

36 Treasury Mountain

Often seen but seldom visited, Treasury Mountain is part of the awesome Raggeds Wilderness. The greatest treasure this mountain offers may be the dramatic views.

Round-Trip Distance	5.6 miles
Hiking Time	4–6 hours
Difficulty	5.5/10
Class	2+
Start Elevation	11,350 ft., at Yule Pass Trailhead
Peak Elevation	13,462 ft.
Total Elevation Gain	2,127 ft.
Terrain	Off-trail ridge walk
Best Time to Climb	July–September
Gear Advisor	Normal gear
Crowd Level	Low

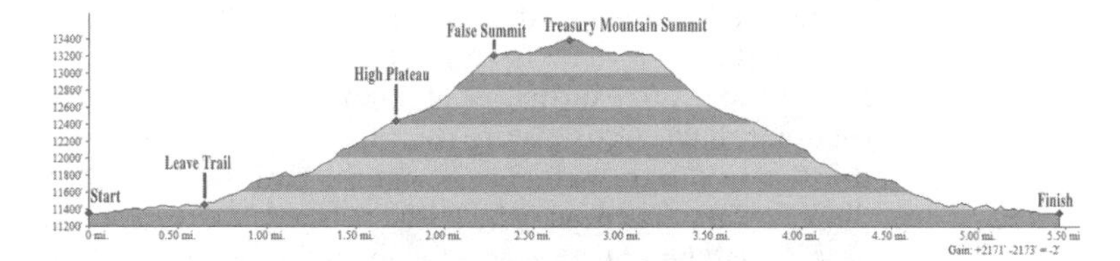

Location Elk Range in the Raggeds Wilderness/Gunnison National Forest and White River National Forest outside of Crested Butte

Intro The Elk Mountains are notorious for harsh weather, often holding onto patches of snow year-round. Treasury Mountain anchors the eastern reaches of a massif that serves as an intermediary between the Elks and the gradual declination of the Rocky Mountains to the west. Treasury is often seen from points in the Maroon Bells–Snowmass Wilderness, notably from West Maroon Pass. A great and little-known hike, Treasury is a part of Colorado that is a little more untamed than other areas.

Why Climb It? Treasury's setting brings to mind visions of the Greek underworld, with dark, stormy mountains and precipitous drop-offs into vertigo-inducing canyons. The area is wild, rugged, and teeming with elemental malice—storms that hit the area often unleash their fury with amplified force. Treasury sits on the edge of the turmoil, offering views to the benevolent Maroon Bells–Snowmass Wilderness peaks to the north and to the more sinister-looking Raggeds Wilderness peaks to the south.

Of course, if you get a blue, sunny day, it's simply a heck of a mountain with incredible views. The ridge is a splendid experience, reaching a broad alpine plateau before the final summit push. The 300-million-year-old marine shale atop the peak is decorated with fossils of fish, plants, and shells—keep your eyes open. These may be the best treasures found on the mountain.

Driving Tough passenger cars can make it to the Yule Pass Trailhead, though it may be a dramatic experience. Schofield Pass is a maintained dirt road; the last 2.5 miles on Paradise Divide Road are rougher. The road is generally passable and in good shape, but there is one particular hill that low-powered vehicles will strain to climb (my Honda Accord barely made it up, floored and in first gear).

How to Get There From Crested Butte, follow Colorado Highway 135 north out of town to Gothic Road (Forest Service Road 317). Pass Mount Crested Butte and continue on Gothic Road, which turns to dirt. Follow this road 10.5 miles to Schofield Pass, bypassing the mysterious town of Gothic en route. At the top of Schofield Pass, 10,707 feet, turn left (west) onto Paradise Divide Road (County Road 734). The road gets a little rougher as it drops down to the flats of Elko Park. Stay left at 0.6 mile, and head up a steep hill that will challenge four-cylinder vehicles. At 1.6 miles, stay right on the main road at the junction with an old 4x4 road. At 2.3 miles, you'll reach the flats of Paradise Divide, where the road splits. The left split will go downhill, and there will be two roads uphill to the right—both lead to Yule Pass Trailhead. Take the one farther right, as the other is a gratuitous 4x4 road. The road will have signs giving the mileage to Yule Pass; note that this is the distance to the actual pass, not the parking area. Proceed 0.2 mile to the Yule Pass Trailhead (which isn't marked; the road reaches a closure gate near a small pond with spaces for about five or six vehicles).

Fees/Camping There are no fees to camp or hike in this area. There are dozens of magnificent camping areas along Schofield Pass and the Paradise Divide Road. You can pitch a tent in the area around the trailhead, but the ground is a bit lumpy.

Route Notes None.

Mile/Waypoint **0.0 mi (1)** Start at the Yule Pass Trailhead and proceed on the Yule Pass Trail. This rocky but solid trail is cut into the hillside and has amazing views of the Slate River Canyon to the left (south).

0.7 mi (2) At the low saddle between Cinnamon and Treasury Mountains, leave the trail and gain the southeast ridge of Treasury Mountain. There is no trail on the ridge, but the spine is easy to follow as it curves northwest. This ridge undulates as it heads toward the mountain's highest point, now visible on the horizon.

1.8 mi (3) After climbing a few hills, you'll come to a broad plateau and slope with very good views. Push northwest up the hill, hiking just to the left (east) of the ridge for the best footing.

2.3 mi (4) Oh, man! After that big push up the long slope, the high point on the ridge turns out to be a false summit at 13,215 feet. Luckily, the plateau over to the summit is mild and has quite an ethereal atmosphere. Follow the plateau to a short, enjoyable scramble to the summit.

2.8 mi (5) Treasury Mountain summit. Look at the rocks beneath your feet—fossils abound. From here, you can continue your trek northeast to the Treasure Mountain massif via the optional northwest ridge. Otherwise, return down the ridge the way you came.

5.6 mi Finish.

Options There are lots of options from Treasury to extend your day. The most obvious side trip is a quick but steep 0.4-mile push up to Cinnamon Mountain summit (only 0.8 mile, round-trip, from waypoint **2**).

From waypoint **2**, stay on the Yule Pass Trail to Yule Pass, and challenge the north ridge of Purple Mountain, a class 3 scramble to Treasury's sister summit.

From the parking lot (or Paradise Divide), it's 1.8 miles one way to the eastern summit of Mount Baldy; this is a nice hike that gives you great views of Treasury.

Finally, traverse northwest from Treasury's summit to point 13,407, one of the high peaks that grace the Treasure Mountain massif to the northwest.

Want to add in a bonus peak? Galena Mountain (12,580 feet) is a fun, class 2+ scramble that is 1.58 miles from the false summit (waypoint **4**). If you don't mind a moderately steep, off-trail descent, you can return to your car via Galena's southeast slopes. Hiking poles are recommended.

Quick Facts Treasury Mountain is so named for the silver mines that were dug into its flanks. There were many mining camps set up in the area, with mixed results.

A few of the features in the area, including Yule Pass and North Pole Basin, are based on a Christmas theme.

Contact Info White River National Forest
Aspen Ranger District
806 W. Hallam Street
Aspen, CO 81611
(970) 925-3445

Gunnison National Forest
Gunnison Ranger District
216 N. Colorado Street
Gunnison, CO 81230
(970) 641-0471

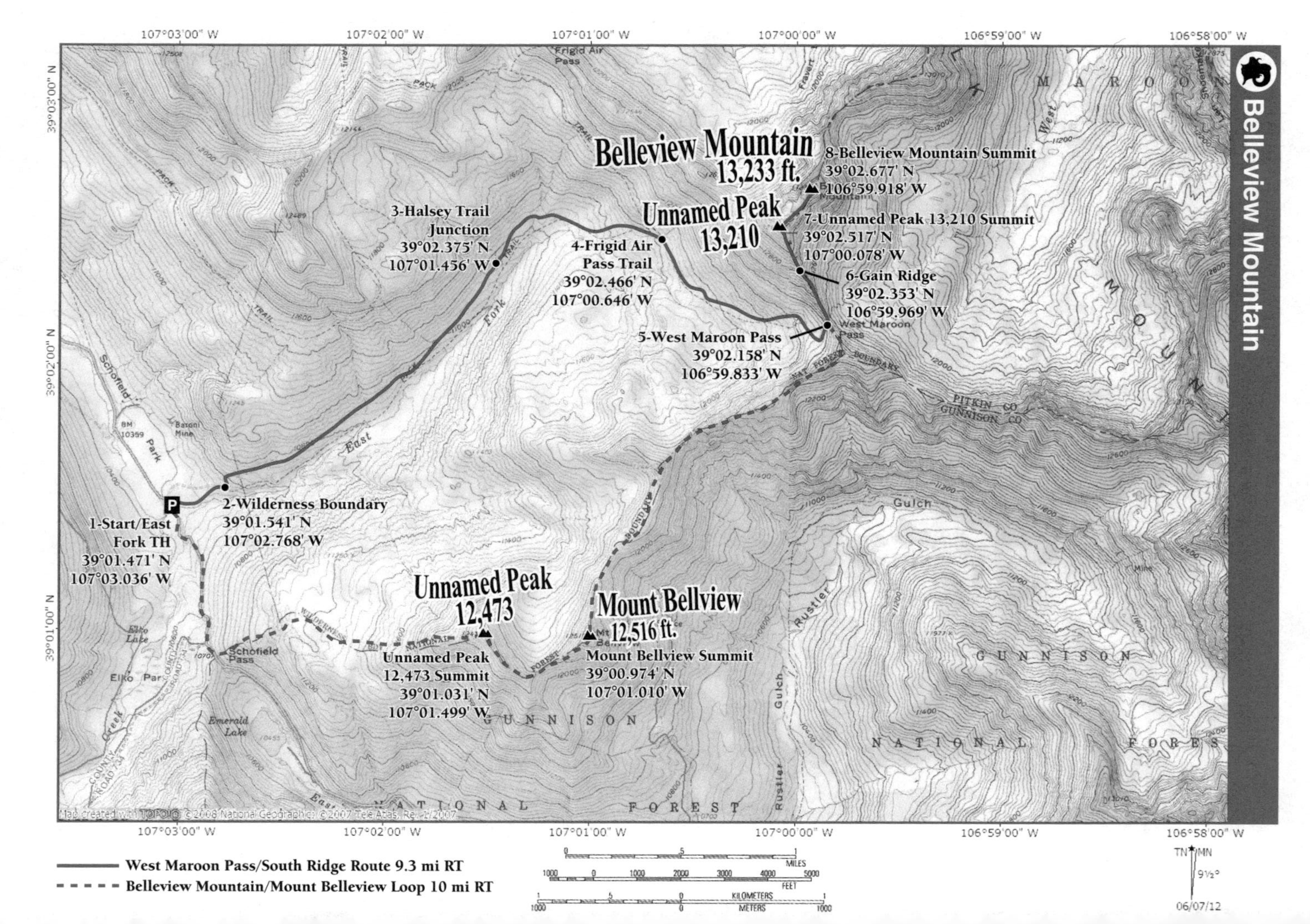

Belleview Mountain
Belleview Mountain 13,233 ft.
8-Belleview Mountain Summit
39°02.677' N
106°59.918' W
Unnamed Peak 13,210
7-Unnamed Peak 13,210 Summit
39°02.517' N
107°00.078' W
6-Gain Ridge
39°02.353' N
106°59.969' W
5-West Maroon Pass
39°02.158' N
106°59.833' W
4-Frigid Air Pass Trail
39°02.466' N
107°00.646' W
3-Halsey Trail Junction
39°02.375' N
107°01.456' W
2-Wilderness Boundary
39°01.541' N
107°02.768' W
1-Start/East Fork TH
39°01.471' N
107°03.036' W
Unnamed Peak 12,473
Unnamed Peak 12,473 Summit
39°01.031' N
107°01.499' W
Mount Bellview 12,516 ft.
Mount Bellview Summit
39°00.974' N
107°01.010' W
Frigid Air Pass
West Maroon Pass
Schofield Pass
Schofield Park
Baroni Mine
Elko Lake
Emerald Lake
East Fork
Rustler Gulch
PITKIN CO
GUNNISON CO
MAROON
GUNNISON NATIONAL FOREST
107°03'00" W
107°02'00" W
107°01'00" W
107°00'00" W
106°59'00" W
106°58'00" W
39°03'00" N
39°02'00" N
39°01'00" N
Map created with TOPO! © 2008 National Geographic; © 2007 Tele Atlas, Rel. 1/2007
TN MN 9½°
06/07/12
MILES
FEET
KILOMETERS
METERS

West Maroon Pass/South Ridge Route 9.3 mi RT
Belleview Mountain/Mount Belleview Loop 10 mi RT

37 Belleview Mountain

Belleview's name doesn't pull any punches: you'll have spectacular views of the fabled Maroon Bell peaks. A fine scramble to the summit has a few hidden surprises as well.

Round-Trip Distance	9.3 miles
Hiking Time	6–8 hours
Difficulty	8/10
Class	3
Start Elevation	10,410 ft., at East Fork Trailhead
Peak Elevation	13,233 ft.
Total Elevation Gain	3,120 ft.
Terrain	Good trail leads to scrambling on crumbly, semisolid rock
Best Time to Climb	Late June–September
Gear Advisor	Boots that do well in loose scree and helmet
Crowd Level	Low on peak; moderate on trail

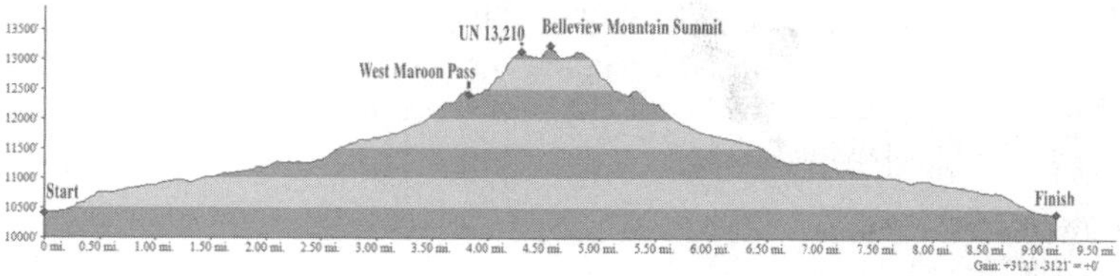

Location Elk Mountains in the Maroon Bells–Snowmass Wilderness/White River National Forest just outside of Crested Butte or Aspen, depending on your approach

Intro The Maroon Bells are among the most popular and photographed mountains in Colorado. When it comes to hiking them, it's a different story. The stratified layers of ruddy rock hide a shell of molting marine shale that makes hiking unstable and loose. Belleview offers a nice change of pace from its more photogenic neighbors to the north. Terrain on Belleview is still loose, but the ridge from West Maroon Pass has good scrambling and less exposure. Views from the summit are incredible, as this peak is centrally located between Aspen and Crested Butte. If you're thinking of challenging the big bells, why not preview this nifty 13er first? You may prefer it to its 14er kin.

Why Climb It? Belleview's south ridge starts from the top of West Maroon Pass, a beautiful trail that runs from Aspen to Crested Butte. No matter which approach you prefer, you're already a winner—views of the Elk Mountains on both sides of the pass are exquisite. The ridge on Belleview has a tricky start, but the scrambling is fun, and you always have an out on the west side of the mountain. Once you clear a trio of rocky obstacles, you have a clean line up to Unnamed Peak 13,210 (a nice peak in its own right). The short stroll between UN 13,210 and Belleview reveals wild rock formations and great views of Halsey Basin and the Maroon Bells. Much of the brown rock you'll see is hardened mud that once lined the bottom of an ancient sea. I have found several fossils in this area, including dozens of seashells.

Driving Tough passenger cars can make it to the East Fork Trailhead. (The dirt road to Schofield Pass was resurfaced in 2011 and is regularly maintained. The only part that was tough on my car was the rutted-out parking lot.)

How to Get There From the town of Crested Butte, follow Colorado Highway 135 north, where it becomes Gothic Road (County Road 317). Pass the resort village of Mount Crested Butte, and stay on Gothic Road north of town as it turns to dirt. This road is maintained and is passable by cars, though in rainy weather it can get mucky. From the start of the dirt road, it's 10.5 miles to the top of Schofield Pass. Note that you'll pass the eerie "research town" of Gothic, which I am convinced is a zombie-testing facility, 4.0 miles up the road.

Go over the pass 1.0 mile north to the large, rutted parking area; East Fork Trailhead is on your right (east) side, just after a shallow stream crossing.

Fees/Camping There are no fees to hike or camp in this area. Campsites abound along Gothic Road, though you'll be fighting with mountain bikers for spots in the summer. More good camping can be found in Elko Park, which is just west of the Schofield Pass summit on Forest Service Road 519 (Paradise Divide Road).

Route Notes None.

Mile/Waypoint

0.0 mi (1) Start at the East Fork Trailhead. Head east on the West Maroon Pass Trail #1970 and begin your adventure.

0.3 mi (2) There's a smashed cabin just before the wilderness boundary; go up a small hill to an expansive meadow. Continue along the West Maroon Pass Trail. A few faint side trails are along the way; just stay the course on the well-worn main trail.

Note: On some maps, this trail appears to follow the flat land directly next to East Fork Creek. Do not go down to the river. The trail is actually side-cut into the slope above the river, as shown on this map.

1.9 mi (3) A small sign in the grass denotes the split of the Halsey Trail to the left (west). Go right and remain on the West Maroon Pass Trail as it begins to arc east.

2.8 mi (4) The junction for Frigid Air Pass Trail cuts in to your left (north). Stay the course and continue on the main trail toward the pass. You won't be able to see Belleview yet, which is to the north (left), but you can see Unnamed Peak 13,210, which looks most impressive from the open alpine valley. The mountain on the ridge to your right (south) is Mount Bellview—not to be confused with Belleview Mountain.

3.9 mi (5) Hike up the mild switchbacks to the top of West Maroon Pass. You finally get your first views of Belleview Mountain from here. The ridge to the summit is on your left. Ditch any trekking poles here and get ready to scramble.

The crux of this scramble is the first 0.3 mile from the pass to waypoint **6**. The terrain is easy class 3 but rather crumbly, so you'll need to be keen in your route finding. Staying to the left (west) side offers the path of least resistance. A brief, grayish scree gully avoids the steepest-looking pinnacle. Don't stray too far from the spine of the ridge, which you will rejoin at waypoint **6**.

4.2 mi (6) After clearing the initial obstacles, gain the broad ridge and enjoy the easy class 2 terrain to the summit of Unnamed Peak 13,210.

4.4 mi (7) Go up and over this fine 13er and continue north to the obvious summit pyramid of Belleview Mountain. Views here are sublime.

As you near the base of the Belleview's final scramble, the way up may not be obvious. If you traverse to the east and northeast faces, you'll find lots of good chutes that will offer easy class 3 scrambles to the top.

4.6 mi (8) Belleview Mountain's summit! You can't beat the views from here. To the north is the enormous bulk of South Maroon Peak (also known as Maroon Peak). To the northeast, Pyramid Peak dominates a striated ridgeline. To the west is the Treasure Mountain massif, including Treasury Mountain, another fine hike (Hike 36) in this book.

Watch your step on the way down, and return the way you came.

9.3 mi Finish.

Options If ridge walks are your thing, try the optional exit that goes south from West Maroon Pass and follows a class 3 ridge over to Mount Bellview and Unnamed Peak 12,473. Follow the southwest ridge of UN 12,473 down to Schofield Pass; almost all of this route will be easy to visually follow. It's possible to intersect with the fabled 401 Trail, one of Colorado's best mountain bike rides. Continue west to Schofield Pass and walk back down to your car. This option is roughly a 10-mile loop.

Quick Facts *Belle vue* in French means "beautiful view." This is a fitting name for the mountain and a double entendre, for Belleview offers great views of the Maroon Bells. Mount Bellview and Belleview Mountain have slightly different spellings, but that doesn't make me any less forgiving of the geographers who were too lazy to come up with original names.

Schofield Pass is named for the immortal B. F. Schofield, who mined for silver in this area in 1879. He ran his camp from Schofield Park, 0.25 mile north of the East Fork Trailhead parking lot.

Contact Info Maroon Bells Wilderness/White River National Forest
Aspen Ranger District
806 W. Hallam Street
Aspen, CO 81611
(970) 925-3445

East Beckwith Mountain–Far East Peak Traverse

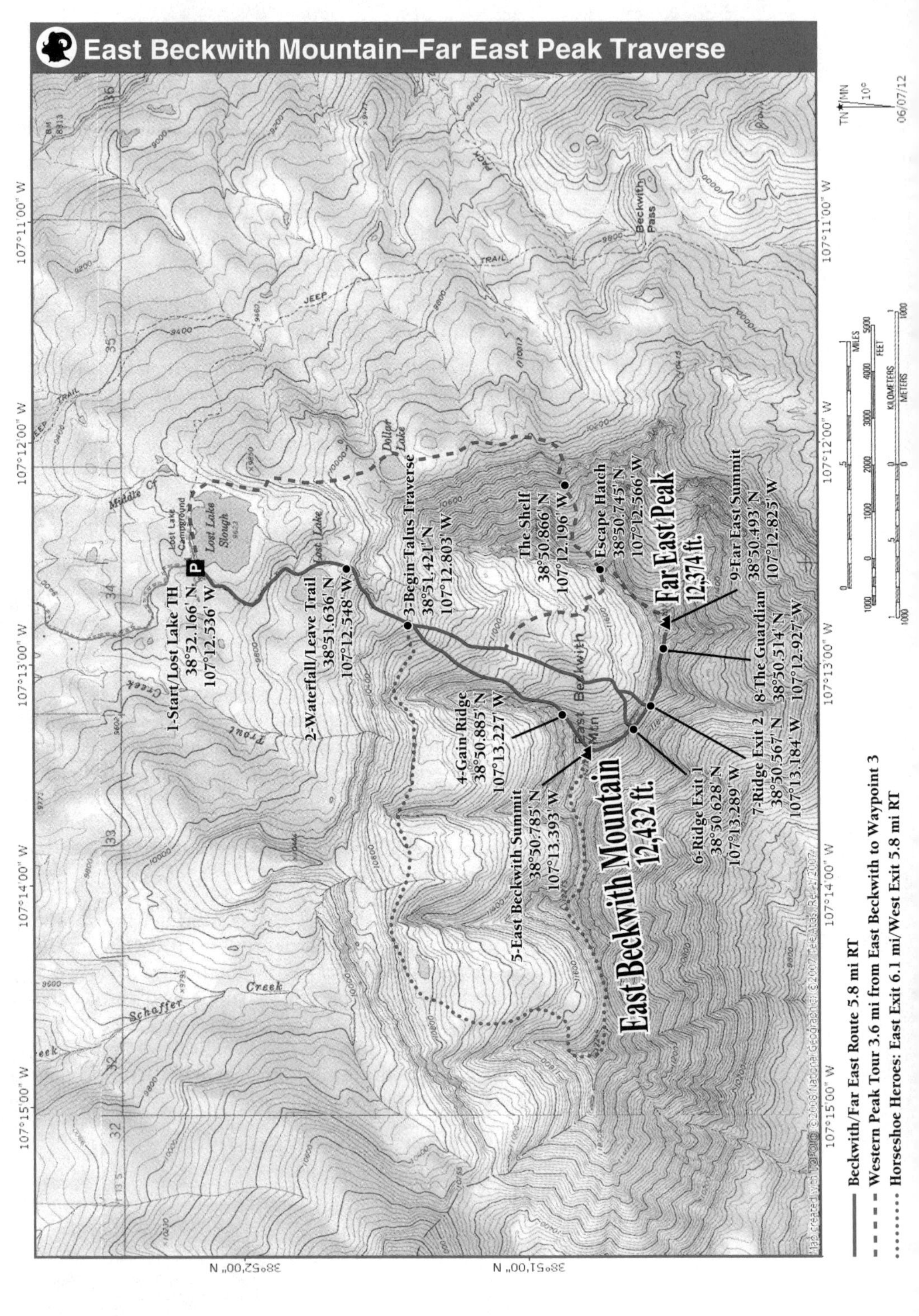

1-Start/Lost Lake TH
38°52.166' N
107°12.536' W
2-Waterfall/Leave Trail
38°51.636' N
107°12.548' W
3-Begin Talus Traverse
38°51.421' N
107°12.803' W
4-Gain Ridge
38°50.885' N
107°13.227' W
5-East Beckwith Summit
38°50.785' N
107°13.393' W
6-Ridge Exit 1
38°50.628' N
107°13.289' W
7-Ridge Exit 2
38°50.567' N
107°13.184' W
8-The Guardian
38°50.514' N
107°12.927' W
9-Far East Summit
38°50.493' N
107°12.825' W
The Shelf
38°50.866' N
107°12.196' W
Escape Hatch
38°50.745' N
107°12.566' W
East Beckwith Mountain
12,432 ft.
Far East Peak
12,374 ft.
Lost Lake Slough
Lost Lake Campground
Lost Lake
Dollar Lake
Middle Cr
Trout Creek
Schaffer Creek
Beckwith Pass
East Beckwith Mtn
JEEP
TRAIL
107°11'00" W
107°12'00" W
107°13'00" W
107°14'00" W
107°15'00" W
38°52'00" N
38°51'00" N
Beckwith/Far East Route 5.8 mi RT
Western Peak Tour 3.6 mi from East Beckwith to Waypoint 3
Horseshoe Heroes: East Exit 6.1 mi/West Exit 5.8 mi RT
TN MN 10°
06/07/12
MILES
FEET
KILOMETERS
METERS
Map created with TOPO! © 2008 National Geographic; © 2007 Tele Atlas Rel 2/2007

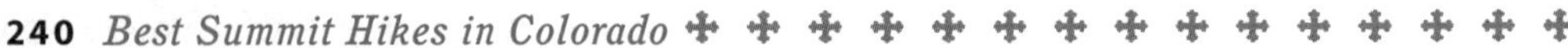

38 East Beckwith Mountain–Far East Peak Traverse

The East Beckwith massif looks as cool in person as it does on the map. Go for the twin summits or saddle up your courage and go for the optional Horseshoe Heroes Loop.

Round-Trip Distance 5.8 miles
Hiking Time 5–7 hours
Difficulty 7.5/10
Class 2+/3
Start Elevation 9,625 ft., at Lost Lake Trailhead
Peak Elevations East Beckwith Mountain: 12,432 ft.; Far East Peak: 12,374 ft.
Total Elevation Gain 3,000 ft.
Terrain Trail to rocky, talus ridge and basin; mostly off-trail
Best Time to Climb July–October
Gear Advisor Normal gear and GPS
Best Time to Climb July–October
Crowd Level Low

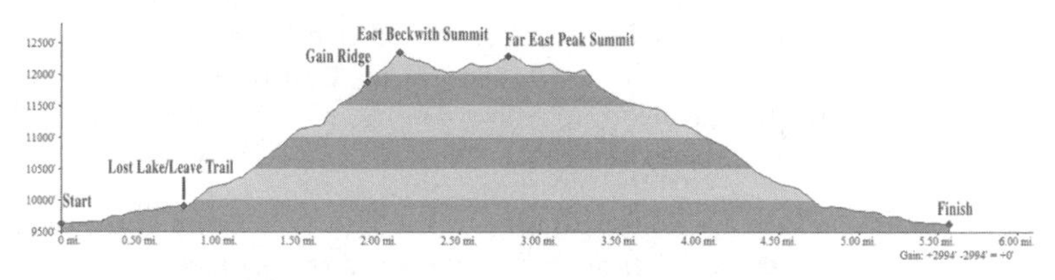

Location Elk Mountain in the Raggeds Wilderness/Gunnison National Forest outside of Paonia/Crested Butte

Intro East Beckwith is a remarkable glacially carved massif that is in the heart of aspen country. Many people consider the drive to the trailhead via Kebler Pass the most scenic in Colorado; it's a favorite of tourists, mountain bikers, campers, and runners. At Lost Lake, East Beckwith's rocky horseshoe of peaks rises to the south like an incredible, natural coliseum. The peak sees few visitors, however, due to a lack of trail and a tough talus field below the ridges. If you're up for a little work, the trip to the top is worth it. And if you're up for some *real* work, try the rough Horseshoe Heroes Loop to get most of the peaks above the basin.

Why Climb It? These peaks give hikers something lacking in most areas: an untamed mountain that is raw, rugged, and challenging—but has easy access. Most of the hike is off-trail, and while it's easy to navigate, it's on some very loose and unsettled talus fields in sections. All that is forgotten once you gain the ridged rim of the horseshoe, which bestows a good class 2+/3 scramble to Beckwith's isolated summit. A short walk over to Far East Peak is part of the standard route. Incredible views are everywhere, especially of the high Elk Range peaks to the north in Aspen (the Maroon Bells, Treasury Mountain, and so on). If you're a fan of truly rugged off-trail mayhem, the Horseshoe Heroes Loop is waiting.

Driving Passenger cars can make it to the trailhead. Kebler Pass is a maintained dirt road with a few rough spots; under normal conditions, all vehicles can make this beautiful drive. This applies to both sides of the pass.

How to Get There The access road to Lost Lake Trailhead is off Kebler Pass Road (County Road 12) on the west side of the pass. It's approximately 15 miles from either entrance on the pass.

To access the trailhead from Crested Butte (east side), take the Kebler Pass Road (County Road 12/Whiterock Avenue) west off Colorado Highway 135; this turn is right in town. Follow the road 16 miles up and over the pass, and turn left (south) onto Forest Service Road 706; follow the signs for LOST LAKE SLOUGH/CAMPGROUND. It's 2.2 miles on FS 706 to the Lost Lake Slough Trailhead and Campground; at 2.0 miles the road forks, and the parking area is to the left.

From the west side, locate the junction of Colorado Highway 133 and CR 12, about 14 miles north of Paonia. This turn is just south of Paonia Reservoir. If you're taking this route from the north, go over McClure Pass and turn east onto CR 12 after the long reservoir. Note that this road has a lot of signs, but none that explicitly say it is CR 12 (look for Kebler Pass signs instead). Follow it 15.2 miles and turn right (south) onto FS 706—again, there will be signs for Lost Lake Campground. It is 2.2 miles to the trailhead on this road; the parking area is to the left at mile 2.0 (where the road forks).

Fees/Camping There are no fees to hike in the area or to camp at the primitive sites. The developed sites at the campground at Lost Lake Slough are $10 per night, though there are plenty of places to pull off on Kebler Pass and car camp for free.

Route Notes None.

Mile/Waypoint **0.0 mi (1)** Start at the Lost Lake Trailhead. Go south on the Three Lakes Trail #843 toward Lost Lake. This is a pleasant introduction on a good trail; note that the large body of water in front of you is Lost Lake Slough, not Lost Lake. (Slough means an area of soft, muddy ground or swamp or swamplike region.)

0.8 mi (2) After a "river" crossing on the north side of Lost Lake, continue to the east shore on trail. At a bend in the trail where a waterfall meets the lake, go off-trail. Cross the waterfall and begin a climb up to the basin. This off-trail section is not difficult, but it is steep. Gradually diverge southwest from the waterfall, where the ridge is easier to hike up. The goal is to get into the basin at this point, not onto the north ridge. The north ridge may look good from here, but just out of view it reaches a broken section that is difficult to climb.

1.2 mi (3) At the base of the talus basin, the real grunt work of the hike begins. Even though the boulders here are a good size, the footing is still bad. A lot of the rocks are unstable, so test your steps. You are better off staying left on the flatter section for the time being and making the push up to the north ridge in one effort. As you get higher, you'll be able to scan the north ridge for a good line up. I waited until I was past the broken gap and then made my way to the ridge via a strong push at mile 1.9. You'll need route-finding skills to find the best way up; it's steep but still class 2 talus terrain.

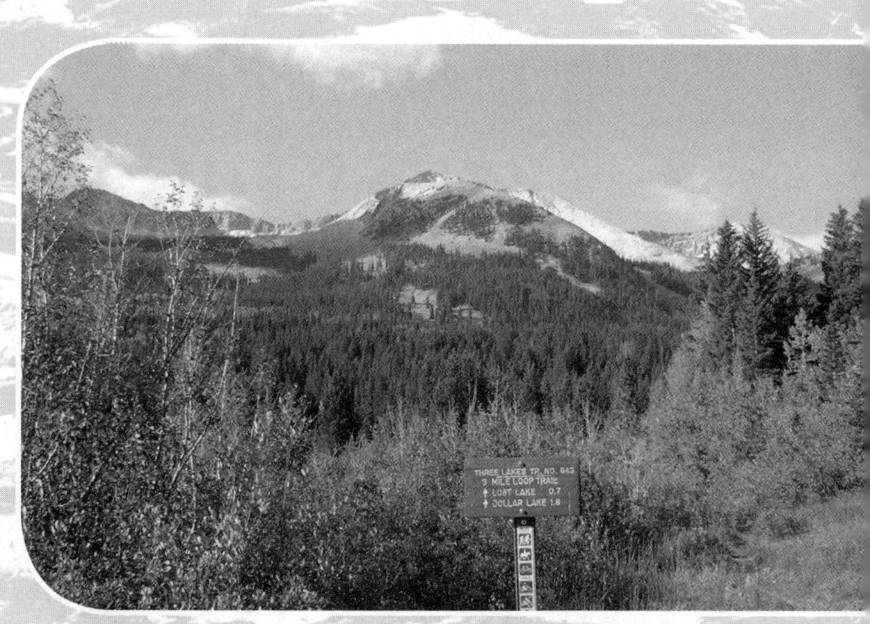

You'll be on trail for the start and finish of the hike, but the bulk of your adventure is off trail.

2.0 mi (4) At 11,880 feet, you're on the ridge proper, and the hard part is an easy class 3 move that will get you over small outcrops. There is some exposure, but the ridge never gets narrow enough to freak out about. Carry on south to the summit.

2.2 mi (5) East Beckwith summit. It's a photographer's dream up here. Continue on toward Far East summit via the southeast ridge.

2.5 mi (6 and 7) In the saddle between East Beckwith and Far East, I have marked two good exit chutes that return to the talus basin. You may want to take one or the other on the way back. These are both easy class 3 scrambles and are preferable to returning to the north ridge to descend.

2.8 mi (8) The Guardian is a formidable-looking rock section that is the last obstacle before Far East's summit. Once you are up close, it turns out to be a piece of cake. Easy class 2 scrambling will grant you passage to the top.

2.9 mi (9) Far East Peak's summit! There are great views of East Beckwith from here. There's no easy way down; returning to the saddle and dropping down at waypoint **6** or **7** (**6** is the easiest) is the way to go. Once you are in the talus basin, return the way you came. You can use the waterfall as a guide to get you back to Lost Lake if you are without a GPS, or if you aren't handy with a compass. Once on the trail, it's an easy hike back.

5.8 mi Finish. The mileage for this hike isn't a lot, but you'll be tired. Why not enjoy the rest of the day at this lovely area? I hear the fishing in these lakes is quite good.

Options From East Beckwith's summit, you have some major options. The first is a westward traverse that goes over several unnamed peaks and drops down in the farthest cirque. From there, skirt east along the base of the massif and return to the top of the waterfall. This option tacks 3.6 miles onto your route, from the top of East Beckwith back to waypoint **3**.

The Horseshoe Heroes route is for expert scramblers only, and you may want to bring a helmet along. Once you get to Far East, continue north to several unnamed peaks that are connected by a sloping, and at times narrow, ridge. This is exciting stuff! You'll pass through a neat rock gap as you descend; it's class 3 down climbing most of the way. The rock is rotten in places, so test all your handholds. At several points, there are steep but feasible scrambles that break off west, back into the talus basin. The best way

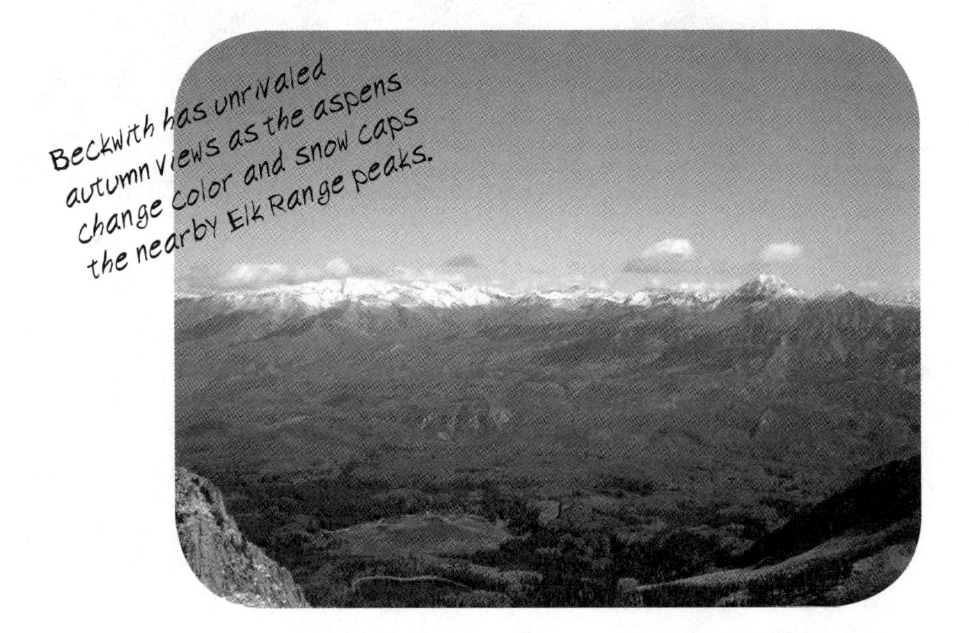

Beckwith has unrivaled autumn views as the aspens change color and snow caps the nearby Elk Range peaks.

back is probably the Escape Hatch waypoint (via the western chutes). Me, I decided to make things difficult for myself and go east.

Note that a straight traverse north over the final northern peak gets into class 3+ or 4 terrain on broken rock—no fun! You'll need to exit the ridge; west is better, but I went east for a steep crawl down to a wide gully. On the map, it looks like a good way to close the loop. If you choose to take the recommended direction to exit, you're wise enough to find your own way down to Lost Lake Slough and back out. On the other hand, if you make the foolhardy choice of following in my misbegotten footsteps, the following account may be useful.

After a steep, knee-grinding descent on snowy talus, I reached the halfway point in the gully, only to find that it's almost entirely cliffed out. At the Shelf, I traversed left (north) into the shrubs, where the terrain is passable—though a hiker needs great route-finding skills to reach the bottom of this gully. At times it was quite fun, sliding through tunnels of shrubs and grabbing their roots to prevent myself from skidding off 10- to 12-foot cliffs. Finally, I made my way down. Looking up at the cliffed-out section, I saw a prime wall for ice climbing come winter . . . interesting. I then skirted northwest to Dollar Lake, where a nice class 1 trail led me home. Do I recommend this route? Not really. Did I have a blast doing it? Absolutely!

Quick Facts

This mountain is named for Lieutenant E. G. Beckwith, who joined Captain John Gunnison on his surveying trip to the area in 1853. West Beckwith Mountain is not connected to the East Beckwith massif; a low saddle separates the two, but it is possible to climb them both in one long day. (While sitting in my car after the hike, I was reading a Dave Barry article about anagrams. Thus inspired, I discovered the letters in "East Beckwith" can be arranged to read "be a thick stew" and "beast chew kit.")

Kebler Pass is named for J. A. Kebler, who served as an official for the Colorado Fuel and Iron Company.

Contact Info

Gunnison National Forest
Paonia Ranger District
P.O. Box 1030
N. Rio Grande Avenue
Paonia, CO 81428
(970) 527-4131

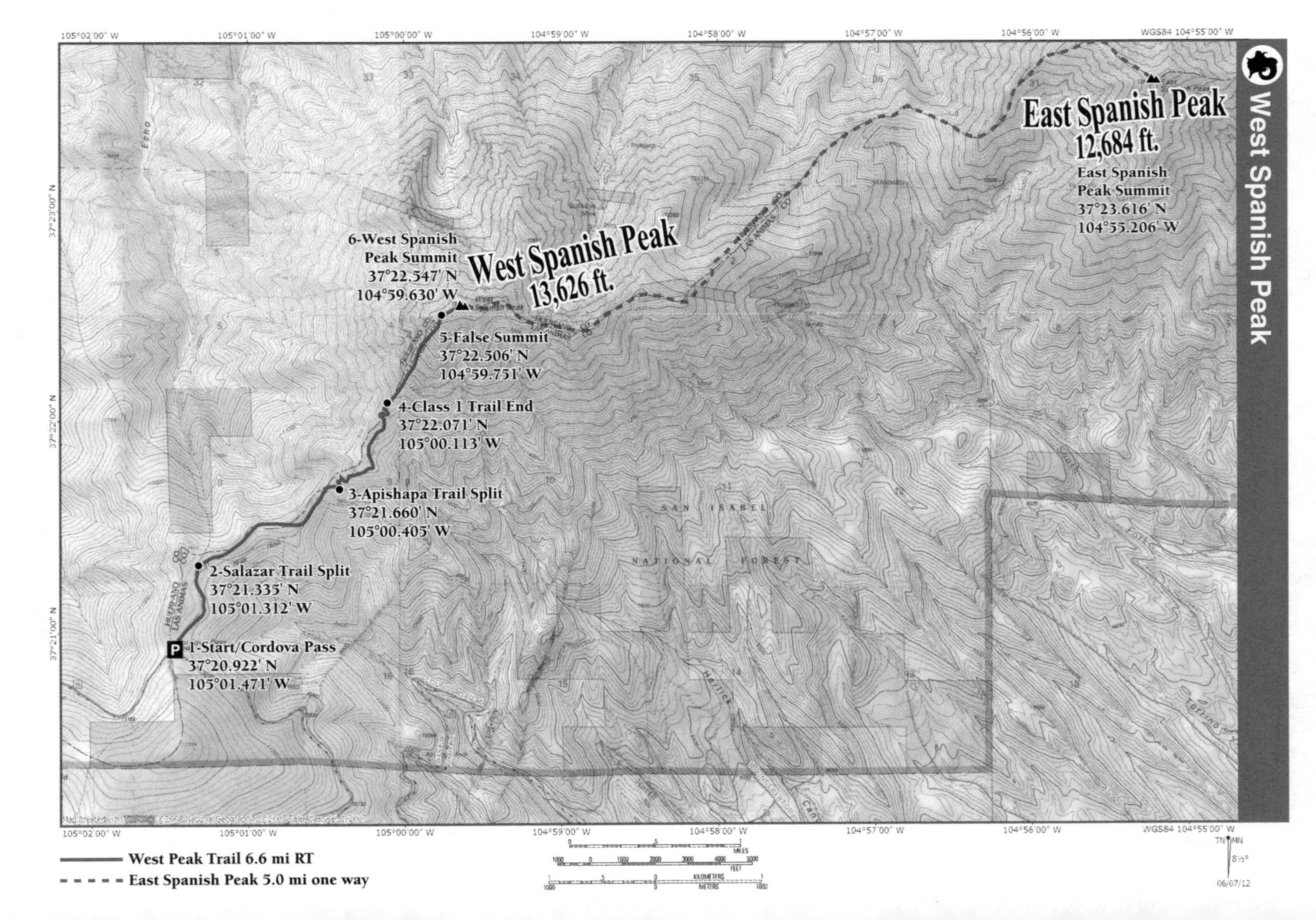

West Spanish Peak
East Spanish Peak 12,684 ft.
East Spanish Peak Summit
37°23.616' N
104°55.206' W
West Spanish Peak 13,626 ft.
6-West Spanish Peak Summit
37°22.547' N
104°59.630' W
5-False Summit
37°22.506' N
104°59.751' W
4-Class 1 Trail End
37°22.071' N
105°00.113' W
3-Apishapa Trail Split
37°21.660' N
105°00.405' W
2-Salazar Trail Split
37°21.335' N
105°01.312' W
1-Start/Cordova Pass
37°20.922' N
105°01.471' W
SAN ISABEL NATIONAL FOREST
West Peak Trail 6.6 mi RT
East Spanish Peak 5.0 mi one way

39 West Spanish Peak

The contrast between the enormous Spanish Peaks and the surrounding farmland is striking. These stand-alone mountains dominate the southern landscape and offer good climbs.

Round-Trip Distance	6.6 miles
Hiking Time	4–6 hours
Difficulty	6/10
Class	2
Start Elevation	11,256 ft., at Cordova Pass
Peak Elevation	13,626 ft.
Total Elevation Gain	2,929 ft.
Terrain	Good trail leading to a rocky summit push
Best Time to Climb	May–September
Gear Advisor	Trekking poles
Crowd Level	Moderate

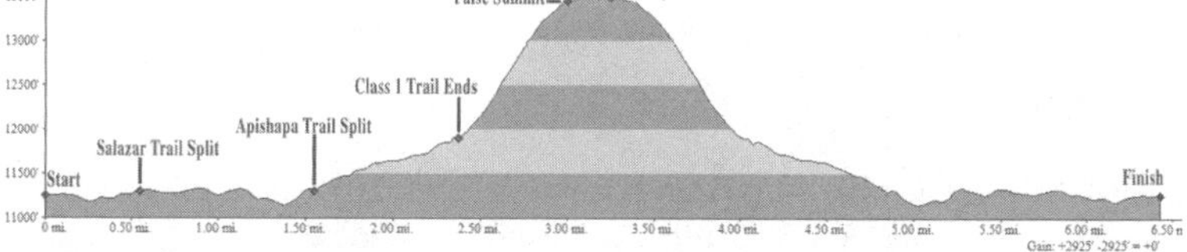

Location Sangre De Cristo Range in the Spanish Peaks Wilderness/San Isabel National Forest south of the small town of La Veta

Intro Gazing at the gargantuan profile of the Spanish Peaks for the first time, I got the "I can't believe I'll be standing on the top of that tomorrow" feeling. The two mountains that make up the Spanish Peaks explode from a flat valley, dominating the landscape with pure, massive, mountain goodness. Only Mount Sopris (which is very similar in design) rivals the Spanish Peaks in perceived height. The entire mountain is flanked on all sides by the Great Spanish Dykes—long walls of rock that fortify the lowlands.

Why Climb It? West Spanish Peak is the lower of the two mountains (the other being 13,683-foot East Spanish Peak). When mountains rise straight out of the ground like West Spanish, you are guaranteed spectacular views. To the south, the views open up into New Mexico, including the distant Wheeler Peak, at 13,161 feet, the state high point. "Forbidden" Culebra Peak and the Culebra Range dominate the western horizon. (Culebra Peak is the only privately owned 14er; the owners charge $100 per person to hike it.) To the north, the fortresslike Mount Blanca group juts into the clouds.

The Spanish Dykes look like man-made walls, but are in fact natural formations (more on this in the "Quick Facts" section). In addition to the views, this is a good hike, with a graceful prelude trail leading to a challenging and steep summit pyramid.

Driving Passenger cars can make it to Cordova Pass without any trouble, thanks to J. J. Cordova's dream come true (read more on him in "Quick Facts"); the dirt road is well maintained.

How to Get There Find the intersection of US Highway 160 west and Colorado Highway 12, roughly 7 miles west of the town of Walsenburg (located in southern Colorado along I-25). Turn left (south) onto CO 12 and stay on this road for 22.3 miles, heading for Cucharas Pass. You will go through the small town of La Veta (follow the signs for CO 12 through town). After passing La Veta, keep your eyes out for the walls of the Spanish Dykes on your left (east). Drive past the village of Cuchara and continue all the way to Cucharas Pass. At mile 22.3, turn left onto the dirt road to Cordova Pass (Las Animas County Road 46). Another 6.0 miles will bring you to the top of the pass and to the trailhead for West Spanish Peak.

Fees/Camping There is a $4 day-use charge for hiking in the Spanish Peaks Wilderness. There is a self-pay box at the trailhead. There are also a few campsites, which are $6 per night; at the time I visited the area, there were only six sites available. Note that if you camp up here, there are no water sources, so bring enough for camping and the hike.

Route Notes None.

Mile/Waypoint **0.0 mi (1)** Start on the north side of Cordova Pass on the West Peak Trail. The first 2.5 miles of this class 1 trail are nearly flat, taking you through forests and open meadows. At the onset of the hike, a plaque on a rock (on the right) proclaims the Spanish Peaks designation as a National Natural Landmark. Stay on the West Peak Trail.

0.3 mi (2) There is a split for the very faint Salazar Trail to the left (west); stay on the main West Peak Trail.

1.5 mi (3) Pay attention at mile 1.5. The Apishapa Trail splits from the West Peak Trail. A hard-to-notice brown forest marker designates the split. The mellow pace of the trail up to this point can lull you into not noticing that the Apishapa Trail goes straight (then turns southeast). You need to turn left (northeast) to remain on the West Peak Trail.

2.4 mi (4) At a clearing with good views, the formal class 1 trail ends. You will be at the base of the southwest ridge, which you will climb to reach the top. Get off-trail and prepare for a 1,500-foot push to the top.

Note that there are a few cairned trails and worn paths on the way up. It gets very rocky; the less crumbly stuff can be found just below the ridge on your left (north) side. If you stay on the southwest face, the rocks will be loose and frustrating. Staying left gives you better footing. About halfway up, there are random wind shelters built into the mountain at various points, some on trails, some not. Continue your push, aiming for the highest point you see.

3.1 mi (5) Surprise! After all that work, you're at a false summit. At 13,450 feet, it really isn't that bad. The remaining 180 vertical feet are on easy, relatively flat terrain.

3.4 mi (6) West Spanish Peak's true summit is the first major rock pile/cairn that you encounter on this summit block. A register is here. I swore that the gleaming, large cairn to the northeast was the top when I first got here. It *looks* higher from the true summit. However, after taking the short walk over to it, my GPS reported it as being slightly lower. And, to add to the optical confusion, now the *real* summit looked higher. Just to be sure you've topped out, visit them both.

Descend the way you came up, picking your best line down the mountain to return to the trees where the class 1 West Peak Trail terminated (waypoint **4**). Pick up the trail again and follow it all the way back.

6.6 mi Finish.

Options The cheese truly stands alone here. There aren't many options off West Spanish Peak. The obvious question is: can you do both peaks in one day? From the summit of West Spanish, you can follow the east ridge to a saddle that connects the two, and then ascend the west ridge of East Spanish Peak (not shown on this map). There is an intermittent trail. This option is class 2, but it's 5.0 miles one way from the summit of West Spanish Peak. Done as an out-and-back, that's more than 17 miles. (If you are creative, you can

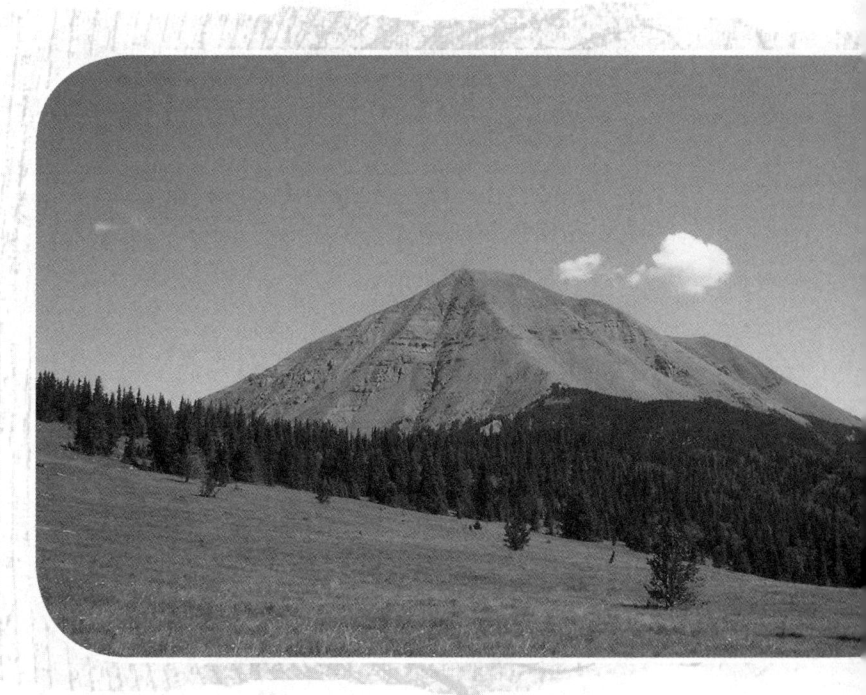

West Spanish Peak cuts an impressive profile.

make a one-way trip using two cars; however, because these peaks are a long drive from most areas, you'll probably only have one car at your disposal.) From the saddle between the two, a pack trail (#1304) heads north to Wahatoya Camp, a possible parking option for a second car if you were trying the two-car idea. It may be more fun to hike East Spanish Peak the next day. You can fill the post-hike afternoon with tours of the Great Spanish Dykes if you'd like more hiking.

Quick Facts When explorer Zebulon Pike first saw the Spanish Peaks in 1806, he called them the Mexican Mountains. At that time, the peaks were still within the boundaries of Spanish-controlled territory; thus the name morphed into its present form.

Native people called the mountains Wahatoya, which translates to "the breasts of the Earth." This proves that the lonely French fur trappers who dubbed the Grand Tetons in Wyoming weren't the only mountain men longing for the company of women.

Native tribes as widespread as the Apache and the Aztecs were familiar with the Spanish Peaks.

The striking geology, including the Spanish Dykes, was formed when continental pressures pushed the entire Sangre De Cristo Range sky high (irregularities in the uplifted plate explain the gaps between mountains in the range). Molten rock cooled in gaps under the Earth, forming granite batholiths known as stocks. (Batholith is a large body of intrusive igneous rock believed to have crystallized at a considerable depth below the Earth's surface.) Some of these stocks formed in narrow veins and cracks in the Earth; when the land was pushed up, these hard igneous batholiths went up as well. Both Spanish Peaks were formed this way; thus they are not true volcanic mountains. The dykes were pushed up with the peaks. When the sedimentary rock eroded, the tougher granite of the dykes remained, creating the long walls we see today.

An interesting sign at the top of Cordova Pass tells the story of Jose de Jesus Cordova and his dream of connecting the town of Aguilar and Cucharas Pass. Spurred on by his vision, the road was completed in 1934 and named after the man himself in 1978. It was a very practical dream, and he made it come true. Three cheers for J. J. Cordova!

Contact Info San Isabel National Forest
Main Pueblo Office
2480 Kachina Drive
Pueblo, CO 81008
(719) 553-1400

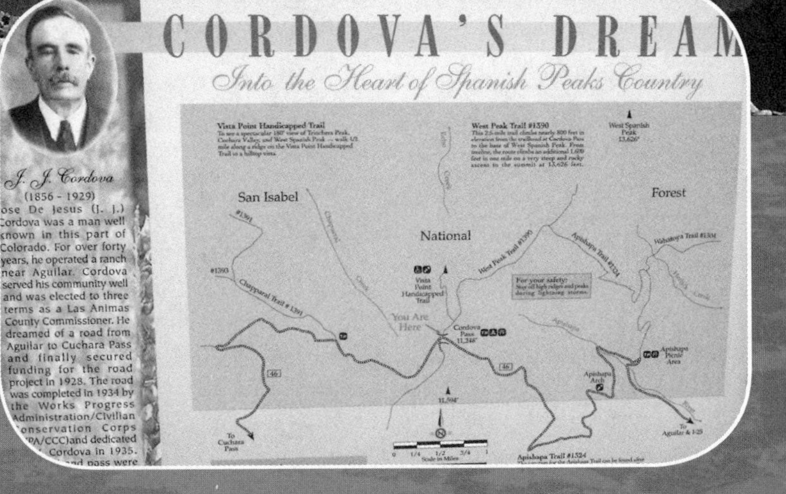

CORDOVA'S DREAM
Into the Heart of Spanish Peaks Country
J. J. Cordova
(1856 - 1929)
ose De Jesus (J. J.) Cordova was a man well known in this part of Colorado. For over forty years, he operated a ranch near Aguilar. Cordova served his community well and was elected to three terms as a Las Animas County Commissioner. He dreamed of a road from Aguilar to Cuchara Pass and finally secured funding for the road project in 1928. The road was completed in 1934 by the Works Progress Administration/Civilian Conservation Corps (WPA/CCC)and dedicated Cordova in 1935.
Vista Point Handicapped Trail
West Peak Trail #1390
West Spanish Peak 13,626'
San Isabel
National
Forest
Vista Point Handicapped Trail
You Are Here
Cordova Pass 11,248'
Apishapa Picnic Area
Apishapa Arch
To Cuchara Pass
To Aguilar & I-25

The Spanish Dykes are amazing examples of Colorado's distinct geology.

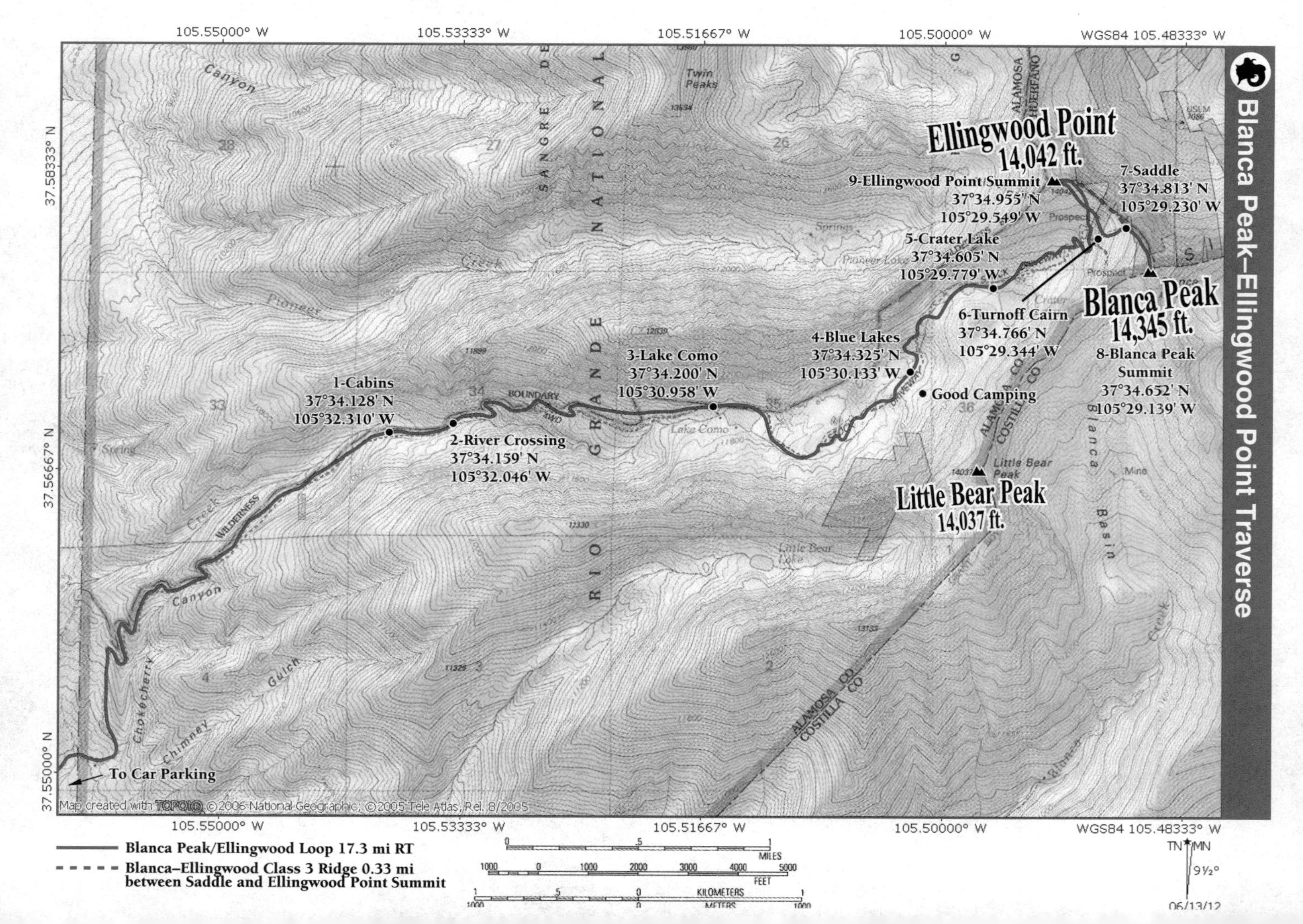

Blanca Peak–Ellingwood Point Traverse
Ellingwood Point
14,042 ft.
9-Ellingwood Point/Summit
37°34.955' N
105°29.549' W
7-Saddle
37°34.813' N
105°29.230' W
5-Crater Lake
37°34.605' N
105°29.779' W
6-Turnoff Cairn
37°34.766' N
105°29.344' W
Blanca Peak
14,345 ft.
8-Blanca Peak Summit
37°34.652' N
105°29.139' W
4-Blue Lakes
37°34.325' N
105°30.133' W
Good Camping
3-Lake Como
37°34.200' N
105°30.958' W
1-Cabins
37°34.128' N
105°32.310' W
2-River Crossing
37°34.159' N
105°32.046' W
Little Bear Peak
14,037 ft.
To Car Parking
SANGRE DE
RIO GRANDE NATIONAL
Twin Peaks
ALAMOSA
HUERFANO
ALAMOSA CO
COSTILLA CO
Lake Como
Little Bear Lake
Blanca Basin
Chokecherry Canyon
Chimney Gulch
WILDERNESS
BOUNDARY
105.55000° W
105.53333° W
105.51667° W
105.50000° W
WGS84 105.48333° W
37.58333° N
37.56667° N
37.55000° N
Map created with TOPO! ©2006 National Geographic; ©2005 Tele Atlas, Rel. 8/2005
Blanca Peak/Ellingwood Loop 17.3 mi RT
Blanca–Ellingwood Class 3 Ridge 0.33 mi between Saddle and Ellingwood Point Summit
MILES
FEET
KILOMETERS
METERS
TN
MN
9½°
06/13/12

40 Blanca Peak–Ellingwood Point Traverse

Good Overnight!

Blanca Peak is the high point of a high alpine oasis featuring a great scramble and magnificent scenery. This hard-earned peak is my favorite climb of all the 14ers.

Round-Trip Distance 17.3 miles
Hiking Time 2 days (13–15 hours of hiking from car parking and trailhead)
Difficulty 7/10
Class 2+
Start Elevation 7,860 ft., at Lake Como Road (4x4s can start a few miles higher)
Peak Elevations Blanca Peak: 14,345 ft.; Ellingwood Point: 14,042 ft.
Total Elevation Gain 7,225 ft.
Terrain Long access road and good scramble to Blanca; loose scramble to Ellingwood
Best Time to Climb May–September
Gear Advisor Bug gear in midsummer, backpacking boots, and sandals for river crossing
Crowd Level Low to moderate

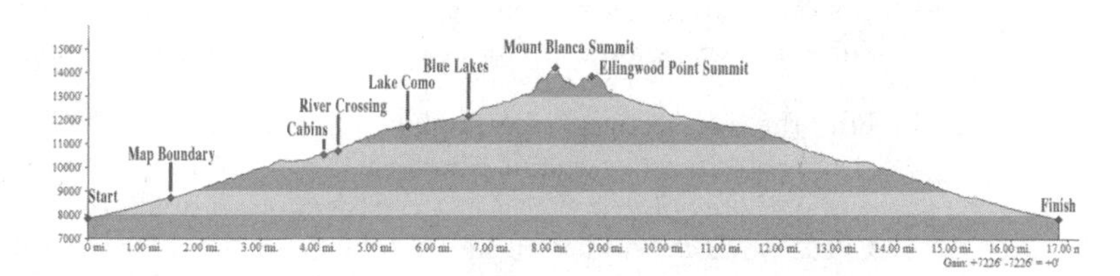

Location Sangre De Cristo Range in the Rio Grande National Forest near the town of Alamosa

Intro Blanca Peak is the sacred mountain of the east to the Navajo people. It's easy to see why Blanca massif, home to three other 14ers, would inspire spiritual awe. At the base of the group, the land is dry and hot, evidenced by the nearby Great Sand Dunes National Monument. Elevated from the scorching heat, the secret alpine garden in the Blanca basin is an oasis of lakes, streams, and snow. Climb to the top of Blanca and traverse over to Ellingwood Point to grab your second 14er in one day.

This is a great overnight trip; the camping in Blanca's basin is incredible (though it may be buggy midsummer). It is possible to climb these two peaks as an epic one-day hike, but you'll be missing out on the extraordinary experience of spending time in Blanca's covert campground.

Why Climb It? Mount Blanca is the highest mountain in Colorado outside of the Sawatch Range. It is the king of the Sangre De Cristos and the fifth-highest peak in Colorado (the eighth highest in the lower 48 states and 27th highest in the US). In the past, many people thought that this was the highest Colorado mountain, and you can't blame them. Blanca cuts a much more regal profile than the state's true high point, the gentle giant Mount Elbert. The Lake Como Road that you'll be hiking up is a test piece for advanced 4x4 drivers. Unlike other 4x4 roads in Colorado, this road is more like a wide class 2 trail that a few maniacs attempt to drive up. The stiff elevation gain (more than 7,000 feet total) has a silver lining—you get to observe ecosystems gradually transform from parched desert land to lush meadows of alpine lakes. The hike up to Blanca's apex is a scrambler's delight, following a rocky but solid ridge to a small summit platform.

I added in Ellingwood Point for those hoping to bag another 14er. The class 2 traverse over from Blanca is a pain. (I find staying high on the ridge, which is a class 3 option, preferable.) The rock is very loose and the angle is steep, meaning that you'll be spinning your wheels all the way up and slippin' and slidin' all the way down. It does have some great views, especially of Blanca, but it's a scrappier climb.

Driving Passenger cars and tough passenger cars should park 1.5 miles up the road, before it gets super rocky. Sport utility cars (SUCs), sport utility vehicles (SUVs), Jeeps, and 4x4s will be able to push it another 2–3 miles before the obstacles get too great—look for good turnoffs to park before it gets too late (see sidebar, "Good Spots to Park SUVs and 4x4s along Lake Como Road" on the opposite page). Only true, dedicated, modified 4x4s with super-high clearance, mega-suspension, and necessary adaptations (such as winches and roll cages) should attempt the drive to reach Lake Como.

How to Get There Find the intersection of US Highway 160 and Colorado Highway 150; this is roughly 26 miles east of Alamosa. Those coming from the metro areas will probably pick up US 160 in the town of Walsenburg. Turn north onto CO 150, which will have a sign for the Great Sand Dunes National Monument. Follow this road for 3.2 miles and turn right (this turnoff is not well marked, so be sure to check your odometer). You'll go over a grate and find yourself in a very sandy lot. This is the start of the fabled Lake Como Road, also known as Forest Service Road 975 and hiking trail #886. All passenger cars can drive to the large lot on the left (north) side of the road at mile 1.5. If you value your car, park here. SUCs and SUVs can struggle up another 2.0 miles and park at one of the pull-offs along the way. Jeeps and 4x4s can likely get to mile 4.5; after that, the only vehicles capable of clearing the road are specialized 4x4s, driven by experienced (that is, crazy) drivers.

Fees/Camping There are no fees to hike and camp in this part of the Rio Grande National Forest. Be aware that if you camp on the lower part of the road, there will be no water sources.

Route Notes This hike begins 1.5 miles up Lake Como Road at the car parking area. From the paved road (CO 150), the road is 7.3 miles to Lake Como. From the car parking area, the first good campsites at Lake Como are at 5.8 miles, though the better spots are a bit higher, around mile 6.0. Please note that mile 0.0 in the hike description is 1.5 miles up Lake Como Road.

For those of you who are curious, the three Jaws obstacles can be found at miles 5.74, 6.31, and 6.64. You'll know them when you see them.

Good Spots to Park SUVs and 4x4s along Lake Como Road

These mileages are measured from the start of Lake Como Road, where it intersects with CO 150.

1.5 mi **Car parking; a good place to drop a trailer if you brought all-terrain vehicles to get up the road: 37° 32.147' N, 105° 34.825' W**

2.5 mi **Parking/camping spot 1: 37° 32.734' N, 105° 33.992' W**

3.1 mi **Parking/camping spot 2: 37° 33.067' N, 105° 33.6' W**

3.8 mi **SUV max camp (farthest recommended point for SUVs and SUCs): 37° 33.413' N, 105° 33.469' W**

4.2 mi **4x4 camp 1: 37° 33.591' N, 105° 33.321' W**

4.8 mi **High 4x4 camp: 37° 33.713' N, 105° 32.99' W**

These are just my suggestions; you are welcome to bash your vehicle as you see fit. Amazingly, the highest "normal" vehicle I saw on the trail was parked at mile 5.5, which is just before the first 4x4-exclusive obstacle, known as Jaws 1. More amazingly, this vehicle was a Suzuki XL7.

Mile/Waypoint **Note:** This description assumes a two-day trip with an overnight in the Lake Como Area.

0.0 mi (off map) Start at mile 1.5 on Lake Como Road. Walk up the road as it starts in shrubs, passes through aspens, and eventually reaches Lake Como. The main road is easy to follow; the few side roads you see are mostly parking areas.

You have at least 5.8 miles to go before reaching comfortable campsites around Lake Como.

4.1 mi (1) At 10,510 feet, you'll pass some cabins on your right. You're getting closer!

4.4 mi (2) A sizable river crossing is here, even if you're on foot. After this, the big rock obstacles in the road seem impossible to pass in a vehicle, but people do it.

5.6 mi (3) Finally, you are at Lake Como. There is decent camping here, but for better sites, look between here and the Blue Lakes at mile 6.7. Just above Lake Como are good sites in the trees. If you prefer to camp above tree line, there are lots of places around the Blue Lakes to pitch a tent. I would not recommend going to Crater Lake, as it is very rocky (though if you are determined to pitch a tent there, look to the south side of Crater Lake for a few flat, grassy spots).

6.7 mi (4) The Blue Lakes region and, incredibly, the formal end of the 4x4 road—at 12,200 feet! The trail finally becomes suitable strictly for foot traffic; follow it northeast and stay on the right (east) side of the Blue Lakes. Past the Blue Lakes, head up the rocky and steep slope to Crater Lake. Stay on the left (west) side of Crater Lake and the small sublake that precedes it.

7.3 mi (5) Crater Lake. From here, you must go northeast toward the saddle between Blanca and Ellingwood Point. The trail has cairns occasionally, but the Colorado Mountain Club has blazed the official trail with whisker markers in the ground. Follow these for the easiest route to the saddle.

7.8 mi (6) Stay right at this cairned intersection and continue toward the saddle. (The left is the class 2 route to Ellingwood Point.)

8.0 mi (7) At 13,700 feet, gain the saddle. Turn east and begin a very enjoyable scramble on class 2+ terrain to Blanca's summit.

8.3 mi (8) Blanca's summit! Amazing, isn't it? It's obvious from this vantage that Blanca is considerably higher than Little Bear Peak and Ellingwood Point. Return down to waypoint **7**. Those comfortable with class 3 scrambling can take the optional (and in my opinion, better) ridge walk to Ellingwood, though it is quite exposed and a little crumbly. Otherwise, return to waypoint **6**.

8.7 mi (6) Back at the turnoff cairn, follow a faint trail north to the east ridge to Ellingwood Point. This slope is loose, and the trail dissolves after a while. Slog up to the ridge, clear a minor false summit, and continue to the true summit of Ellingwood.

9.0 mi (9) Ellingwood's summit! The hike up isn't pretty, but the views sure are. Brace your knees for the descent on the loose rock and scree; find the best line down, and rejoin the main trail above Crater Lake. From Crater Lake, reverse your route back to your car.

17.3 mi Finish at the car parking lot. With luck, you were able to cut a few miles from this hike by driving to a higher starting point than I could reach in my Honda Accord.

Options This is such a long hike that you probably won't want to do much more. There is an option to climb 14,037-foot Little Bear Peak from the basin. It is a class 3+/4 route and, given its technical nature, is not covered in this book.

The option to stay high on the ridge between Blanca and Ellingwood has some good but exposed scrambling. This high traverse is only 0.33 mile one way from the saddle waypoint to Ellingwood's summit.

Quick Facts Blanca is one of the four sacred mountains of the Navajo. (Read more about the sacred mountains in the "Quick Facts" section for Hike 34 on page 227.) Blanca is Spanish for "white," a name that reflects the peak's often snowy summit.

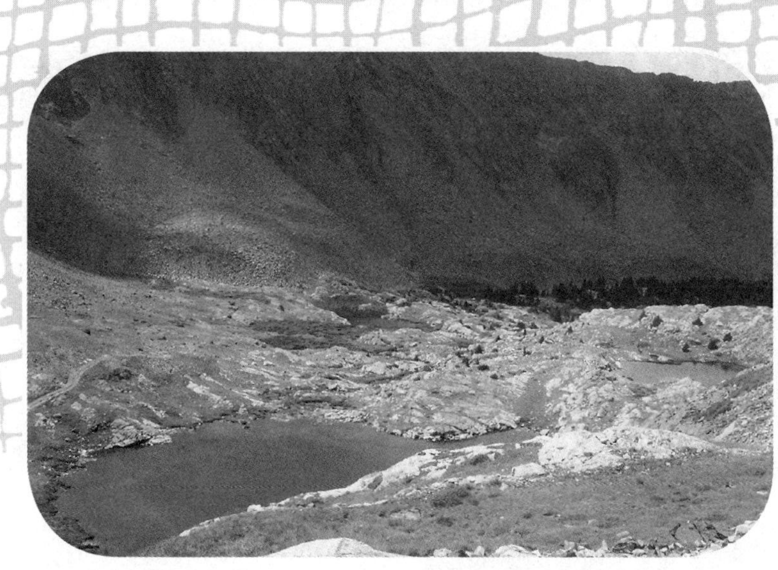

Camping in Blanca's basin is a pleasure. The best campsites can be found around Lake Como.

Ellingwood Point was officially ratified as a 14er in 1990; before then, some considered it a mere subpeak of Blanca. The rule to determine if a peak is an official 14er is that the summit must be at least 0.25 mile from the "mother" peak, and there must be a saddle that drops at least 300 feet between the two. After enough surveying, Ellingwood was welcomed into the club.

Ellingwood is fittingly named after Albert R. Ellingwood, a truly innovative and bad-ass climber. He was one of the first three people to scale all the 14ers, including first ascents of Crestone Needle, Crestone Peak, and Kit Carson Peak—in 1916! Even more impressive was his gutsy ascent (with Barton Hoag) of the crumbling Lizard Head formation in 1920, an incredible feat at the time, as the 400-foot tower had to virtually be free-climbed. He also pioneered two major routes on 14ers: Ellingwood Ridge on La Plata Peak and Ellingwood Arete on Crestone Needle.

When he wasn't putting up routes, this Rhodes scholar taught political science at Colorado College. He died at the young age of 46, having lived more than most men twice his age.

Contact Info

Rio Grande National Forest
1803 W. Colorado Highway 160
Monte Vista, CO 81144
(719) 852-5941

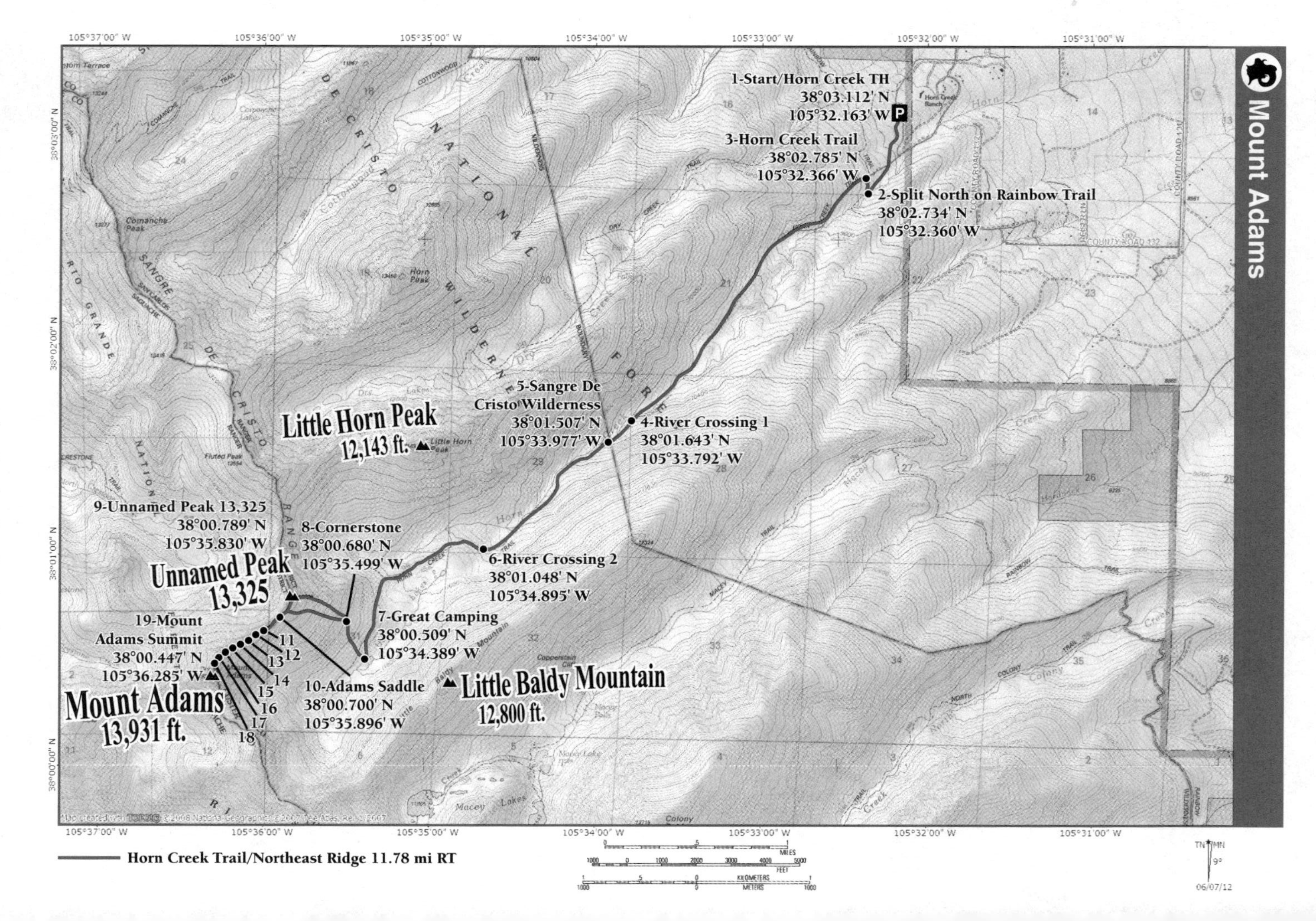
Mount Adams
1-Start/Horn Creek TH
38°03.112' N
105°32.163' W
2-Split North on Rainbow Trail
38°02.734' N
105°32.360' W
3-Horn Creek Trail
38°02.785' N
105°32.366' W
4-River Crossing 1
38°01.643' N
105°33.792' W
5-Sangre De Cristo Wilderness
38°01.507' N
105°33.977' W
6-River Crossing 2
38°01.048' N
105°34.895' W
7-Great Camping
38°00.509' N
105°34.389' W
8-Cornerstone
38°00.680' N
105°35.499' W
9-Unnamed Peak 13,325
38°00.789' N
105°35.830' W
10-Adams Saddle
38°00.700' N
105°35.896' W
19-Mount Adams Summit
38°00.447' N
105°36.285' W
Little Horn Peak
12,143 ft.
Little Baldy Mountain
12,800 ft.
Unnamed Peak
13,325
Mount Adams
13,931 ft.
Horn Creek Trail/Northeast Ridge 11.78 mi RT
SANGRE DE CRISTO NATIONAL FOREST
SANGRE DE CRISTO WILDERNESS
RIO GRANDE NATIONAL FOREST
SANGRE DE CRISTO RANGE
105°37'00" W
105°36'00" W
105°35'00" W
105°34'00" W
105°33'00" W
105°32'00" W
105°31'00" W
38°03'00" N
38°02'00" N
38°01'00" N
38°00'00" N
06/07/12

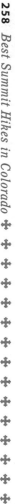

41 Mount Adams

Good Overnight!

Adams is located in the heart of the Sangre De Cristo Range yet remains relatively unknown. Adams is a great adventure, with one of the best ridge scrambles in Colorado.

Round-Trip Distance	11.78 miles
Hiking Time	10–12 hours/2-day option
Difficulty	9/10
Class	3; class 2 hike in
Start Elevation	9,095 ft., at Horn Creek Trailhead
Peak Elevation	13,931 ft.
Total Elevation Gain	4,898 ft.
Terrain	Rugged, steep, solid rock scramble on long ridge
Best Time to Climb	July–September
Gear Advisor	Trekking poles, gaiters, and sandals: there are two or three river crossings, plus mud.
Crowd Level	Low on Horn Lakes Trail; hermit on the peak

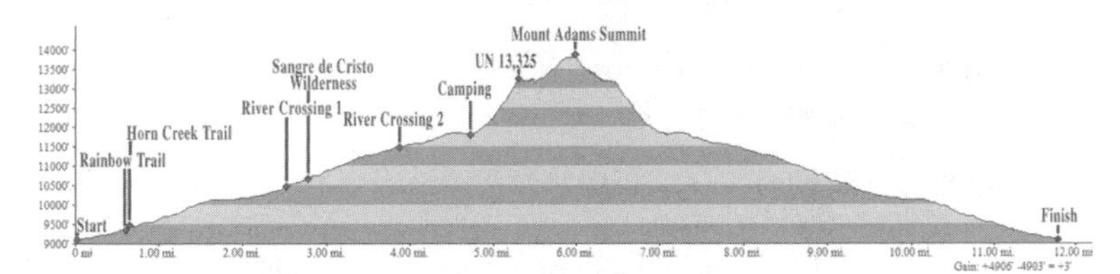

Location Sangre De Cristo Range in the Sangre De Cristo Wilderness/San Isabel National Forest outside of Westcliffe

Intro If it were a little bit taller, Adams would be one of the most talked about peaks in Colorado. Measuring in at 13,931 feet, Adams is just a 69-foot whisker short of 14er status. It also has a rather generic name: there are two Mount Adams in the state (the other is in Rocky Mountain National Park), and dozens of other Adams features—lakes, rivers, towns, and so on. Nonetheless, this is an Adams you should get to know. Not only do you get to scramble a premier class 3 ridge to the summit, but your path to the mountain also takes you to the beautiful Horn Lakes Basin. Be ready for some steep hiking and amazing views.

Why Climb It? The northeast ridge of Adams is an absolute delight. The scramble is roughly 0.25 mile on classic Crestone-style conglomerate and granite rock; that means lots of knobby holds. From the base of the ridge, finding the line looks like a thoroughly daunting prospect. Once on the ridge, however, the line becomes apparent, as the mountain reveals its best route. The exposure is diminished by switching from the south side of the ridge to the north and back; there is always a safe class 3 option to negotiate obstacles.

The hike/backpack in is very scenic. Camping at Horn Lakes is awesome. The amphitheater of enormous peaks surrounds you to the southwest, while your view to the northeast shows the flat, peaceful farmland and city lights of Westcliffe. This is a perfect late-summer or early-autumn trip, best done as a two-day adventure. It is certainly possible as a hearty day hike, but the area is so pristine and beautiful that I see no reason to rush the experience.

Driving The Horn Creek Trailhead is off a paved road and is reachable by any vehicle.

How to Get There From the town of Westcliffe, take Colorado Highway 69 south out of town. Drive 2.8 miles south, and turn right (west) onto Schoolfield Road (County Road 140). Go west 1.8 miles and turn left (south) onto Macey Lane (County Road 129). Go south 1.9 miles and turn right onto Horn Road (County Road 130). It is 2.97 miles west on Horn Road to the Horn Creek Trailhead; signs for the trailhead are well marked. Stay on Horn Road after you pass Horn Ranch Creek (which will have you bearing right at an intersection). As you come up the road, you may see a small parking area with a sign for the Rainbow Trail on the right; bypass this parking area and continue to the end of the road, where you will come across a large parking area with a sign kiosk, restroom, and ample space for horse-trailer parking.

Fees/Camping There are no fees for hiking Mount Adams or for camping in this section of the San Isabel National Forest.

Route Notes The Horn Creek Trail #1342 follows a canyon that begins in conifer trees and eventually passes through a striking aspen stand. As you near Horn Lakes, you'll pass into the Sangre De Cristo Wilderness. Upon reaching the open lakes area, you'll have a stunning view of the black wall between Fluted Peak and Unnamed Peak 13,325—Adams will still be blocked. There are three sections of lakes here; the middle and upper lakes are optimal campsites.

To reach the northeast ridge, you have to march directly up a more than 1,500-foot slope, which is grassy and steep but has excellent footing. The route described here includes the summit of Unnamed Peak 13,325, though it's possible to shortcut from the slope to the saddle between it and Adams (the footing is actually better if you scale UN 13,325, but the choice is yours). From the saddle, the ridge is a fine scramble to the blocky summit of Adams. Views to the south include the epic profiles of three breathtaking 14ers: Kit Carson Peak, Crestone Peak, and Humboldt Peak.

Mile/Waypoint **0.0 mi (1)** From the Horn Creek Trailhead, take the obvious marked trail into the woods. Note that this connector will bring you to the Rainbow Trail, your first goal. There are some trails that come in from the north before you intersect the Rainbow Trail; stay on the large obvious trail bearing southwest.

0.5 mi (2) Here you intersect with the actual Rainbow Trail, which runs north and south. Head right (north), following the signs for Horn Lakes

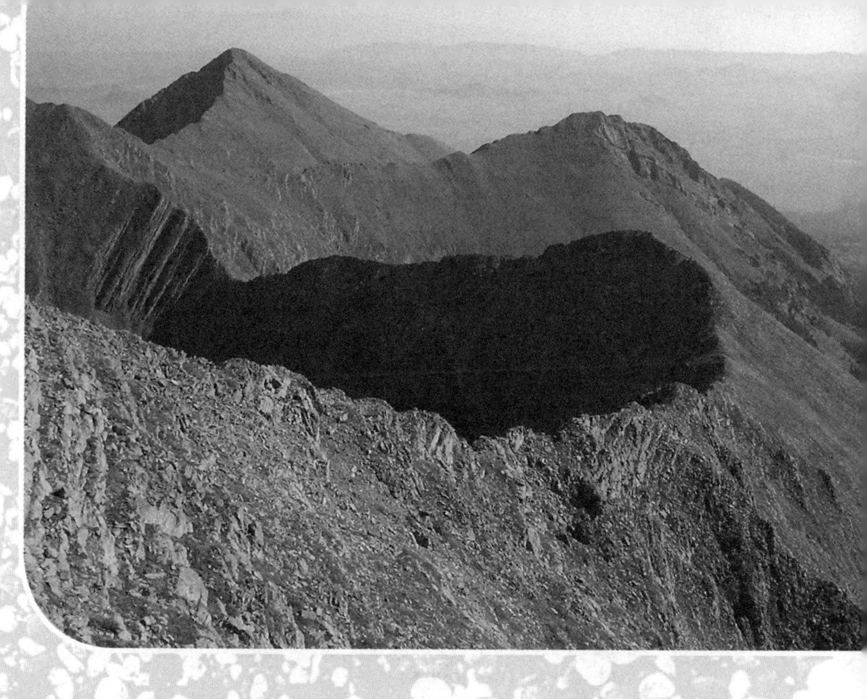

The ridgeline on Adams can be intimidating until you unlock its secrets.

and Horn Creek Trail. Do not head toward Macey Lakes, even though you may be lured by the nearby sound of rushing water.

0.6 mi (3) Your stay on the Rainbow Trail is short-lived. Turn left (west) onto Horn Creek Trail #1342; the marked sign also mentions the Horn Lakes. From here on out, the trail is class 2, with rocks, roots, and mud. Despite the obstacles, this is still a maintained trail that is good for backpacking. Elevation gain is gradual, and it's easy to set a good pace on the lower section of the trail.

2.6 mi (4) River crossing number one. In early spring, this stream can flow quite high.

2.8 mi (5) Cross into the Sangre De Cristo Wilderness. From here, the trail gets muddier and has steeper sections. In other words, it's time to get dirty and sweaty.

4.0 mi (6) As you finally begin to emerge from the trees, you'll be surrounded by Little Baldy Mountain on your left and Little Horn Peak on your right. As you reach a clearing, you'll come to your biggest river crossing (which is also at the base of the first of the Horn Lakes). Check out the incredible blackish eastern wall of Fluted Peak to your right.

4.8 mi (7) Here you reach the middle group of the Horn Lakes; this is a great place to set up camp. Camping at the largest Horn Lake is an option, too; in fact, you'll have to pass just over 5.0 miles to actually see the summit block of Adams, to the northwest.

Right around this area, you'll want to get off-trail and begin the grueling push up the giant grassy slope to Unnamed Peak 13,325. Consult the Adams Ridge map for this and the rest of the route. From camp, at around 11,800 feet, it is 1,525 feet straight up to UN 13,325's summit. I found that staying north on the slope offered much better footing, mostly grass. While the lines may look more direct to the south, the terrain is talus-filled and rocky. Set the line of your ascent north to the next waypoint, a small rock outcrop I call the Cornerstone.

5.1 mi (8) Reach the Cornerstone, and head directly for the summit of UN 13,325. If you don't mind off-camber hiking (or you want to bypass UN 13,325), you can traverse diagonally to the saddle of Adams.

5.4 mi (9) Reach the summit of UN 13,325. You'll have a stunning, somewhat intimidating view of the ridge to Adams. Drop down southwest to the saddle and get ready to scramble.

5.6 mi (10) The saddle is a good place to ditch your trekking poles. From here, it's a mere 0.4 mile and 800-plus vertical feet to the summit—this is where the fun begins.

Navigating the northeast ridge of Adams is not as hard as it looks. It will take some route finding, but the challenge is never overwhelming. I offer the following tips.

You can stay on the spine of the ridge for most of this climb, but there are a few sections where you may want to diverge. Pinnacle 1 **(11)** will be easy to scramble up and maintain the ridge. Get up the pinnacle notch **(12)** and stay on the ridge to Pinnacle 2 **(13)**.

Pinnacle 2 is your first real challenge. If you are feeling bold, scramble directly up (class 3+) and walk on a short, exhilarating section that I call the Adams Skyway. If you prefer a safer traverse, divert to the right (north) side of the ridge, which will likely be in shadows and has snow year-round. Here, you'll find a nice detour with solid terrain. Rejoin the ridge **(14)**, where you'll exit the skyway.

Next, you'll encounter Pinnacles 3 **(15)** and 4 **(16)**. You again have the option of a direct scramble or an easier detour; this time, the detours are safer on the left (south) side of the ridge. Once you climb Pinnacle 4 or detour around it, get back up on the ridge for the best part of the hike. It may be tempting to head for the loose, rocky slopes on Adams's east face, but stay on (or close to) the ridge.

Pinnacle 4 may have seemed tough, but once you are atop it, you have it free and easy to the summit. Begin Skyway 2 **(17)** and follow it to Adams Side summit **(18)** at mile 6.0 of your hike.

From Side summit, head south to the prized main summit. I found it easiest to divert left (southeast) of the ridge and get out a bit on the east face, where a faint path zigzags up to the summit block proper. Enjoy the awesome views, especially those to the south. You've earned it!

6.1 mi (19) Mount Adams's summit! Take your photos and return down to the saddle.

6.6 mi (10) Once at the saddle, pick up any jettisoned gear and begin your descent; there's no reason to revisit UN 13,325. The off-camber route is easier to descend than to ascend, so I recommend it for the way down. Aim for Cornerstone and regain the Horn Creek Trail at mile 7.1. Walk out the way you came.

11.8 mi Finish.

Options The Sangre De Cristos rise from the plains like a giant, natural amusement park. There's always a lot to see and explore in each distinct basin. Because Adams is such a demanding route, it will probably be the focus of your trip, but if you are feeling robust, you can go for Little Horn Peak and connect it to Fluted Peak. The ridge between UN 13,325 and Fluted Peak looks possible, but you drop down quite a bit in the saddle. Little Baldy Mountain has several summits that you can scale, most easily by slogging up the northeast slopes that begin at the lower section of Horn Lakes. Also note that Adams has an easier ascent route from the west side, starting at Willow Creek Trailhead—but the northeast ridge is much more fun.

Quick Facts The origin of Mount Adams's name is somewhat shrouded in mystery, as there were a few notable Adams from which to choose. Most think that the peak is named for Colorado Governor Alva Adams, who served two full terms and won the election in 1904; the third term was contested by legislature, and Adams was forced out. Oddly, there was a second Colorado politician named Alva Adams (Alva B. Adams), a senator for whom the *other* Mount Adams is named.

Sangre De Cristo, which translates to "the blood of Christ," is rumored to have been uttered by a Spanish missionary upon his first sight of the deep red alpenglow over these impressive peaks.

Contact Info San Isabel National Forest
2480 Kachina Drive
Pueblo, CO 81008
(719) 553-1400

Eureka Mountain–Hermit Peak

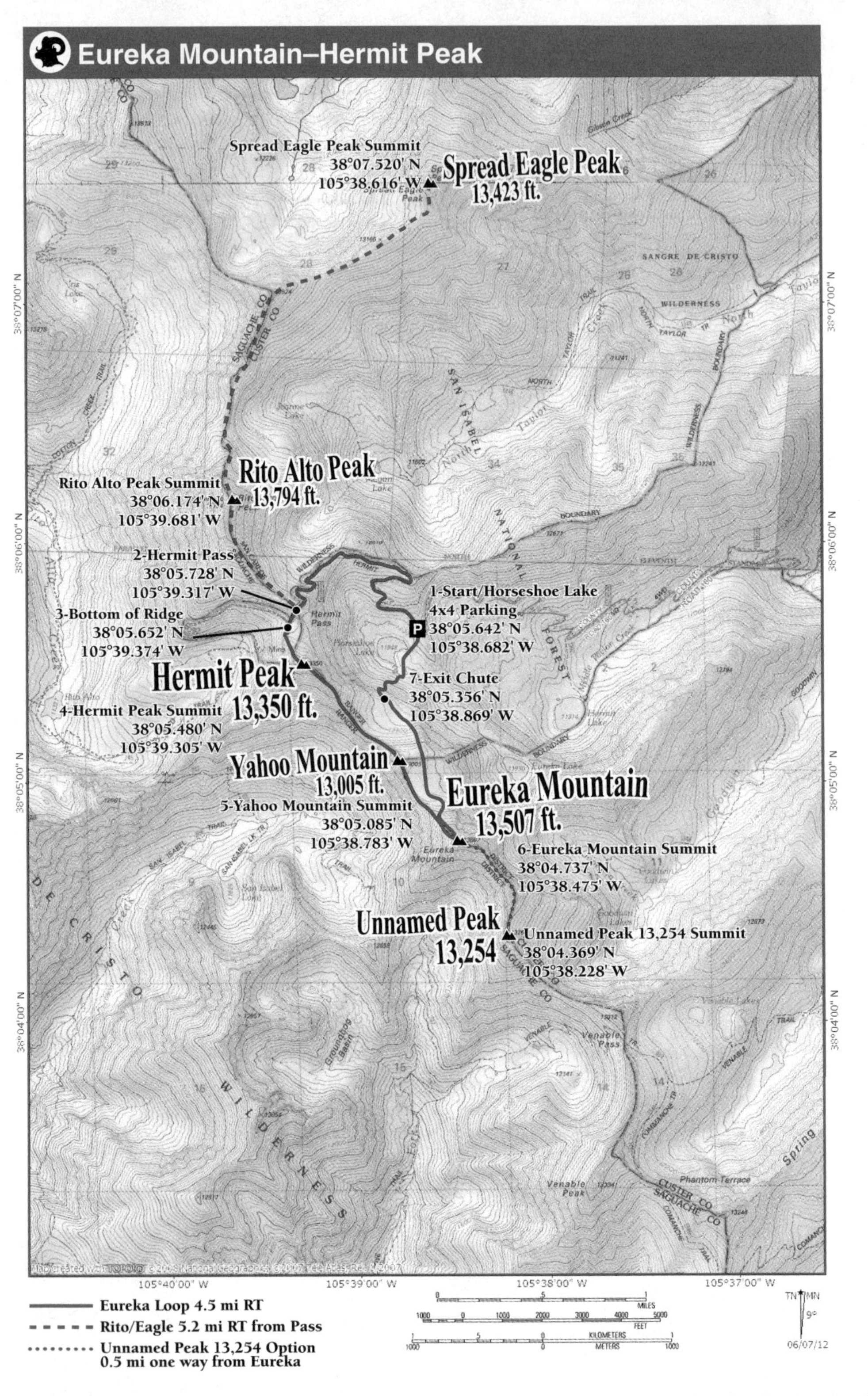

Spread Eagle Peak Summit
38°07.520' N
105°38.616' W
Spread Eagle Peak
13,423 ft.
Rito Alto Peak
13,794 ft.
Rito Alto Peak Summit
38°06.174' N
105°39.681' W
2-Hermit Pass
38°05.728' N
105°39.317' W
3-Bottom of Ridge
38°05.652' N
105°39.374' W
1-Start/Horseshoe Lake
4x4 Parking
38°05.642' N
105°38.682' W
Hermit Peak
13,350 ft.
4-Hermit Peak Summit
38°05.480' N
105°39.305' W
7-Exit Chute
38°05.356' N
105°38.869' W
Yahoo Mountain
13,005 ft.
5-Yahoo Mountain Summit
38°05.085' N
105°38.783' W
Eureka Mountain
13,507 ft.
6-Eureka Mountain Summit
38°04.737' N
105°38.475' W
Unnamed Peak
13,254
Unnamed Peak 13,254 Summit
38°04.369' N
105°38.228' W
Eureka Loop 4.5 mi RT
Rito/Eagle 5.2 mi RT from Pass
Unnamed Peak 13,254 Option
0.5 mi one way from Eureka

42 Eureka Mountain–Hermit Peak

BONUS PEAK: YAHOO MOUNTAIN

Shouts of joy are commonplace on these two picturesque Sangre De Cristo peaks. Snag a bonus summit en route from Hermit to Eureka's grand apex.

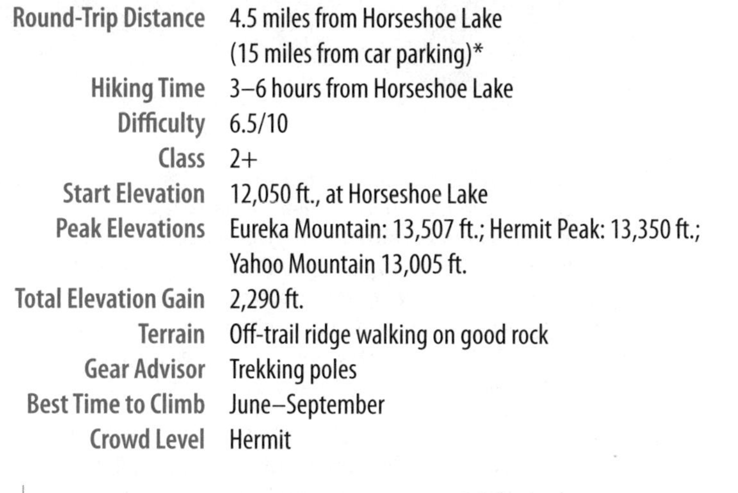

Round-Trip Distance	4.5 miles from Horseshoe Lake (15 miles from car parking)*
Hiking Time	3–6 hours from Horseshoe Lake
Difficulty	6.5/10
Class	2+
Start Elevation	12,050 ft., at Horseshoe Lake
Peak Elevations	Eureka Mountain: 13,507 ft.; Hermit Peak: 13,350 ft.; Yahoo Mountain 13,005 ft.
Total Elevation Gain	2,290 ft.
Terrain	Off-trail ridge walking on good rock
Gear Advisor	Trekking poles
Best Time to Climb	June–September
Crowd Level	Hermit

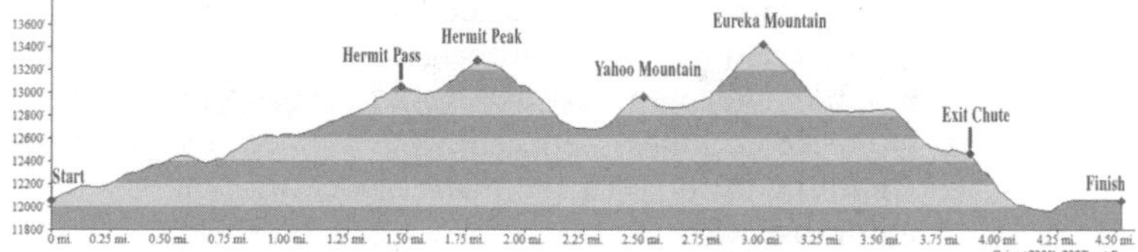

* **Note on Hiking Distance:** The road to Horseshoe Lake is very rocky and rough. Passenger cars will be lucky to make it to the first parking area. Sport utility cars (SUCs) can get higher but are better off not pushing it on the higher parts of the road (the same may be said for sport utility vehicles [SUVs]). Those 4x4s with good clearance will be able to slowly claw their way up to Horseshoe Lake. It is 5.5 miles one way from the wilderness boundary (where the road gets bad) to Horseshoe Lake.

The road is actually a very nice hike in itself. Unlike other roads, which can be tedious, this feels more like a wide hiking trail. I did this hike from the very bottom of the road and enjoyed it. SUVs and SUCs can brave the road at their own discretion, resulting in a 7- to 9-mile round-trip hike, depending on where you park.

Location Sangre De Cristo Range in the Sangre De Cristo Wilderness/San Isabel National Forest outside of Westcliffe

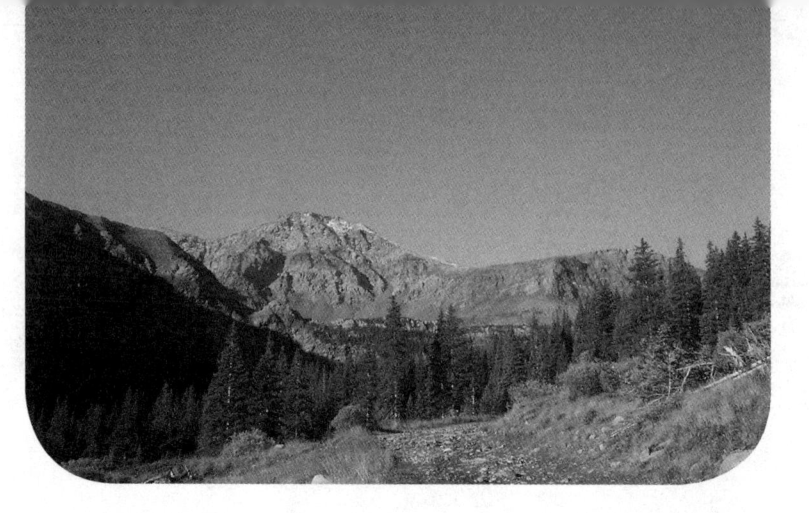

Eureka Mountain as seen from the rugged Hermit Pass Road

Intro Eureka and Hermit are often overlooked in favor of more glamorous 14ers of the Sangre De Cristo Range. Isolation has its benefits, however; a pristine wilderness is yours to discover when you undertake this hike. Eureka is an especially photogenic peak. Mountaineering fans will notice that the striated northeast face bears a strong resemblance to Mount Everest's summit pyramid. The route between these two mountains is a fun class 2+ traverse that doesn't have high exposure. Optional routes can make this a very full day from Hermit Pass.

Why Climb It? Relatively unknown peaks with fun, beautiful traverses are my favorite mountains to climb. Taken from Horseshoe Lake, this isn't a strenuous loop, but it still gives you a good workout. Views to the south from Eureka are marvelous. The Crestone group (as well as Mount Adams, Hike 41) rise like enormous tombstones. As far as Sangre hikes go, these peaks are more for hikers than technical climbers, so everyone can enjoy them. Camping in the area is a distinct pleasure and a great way to spend an autumn weekend.

Driving You're going to need a high-clearance 4x4 vehicle or a beefy SUV to make it to Horseshoe Lake. The way up is extremely rocky in places, especially on steep sections of the road. It's a bit frustrating that many of the rugged sections are followed by long stretches of perfectly smooth dirt roads. SUCs that put up a good fight can make it 2.1 miles up the road. One good thing is that there are plenty of good primitive campsites along the way. SUVs with good clearance and a strong low gear can make it up to Horseshoe Lake. As mentioned before, hiking this road isn't a miserable experience; in fact, you may enjoy the hike more by starting it a bit lower, such as at the trailhead for Hermit Lake.

How to Get There From Colorado Highway 69 in the town of Westcliffe, turn west onto County Road 160, also known as Hermit Road and Hermit Pass Road. This road begins as pavement and then turns into a well-maintained dirt road, passable for all. Old-timers (well, not that old) may recognize this as the way up to the extinct Conquistador Ski Area. Stay on CR 160 for 7.2 miles to the wilderness boundary. Once you reach the boundary, CR 160 turns into

Forest Service Road 301 (Hermit Pass Road) and becomes an utter mess. Rocks galore litter this part of the road. Tough passenger cars may end up sacrificing parts struggling 0.1 mile up to the parking area on the right (when the road turns left).

SUCs, SUVs, and 4x4s can continue on for varying distances. Several side roads split off to campsites, but the main road is obvious—stay on it. One tricky section comes at mile 2.1, where the road splits into two seemingly good sections (there is also a wilderness preservation sign). Go right, up a very rocky hill. Note, however, that the smooth, sandy flat road to the left is a great place for SUCs to park/camp. Keep fighting up this road, passing the Hermit Lake Trailhead at mile 4.0, until you reach a small parking area at Horseshoe Lake, at mile 5.5 (elevation 12,050 feet). The road keeps going up, 1.5 miles to Hermit Pass, but because the loop ends at Horseshoe Lake, do not park there (unless you want to climb back up over Hermit Peak, which is another 800 feet of elevation gain). Horseshoe Lake has several parking spots and good areas to pitch a tent.

Fees/Camping There are no fees to hike or camp in this area; please do not camp before reaching the wilderness boundary.

Route Notes The route detailed here does not include the mileage you may incur hoofing it up Hermit Pass Road from parking areas before Horseshoe Lake.

Mile/Waypoint

0.0 mi (1) Start at the parking area at Horseshoe Lake. Hike up the wide switchbacks on Hermit Pass Road up to Hermit Pass—this is a good warm-up.

1.5 mi (2) Reach the top of Hermit Pass, at 13,050 feet. There's a sign-in register here. Fill out your information and start south toward Hermit Peak, just off to your left.

1.6 mi (3) Here, at the bottom of the ridge, leave the road and scramble directly up to the summit of Hermit Peak. This short ascent covers about 270 vertical feet, depending on where you begin on the ridge.

1.8 mi (4) Hermit Peak summit. Getting here was the easy part; now you have to down climb over to Yahoo Mountain (which looks like a real mountain from here). Stay due south and climb all the way down to the saddle (at 12,680 feet) between Hermit and Yahoo. Hike/scramble the ridge up to the top of Yahoo.

2.6 mi (5) Yahoo Mountain summit! Now that you are up here, you realize that this isn't so much a mountain as it is a raised shoulder of Eureka Mountain. Drop down into a saddle at 12,870 feet, and get ready to ascend Eureka's northwest ridge. Staying on the spine of the ridge is the most fun. There are plenty of handholds on this class 2+ scramble, and they are made of knobby Crestone conglomerate rock. If you feel a bit uneasy on the ridge, stay to the left and ascend the rocky slope. The higher you get on this ridge, the less humble Yahoo Mountain looks like a mountain.

3.1 mi (6) Eureka's summit! Views to the south will make your jaw drop. When you descend, it's faster to storm down the north slope to the plateau between Yahoo and Eureka. Stay on this plateau and descend, slightly rising to pass a bump that is lined up with Yahoo Mountain. Continue down to the Exit Chute, where you'll have a good view of Horseshoe Lake and your vehicle below.

4.0 mi (7) At the Exit Chute, find a good line down the scree hill and make your way back to Horseshoe Lake. The upper parts of this descent are loose, so be careful. Going a bit farther north will bring you to the exact chute listed on the map (waypoint **7**), which is a relatively easy class 2+ descent.

4.5 mi Finish.

Options The short, 0.5-mile traverse (one way) to Unnamed Peak 13,254 from Eureka's summit gives good views of Eureka to the north and Venable Pass to the south. It's not mind-blowing, but it is a good way to extend your day if you parked at Horseshoe Lake.

A good secondary hike is the out-and-back trip north from Hermit Pass (waypoint **2**) to Rito Alto and Spread Eagle Peaks (5.2 miles). This is a class 2 hike on similar rock that you can do as one long day (roughly 11 miles if you do them all). On this route, you'll also summit two unnamed 13ers—meaning that if you do the full loop in a day (not including UN 13,254), you'll summit seven 13ers. Wow! On the other hand, if you are spending a weekend up here, why not do this trek on your second day?

Quick Facts Eureka is Greek for "I found it!" This was a buzzword of the late 1800s, and the peak was named in honor of this exclamation. Hey, it's better than Consarnit Mountain.

One last interesting note concerns the short-lived Conquistador Ski Area that once operated east of the spot where County Road 160 crosses the wilderness boundary. Westcliffe residents resisted the development, knowing full well that there wasn't enough snow to make the area worthwhile. Nonetheless, developers tried. From 1978 to 1988, the ski area operated four lifts. The resort last operated in 1992. A comeback in 1996 fell short, and the lifts were removed forever. The current owner plans to make the area a mountain resort not focused on skiing.

Contact Info San Isabel National Forest
Salida Ranger District
325 W. Rainbow Boulevard
Salida, CO 81201
(719) 539-3591

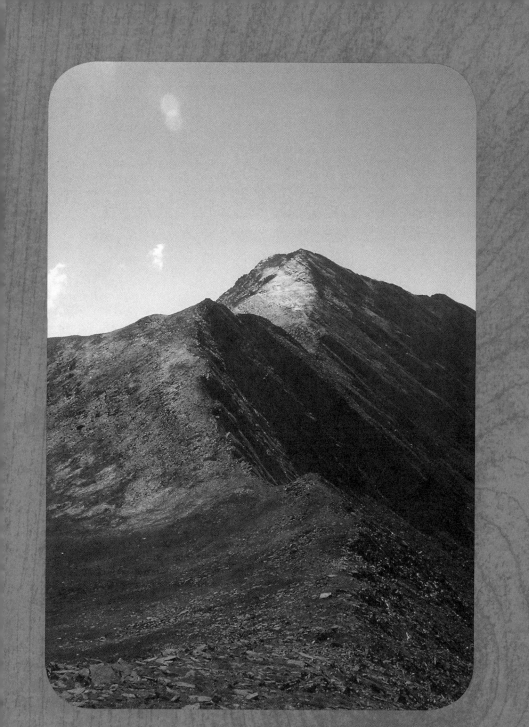

A great look at the traverse to Yahoo Mountain with Eureka Mountain in the background

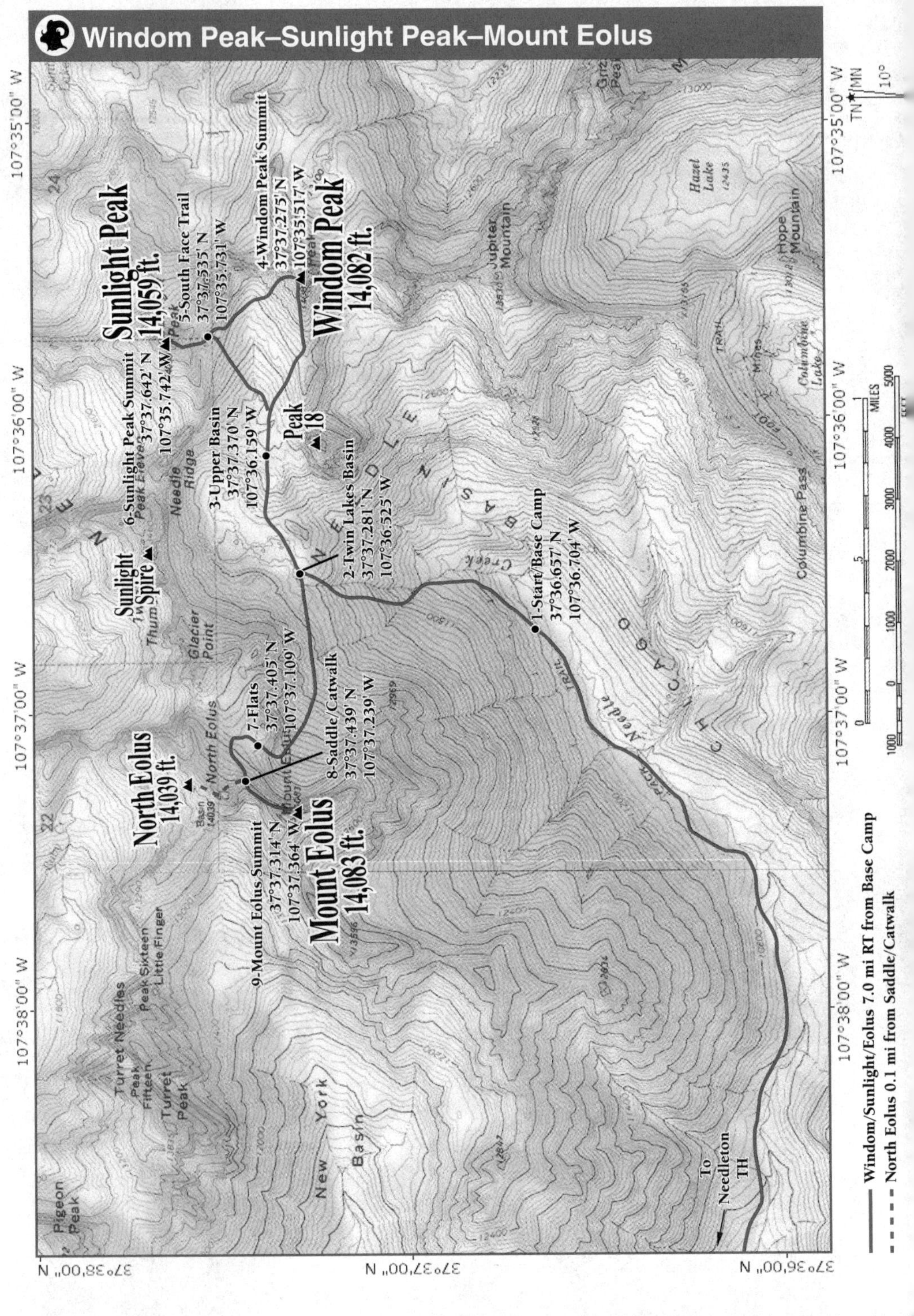

Windom Peak–Sunlight Peak–Mount Eolus
Sunlight Peak
14,059 ft.
Windom Peak
14,082 ft.
Mount Eolus
14,083 ft.
North Eolus
14,039 ft.
Sunlight Spire
Peak 18
1-Start/Base Camp
37°36.657' N
107°36.704' W
2-Twin Lakes Basin
37°37.281' N
107°36.525' W
3-Upper Basin
37°37.370' N
107°36.159' W
4-Windom Peak Summit
37°37.275' N
107°35.517' W
5-South Face Trail
37°37.535' N
107°35.731' W
6-Sunlight Peak Summit
37°37.642' N
107°35.742' W
7-Flats
37°37.405' N
107°37.109' W
8-Saddle/Catwalk
37°37.439' N
107°37.239' W
9-Mount Eolus Summit
37°37.314' N
107°37.364' W
Needle Ridge
Glacier Point
Jupiter Mountain
Hope Mountain
Hazel Lake
Columbine Lake
Columbine Pass
Needle Creek
Chicago Basin
Turret Needles
Turret Peak
Peak Fifteen
Peak Sixteen
Little Finger
Pigeon Peak
New York Basin
To Needleton TH
107°35'00" W
107°36'00" W
107°37'00" W
107°38'00" W
37°38'00" N
37°37'00" N
37°36'00" N
TN MN 10°
MILES
Windom/Sunlight/Eolus 7.0 mi RT from Base Camp
North Eolus 0.1 mi from Saddle/Catwalk

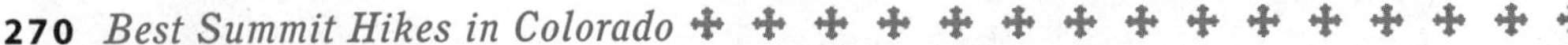

43 Chicago Basin 14er Circuit: Windom Peak–Sunlight Peak–Mount Eolus

Good Overnight!

A trip to Chicago Basin is an unforgettable experience. Ride the Durango & Silverton train to a remote stop in the San Juans and prepare to embark on an amazing journey.

Round-Trip Distance	21 miles from Needleton Trailhead; 7-mile loop when camping in Chicago Basin
Hiking Time	3–4 days; depends on route, but expect 10–12 hours for the three 14ers in one day from camp
Difficulty	8/10
Class	2+/3
Start Elevation	8,233 ft., at Needleton Creek Trailhead
Peak Elevations	Windom Peak: 14,082 ft.; Sunlight Peak: 14,059 ft.; Mount Eolus: 14,083 ft.
Total Elevation Gain	8,220 ft.
Terrain	Train ride; long class 1 trail to Chicago Basin; class 2+/3 scrambling
Best Time to Climb	July–September
Gear Advisor	Camping gear, GPS, quad maps, trekking poles, camera, and helmet
Crowd Level	Moderate

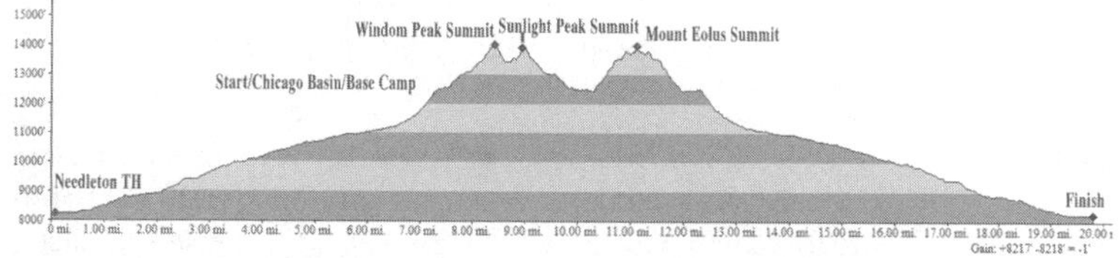

Location San Juan Mountains in the Weminuche Wilderness/San Juan National Forest outside of Durango and Silverton

Intro There's nothing like the feeling of taking the old steam train to Needleton Trailhead, grabbing your pack, and watching the old locomotive chug away. All grows quiet except the soothing rush of water in the Animas River. From here, you're in the backcountry. A 5- to 6-mile approach (depending on where you set up camp) lets you set up a real, honest-to-goodness base camp, from which you'll have many options regarding how to climb these mountains. Your 14ers on this hike come in three different flavors—quite a nice bit of diversity for three peaks so close to one another. Gear up and get ready to get away from it all.

Why Climb It? The train ride to Needleton is obviously a nice touch, but you're here for the hiking, not the choo-choo. The great part about hiking these three mountains is that they sample different climbing styles. Windom is class 2/2+ on big, blocky boulders. Sunlight has a good class 3 route that culminates with a fun scramble to an exposed summit. Eolus has sustained class 3 scrambling along narrow catwalks and rocky ledges. Some people do all three in one day (about 10 miles round-trip from camp), but my preferred option is to hike Windom and Sunlight in one trek (about 5.3 miles round-trip from camp), and on a second day to hike Eolus and optional North Eolus (about 4.2 miles round-trip from camp).

Driving Needleton Trailhead is accessed by train, specifically the Durango & Silverton Narrow Gauge Railroad. Costs for tickets are $83 per person round-trip (for the year 2012), and you must make reservations. You can start from either of the two train stations, though most prefer to start in Durango (parking is $7 per day, so factor that into your expenses as well). The Durango station is at the intersection of US Highway 550 and US Highway 160 in the south part of town and is very well marked. The Silverton station is off Colorado Highway 110 and is also well signed. To make your reservations, or for any other questions, contact the train service:

Durango & Silverton Narrow Gauge Railroad
479 Main Avenue
Durango, CO 81301
Reservations and General Information: (970) 247-2733
Toll Free: (877) 872-4607
durangotrain.com

For those who are wondering, there is a very long trail, aptly named the Purgatory Trail, that you can take to avoid the train. It is 9.0 miles one way to the Needleton Trailhead (then another 5–6 miles to camp) from this route—more than 30 miles of approach hiking. Not much fun, but it's a possibility if you have lots of time and no money.

How to Get There Needleton Trailhead is almost exclusively accessed by train. Check the schedule, and make sure that you are on a train that stops at Needleton. The folks who work for the train service are used to backpackers and will answer any additional questions that you may have.

Fees/Camping There are no fees for hiking or camping in the area. Train tickets are $83 per adult (in 2012); parking on-site at the train station is $7 per day.

Route Notes The mileage for the first waypoint is approximate, based on where you camp in Chicago Basin, which may be in any number of places. My camp was at the flat north end of the basin just before the steep hiking begins. I would advise hiking into the basin for better camp spots; the good ones start once the basin opens up, about 5.3 miles in. Be prepared, as this is truly a backcountry area. There will be other people around, but you must be self-reliant.

As mentioned, I recommend hiking Windom and Sunlight in one day and Eolus and North Eolus on another day. The route description below follows that itinerary. Spending three to four days in the area is the best plan, taking a whole day each for the hike in and hike out. The less rushed you are, the more you'll enjoy the area. Make enough time to catch the train home by not overwhelming yourself with too much on your last day.

Note: If you go for all three 14ers in a day, get a very early start.

The mountain goats in the basin are numerous and nearly domesticated. Do not feed, ride, pet, chase, tackle, groom, wrestle, snuggle, touch, or engage the goats. They are wild animals that are capable of inflicting some serious damage on hikers who get too close.

A final note: U.S. Geological Survey (USGS) quad maps are *highly* advised for this hike. You'll need the following quads: *Columbine Pass, Mountain View Crest,* and *Snowdon Peak.*

Mile/Waypoint

Day 1: The Hike In
Mileage from Needleton Trailhead: 5–6 miles

0.0 mi Get off the train at the Needleton Trailhead, and get on the Chicago Basin pack trail that crosses over the bridge spanning the river. Follow this well-worn class 1 trail up to Chicago Basin. The way up is very well marked and easy to follow. The few intersections are well marked. As you begin to get closer to the basin, views will open up and you'll be in another world. You will slowly gain about 3,000 feet of elevation. I would suggest camping around mile 5.5, at roughly 11,150 feet.

5.5 mi (1) Find a good campsite. We'll reset the trip mileage here.

Day 2: Windom and Sunlight from Chicago Basin
Round-trip mileage from camp: 5.4 miles

0.0 mi (1) From camp, get back on the main trail and follow it north up the steep slopes that lead to the high basin west of Sunlight and Windom. This trail crosses the stream/waterfall and pushes straight up to the Twin Lakes, at 12,560 feet.

0.8 mi (2) You've reached the flat Twin Lakes Basin. The trail here goes right (east) to a still higher basin. There is a cairned trail as well as a few other faint trails. As you gaze up, Windom is the big block to your upper right. That's your first goal, so keep moving east in its direction.

1.3 mi (3) The upper basin has one tiny lake and many boulders. From here, gain the saddle between Peak Eighteen and Windom at its lowest point, which will be on your right. You can get to the saddle by staying on the cairned trail or by scrambling up off trail.

Once you gain Windom's west ridge, the way up is obvious (and there's a faint trail). As you near the summit, the blocks become giant cubes. Have fun on this class 2 terrain until you reach the highest point.

2.0 mi (4) Windom Peak's summit! To traverse over to Sunlight Peak's south face, you have a few options. This route follows a steep scree gully that eliminates the need to drop back into the high basin. It begins northwest of the summit and is a bit slowgoing in places, but it's quicker in the long run, if you have the knees for it. The other option is to drop back down Windom's west ridge and traverse north to the basin from the saddle of Windom and Peak Eighteen.

2.5 mi (5) If you are unsure where to start the climb on Sunlight, look for the red, rocky gully east of the slopes to Sunlight Peak. From here, a whisker-marked trail goes into the south face and works its way up a series of rocky ledges. You may lose the trail or prefer to scramble up at your own pace; in any case, it's class 3 terrain. As you get higher, start heading to the left (west) and work your way over to a saddle between Sunlight and Sunlight Spire. The climbing narrows considerably and gets harder from here. Continue west by following rocky (and somewhat exposed) ledges or by walking to the west edge of the saddle and scrambling up (north) from there. Stop when you are about 20 feet from the ridge and turn right, choosing a good class 3 route to ascend.

The best way is the famous Keyhole, a 30-foot section that is enclosed by a boulder. Scramble east up the Keyhole and toward the summit, which will be very close. The summit register and USGS marker will be on a flat section below the final summit block. It doesn't look so bad from here, does it?

2.8 miles (6) Sunlight Peak's perilous summit! The move to reach the high point of Sunlight is a dangerous, exposed move that you must commit to; do not climb it if you are unnerved. (And don't feel bad about it if you don't: it's a dangerous, high-risk, class 4 move.) The summit block is about 30 feet tall; go up and over to your right to reach the "launching pad," a sloped rock linking the last few boulders. The gap you need to clear drops about 12 feet in front of you and about 1,200 feet on the right side. This gap is only about 2.5 feet across, and to clear it you must jump onto a sloped, polished rock. Once you clear the gap, it's a quick hop (or belly crawl) to the summit. Getting down is the hardest part; the jump to clear the gap is tough because you land on a downhill-sloped boulder. There is a rock in the gap that you can hop onto, but this may be even harder to land on. Having a friend spot you is a good idea.

It isn't necessary to claim the summit. If you really want to, however, you may want to bring along a pair of rock climbing shoes for extra grip (and a mental boost). It's a tough move to protect, so if you want to belay a friend, bring a 100-foot (or longer) length of static rope and set an anchor by looping it around the summit boulder.

To return, drop down the south face again, taking your time and making your way back to the lakes area (waypoint **2**). Rest up. You have another summit ahead of you tomorrow (or later today, if you're linking them).

5.3 mi Finish the Windom and Sunlight hike.

Day 3: Mount Eolus

Round-trip mileage from base camp to summit and back: 4.2 miles

0.0 mi (1) Start as you did for the Windom/Sunlight hike, going back up to the top of the waterfall just before Twin Lakes.

0.8 mi (2) Below (south of) the Twin Lakes, a trail hops over the stream (before it becomes a full-fledged waterfall), and heads west toward Eolus. This trail is well worn and goes up into a sloped basin. Follow it all the way to a flat section below North Eolus.

1.7 mi (7) From the flats, you'll need to scramble up to the north ridge; it's also a good place to ditch your trekking poles. There is a cairned trail, but you can also pick your own line. (Once you are in the saddle, it's a quick class 3 optional traverse up to 14,039-foot North Eolus summit.) If your sights are set squarely on Mount Eolus, get on the ridge and head south.

1.9 mi (8) On the ridge at 13,800 feet, you'll encounter a narrow, 15-foot-long-by-2-foot-wide section known as the Catwalk. There's nothing hard about it, but the exposure is high; some prefer to unleash their inner felines and cross it on all fours. Once you clear it, continue on to the east face.

From here, the route is semicairned. The cubic piles of rock on this mountain seem intimidating, but you can find many safe paths up the east face, where series of ledges and traverses will bring you to the summit. This requires some route finding, so plot out your path with care. The cairns are useful but seem to trace several different routes. A helmet is suggested for this section.

2.1 mi (9) Mount Eolus's summit! Notice that the USGS marker up here uses the Greek spelling Aeolus. The hardest part of the climb may be returning the way you came. Take your time and pick good lines back to the ridge. Retrace your path back to camp.

4.2 mi Finish.

Now that the work is done, you can head out whenever you please—just make sure that you catch your train on time.

Options The short scramble up to North Eolus is a mere 0.1 mile from waypoint **8**. It's a nice peak, and if it were a bit farther north of Eolus, it would be distinct enough to be a ranked 14er.

Quick Facts Windom is named for politician William Windom, a senator from Minnesota who went to serve as the US secretary of the Treasury from 1889–91. Sunlight Peak was named by surveyor Whitman Cross in 1902; it must have been a sunny day. Mount Eolus was named after the Greek god of wind. After initially being named Mount Aeolus by the Hayden survey of 1874, the Wheeler survey inexplicably changed the spelling to Eolus on its 1878 maps.

Contact Info Information for the Durango & Silverton train is listed on page 272.
San Juan National Forest
15 Burnett Court
Durango, CO 81301
(970) 247-4874

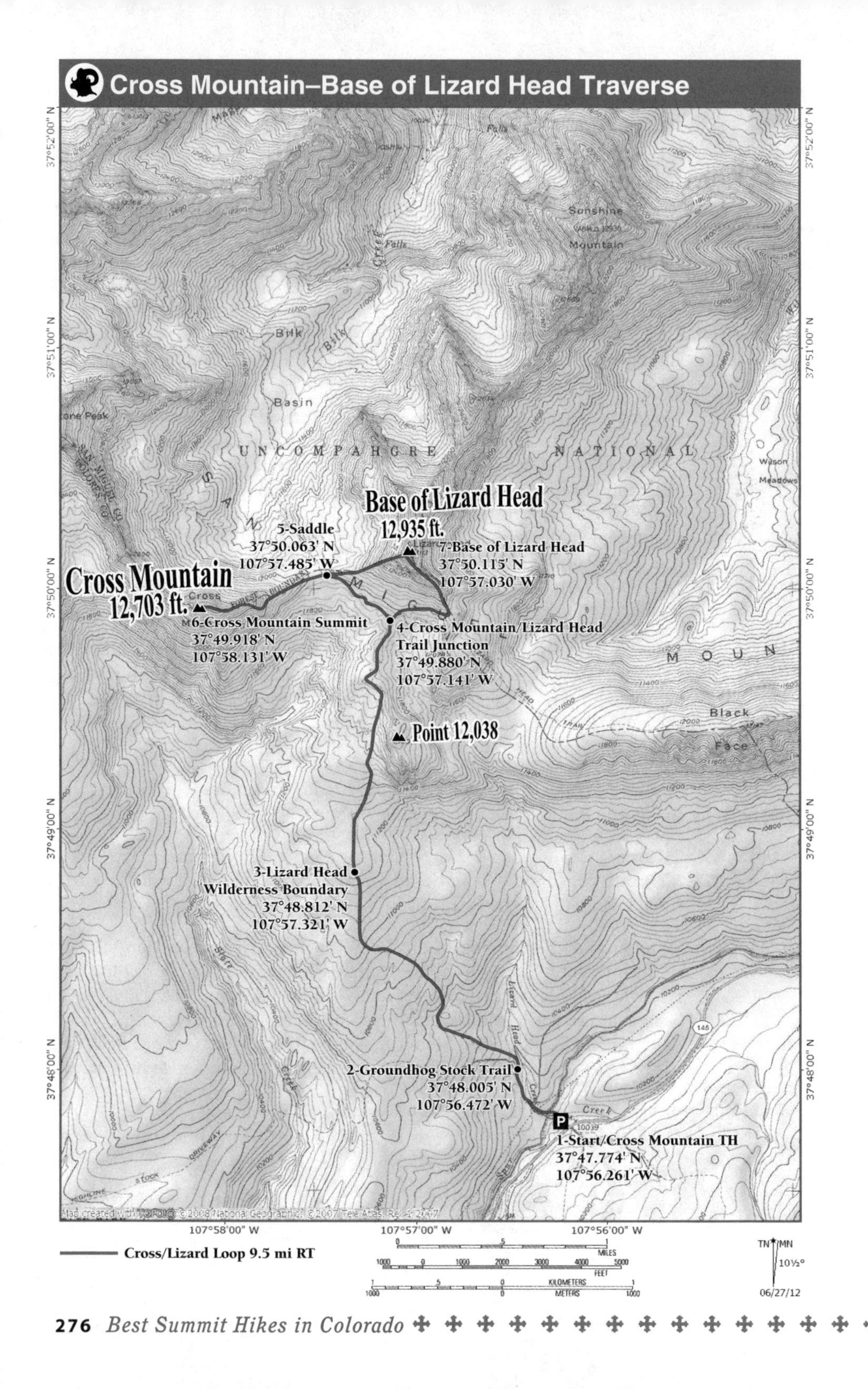

Cross Mountain–Base of Lizard Head Traverse
Base of Lizard Head
12,935 ft.
5-Saddle
37°50.063' N
107°57.485' W
7-Base of Lizard Head
37°50.115' N
107°57.030' W
Cross Mountain
12,703 ft.
6-Cross Mountain Summit
37°49.918' N
107°58.131' W
4-Cross Mountain/Lizard Head Trail Junction
37°49.880' N
107°57.141' W
Point 12,038
3-Lizard Head Wilderness Boundary
37°48.812' N
107°57.321' W
2-Groundhog Stock Trail
37°48.005' N
107°56.472' W
1-Start/Cross Mountain TH
37°47.774' N
107°56.261' W
Sunshine Mountain
Bilk Basin
UNCOMPAHGRE NATIONAL
Wilson Meadows
Black Face
107°58'00" W
107°57'00" W
107°56'00" W
37°52'00" N
37°51'00" N
37°50'00" N
37°49'00" N
37°48'00" N
Map created with TOPO!® ©2008 National Geographic; ©2007 Tele Atlas, Rel. 1 2007
Cross/Lizard Loop 9.5 mi RT
MILES
FEET
KILOMETERS
METERS
TN MN
10½°
06/27/12

44

Cross Mountain–Base of Lizard Head Traverse

Take a tour of two mystical mountains. Cross stands like an altar before a council of mountain gods while Lizard Head has dimensions that defy conventional form.

Round-Trip Distance	9.5 miles
Hiking Time	5–7 hours
Difficulty	6.5/10
Class	2
Start Elevation	10,040 ft., at Cross Mountain Trailhead
Peak Elevations	Cross Mountain: 12,703 ft.; Base of Lizard Head: 12,935 ft.
Total Elevation Gain	3,565 ft.
Terrain	Class 1 trail leads to rocky scramble to Cross summit and base of Lizard Head
Best Time to Climb	June–September
Gear Advisor	Normal gear
Crowd Level	Low/moderate

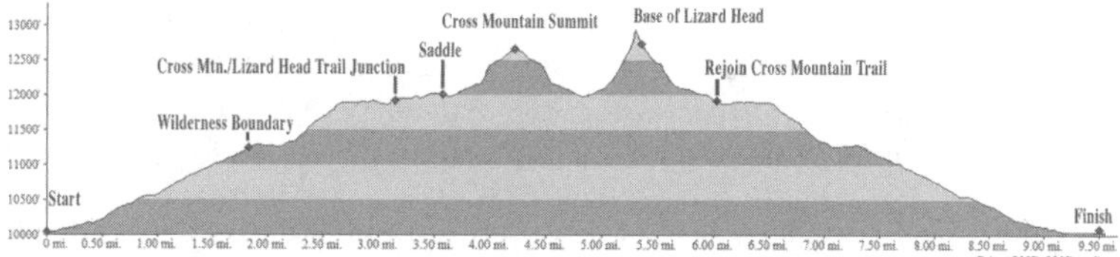

Location San Juan Mountains in the Lizard Head Wilderness/San Juan National Forest outside of Telluride

Intro Cross Mountain's unique position among a crowd of 14ers and high 13ers offers a rare perspective of the mighty San Juan Mountains. Atop its modest summit, I felt like a traveler who had come to seek the advice of a sagacious council. Cross is dwarfed by peaks from the Wilson group to the west; the effect of gazing at these enormous mountains is mesmerizing. Across the way is Lizard Head, indisputably the most difficult summit to ascend of any mountain higher than 13,000 feet in Colorado. This crumbling, 400-foot, sheer monolith is the enduring throat of an extinct volcano. This hike tours the platform beneath the cracking bust, giving you views to its upper reaches that will send chills down your spine and into your knees.

Why Climb It? While erosion has had its way with the rock spewed forth from Lizard Head (which looks remarkably like a giant Atari joystick), the granite pipes that siphoned magma from the center of the Earth have defiantly remained intact. As a result, this amazing tower is visible from many places in the San Juans (I could clearly make it out from the faraway summit of Redcloud).

Fewer people have reached its summit than have climbed Mount Everest. The technical climb to the top is only graded class 5.7–5.8, but the entire edifice is falling apart, making every handhold suspect and placements for protective gear purely ornamental. A trip to the base of Lizard Head will give you a gander at the intimidating tower from up close, and a new appreciation for Albert Ellingwood and Barton Hoag's first ascent—in 1920!

Cross Mountain has a different feeling than any mountain I have ever climbed. It's a fun scramble in its own right, and the views from the top are incredible. If I had a say, I would rename it the Altar for the way that it pays homage to nearby high peaks. I wish that everyone could have the experience that I did when climbing the peak: a full-grown bald eagle lifted off from the summit when I was less than 20 feet away.

Driving Any vehicle can reach the Cross Mountain Trailhead. The road is paved the entire way (though the parking lot is not).

How to Get There Cross Mountain Trailhead is 2.0 miles south of Lizard Head Pass off Colorado Highway 145; this is roughly 15 miles south of Telluride. The large parking area is on the west side of the road and is marked by signs for Cross Mountain Trail at the turnoff. If you are coming from the south, the trailhead turnoff is approximately 12 miles north on CO 145 from the town of Rico.

Fees/Camping There are no fees to hike or camp in this area. Please note that camping in the parking area is illegal. You must pass the wilderness boundary to legally camp in the area. Just south of Lizard Head Pass are dozens of good primitive campsites on the east side of the road. These unmarked areas can be found off many of the dirt roads to the east a few miles after the pass.

Route Notes I suggest making the loop by climbing Cross first and returning with the tour of Lizard Head's base.

Mile/Waypoint

0.0 mi (1) Start at the Cross Mountain Trailhead and head west on the Cross Mountain Trail (#637). Lizard Head stands like a granite lighthouse in the distance, serving as your beacon. When you start on this trail, make sure not to turn left or right onto the dirt road that intersects the trail very early on. The correct way is lined with a series of wooden fence posts (but no fence). A US Forest Service marker at the start of the woods confirms that you're on the correct trail.

0.4 mi (2) There is a split here for the bizarrely named Groundhog Stock Trail. (Are they stocking groundhogs these days?) Avoid this trail and stay the course on the Cross Mountain Trail. After this intersection, the class 1 trail is obvious. Hiking into the shadows of the pine forest is a treat and a nice way to set up the next part of the hike.

1.8 mi (3) Pass the official wilderness boundary into the Lizard Head Wilderness.

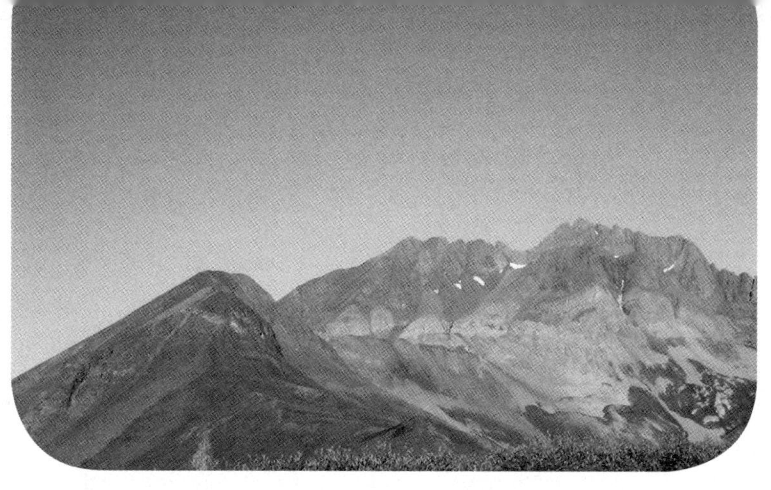

Cross Mountain, on the left, isn't the highest peak in the area but has some of the very best views.

3.2 mi (4) When you clear timberline, things begin to open up. Cross Mountain is the reddish "hill" off to the west. At this point, you are at the pedestal of Lizard Head and at the junction of the Cross Mountain Trail and the Lizard Head Trail. (This is just after you hike on a short section of powdery, fine black rock.) Go left (west) on the Cross Mountain Trail to the western saddle between Lizard Head and Cross.

3.6 mi (5) At the saddle, get off the trail and head west onto the northeast ridge of Cross. Stay on the ridge spine while it is grassy. When the slope morphs to rock, hike onto the south side of the mountain, below the ridge. A faint trail leads out to a brief class 2+ scramble where the northeast and east ridges intersect. Note that staying on the spine of the ridge is a class 3 option and is perfectly acceptable. Do not attempt to climb the grayish gully; pass it and then scramble right onto steep scree to gain the ridge.

4.0 mi You're on the ridge (where you ascended determines the exact spot that you've topped out). This ridge walk turns out to be quite a thrill. It has just enough exposure to keep your adrenaline glands on standby. Follow it to its western terminus.

4.3 mi (6) Cross Mountain summit! Behold the mighty peaks to the west (from left to right): El Diente, Mount Wilson, Gladstone Peak, and Wilson Peak. From here, Lizard Head looks less saurian and more like the rotten fang of an aged predator. Return back to the saddle (waypoint **5**).

5.0 mi (5) From the saddle, hike off-trail and gain Lizard Head's west ridge. This steep climb has a faint trail that switchbacks up to the base of the peak. The preview from the base may look scary, but this is a low-exposure class 2 trail, which becomes obvious when you actually get on it. Despite the fact that it doesn't reach a summit, the elevation here is higher than on Cross Mountain.

5.4 mi (7) The base of Lizard Head! Be careful of falling rock; as Albert Ellingwood put it, "pebbles rain down from the sides as readily as needles from an aging Christmas tree." The sheer profile of Lizard Head will make your knees knock. Once you've seen your fill, finish this side loop by traversing down the rocky southeast ridge and drop to your right (south) to intersect the Lizard Head Trail, which will be visible from here. Take your time on the loose terrain. Once you gain the Lizard Head Trail, follow it a short distance west to its junction with the Cross Mountain Trail.

6.2 mi (4) At the trail junction, return south the way you came on the Cross Mountain Trail.

9.5 mi Finish.

Options If you want to hike down to Bilk Basin by remaining on the Cross Mountain Trail, you'll get a good look at the 14ers as well as the couloirs on the north face of Cross. There are no other close summits, though you could scramble around on the hills south of Lizard Head (for example, point 12,038) to get some different looks at the area.

Quick Facts Albert Ellingwood (of Ellingwood Point fame) and his inexperienced but willing partner Barton Hoag made the first ascent of Lizard Head in 1920, an incredible feat given the technology at the time. Unlike most mountains in Colorado, this first ascent probably was a first ascent by men of any skin color. Modern gear has made the climb more accessible and marginally safer. It is estimated that about 10–20 climbers a year make their way to the summit of Lizard Head. If you'd like to try it, consult a technical climbing guidebook and wear a helmet.

Contact Info San Juan National Forest
San Juan Public Lands Center
15 Burnett Court
Durango, CO 81301
(970) 247-4874

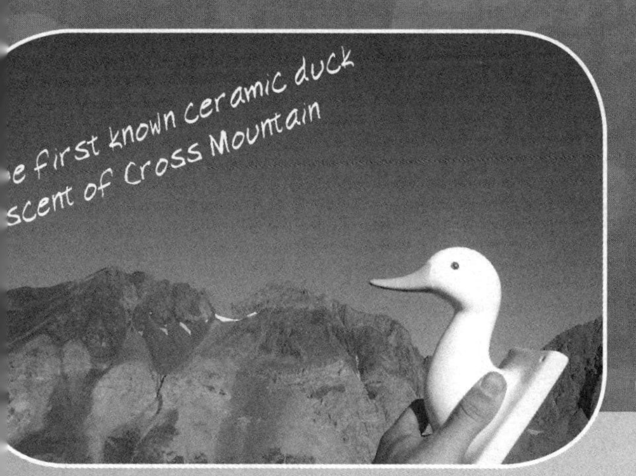

Lizard Head stands guardian over the land.

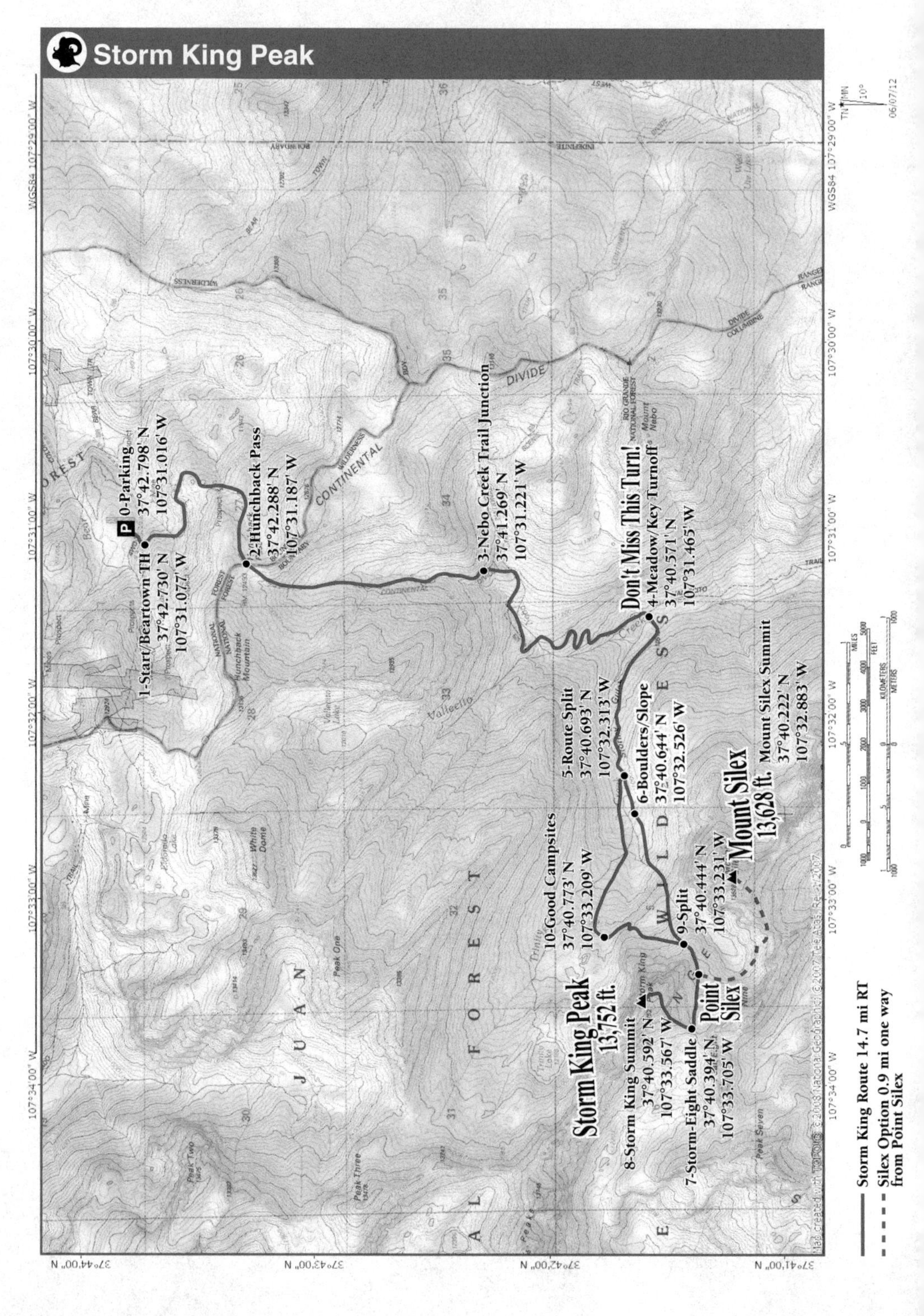

Storm King Peak
0-Parking 37°42.798' N 107°31.016' W
1-Start/Beartown TH 37°42.730' N 107°31.077' W
2-Hunchback Pass 37°42.288' N 107°31.187' W
3-Nebo Creek Trail Junction 37°41.269' N 107°31.221' W
Don't Miss This Turn!
4-Meadow/Key Turnoff 37°40.571' N 107°31.465' W
5-Route Split 37°40.693' N 107°32.313' W
6-Boulders/Slope 37°40.644' N 107°32.526' W
Mount Silex Summit 37°40.222' N 107°32.883' W
Mount Silex 13,628 ft.
9-Split 37°40.444' N 107°33.231' W
10-Good Campsites 37°40.773' N 107°33.209' W
Storm King Peak 13,752 ft.
8-Storm King Summit 37°40.592' N 107°33.567' W
7-Storm-Eight Saddle 37°40.394' N 107°33.705' W
Point Silex
Hunchback Mountain
Vallecito
White Dome
Peak One
Peak Two
Peak Three
Peak Seven
CONTINENTAL
DIVIDE
Mount Nebo
Storm King Route 14.7 mi RT
Silex Option 0.9 mi one way from Point Silex

45 Storm King Peak Good Overnight!

All hail the king! Storm King Peak in the Grenadier Range is as good as it gets; this is my favorite summit hike in Colorado. Get ready for a wild experience that you'll never forget.

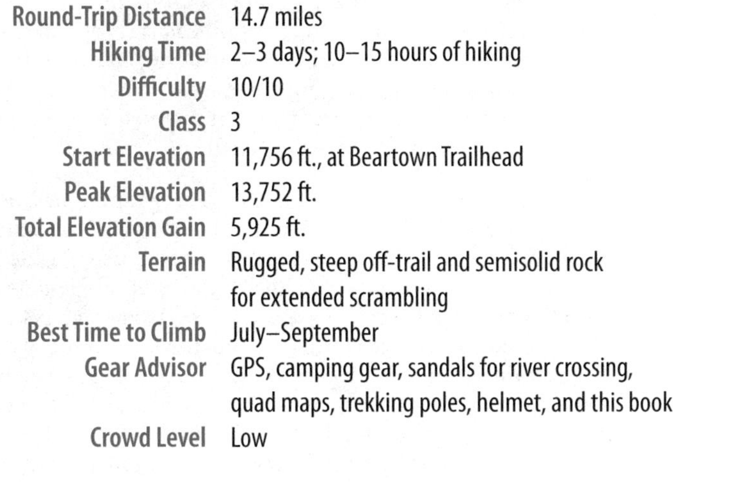

Round-Trip Distance	14.7 miles
Hiking Time	2–3 days; 10–15 hours of hiking
Difficulty	10/10
Class	3
Start Elevation	11,756 ft., at Beartown Trailhead
Peak Elevation	13,752 ft.
Total Elevation Gain	5,925 ft.
Terrain	Rugged, steep off-trail and semisolid rock for extended scrambling
Best Time to Climb	July–September
Gear Advisor	GPS, camping gear, sandals for river crossing, quad maps, trekking poles, helmet, and this book
Crowd Level	Low

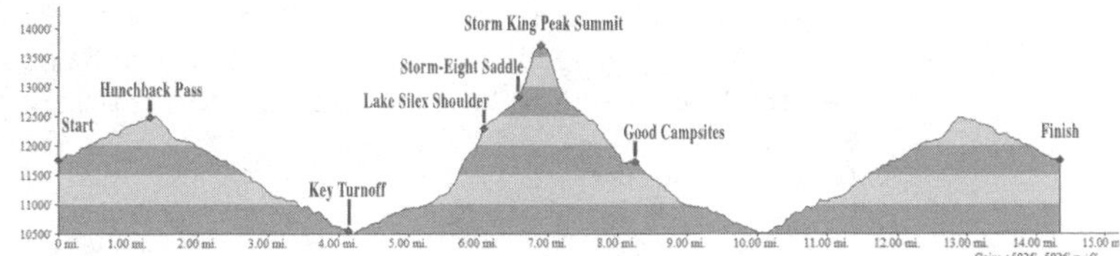

Location Grenadier Range in the Weminuche Wilderness/San Juan National Forest outside of Lake City, Creede, and Silverton

Intro This is the best summit hike that I've done in Colorado. The Grenadier Range is the best-kept secret in the state; I actually feel a little guilty getting the word out. There were several other peaks in the Grenadiers that could have easily made this book; Storm King and the optional trek to Mount Silex are the best of the bunch. The difficulty rating on this hike pertains to the overall experience; just getting to the trailhead is an epic journey. Once you are there, you'll need solid backcountry navigation skills, strong legs, and good scrambling ability. This is a fantastic overnight, though it is possible as a day hike—as a very long day hike (that's how I did it while researching for this book). The Grenadiers feel like nothing else in Colorado—possibly like nowhere else in the world. Come see the secrets waiting for you in the wild, wonderful Weminuche Wilderness.

Why Climb It? Besides the pleasure of seeing an area known to only a few, Storm King's scramble has the perfect balance of challenge, exposure, and scenery. It is similar in feel to the Keyhole route on Longs Peak, except that Storm King is unmarked, so you'll need decent route-finding skills. The ridge up is airy but never exceeds class 3 (not even 3+), and the summit is a truly divine experience. Camping is great, and the optional climb over to Mount Silex is just as fun. I hope that this adventure will intrigue you to visit other great Grenadier climbs: Arrow, Vestal, the Guardian, the Numbers Peaks, Greystone, and so on. You'll have to work hard on this hike; the elevation gain is over 5,000 feet, and that is from a trailhead start of 11,700 feet.

I have not had the time to do this (yet), but the ultimate Colorado backpacking/summit-bagging trip may start here and conclude in nearby Chicago Basin—the two areas are linkable via the Vallecito Creek Trail to Columbine Pass and then out to Needleton Trailhead.

Driving Passenger cars and sport utility cars: Forget about it. Don't even try. The access road to the Beartown Trailhead requires a high-clearance 4x4 with a powerful low gear. There is also a true river crossing, which may be high in the spring. You'll be on rocky, rutted, and steep single-lane 4x4 roads. Sport utility vehicles (SUVs) that are geared toward actual 4x4 use (for example, Nissan Xterras, Dodge Durangos, and Toyota 4Runners) will be able to get up just fine. Hikers with good 4x4 trucks or Jeeps—you're going to thoroughly enjoy the eastern approach. It's what your truck was made for. At the trailhead (which I reached in a Toyota Tacoma) I saw several Tacomas, a few Dodge Rams, a Nissan Xterra, and a Ford Explorer.

If you don't have access to a car, there is a service available out of Silverton that serves to drop off and pick up hikers at the Beartown Trailhead. Rates vary, but if you don't have access to a 4x4, give them a call:

San Juan Backcountry
P.O. Box 707
Silverton, CO 81433
(800) 494-8687
sanjuanbackcountry.com

How to Get There There are two ways to get to Beartown Trailhead/Kite Lake. Both require 4x4 vehicles with good clearance. SUVs are better off when approaching from Silverton. All these roads are rough, so make sure that your tires and brakes are up to the task. Call the ranger station (numbers follow in the "Contact Info" section) to ensure that the roads are open and passable.

From Silverton: Drive northeast out of town on Colorado Highway 110 toward Howardsville. Turn right (southeast) about 5 miles out of town onto County Road 4; this is the road to Stony Pass. From here it is 11.84 miles to the intersection of Forest Service Road 506. Follow the signs to Stony Pass. Turn left onto County Road 3/Forest Service Road 520 and climb up to Stony Pass. Drive down the other side and reach FS 506, the road to Beartown/Kite Lake. Directions from Beartown continue after the following paragraph.

From Lake City/Creede: Take Colorado Highway 149 to Forest Service Road 520 and turn west (toward Rio Grande Reservoir). This is an easy, car-friendly dirt road for about 17 miles. At mile 18.5, you get into real 4x4 terrain. There are several river crossings, deeply rutted sections, and the rock-filled fiasco of Timberhill, a very steep hill strewn with rocks of all sizes. Stay the course for an additional 6.5 miles (making it 25 miles total from the start of FS 520), to the junction of FS 520 and Forest Service Road 506.

Once you've reached FS 506, the road to Beartown goes west 6.5 miles and terminates at Kite Lake. The Beartown Trailhead is at mile 6.0. Immediately, you are forced to cross Bear Creek. In the early spring, this waterway can run high enough to prevent passage. Clear Bear Creek and the road becomes milder, passing through grazing lands.

Eventually, the road goes up some rough and rocky hills; claw your way up and reach the Beartown Trailhead (without ever seeing Beartown) on your left at mile 6.1. There is a sign/kiosk and a trail sign for Trail #787. If you reach Kite Lake (which is worth checking out), you've gone 0.5 mile too far. Kite Lake is the end of the road.

Important Note: Don't expect to actually see Beartown. The few ruins that remain are not visible from the road, and there is little more left than old foundations and rusty nails. For all the signs, you'd think that there would be something to see.

Fees/Camping

There are no fees to hike or camp in the area. There are plenty of places to camp along FS 506 and at the trailhead. Backcountry campers can stay at dozens of places. On Trail #787, once you clear Hunchback Pass and reenter the woods, there are lots of very nice sites next to the creek. The best camping is above Stormy Gulch, which requires a good effort to reach (it's marked on the map). Camping there gives you an easier shot at climbing both Storm King and Silex.

Route Notes

The trail maps on the sign and on topographical maps are pure confusion. In the following route description, I use the trail signs that are given along the way to avoid mixing up the routes. Even rangers were confused about the actual trail designations.

Mile/Waypoint

0.0 mi (1) At the Beartown Trailhead, Trail #787 begins from the lot behind the sign and proceeds south and uphill to Hunchback Pass. The trail is well worn and easy to follow up to the pass.

1.3 mi (2) The top of Hunchback Pass (12,496 feet) gives you amazing overviews of the area. The Guardian stands out from the peaks in the area; if your jaw drops, kindly close it and continue downhill.

Note: Once you are on the south side of the pass, consider this the Vallecito Trail (it will be referred to as such below).

2.6 mi (3) The Nebo Creek Trail intersects on the left. Stay on the Vallecito Trail. Between here and the next waypoint, at 4.1 miles, there are lots of campsites. Yes, you're going to have to make up all this elevation you're losing later.

4.1 mi (4) This is the key to your hike. Once you bottom out at about 10,500 feet, you will need to get off the Vallecito Trail. There will be an open meadow on your right with a faint hiker's trail that goes to the river and the forest beyond. Get off-trail, cross the meadow and make a river crossing at Vallecito Creek. In the spring, this creek can really get moving, so be careful. Use your sandals here.

4.2 mi Once you have crossed the river, you should see a trail leading up to Stormy Gulch. There is a comically small hand-carved sign, but don't expect the trail to be easy to follow. There *is* a trail, but it is faint. Consider this off-trail terrain. Still, do your best to pick up the trail where you can.

5.1 mi (5) At 10,940 feet (approximately) you will have a choice. If you've followed the trail, it goes down to a river crossing that looks as though it leads into weeds. If you are camping or want a longer, less direct ascent of the peak, cross the river here and snoop around for the trail on the other side. At about 11,200 feet, the weeds clear out, and there are lots of good camp possibilities about 200 feet southwest of the creek (see waypoint **10**). The higher you head up, the more level ground there is. You can follow the trail up to a less direct route to reach Storm King; check out the descent on the main route and take the same directions—but in reverse. Also, though camping at Lake Silex looks good on a map, in reality it's not: the entire place is a huge boulder field. Camp lower, in the shelter of trees.

The direct ascent (which is what this route details) stays on the left (south) side of the creek, where there is no real trail.

5.4 mi (6) As you clear tree line, you'll see a very steep grassy slope heading up toward Lake Silex. It's a big push, but you can do it! Work southwest up the slopes. The creek listed on the map may or may not be running when you hike. Note that your goal is not Lake Silex but the boulder field higher and north of the lake. Keep heading right (southwest). **Note:** Storm King is the peak on the right of this slope; Silex is the one directly above and to the left.

6.2 mi Keep going southwest and you'll reach a boulder field below Storm King's southeast ridge. Your goal is to climb the southwest ridge, so skirt the peak and head west to Storm-Eight Saddle. When you are closing in on the saddle, it is easier to stay low and reach the low point in the saddle instead of trying to intercept the southwest ridge higher up. The footing below Storm King's south face is off-camber, loose, and cruddy. The choice is yours, but I found it quicker to stay lower and reach the saddle on better footing.

6.7 mi (7) Finally, you're at Storm-Eight Saddle (between Storm King and Peak Eight). You are within striking distance of the summit. The southwest ridge is pure, unfettered scrambling on good rock. It's all class 3, and you can stay fairly close to the spine most of the way up; staying on the left (west) side offers safer options if the ridge gets too airy. Those with good route-finding skills will blaze up this rock like a jungle gym, linking together fun scrambling sections and indulging in the thrill of the climb. Once up high, a fitting catwalk goes northwest like a red carpet to the summit of this awesome mountain.

7.07 mi (8) You are among royalty: Storm King's summit! Enjoy! On the descent, you will return to the saddle (waypoint **7**) and to the shoulder of boulder (Point Silex) above Lake Silex and take a slightly different route back.

8.0 mi (9) At the trail split, go northwest on a trail that stays below the east side of Storm King's northeast ridge. There is an actual path that goes near the lower Trinity Lakes and then follows a trail to waypoint **5** at the top of Stormy Gulch. If it's faded, just work down to Trinity Creek, and follow it to the top of the gulch.

8.3 mi The trail cuts through a big notch—more like a gash—and goes into tree line.

8.5 mi (10) This is the camping waypoint. To get back to your vehicle, follow the creek (or the faint trail) back to the top of Stormy Gulch. Again, if you have GPS, retracing your tracks is a lot easier.

10.3 mi (4) It's a bittersweet moment when you cross over the creek and return to the Vallecito Trail; not just because the fun is over, but also because you now have to hike uphill another 2,000 feet to Hunchback Pass (waypoint **2**). Oy! Hey, if you're lucky, you'll be on Hunchback Pass just in time to see a beautiful sunset. Continue on over the pass to your car.

14.7 mi Finish.

Options There is so much to do here. Mount Silex (13,628 feet) is just one option. From above Lake Silex, go to the saddle between Silex and the northeast shoulder of Peak 9. Once on the southwest ridge, stay about 200 feet below the top for a class 3 scramble to Mount Silex summit, similar to the one on Storm King. Bolder scramblers can stay on the ridge proper, which is a class 4 route. This route is 0.9 mile one way from Point Silex (between waypoints **7** and **9** on the mapped route).

The other peaks in the area are similar scrambles waiting to be discovered. Get out there, have fun, and be safe. One route that looks fun on the map (though I haven't done it personally) is the traverse from Mount Silex's south side to the Guardian. Rock climbers take note: the quartzite rock here has several classic multi-pitch routes, some up to 1,500 feet.

Quick Facts Storm King is one of four peaks in the state with this same name; this one is the highest (and the best!). *Silex* is the Latin word for "silicon." The Grenadiers are one of the few ranges in Colorado not explored by the Hayden or Wheeler surveys. Two climbers (William S. Cooper and John Hubbard) ventured into the area in 1908 and made many first ascents in the region.

With all the signs and its name still on the map, you'd think that Beartown would be a bigger deal. It was founded in 1893 and brought more than 400 prospectors to the area. The Sylvanite Mine yielded a great deal of ore and was worked well into the 20th century. However, today, even the ruins are hard to find, making Beartown a true ghost town.

Contact Info San Juan National Forest
Columbine West Ranger District
110 W. 11th Street
Durango, CO 81301
(970) 884-2512

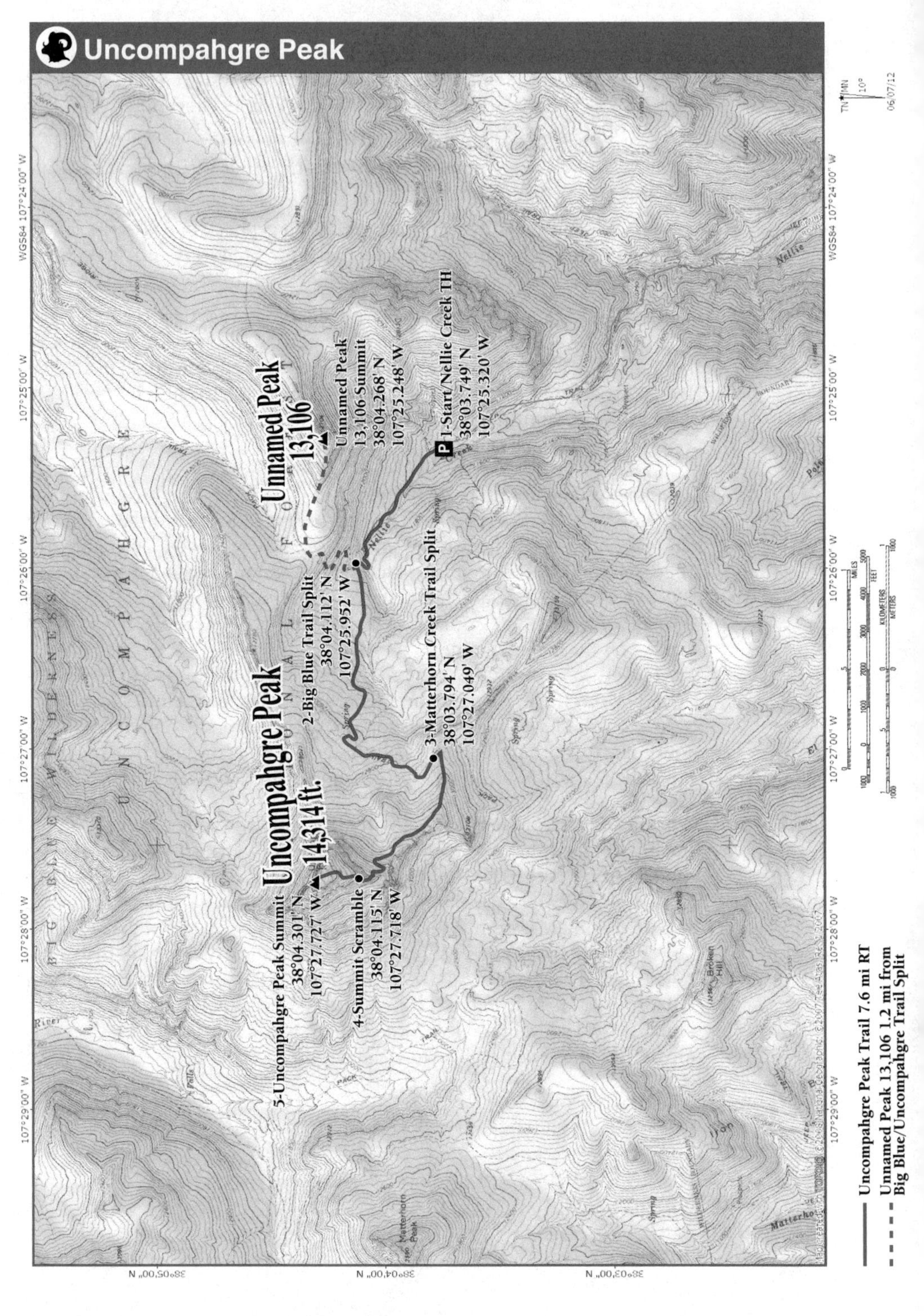
Uncompahgre Peak
Uncompahgre Peak
14,314 ft.
Unnamed Peak
13,106
5-Uncompahgre Peak Summit
38°04.301' N
107°27.727' W
4-Summit Scramble
38°04.115' N
107°27.718' W
3-Matterhorn Creek Trail Split
38°03.794' N
107°27.049' W
2-Big Blue Trail Split
38°04.112' N
107°25.952' W
Unnamed Peak
13,106 Summit
38°04.268' N
107°25.248' W
1-Start/Nellie Creek TH
38°03.749' N
107°25.320' W
BIG BLUE WILDERNESS
UNCOMPAHGRE
NATIONAL FOREST
Uncompahgre Peak Trail 7.6 mi RT
Unnamed Peak 13,106 1.2 mi from Big Blue/Uncompahgre Trail Split

46 Uncompahgre Peak

Colorado's sixth-highest mountain dominates the open plains of the San Juans, rising from the land like the bow of a sinking ship. Most of this scenic hike is above tree line.

Round-Trip Distance	7.6 miles
Hiking Time	4½–6 hours
Difficulty	5/10
Class	2
Start Elevation	11,410 ft., at Nellie Creek Trailhead
Peak Elevation	14,314 ft.
Total Elevation Gain	2,911 ft.
Terrain	Good trail with some easy scrambling toward the summit
Best Time to Climb	June–September
Gear Advisor	Normal gear
Crowd Level	Low due to tough access road

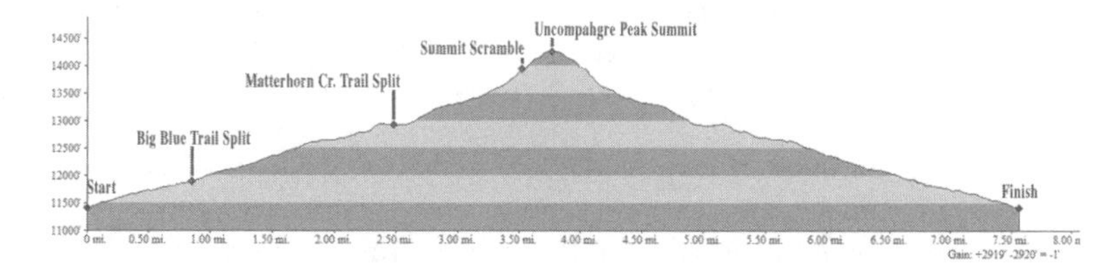

Location San Juan Range in the Uncompahgre Wilderness/Uncompahgre National Forest near Lake City

Intro The name alone is enough to inspire curiosity. Uncompahgre Peak is the highest mountain in the San Juan Range in southwest Colorado. The San Juans receive more precipitation than central and southern ranges, tinting the tundra with flora of green, yellow, red, and blue. There is something that draws you into Uncompahgre; perhaps it is the colorful burst of life that contradicts the apocryphal notion of mountains as barren, grim places. On clear-blue-sky days, the vivid hues and spacious views embody the refreshing rewards of being in the mountains.

Why Climb It? The colors, the views, and Uncompahgre's distinct wedding cake shape will elevate your senses and psych you up to climb this peak. Most of this trek is above tree line on gentle, rolling alpine tundra. You'll be in spacious, wide-open land the entire hike. The trail is well maintained and easy to follow. After a long, gradual ascent, there are a few moderate switchbacks and a brief, easy scramble to the flat and accommodating summit. It's not a very long or difficult hike, but every foot of the trail will enliven your senses with incredible views and fresh mountain air.

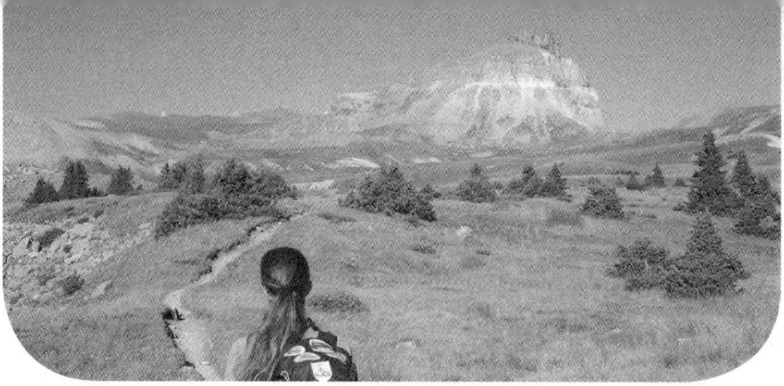

Uncompahgre's famous sinking ship profile

Driving You'll need a high-clearance SUV or 4x4 to get up the tough Nellie Creek Road. Sport utility cars with good clearance and a strong low gear have a shot at making the whole road (I saw a Honda CRV at the trailhead when I was there). The road is steep with very sharp turns; it has some rocky sections and some major ruts. There are two stream crossings as well. If you have a car, you'll have to park at the base of the Nellie Creek Road and hoof it—making this a 16-mile hike with more than 5,000 feet of elevation. The road and trail are easy to hike, so if you have the time and endurance (especially during a monotonous walk up/down the 4x4 road), give it a shot.

How to Get There From County Road 149 in Lake City, follow the signs for Engineer Pass. Turn west off CR 149 onto Second Street. Drive a short 0.1 mile, and you'll begin the road up Engineer Pass (also known as Alpine Loop Scenic Byway/ Henson Road/20 Road). Drive 5.0 miles up this well-maintained dirt road to Nellie Creek Road, passable by all vehicles. Keep an eye out on the left (south) side of the road for an old, amazing abandoned mine operation built into the canyon (there are a few informative plaques to learn about the area). This is a good place to stop on your way home.

At mile 5.0, you'll reach the intersection for the Nellie Creek Road (#877) on your right. Cars and low-clearance sport utility cars will have to stop here and walk up. Nellie Creek Road is 4.0 miles and ends at the Nellie Creek Trailhead and wilderness boundary. This road is rugged, steep, rocky, rutted, and tight. At mile 2.3, there is a junction on a turn. Stay left on the main road here. Cross two streams, muscle your vehicle up the road, and at mile 3.7, you'll come to a flat section ideal for camping. The trailhead is just beyond at mile 4.0; it has ample parking, a restroom, and a small sign kiosk.

Fees/Camping There are no fees to hike Uncompahgre Peak. There are no fees to camp at the unimproved sites along the access road or in this area of the San Juan Mountains.

Route Notes None.

Mile/Waypoint

0.0 mi (1) Start at Nellie Creek Trailhead. Get on the well-marked, well-worn Uncompahgre Peak Trail. Note that the large, impressive mountain to your right (north) is Unnamed Peak 13,106, an optional summit.

0.8 mi (2) As you come up a small hill, a field of green opens up with Uncompahgre's imperial shape finally coming into view. There is an intersection for the Big Blue Trail here; stay left on the Uncompahgre Peak Trail. Continue over the tundra on trail.

2.5 mi (3) After climbing another short hill, you'll intersect with the Matterhorn Creek Trail at 12,920 feet. Stay right on the Uncompahgre Peak Trail. This semi-flat ridge has great views of rock formations to the left and San Juan vistas to the right.

3.2 mi At 13,460 feet, begin a brief, steep section of dusty switchbacks.

3.6 mi (4) Atop the switchbacks, at 13,930 feet, the trail splits into several worn paths (all of them with cairns). My preferred route is to bear right (which is more straight than right) and make the class 2+ scramble up. If you go left, you'll be fine—it's a similar trail that goes onto the west face of the mountain and scrambles up.

3.8 mi (5) Uncompahgre's broad summit. There are several summit markers on the summit. The highest point will be obvious. Return the way you came.

7.6 mi Finish.

Options The wide-open, rolling terrain makes hiking and scrambling to the unnamed hills around Uncompahgre a fun diversion. There are a few 14ers and high 13ers in the area, notably 14,017-foot Wetterhorn Peak to the northwest, not on the map. For those looking for a burly challenge, try linking Uncompahgre and Wetterhorn by splitting off the Matterhorn Creek Trail at waypoint **3** after climbing Uncompahgre. (Or camp down in the basin northeast of the Wetterhorn/Matterhorn ridge, and bag the peak the next day.)

A more modest peak to grab is Unnamed Peak 13,106 (which is looming to the northwest from the Nellie Creek Trailhead parking area). Turn right (at waypoint **2**) onto the Big Blue Trail for 0.5 mile, and then get off-trail and scramble up the class 2 ridge to the top. This is 1.2 miles one way from the intersection of the Big Blue and the Uncompahgre Peak Trails.

Quick Facts Unlike many other names in the San Juans, Uncompahgre is not Spanish in origin. Rather, the word comes from the native Ute people, who used the term Ancapagari (translated: "red lake" or "red water") to describe a reddish hot spring near the mountain. The name was first applied to the Uncompahgre River; the mountain was named shortly thereafter. Despite some resistance, the native title stuck, albeit with a European phonetic twist.

Contact Info Uncompahgre National Forest
Gunnison Ranger District
P.O. Box 89
Lake City, CO 81230
(970) 641-0471

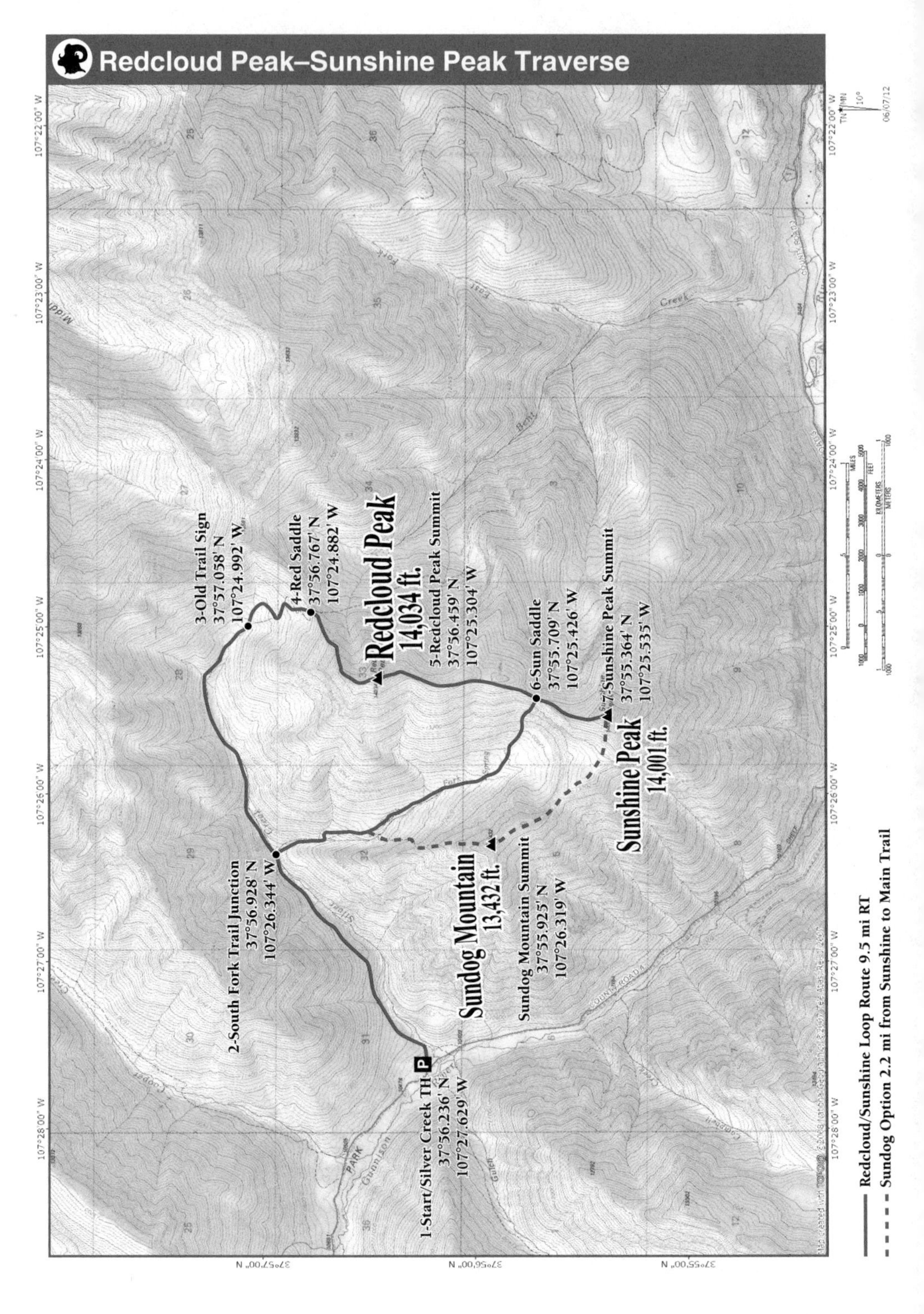

Redcloud Peak–Sunshine Peak Traverse
1-Start/Silver Creek TH
37°56.236' N
107°27.629' W
2-South Fork Trail Junction
37°56.928' N
107°26.344' W
3-Old Trail Sign
37°57.058' N
107°24.992' W
4-Red Saddle
37°56.767' N
107°24.882' W
Redcloud Peak
14,034 ft.
5-Redcloud Peak Summit
37°56.459' N
107°25.304' W
6-Sun Saddle
37°55.709' N
107°25.426' W
7-Sunshine Peak Summit
37°55.364' N
107°25.535' W
Sunshine Peak
14,001 ft.
Sundog Mountain
13,432 ft.
Sundog Mountain Summit
37°55.925' N
107°26.319' W
Redcloud/Sunshine Loop Route 9.5 mi RT
Sundog Option 2.2 mi from Sunshine to Main Trail

47 Redcloud Peak–Sunshine Peak Traverse

How can you go wrong with mountains that are red and sunny? Green San Juan meadows and rusty crimson rocks give a burst of color to this beautiful landscape.

Round-Trip Distance	9.5 miles
Hiking Time	5–7 hours
Difficulty	5/10
Class	2
Start Elevation	10,438 ft., at Silver Creek/Grizzly Gulch Trailhead
Peak Elevations	Redcloud Peak: 14,034 ft.; Sunshine Peak: 14,001 ft.
Total Elevation Gain	4,100 ft.
Terrain	Good trail to summits; rocky descent on medium talus
Best Time to Climb	June–September
Gear Advisor	Normal gear; trekking poles if doing the loop descent
Crowd Level	Low

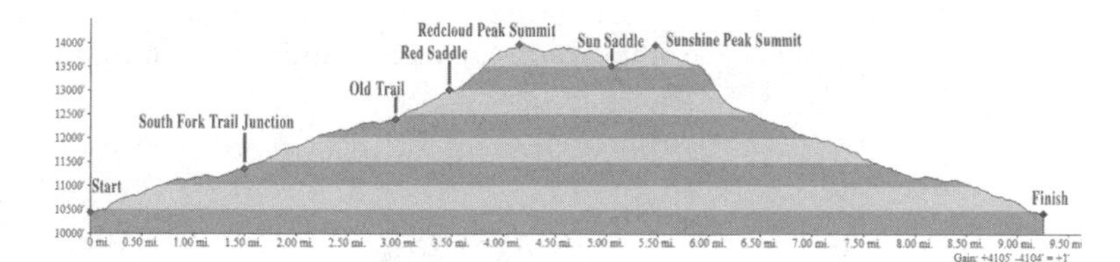

Location San Juan Range in the Uncompahgre Wilderness/Bureau of Land Management lands west of Lake City

Intro The San Juan Mountains owe most of their color to the precipitation that targets southwest Colorado. The increased flora is especially scenic when paired with natural red rocks that compose the upper reaches of these two peaks. Taken as a pair, they are very welcoming summits, reached by a well-maintained, nontechnical trail. Sunshine Peak is the lowest of the 14ers, clearing the height requirement with just a foot to spare!

Why Climb It? The colorful palette of the San Juans is on display, so bring your camera. Even the clear waters of Silver Creek contribute, illuminating the gray and white rocks of the streambed with flashes of silver when the sun shines. All the natural beauty is easy on the eyes (and the knees, thanks to a well-made trail). The loop described includes a shortcut down rocky talus that eliminates the need to reverse your route. If you are hesitant to plod down a loose, rocky slope, it's easy enough to go back the way you came. No matter how you visit these two 14ers, it's a trip well worth taking.

Driving Tough passenger cars can make it to the trailhead in normal conditions. The road is rough in places, and the shelf-road section is exciting. I was able to make it to this trailhead with my Honda Accord, but I had a few minor scrapes on the way up.

How to Get There From Lake City (which is roughly 50 miles south of Gunnison), find the intersection of Colorado Highway 149 and Hinsdale County Road 30. There will be a large sign for the Alpine Loop and Cinnamon Pass. Turn onto CR 30, which is a paved road at this point. It is 16.6 miles from here to the trailhead. Pass the beautiful Lake San Cristobel, staying on CR 30. Stay right at the southern terminus of the lake (or else you'll just loop around the east shore). CR 30 is paved for 4.2 miles and then becomes a well-maintained dirt road that passes Williams Creek and Mill Creek Campgrounds. At mile 12.4, you'll come to a fork in the road; go right to start the more rugged part of your drive up to Cinnamon Pass Road (County Road 4). (Note that going left here takes you to the ghost town of Sherman.)

You'll climb on a shelf road that is washed out in places but passable by a carefully driven car. Continue along this road for 4.0 miles to the trailhead (look for mile marker 16; the trailhead is 0.6 mile after it). There are some campsites and a toilet on the left-hand side; your trailhead starts from the right-hand (northeast) lot.

Fees/Camping There are no fees for hiking or camping in this area; many parties camp at or just outside of the trailhead. Please minimize your impact.

Closing in on the summit of Redcloud

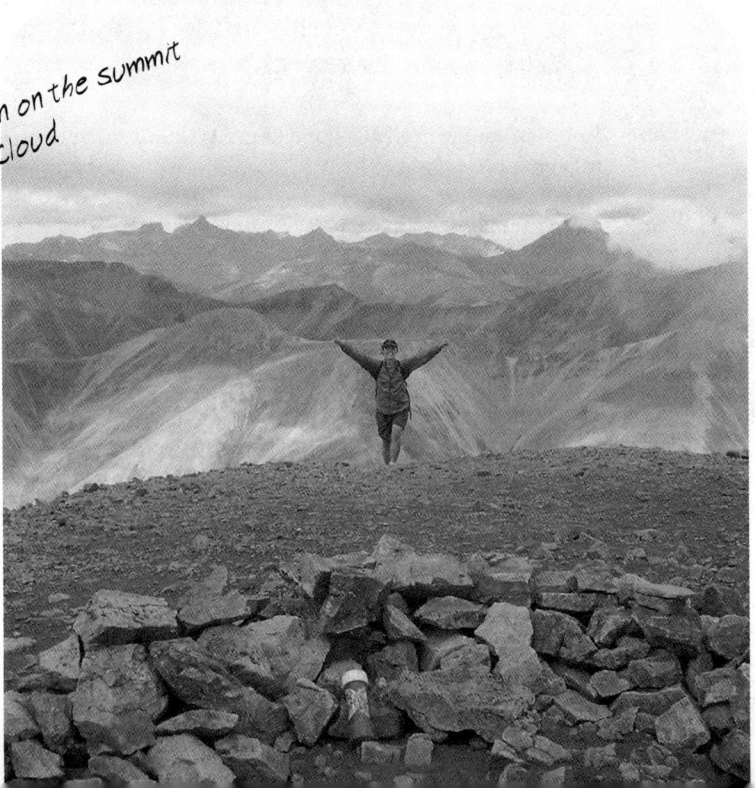

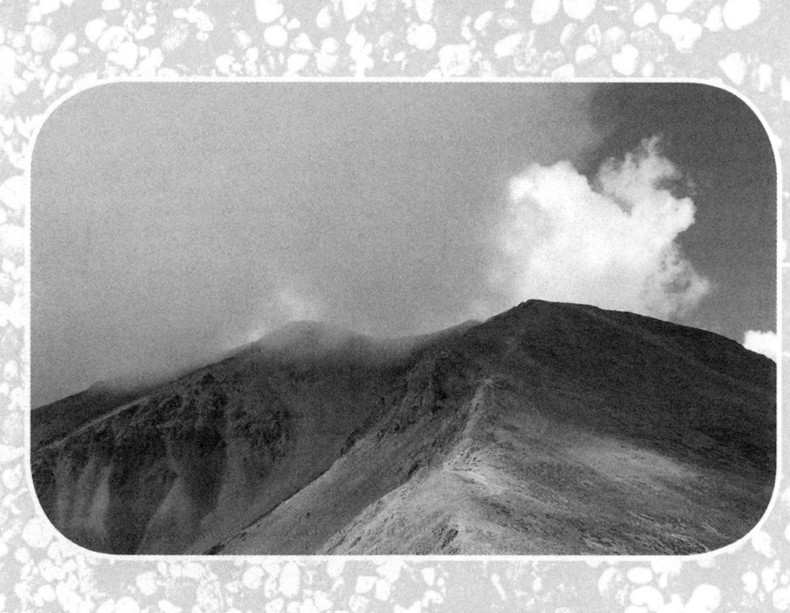

Redcloud Peak surrounded by white clouds

Route Notes None.

Mile/Waypoint

0.0 mi (1) Start at the Silver Creek Trailhead. Go east on the two-lane trail that heads uphill into the woods. You'll soon parallel Silver Creek; for the ascent, stay on the left (north) side of the creek on the obvious trail.

1.5 mi (2) You'll now be hiking next to Silver Creek. This is where you will exit South Fork Basin on your descent. There is a hard-to-see cairn designating the faint trail to the right (south-southeast) that you will be following on the way back. Note, however, that this is a poor ascent route and should be avoided for the time being. Stay on the main trail as it cuts northeast. When you get into the high part of the basin, doesn't it seem like something is missing? Unlike most mountain basins, this one has no lakes or ponds.

3.0 mi (3) As you begin to climb to Red Saddle, you'll see a sign politely asking you to use the switchbacked trail instead of the older, more direct trail. Help lessen erosion by going on the switchbacks.

3.5 mi (4) On top of Red Saddle (13,000 feet) you have a 1,000-foot climb to reach the top of Redcloud. The mountain looks every bit a 14er, looming to the southeast in all its crimson glory. You have two options here: attack the ridge directly by staying on the steep, rocky spine trail, or go out onto the northeast face and take the switchbacks up. Both trails go to the top and merge at a level section just before the final summit push.

4.2 mi (5) Redcloud Peak's very red summit is beneath your boots. The trail that traverses to Sunshine is easy to follow. Head south to the Sun Saddle en route to Sunshine Peak.

5.2 mi (6) The low point of the traverse is Sun Saddle, at 13,500 feet. The switchbacks that climb to the summit are easier than they look. The trail is still evident and easy to follow.

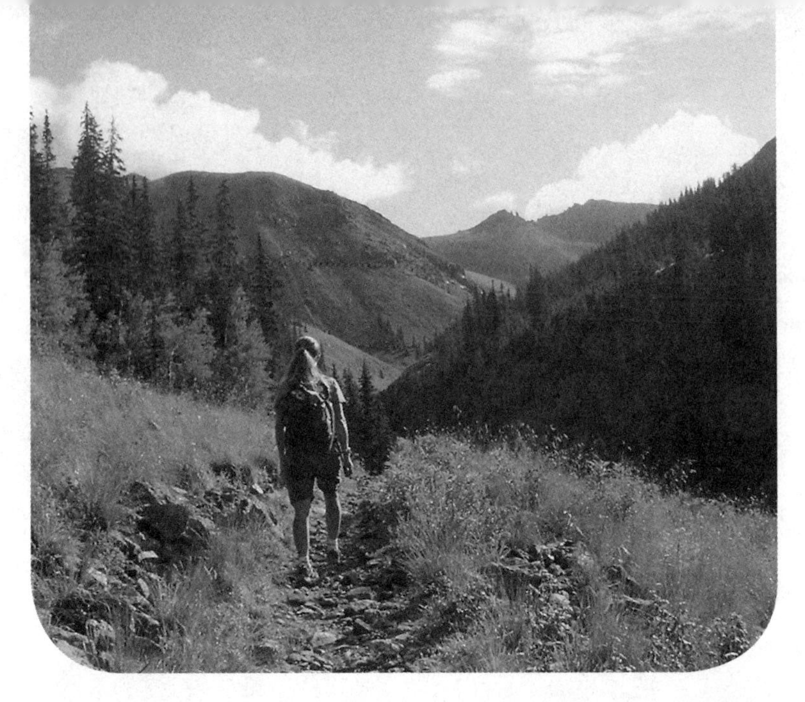

The San Juan mountains are known for their lovely approach trails.

5.6 mi (7) Sunshine Peak's flat summit has a nice wind shelter and great views. Don't rest too long if you want to try the Sundog Mountain option to the northwest. If you are following the standard route, return to Sun Saddle.

6.0 mi (6) A trail to the left (northwest) descends the scree into South Fork Basin. A sign warns that this trail is dangerous. The terrain is not difficult (though it is a little annoying)—the danger is more from rocks that may get kicked down on you by other hikers. If you are in a group, stay close together so rocks don't have time to gain momentum. If others are on the trail below you, wait until they are out of the fall line before you continue down.

Once you get down the steepest section, a cairned trail through the talus leads you to the South Fork Creek. A spring supplies much of the creek's water, which seems to magically flow from the Earth; it's a curious sight. Stay close to the creek as you hike out to the north. The trail fades in and out; you'll know that you are out of the basin when you cross Silver Creek and the well-worn access trail reappears. (This is the trail that you avoided on the way up.)

8.0 mi (2) Return to the main trail (Silver Creek Trail) and follow it out to the trailhead.

9.5 mi Finish.

Options The Sundog Loop is a popular alternative for those who don't want to fumble down scree nor return via Redcloud. Follow the northwest ridge of Sunshine (class 2) for 1.0 mile to the 13,432-foot summit of Sundog Mountain. This is the 299th-highest peak in the state. To descend, take the northeast ridge down. Before you get into tree line, go north toward South Fork Creek. Cross the stream (possibly gaining the South Fork Trail, if it's visible), and rejoin the main trail at waypoint **2**. It is 2.2 miles from Sunshine's summit to the main trail if you take this option.

Quick Facts

Sunshine Peak's elevation has been accurately measured several times, and with each survey, it remains in the elite 14ers club. Sunshine Peak was named by the U.S. Geological Survey in 1904; before then it was known variously as Niagara Peak or Sherman Peak. Redcloud was named in 1874 by the Hayden survey, whose members thought that the red rocks resembled scarlet clouds from a distance.

There are two Sunshine mountains in Colorado. The other is located just outside of Telluride; despite standing only 12,930 feet, it is a very visually impressive peak that is often mistaken for a 14er.

Contact Info

Bureau of Land Management
Gunnison Office
216 N. Colorado Street
Gunnison, CO 81230
(970) 641-0471

Bureau of Land Management
Lake City Office
(970) 944-2344

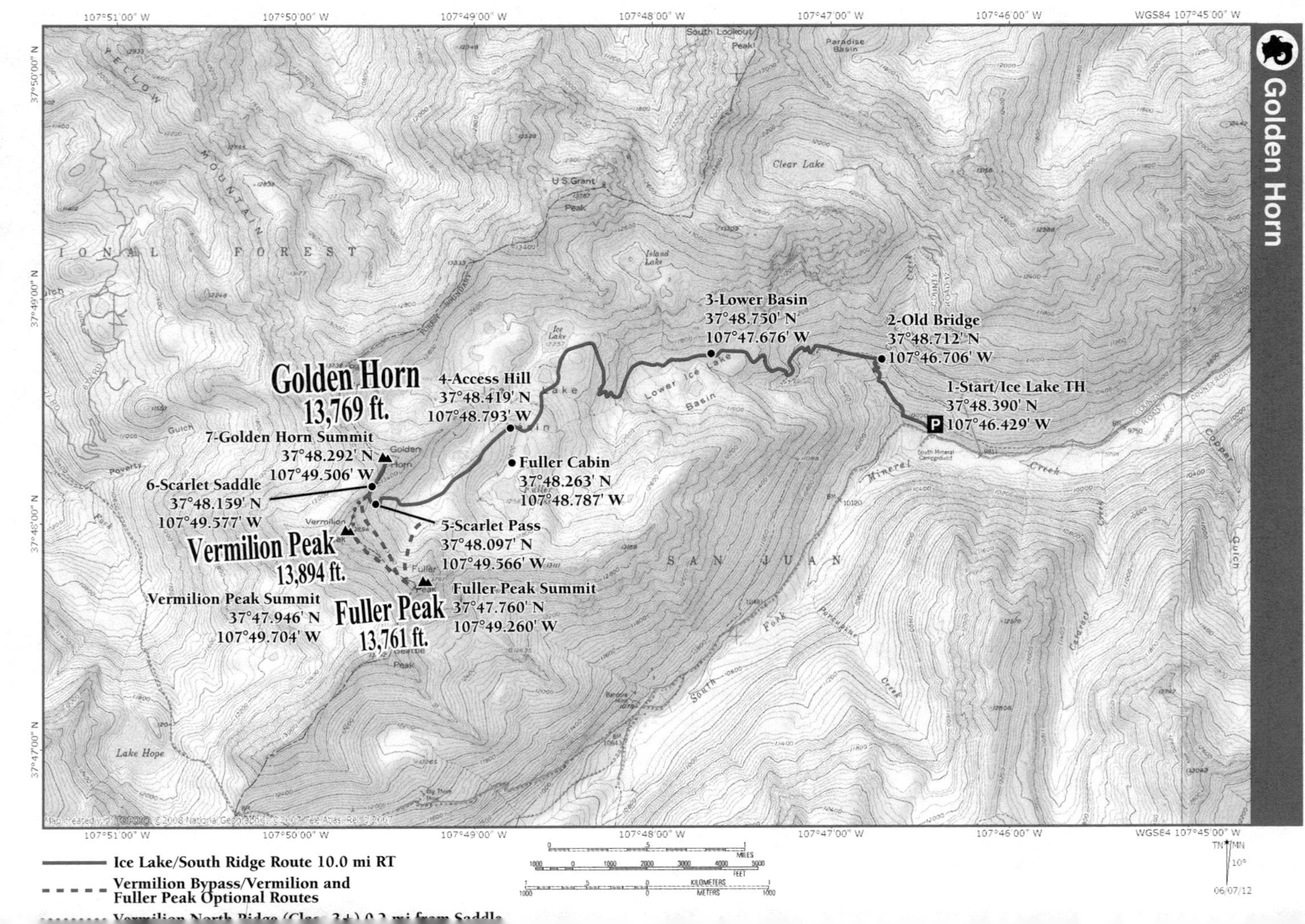
Golden Horn
Golden Horn
13,769 ft.
4-Access Hill
37°48.419' N
107°48.793' W
3-Lower Basin
37°48.750' N
107°47.676' W
2-Old Bridge
37°48.712' N
107°46.706' W
1-Start/Ice Lake TH
37°48.390' N
107°46.429' W
7-Golden Horn Summit
37°48.292' N
107°49.506' W
Fuller Cabin
37°48.263' N
107°48.787' W
6-Scarlet Saddle
37°48.159' N
107°49.577' W
5-Scarlet Pass
37°48.097' N
107°49.566' W
Vermilion Peak
13,894 ft.
Fuller Peak Summit
37°47.760' N
107°49.260' W
Vermilion Peak Summit
37°47.946' N
107°49.704' W
Fuller Peak
13,761 ft.
Clear Lake
Island Lake
Ice Lake
Lower Ice Lake Basin
U.S. Grant Peak
South Lookout Peak
Paradise Basin
Lake Hope
S A N J U A N
Mineral Creek
Copper Gulch
Ice Lake/South Ridge Route 10.0 mi RT
Vermilion Bypass/Vermilion and Fuller Peak Optional Routes

48 Golden Horn

Answer the call for adventure by scaling the best horn in Colorado. Ice Lake Basin is your gateway to this finely crafted mountain, whose profile dominates the western skyline.

Round-Trip Distance	10.0 miles
Hiking Time	6–8 hours
Difficulty	8/10
Class	2+/optional class 3 moves on summit
Start Elevation	9,840 ft., at Ice Lake Trailhead
Peak Elevation	13,769 ft.
Total Elevation Gain	3,890 ft.
Terrain	Good trail to rocky basin; loose but fun scramble to summit
Best Time to Climb	July–September
Gear Advisor	Normal gear
Crowd Level	Low

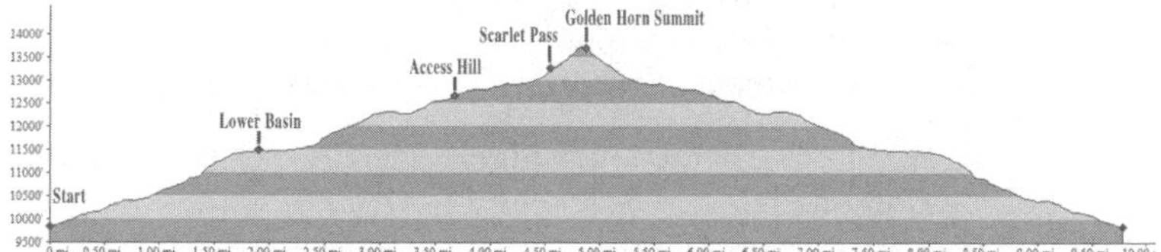

Location San Juan Mountains in the Weminuche Wilderness/San Juan National Forest outside of Silverton

Intro Ice Lake Basin (and the approach to reach it) is a feast for your senses. Dazzling waterfalls thunder down sheer cliffs, and colossal mountains partition the beauty into distinct compartments. At the center of it all is Golden Horn, rising like a rusty Gothic castle. Your camera will be working overtime as you make your way up to the summit. Views from the top look out into the Lizard Head Wilderness and the Grenadier Range, as well as at several other San Juan beauties.

Why Climb It? Golden Horn looks like a miniature version of Uncompahgre Peak, but the climbing is much different. As you can tell by its crumbly appearance, rock in this area is constantly being shed from the shattered peaks. Despite the ruinous appearance, the route to Golden Horn is on mostly solid rock. The only loose slope is found on a short scree section just below the summit. Once you get to the top, there are several places where fun scrambling offers new vantage points of the area. Bring a friend along and take photos of one another on opposing summit blocks.

Driving Mineral Creek Road (Forest Service Road 585) is a very well-maintained dirt road and is passable by all vehicles under normal conditions.

How to Get There From Silverton at the junction of Colorado Highway 110 and US Highway 550, drive 2.0 miles south on US 550 and turn right onto Mineral Creek Road (Forest Service Road 585). If you are approaching from the south, this turn is 7.8 miles from the summit of Red Mountain Pass. There is a sign for Mineral Creek. Once on this dirt road, follow it 4.0 miles west to the South Mineral Campground. Do not take any side roads that disappear into the woods. The Ice Lake Trailhead has lots of parking and is directly across the road from the campground on the right (north) side of FS 585.

Fees/Camping There are no fees to hike or camp in the wilderness area. Camping at South Mineral Creek Campground is $14 per night; the 26 sites fill up quickly on weekends. There are several pull-offs that offer free camping on FS 585, but good luck beating the hoards of RVs to a good spot. Lower Ice Lakes Basin is the best place to set up camp if you prefer a backcountry alternative.

Route Notes None.

Mile/Waypoint **0.0 mi (1)** Start at the Ice Lake Trailhead and get on the Ice Lake Trail. This is a well-traveled path that is easy to follow. Enjoy the experience as the secrets of the Ice Lake Basins unfold before you. Stay on the path that switchbacks near the waterfall. Don't take any of the faint shortcuts. There is an easy river crossing along the way. At the top of the switchbacks, you'll see a dilapidated bridge spanning the waterfall. It looks like something out of *Indiana Jones!* Luckily, you don't have to cross it.

0.7 mi (2) At the old bridge, go left (west) and continue on-trail to the lower basin.

2.0 mi (3) The spacious Lower Ice Lake Basin is amazing. If you want to camp in the area, this is the place to do it (though in midsummer, the bugs are fierce). Higher up, things are very exposed. Stay on-trail as you gaze at several waterfalls—many cut into notches in the cliffs that section off this area from the upper basin. Carry on toward Ice Lake and the upper basin.

3.1 mi Ice Lake is before you when you get to the top level of the upper basin. The trail fades out in this area. Continue south to the hill west of Fuller Lake (at a large boulder, a faint, cairned trail is to the right—this is the path of least resistance).

3.7 mi (4) You're on the hill, and you can now see Scarlet Pass. If you want to align yourself a little better, continue to hike south until Fuller Lake and the Fuller Cabin are in sight. Go right (west) from these landmarks to gain the little ridge at 12,900 feet. Once you are on the ridge, drop down into a flat "talus lake" that borders Scarlet Pass. There is a tiny lake and some old wood planks down to your right—go past these to the flat part of the talus field. Traverse this patch of rocks, checking out some of the unique boulders and old mining debris. Scarlet Pass between Vermilion Peak and Golden Horn looks tricky, but it reveals its lines when you actually get there.

4.6 mi (5) Scarlet Pass. This hill to the saddle is much shorter than it looks from a distance. The base is at 13,250 feet. As you look at it, there are a lot of run-out routes on the right (north) side. Ignore these and head to the left (south), where a series of ledges makes travel to the saddle a class 2+ walk. A good place to find your starting point is close to where the gray rocks of Vermilion merge with the reddish stone of Scarlet Pass. A few old cairns are along the way, but you shouldn't need them.

4.7 mi (6) Scarlet Saddle, the high saddle at 13,560 feet, opens up western views. Your remaining scramble follows this south ridge to the summit. You may want to ditch your trekking poles here. The scramble up is loose in places, a little more solid and exposed as you stay toward the left side. If the climbing is getting too difficult, stay right on the sandy slopes and angle up. Eventually you'll reach a notch that splits the two tops of Golden Horn. Go left to make the easier scramble to an airy summit block for the true apex.

5.0 mi (7) Golden Horn's summit! What views! This, the west summit, has a register. You can scramble around up here as you see fit. However, if you want to visit the east summit as well, there is a wiggle notch that you'll have to jam yourself into and then squirm up and through (a class 3 move) to get there. These two summits are the two photograph points that I mention in the "Why Climb It?" section.

Return the way you came. The descent back to the talus field is fast. On the way down, you may want to detour over to Fuller Lake and the old Fuller Cabin. This is a good place to take shelter if storms move in before you can make it to timberline.

10.0 mi Finish.

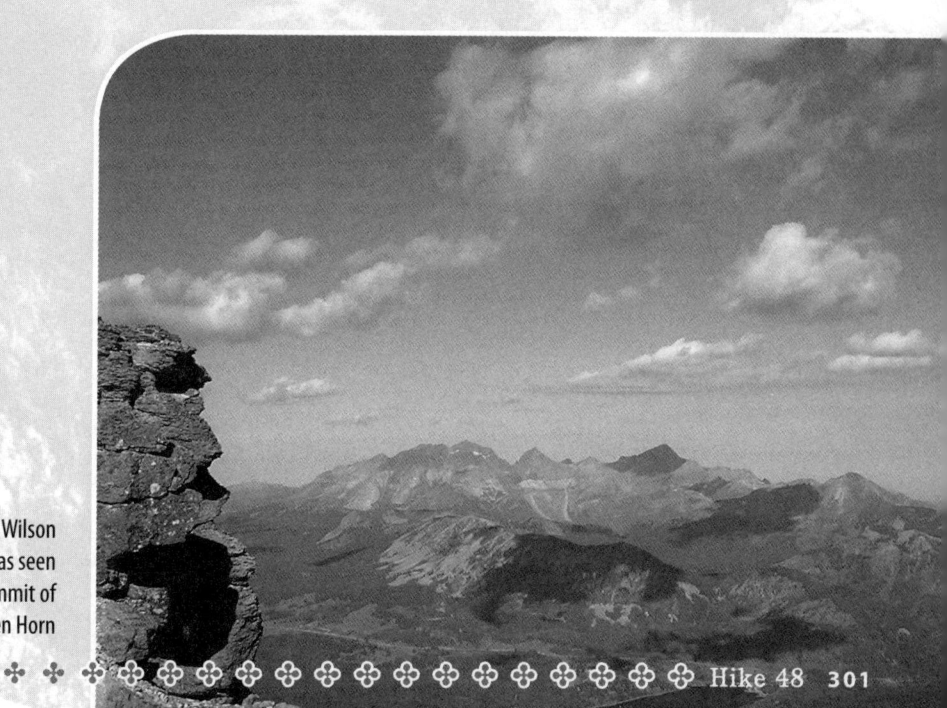

The impressive Wilson group of 14ers as seen from the summit of Golden Horn

Options From Scarlet Pass (waypoint **5**), it's a mere 0.23 mile to Vermilion Peak, but the ridge is a class 3+/4 adventure with some very exposed moves on rotten rock. A lower route on sandy slopes leading to a steep, loose gully is less exposed but still difficult. Either way, the easiest way to get atop this 13,894-foot peak is to follow the sandy notch on the east face to the summit. This traverse is tougher than it may seem, and I only include it for more experienced scramblers. From Vermilion, it's a class 2+ trek of 0.5 mile over to the shapely cone of Fuller Peak (13,761 feet). Descend via the slope between Vermilion and Fuller for a 1.6-mile loop from Scarlet Pass to the small ridge and waypoint **4**.

If you'd rather not go for the scramble on the north ridge of Vermilion but want to bag these two peaks, you can traverse a shelf on the east face of Vermilion Peak, at 13,400 feet, to the saddle between Fuller and Vermilion. Taking the southeast ridge up to Vermilion is much easier than the higher north ridge traverse.

Quick Facts Vermilion Peak is the highest point in San Juan County. The Ice Lake Basins hold their snow into the summer, which is why I'd suggest waiting until July to try the peaks. The slopes are prime avalanche terrain. Even in July, bringing an ice ax may not be a bad idea. The cabin by Fuller Lake used to host winter trips, but it has fallen into disrepair in recent years.

Pilot Knob and other peaks in this area are technical ascents that require ropes and belays.

Contact Info San Juan National Forest
San Juan Public Lands Center
15 Burnett Court
Durango, CO 81301
(970) 247-4874

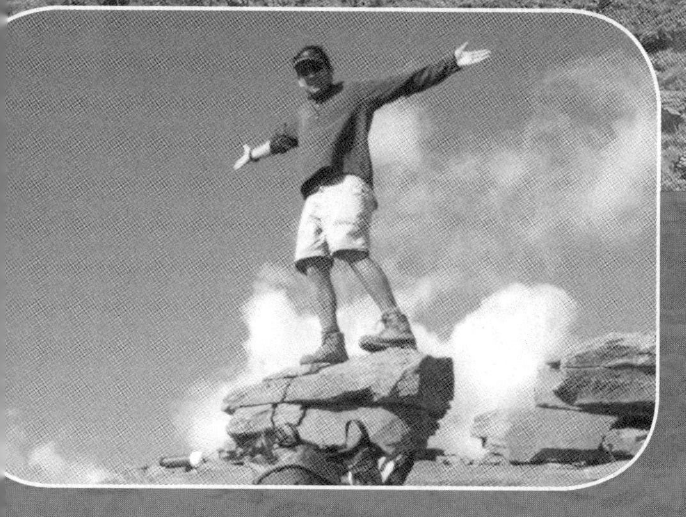

The Ice Lakes Basin is one of my favorite backcountry areas in Colorado.

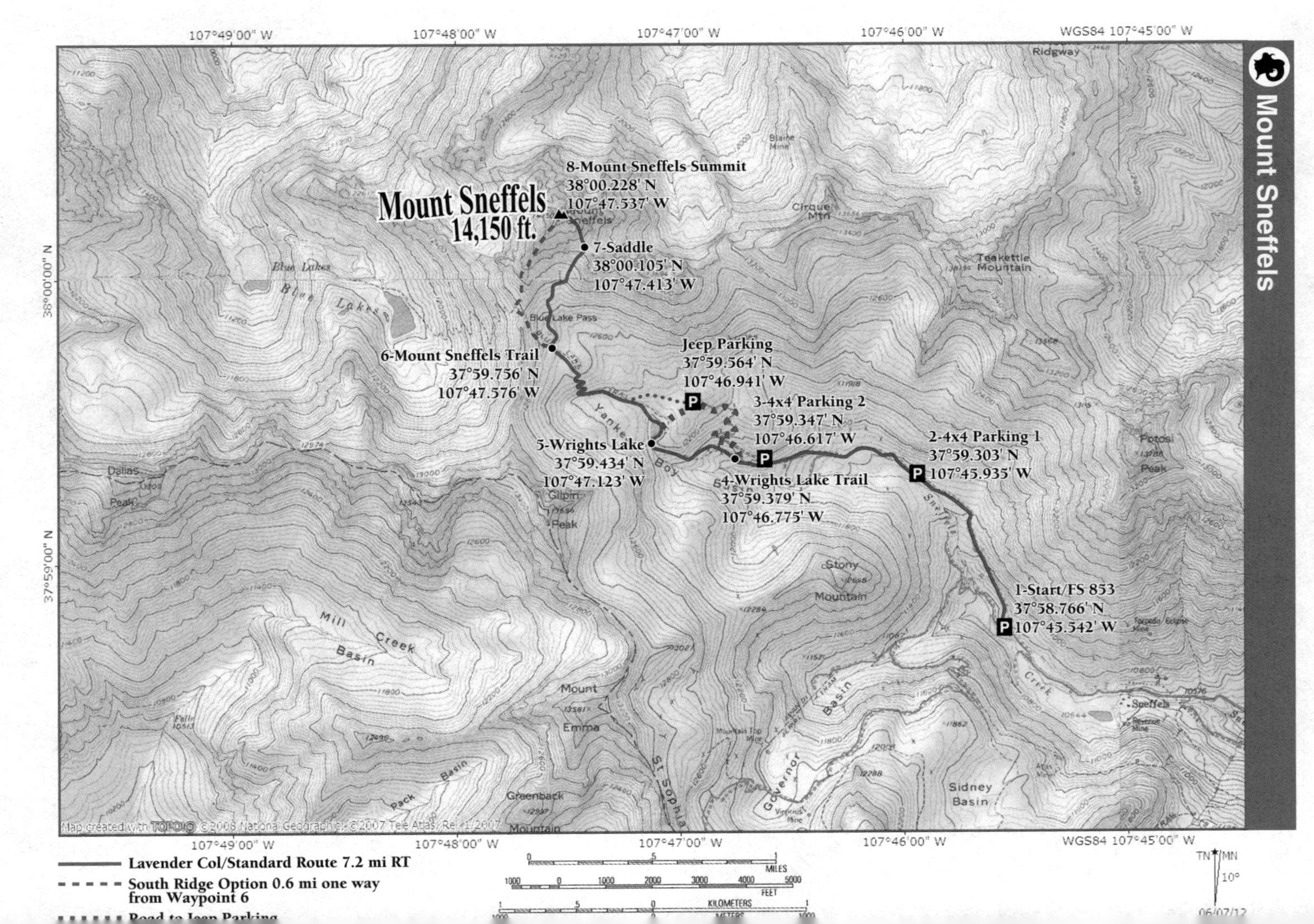

Mount Sneffels
Mount Sneffels 14,150 ft.
8-Mount Sneffels Summit
38°00.228' N
107°47.537' W
7-Saddle
38°00.105' N
107°47.413' W
6-Mount Sneffels Trail
37°59.756' N
107°47.576' W
Jeep Parking
37°59.564' N
107°46.941' W
3-4x4 Parking 2
37°59.347' N
107°46.617' W
5-Wrights Lake
37°59.434' N
107°47.123' W
4-Wrights Lake Trail
37°59.379' N
107°46.775' W
2-4x4 Parking 1
37°59.303' N
107°45.935' W
1-Start/FS 853
37°58.766' N
107°45.542' W
Blue Lakes
Blue Lake Pass
Cirque Mtn
Teakettle Mountain
Potosi Peak
Ridgway
Yankee Boy Basin
Gilpin Peak
Dallas Peak
Stony Mountain
Mill Creek Basin
Mount Emma
Greenback Mountain
Pack Basin
St Sophia
Governor Basin
Sidney Basin
Sneffels Creek
Sneffels
107°49'00" W
107°48'00" W
107°47'00" W
107°46'00" W
WGS84 107°45'00" W
38°00'00" N
37°59'00" N
Map created with TOPO!® ©2006 National Geographic; ©2007 Tele Atlas, Rel. 1/2007
Lavender Col/Standard Route 7.2 mi RT
South Ridge Option 0.6 mi one way from Waypoint 6
MILES
FEET
KILOMETERS
TN MN 10°
06/07/12

49 Mount Sneffels

Mount Sneffels is a photographer's favorite, but it's not just another pretty face. With great scrambling and fantastic views, you'll be salivating for Sneffels.

Round-Trip Distance	7.2 miles
Hiking Time	4–6 hours
Difficulty	6.5/10
Class	2+
Start Elevation	10,784 ft., at Yankee Boy Basin Road
Peak Elevation	14,150 ft.
Total Elevation Gain	3,250 ft.
Terrain	Good trail leads to scree slope and solid, scrambly gully to summit
Best Time to Climb	June–September
Gear Advisor	Ice ax in early spring, trekking poles, and boots for scree
Crowd Level	Moderate

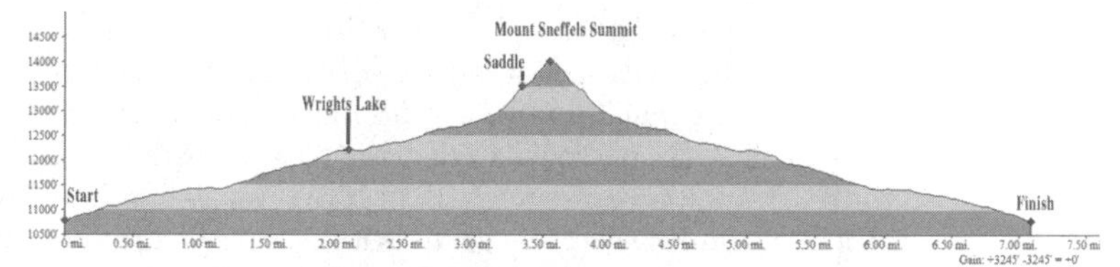

Location San Juan Range in the Mount Sneffels Wilderness/Uncompahgre National Forest outside of Ouray

Intro When you hike Mount Sneffels, you'll literally be climbing on a mountain of gold. Mines from its ore-rich flanks have produced more valuable gold than any other peak in the nation—and the deposits have yet to give out. Who knows—maybe you'll find a nugget or two on your hike. As is the norm in the San Juans, mountain views are tinged with green and orange, making for some of the best hiking pictures in Colorado. The scramble up Lavender Col is a solid and fun way to top out.

Why Climb It? Yankee Boy Basin is a beautiful place to spend an afternoon. The colors of the San Juans and the views of surrounding mountains are spectacular. Many peaks in the region are over 13,000 feet; they sprawl out like a legion of stoic giants. Many wild animals call the area home. A black bear, a coyote, and several elk said hello to me the last time I was in the basin. The gully that exits just below the top is a great finishing touch. Sneffels is a good hike for people who want to try their first rugged 14er.

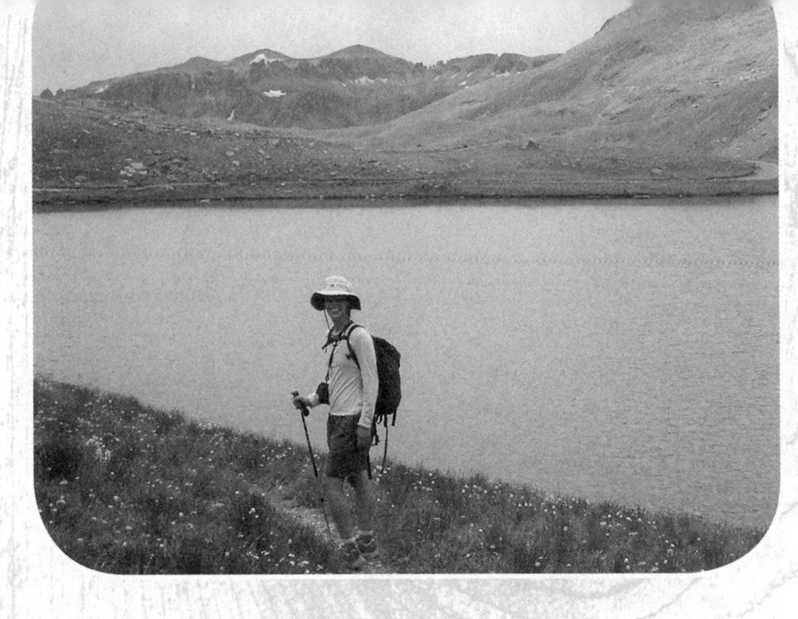

On the way to Sneffels

Driving Driving to the parking areas on Sneffels can be a fun and scenic ride or a sphincter-clenching thrill ride, depending on what kind of vehicle you have. For the record, tough passenger cars can make it to the lower part of Yankee Boy Basin—my Honda Accord made it to the junction of Sneffels Road (Forest Service Road 853) and County Road 26. For those with low-clearance vehicles, there is a section on the shelf road that is cut into solid rock and is just wide enough for one car. It's like driving through a tunnel with one open side. Cars will have to take the rock steps in the road head-on—you will have nowhere else to go. Expect to scrape—hard—a few times. When it's been raining, you may get to exit this cave by driving under a waterfall. The rest of the road is rough but passable to the aforementioned junction.

Of course, if you're driving a sport utility car (SUC), sport utility vehicle (SUV), or 4x4, the road is fun. These vehicles can continue up the road, past the CR 26/FS 853 junction to two different parking areas. Jeeps or 4x4s with a short wheel base can drive up to a high parking area at 12,314 feet.

How to Get There From Ouray, drive 0.5 mile out of the southern end of town on US Highway 550 and turn right onto Ouray County Road 361; the turn is after a sharp left curve and has signs for Yankee Boy Basin. Follow this road as it gets progressively rougher, and make sure to stay right when the road intersects with mining roads down to Camp Bird. Cars that have the guts to brave the Sneffels Cave (see above) can drive 6.8 miles and park at the junction of CR 26 and FS 853 (or just below, in parking areas past the ghost town of Sneffels). SUCs, SUVs, and 4x4 vehicles can stay right on FS 853 and work up the road. Several parking pull-offs are along the way. Some of the rocky stream crossings will challenge SUCs. You will come to a sign warning vehicles with long wheel bases against proceeding. Jeeps and smaller 4x4s have the option of taking the road shown on the map to a high parking area, where a connector trail joins the main route. This takes a mile or two off the route.

Fees/Camping There is no fee to hike here, but camping is restricted to designated areas. Most of the land is privately owned (mostly by mining interests) and must be respected. Call for more information, as regulations regarding camping are subject to change.

Route Notes The route described here starts from the junction of CR 26 and FS 853. If you drive to the 4x4 parking area, there is an easy-to-follow, signed connector trail.

Mile/Waypoint

0.0 mi (1) Start at the CR 26/FS 853 junction. Stay right (on FS 853) and hike up the road, which is quite scenic. Drivers of tougher vehicles can pull off in any number of small parking areas along the way. I've marked two on the map: at mile 0.78 **(2)** and at mile 1.47 **(3)**.

1.6 mi (4) When the road curves to the right, go straight on the footpath to the Wrights Lake Spur/Wrights Lake Trail. It is 0.5 mile to tiny Wrights Lake.

2.1 mi (5) The trail forks as you near the lake. Go right, and avoid the trail on the rocks to the left (it goes to a mine). Go along the east side of the lake and stay on the footpath by turning left at the sign (west), passing the north shore of the lake. A jeep road goes north from the lake; do not take it (though if you do, it simply leads to the 4x4 parking area).

2.9 mi (6) It's a sign! At this junction, go right (north) on the MOUNT SNEFFELS TRAIL NO. 204. There is a semi-visible trail through the boulder field. Following the intended trail may not be feasible, but it lines you up for the steep scree gully that you must climb to reach a saddle at 13,530 feet. This is where trekking poles are a big help.

3.4 mi (7) From the scenic saddle, there's an impressive gully to the top on your left (northwest). Thankfully, this gully is more solid than the scree slope you just came up. A trail reappears and zigzags up. At the top, you have two options to exit. Both are class 2+ or easy class 3 moves. The first option: You can simply top out and scramble left on semi-exposed rock to the summit. The second option is a slightly easier variation: take a small chute left, just below the top—a single tricky move that leads to an easy and fun scramble on ledges to the summit.

3.6 mi (8) Mount Sneffels's sumptuous summit! What views! You can return the way you came, or if you're up for scrambling, take the class 3 south ridge down to Blue Lake Pass. Either way, the descent is a little rough on the knees.

7.3 mi Finish at the CR 26/FS 853 junction.

Options If you continue to Blue Lake Pass instead of turning right at waypoint **6**, you can attempt Sneffels's south ridge. This class 3 route has some exposure on solid rock and is cairned all the way to the top. Descend the standard route for a great loop.

Quick Facts Sneffels's name has been a source of contention for years. The story that has the most artistic merit alludes to novelist Jules Verne's book *A Journey* *to the Centre of the Earth.* In that book, Verne refers to a real-life volcanic mountain in Iceland, known as Snæfellsjökull, as the gateway to the center of our planet. I have no idea how to say that name, and neither did the geographers of old because they condensed it to Sneffels. Other rumors persist that a Mr. Sneffels existed, though if that entity was a man, a hamster, or a stuffed animal is unknown. A third explanation is that miners who worked on the mountain called it Mount Sniffles due to the cold-inducing conditions of the chilly tunnels. It's just as well because many people call it Sniffles anyway.

Speaking of mines, Sneffels sits atop some of the most prolific veins of gold and silver ever mined. Even before the turn of *last* century (1900), the mines had already produced more than $35 million worth of ore. The Camp Bird Mine is still plugging away at the remaining ore. Thomas Walsh made his fortune from the bounty of the Earth here; his daughter, Evalyn Walsh McLean, gained fame by being the last private owner of the supposedly hexed Hope Diamond. She was famous enough to be mentioned in the famous Cole Porter tune "Anything Goes." The reference to her goes as follows:

When Missus Ned McLean (God bless her)
Can get Russian reds to "yes" her,
Then I suppose
Anything goes.

These lines probably made a lot more sense in 1934; the best I can come up with is that "yes" in this context means something very naughty.

Contact Info

Uncompahgre National Forest
Ouray Ranger District
2505 S. Townsend Avenue
Montrose, CO 81401
(970) 240-5300

Additionally, The Yankee Boy Conservation Alliance works with private land owners to manage and maintain access to this beautiful spot. Read about them online at **yankeeboy.org** or contact them at:

YBCA
P.O. Box 1448
Ouray, CO 81427
(970) 325-4116

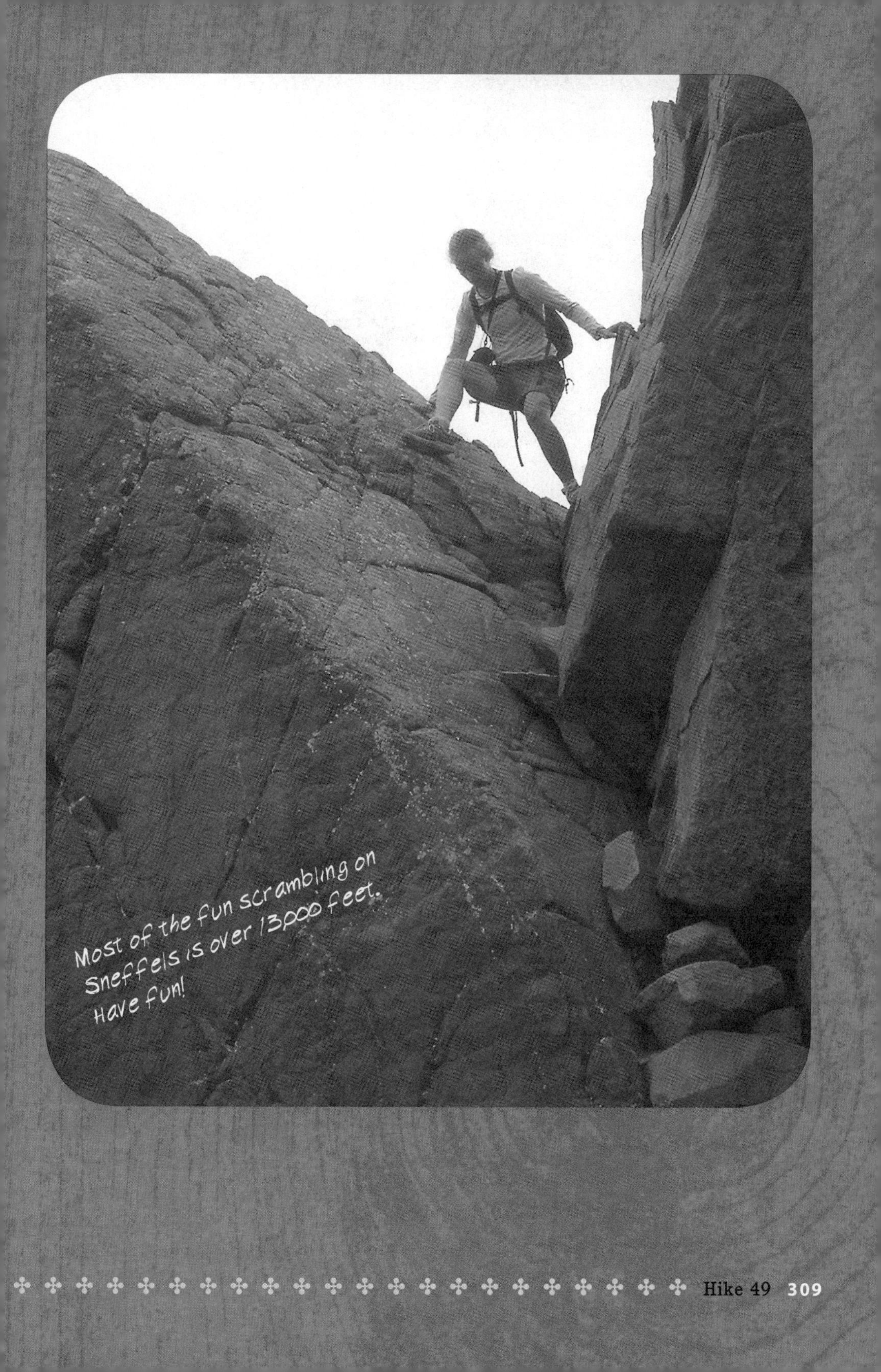
Most of the fun scrambling on
Sneffels is over 13,000 feet.
Have fun!

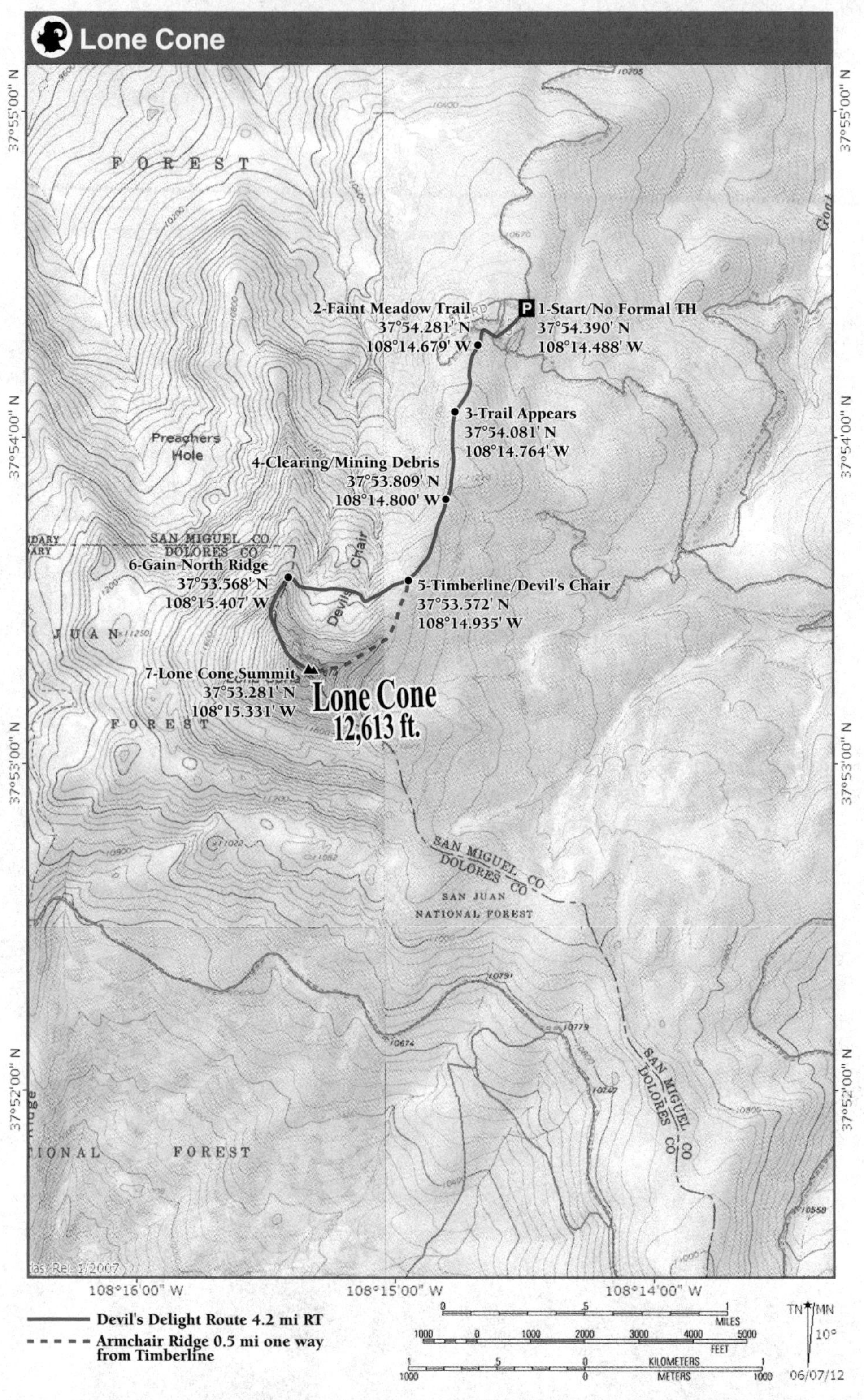

Lone Cone
FOREST
Preachers Hole
SAN MIGUEL CO
DOLORES CO
JUAN
FOREST
Devils Chair
1-Start/No Formal TH
37°54.390' N
108°14.488' W
2-Faint Meadow Trail
37°54.281' N
108°14.679' W
3-Trail Appears
37°54.081' N
108°14.764' W
4-Clearing/Mining Debris
37°53.809' N
108°14.800' W
5-Timberline/Devil's Chair
37°53.572' N
108°14.935' W
6-Gain North Ridge
37°53.568' N
108°15.407' W
7-Lone Cone Summit
37°53.281' N
108°15.331' W
Lone Cone
12,613 ft.
SAN JUAN
NATIONAL FOREST
IONAL FOREST
37°55'00" N
37°54'00" N
37°53'00" N
37°52'00" N
108°16'00" W
108°15'00" W
108°14'00" W
Devil's Delight Route 4.2 mi RT
Armchair Ridge 0.5 mi one way from Timberline
MILES
FEET
KILOMETERS
METERS
TN MN
10°
06/07/12

50 Lone Cone

Lone Cone beckons like an oracle. This remote, stand-alone mountain is the last high peak in western Colorado, signaling an end of the mountains and the start of the desert.

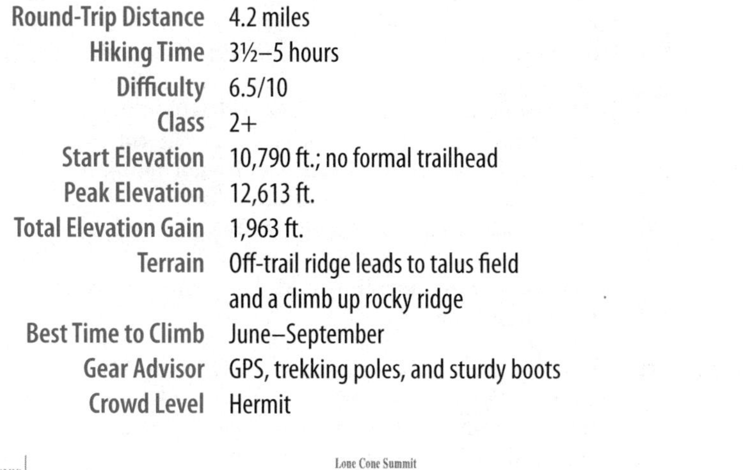

Round-Trip Distance	4.2 miles
Hiking Time	3½–5 hours
Difficulty	6.5/10
Class	2+
Start Elevation	10,790 ft.; no formal trailhead
Peak Elevation	12,613 ft.
Total Elevation Gain	1,963 ft.
Terrain	Off-trail ridge leads to talus field and a climb up rocky ridge
Best Time to Climb	June–September
Gear Advisor	GPS, trekking poles, and sturdy boots
Crowd Level	Hermit

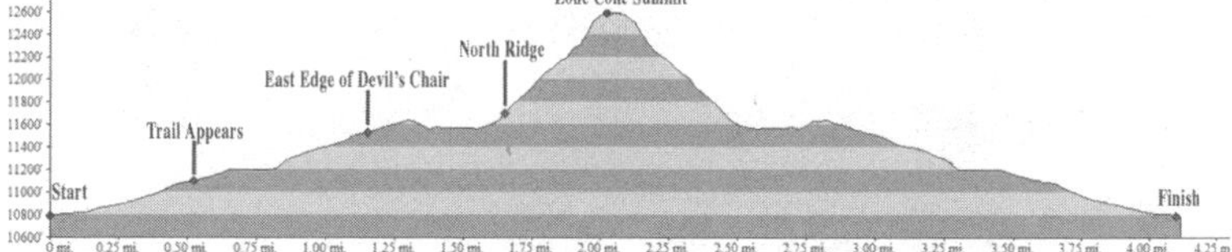

Location Uncompahgre National Forest in the San Miguel Mountains outside the town of Norwood

Intro There is something mystical about Lone Cone. Perhaps I've been in Boulder too long, but I sense that this mountain exudes a strange energy, a kind of surreal force whose effect is amplified by its remote and isolated nature. Crossing the Devil's Chair and gaining the north ridge reminded me of the knights of old journeying to reach a wise hermit in forbidden lands. And yet, the mountain is not far from Telluride and the Lizard Head Wilderness. Summiting Lone Cone puts you in an exclusive club of enlightened trekkers who have gained wisdom from this lonely peak.

Why Climb It? Never mind all my metaphysical mumbo jumbo. Lone Cone is a great climb. Mileage-wise it's short, but you'll be navigating off-trail in pine forests and rocky boulder fields, and focusing on navigation takes time. On the map, the cone rises from the flat land and stands as the final, western vestige of the Colorado Rockies. If you like to get away from it all, this is your hike. The class 2+ scrambling is actually quite enjoyable (comparable to the summit scramble on the standard route on Mount of the Holy Cross). The Devil's Chair is an impressive sight—the entire northwest face is carved out, resembling the perfect recliner for ol' Beelzebub. Those who would deny the Devil a chair anywhere but in hell (even if the chair is metaphorical) may prefer to say that it's simply a stunning natural feature. The climb seems to be inspirational, as many hikers have expressed some very personal and touching emotions in the register at the top.

Driving

Tough passenger cars have a shot at making it to the start of the hike. The roads are fine up until Forest Service Road 612, which is especially troublesome if there has been a lot of rain. The road is rutted and washed out in spots, rocky and steep in others. A carefully driven car in good conditions could make it to the top. Don't be discouraged if you only have a passenger car—you can park 1.6–2.4 miles up the road and just hike or bike up the hill. It's a short distance, so it's not a huge deal.

Sport utility cars, sport utility vehicles, and 4x4s should have no trouble making it up to the parking area. The only real obstacle may be the huge mud puddles that form on the road. Taken too slowly, they will mire your vehicle in their slimy grasp. (Note to passenger cars: If you're gonna try 'em, get some speed.)

How to Get There

Near the town of Norwood, at the junction of Colorado Highway 145 and County Road 44.Z, turn south on CR 44.Z (there will be a sign as you start down the road for the reservoirs and forest access). Stay south on this scenic, paved road. At mile 10.0, the road enters Uncompahgre National Forest, turns to dirt, and becomes known as CR 44.Z/Forest Service Road

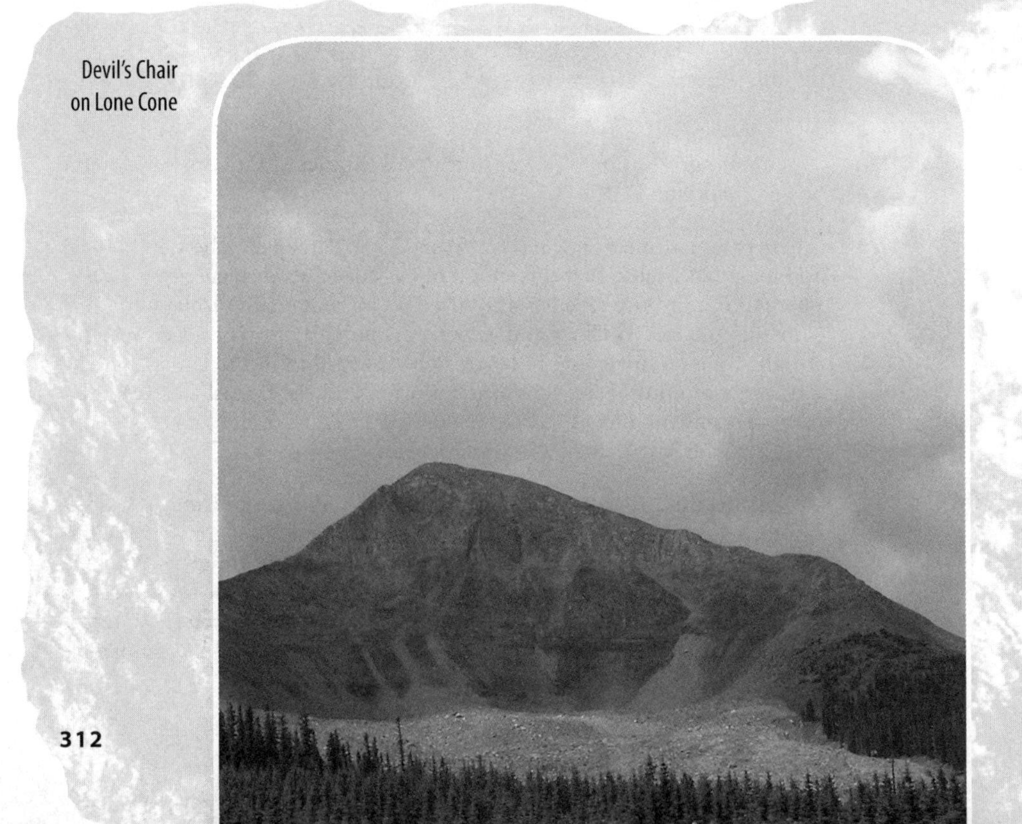

Devil's Chair on Lone Cone

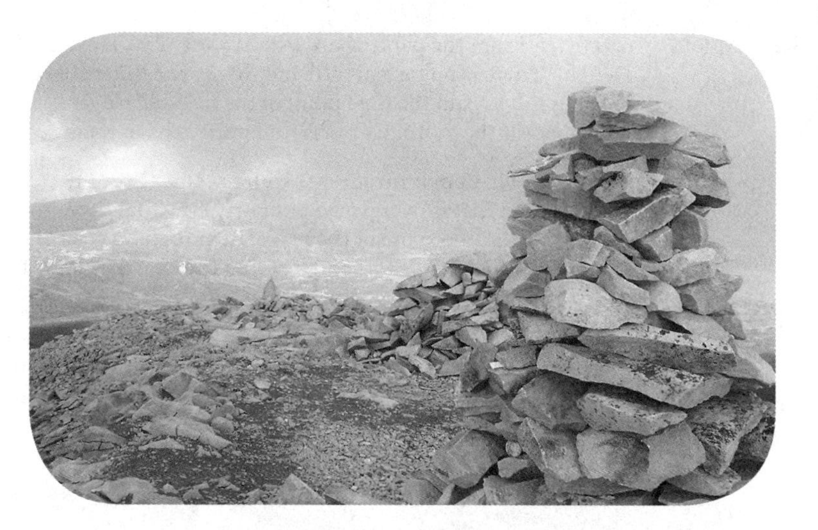

Despite being an isolated peak, the summit of Lone Cone has some nice cairns.

610. Follow this road 2.0 more miles south (as it exits the national forest, it becomes CR 44.Z again—it's still the same road). Just past mile marker 12, turn left onto my favorite road in this whole book, Beef Trail Road (also known as County Road M44). As you start up this road, at mile 0.2, look to your right (south) at the beautiful metalwork on the sign for the Halsey Ranch. Ride the Beef Trail Road 2.5 miles to the intersection with County Road 46M/Forest Service Road 611 and turn right. This is an easy road to miss, so slow down when you near it. The road starts at a gap in a fence with NO TRESPASSING signs; there is also an old wood sign on the left (north) side announcing the mileage to Norwood and Beef Trail Road. You'll know that you've gone too far if you start driving downhill.

Go south on FS 611 for 2.2 miles to Forest Service Road 612 on your right (the turn is 0.1 mile after the WELCOME sign for Uncompahgre National Forest). FS 612 is a fairly uninviting road and will jostle the plucky passenger cars that attempt to climb it. Follow this road 4.4 miles; cars may be forced to park around mile 1.6. At mile 2.5 there is another parking area at a gate, which may serve as a good campsite. Just after this, the road starts a series of switchbacks. There are parking spots at the top of the hill at 10,780 feet. Note the GPS point if you have one with you. There is no trailhead.

Fees/Camping There are no fees to hike or camp in the area. If you do overnight here, make sure that you are within the boundaries of Uncompahgre National Forest and not on private land. The best places are along FS 612 and on the brief section of CR 44.Z/FS 610 before the turn onto the Beef Trail Road.

Route Notes The entire route is technically off-trail, but there are old roads and a faint path through the woods to guide you, to a small degree. Don't rely on them, but note that they are there. Once you clear tree line at the base of the Devil's Chair, the navigation is much easier.

Mile/Waypoint

0.0 mi (1) From the parking area, head west. This is the route I call Devil's Delight. There is no formal trail, but there are a bunch of old logging roads. Head uphill to gain the high point of the forested ridge—you can follow the faint roads if the footing is easier, but don't rely on them.

0.3 mi (2) This open meadow is quite scenic. From here, there is an old logging road that is overgrown but fairly easy to follow. You can use it as a guide to get to the spine of the ridge. Aim high on the ridge and continue south, leaving the meadow and heading into the dark forest.

0.5 mi (3) As if by divine intervention, a trail materializes on the top of the ridge. It has some survey tags here and there. Again, remain on the high point of the ridge and don't be tempted to take any of the faint animal trails that go off into the woods. If the trail is not visible, don't be discouraged—continue along the high point of the ridge, heading south.

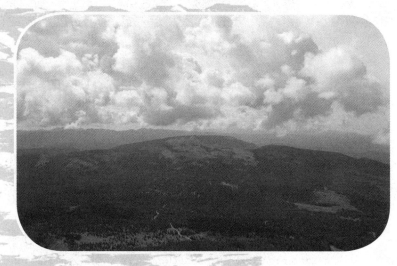

Lone Cone is Colorado's westernmost 11,000-foot summit.

0.9 mi (4) In a flat saddle clearing, there are the remnants of some old mining or survey equipment. There are also good views of Lone Cone. Continue south and uphill on the ridge.

1.2 miles (5) Exit the trees at timberline, at 11,530 feet. Depending on your navigation savvy, that first section was either very easy or very difficult. From here you have a clear visual of Lone Cone, with the north ridge to the west, across the "seat" of the Devil's Chair.

Boulder-hop west across the semi-stable rocks of the seat, taking in wicked views of the chair to your left. Find a spot on the north ridge that suits you and climb to it (the easiest way to gain the ridge is by staying slightly to the north side).

1.7 mi (6) Gain the north ridge and follow its rocky spine south/southeast to the high summit of Lone Cone.

2.1 mi (7) Lone Cone's secluded summit! There's a big cairn on top, as well as a summit register. Views to the east look out at the Lone Cone's partner, Little Cone, and at the high Wilson Peaks in the distance. Return the way you came. Navigation will be a little easier on the way down.

4.2 mi Finish.

Options The east ridge of Lone Cone, also known as Armchair Ridge, is a decent scramble that is 0.5 mile southwest one way from waypoint **5** to the summit. It is a class 3+ route with some exposed moves, but if you're up for some scrambling, it's the way to go.

It took me a few tries to realize that Devil's Delight is the best route up Lone Cone; previously I had entered at the gate 2.5 miles up FS 612 and taken a convoluted and difficult bushwhack through some ugly terrain. Forest sections were dark and eerie, and the landscape was littered with fallen trees and animal skulls. Other fearsome experiences along that route included a fast-moving lightning storm and a mad dash to escape a furious herd of angry, rogue, alpine cows. (This was the second time I was almost mauled by these supposedly peaceful ungulates. I also had to hop a cattle gate while running full speed to escape an ornery cow gang near Summit Peak. In retrospect, it may have been a couple of bulls leading the charge.) In other words, don't go this way. On the way down this bad route, I found the trail and an easier exit to the road, though I logged more than 8 miles figuring this out. Live and learn, right? Better yet, read and beware.

Quick Facts Lone Cone is the most fitting name for any mountain in Colorado. It's a forlorn peak, cast off from the social giants of the Sawatch or the conjoined legions of the San Juans. Technically, the San Miguel Mountains are part of the San Juans, but Lone Cone is a volcanic relic that is not attached to any other mountain.

Contact Info Uncompahgre National Forest
Norwood Ranger District
P.O. Box 388-1150 Forest
Norwood, CO 81423
(970) 327-4261

Afterword

Hike Your Heart Out

I've made the error of thinking that the mountains serve to soothe the sting of my very human blunders. When seeking solace from the troubling architecture of man-made existence, I've run like a child into mother mountain's arms. I've wanted to close my eyes and feel nothing but the pure, sweet singular embrace.

And there I am greeted with dark clouds. My quest for grace is intercepted by something wicked.

I've endured withering heat and marrow-chilling cold. I've run from lightning until my lungs turned to ice on the verge of shattering. I've been lost in the fearful night. I've purpled my skin with bruises, and swollen my wrists and ankles countless times. I have felt the still malice of lurking forces intent on inflicting injury and dread. I have failed to reach summits. I've fantasized about warm meals, women, and soft beds. When I have sought comfort from the mountains, I have often made the mistake of not bringing anything to share but my self-pity. I have seen my troubles brought to life in fast-building storms, high-running rivers, and sheer cliffs.

And yet, even in my most selfish hour, even when I threaten to abandon this life of adventure for a plush couch and plasma screen TV, the mountains have imparted their wisdom. Even when my eyes have welled with tears of frustration, I have returned home again to find that the food tastes sweeter, sleep comes easier, and the body feels lighter. I have faced hardship with meaning, struggled in an honest kingdom, and been humbled by a much wiser teacher. I have endured the tough love of the mountains, and I am made better for it.

I grow. I return to the mountain wiser. I bring a gift of joy. Perhaps this solemn body of rock is curious of the ways of those who seek its heights. Instead of demanding spiritual enlightenment from the mountain, I converse with the details. I appreciate a good storm as much as the clear blue sky. And as I learn to love those details, funny things happen. The brain reprioritizes all the clutter banging around in my head, preferring to focus on faces in the rock and the symmetry of flowers. My heart pounds and my legs burn, with every vessel a throbbing affirmation of life. My legs feel the cold mud and the warm sun. When finally willing to yield my senses to the alpine world, I have received that long-sought embrace.

I admit that I'm not all that savvy in the frontcountry. Material wealth has yet to impress me enough for me to master the means by which many keep score. My ability to relate to this system has been just adequate enough to get by. Ask me what my favorite movie is and I'll struggle and stumble; to me, watching a movie is a last resort. I've found equal inspiration and despair in Eastern and Western beliefs, and I've built a totem pole from the best values extracted from each. I'm at best a clumsy citizen of the world.

But talk with me of mountains and my eyes light up. Suddenly, I can relate and I am connected. I do not care if your journey was a 0.25-mile walk to examine an alpine lake or a harrowing climb of a Himalayan peak; it is a language I understand. And while my fluency may not be as elegant as more enlightened climbers, I can finally listen and speak of an authentic world of triumph and tragedy.

I am made better by mountains. Each visit replenishes me just enough to get by until the next great adventure. Somehow, even the real world becomes more enjoyable and manageable when infused with the afterglow of a good summit hike. I hope that this book gives you a chance to harvest from the mountains the goodness of life and the lessons of Mother Nature. For my own case, I will remain eager to learn from the mountains and revel in the joy of their trails and trials. When given a choice of investments during my short stint on this beautiful planet, the wealth I've received from my time in the hills has proven to be a far superior currency than any I've yet to uncover.

Beyond the Book

Want more hikes? Need trailhead updates? Want to know the best gear to use on Colorado's summits? Visit *Best Summit Hikes in Colorado* online at **updates.WildernessPress.com** for ongoing updates on the hikes in this book, plus links to free maps, hikes, and scrambles from the author's website. See photos from all the summits in the book, stories of adventure (and misadventure), and other behind-the-scene tales.

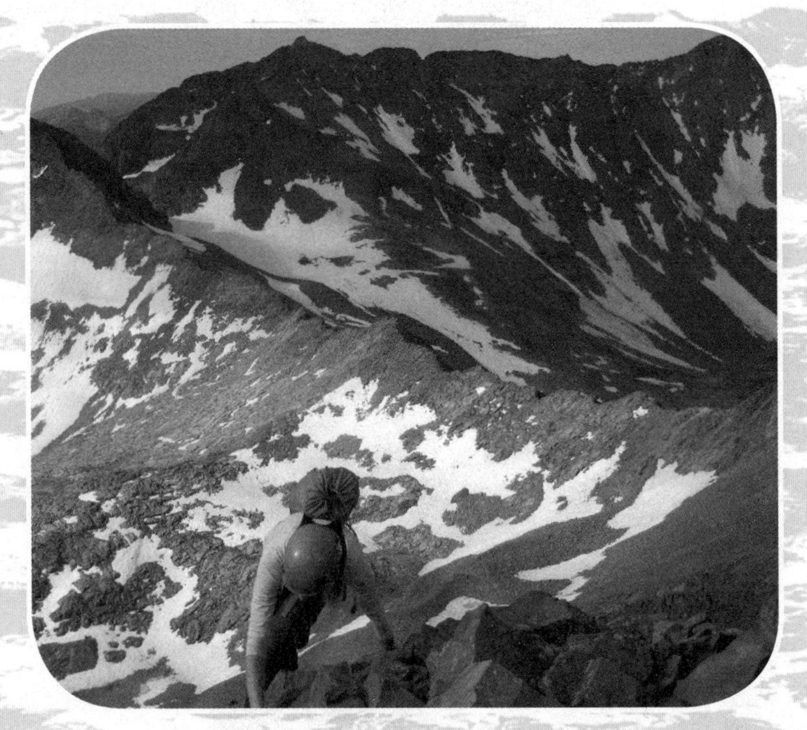

Jenny Salentine scrambling on Wilson Peak

Appendix A

"Best" Hikes and Others of Note

Only have a half day to hike? Have friends from out of town looking to snag a summit or two? Trying to get away from the mind-numbing pace of everyday life? Here are a few suggestions for these and other situations.

Best day hikes for out-of-town friends who aren't hardcore hikers but still want a good summit Mount Sniktau, Mount Elbert, Guardians of the Flatirons, Mount Thomas, Mount Sherman, Geissler Mountain, Treasury Mountain, and Cross Mountain–Lizard Head Traverse

Best overnight adventures Fools Peak, Mount Zirkel, Storm King Peak, Chicago Basin 14er Circuit, Mount of the Holy Cross, Mount Adams, Mount Alice, and Summit Peak

Best from the Denver/Boulder/Golden metro area when you have plans later that night The Citadel, Peak 1/Tenmile Peak, Mount Sniktau, Pacific Peak, James Peak, Mount Chapin group, and Mount Ida group

Best hikes that get away from the crowds Lone Cone, Storm King Peak, Fools Peak, Summit Peak, East Beckwith Mountain, Golden Horn, Hesperus Mountain, Mount Powell, and Mount Alice

Best hikes with excellent scrambling Navajo Peak, Lead Mountain, Mount Richthofen, Longs Peak, Mount Alice, Fools Peak, Belleview Mountain, Mount Blanca, Mount Eolus, Storm King Peak, and Mount Sneffels

Best hikes for wildflowers (in season, of course) Stanley Mountain and Vasquez Peak, Treasury Mountain, Belleview Mountain, Mount Sherman, Mount Thomas, Mount Adams, Deming Mountain, Mount Hope, and Mount Zirkel

Best hikes to do with your dog Huron Peak, James Peak, Clark Peak, Mount Sherman, Mount Zirkel, Mount Sopris, Uncompahgre Peak, Guardians of the Flatirons, Mount Thomas, and Hahns Peak

Best hikes that stay above tree line most of the time Mount Sniktau, Stanley Mountain and Vasquez Peak, Mount Ouray, West Spanish Peak, Eureka Mountain–Hermit Peak, and Uncompahgre Peak

Best off-trail adventures Jasper Peak, Lone Cone, Navajo Peak, Fools Peak, Mount Ouray, Golden Horn, Storm King Peak, Mount Adams, Treasury Mountain, Hesperus Mountain, Mount Powell, Mount Richthofen, and Clark Peak

Best lung busters Mount Powell, Lead Mountain, Peak 1, Stanley's Wall, Mount Sneffels, Storm King Peak, Mount Adams, Mount Sniktau, Navajo Peak, Pacific Peak, Fools Peak, West Spanish Peak, and Mount Richthofen

Best hikes to do when there is still spring snow Navajo Peak, Jasper Peak, Clark Peak, James Peak, Bison Peak, Hahns Peak, Mount Sniktau, and Mount Sherman

Best hikes for autumn leaves and colors Mount Hope, East Beckwith Mountain, Belleview Mountain, Huron Peak, Uncompahgre Peak, Mount Powell, Mount Sopris, and Fools Peak

Best social hikes (lots of people to chat with, observe, and so on) Longs Peak, Mount Elbert, James Peak, Huron Peak, Mount of the Holy Cross, Chicago Basin 14er Circuit, and Redcloud Peak–Sunshine Peak

Best hikes with crazy and cool natural rock formations Bison Peak, Summit Peak, Belleview Mountain, Mount Zirkel, Uncompahgre Peak, Golden Horn, the Citadel, Guardians of the Flatirons, Hesperus Mountain, Mount Adams, Storm King Peak, and Lone Cone

Best hikes to see wildlife Mount Sneffels, Mount Ida group, Mount Chapin group, Mount Thomas, Clark Peak, Chicago Basin 14er Circuit, Storm King Peak, and Summit Peak

Best hikes to see mining ruins and ghost towns Mount Sherman, Huron Peak, Pacific Peak, Peak 1, James Peak, Golden Horn, and Hahns Peak

Hikes with airplane wreckage Navajo Peak, Mount Yale, Jasper Peak, and Lead Mountain

Best on-trail summit hikes Mount Elbert, Huron Peak, Guardians of the Flatirons, Longs Peak, Peak 1, Mount Sopris, Uncompahgre Peak, Redcloud Peak–Sunshine Peak, Mount Thomas, and Mount Ida group

Best hikes that are named after characters in *Street Fighter 2* Mount Blanca and Bison Peak

Best hikes that you can't pronounce properly Tabeguache Peak and Mount Ouray

Best hikes with names that best suit a Muppet Sneffels, Zirkel, Elbert, Stanley, Sniktau, Jasper, Hahns, Eureka, and Chiquita

And finally: Best hikes with the author's name or the author's cat's name in the title James Peak and "Mount Bruplex"

James Dziezynski's Top 10 Hikes

It's a question that is best asked spontaneously—what are your favorite hikes in the book? When given too much time to ponder the question, I could make a diplomatic argument for any of the 50. However, if budget cuts had reduced this book to the 10 best summit hikes in Colorado, I'd have a list ready to go without second thought. Obviously it's a partisan list; the mountains included have just the right amount of all the things I like to experience on a good summit hike.

If you're like me, and I know I am, there's nothing better than a long day in the mountains. Give me steep hills, good scrambling, and great views, and I'm in heaven. Combine that with a scenic approach and good weather, and you have the perfect hike. These 10 hikes have all that plus a special something that makes them linger in my memory.

1. Storm King Peak

A trip to Storm King is part heart-pounding climbing, part exhilarating scrambling, and part mystical spirit quest. The remote setting is an all-natural Shangri-la, a place where the trappings of mankind are left far behind. There's no place like the Grenadier Range, and Storm King reigns supreme as the monarch of these wonderful mountains.

2. Golden Horn

The Ice Lakes Basin is gorgeous, and the Horn serves as the centerpiece. A fine approach followed by good scrambling leads to a nifty summit.

3. Chicago Basin 4er Circuit: Windom, Sunlight, and Eolus

Amplify the exotic nature of this adventure by taking the old narrow-gauge train to the trailhead. You'll feel as though you're in a new frontier when you disembark for these three 14ers. The best part: All three are great climbs with distinct personalities.

4. Fools Peak

Even though the rule in Colorado is that everything that can be climbed has been, you'll feel like the first person to ever stand on Fools summit. I hope no one ever puts a register on top—it would ruin the wild feeling of this marvelous mountain.

5. Mount Adams

What a ridge walk! Adams always feels as though it's on the verge of being unclimbable, only to reveal its secrets upon closer inspection. You never get hung out to dry, and the views are spectacular.

6. Lead Mountain

Another thrilling ridge walk, this time with more exposure and less obvious route finding. You'll have to stay on your toes, but there are always bailout points if you need them. Linking up to neighboring peaks adds to the fun.

7. Longs Peak

It's a classic Colorado climb, with prolonged scrambling and a flat, spacious summit. I'm just one of its countless fans, but it really is a must-do hike.

8. Blanca Peak

The approach alone is worth the adventure. Watching the land change from smoldering desert to a lush basin is incredible! As if that weren't enough, the scramble up to Blanca's summit is solid, with breathtaking views along the way. A tried-and-true winner.

9. Bison Peak Sometimes you have to sit back and wonder how Mother Nature was able to build such impressive monuments. Bison's rock garden is unique and inviting—and you can visit it year-round. It must be seen in person for one to appreciate its fabulous formations.

10. Peak 1 and Tenmile Peak Even though I've already hiked these two, every time I drive by on I-70, I want to stop what I'm doing and climb 'em again. Too often, mountains with good profiles lack the high-quality climbing to match—not the case with these classics. Easy to access and a blast to climb, this summit hike certainly merits a spot in my top 10.

Good Weekend Getaways

All right! You have a long weekend to go out hiking. Try pairing up the suggested hikes or go for a nice overnight in the following areas:

Good hike pairings for a long weekend:
Hope and Huron
Richthofen and Clark
Yale and Carbonado/Tabeguache
Fools and Thomas
The Citadel and Peak 1/Tenmile
The Citadel and James
Yale and Geissler
Treasury and Belleview
Uncompahgre and Redcloud/Sunshine
Stanley/Vasquez and Deming
East Beckwith and Treasury or Belleview

Great two-night trips—leave Friday and return Sunday:
Deming Mountain
Lead Mountain
Clark Peak
Mount Alice
Mount of the Holy Cross
Blanca Peak
Uncompahgre Peak
Mount Adams
Fools Peak
Summit Peak
Mount Zirkel
Eureka Mountain/Hermit Peak

Additional hikes with very good backcountry camping or extended camping:

Storm King Peak

Chicago Basin 14er Circuit

Golden Horn

Mount Sopris

Mount Blanca

Honorable Mention Hikes

Following are some outstanding hikes that could have made the book but didn't quite fit the criteria for the top 50 Colorado summit hikes for one reason or another. However, each of them is definitely worth checking out—once you've finished all the hikes in this book!

Mount Audubon A nice walk up in Indian Peaks but a bit too "normal" for this book.

Twilight Peak Access is too rough on unmaintained roads for this otherwise great San Juan hike.

Vestal and Arrow Peaks Two awesome scrambles in the Grenadiers; route finding pushes them a little into class 4 territory (though both have established class 3 routes—if you can find them).

Ice Mountain A very visible peak with a good hike but lacks that certain zing of other Sawatch hikes.

Mount Massive Same as Ice Mountain; a good hike but it can feel very long and a bit tedious.

Pikes Peak Famous but a rather straightforward hike without a lot of bells and whistles—except for those on the cog railroad to the top!

Maroon Bells Class 4 and crumbly. The Bells are dangerous for inexperienced hikers and the terrain is unstable and exposed.

Crestone Peak Excellent class 3 route but a lot of rockfall present.

Sheep Mountain A good mountain to hike in Telluride, but the Cross–Lizard Head loop is better!

Wilson Group These 14ers, also outside Telluride, include Mount Wilson, Wilson Peak, and El Diente Peak. They are good hikes, but the talus sections are quite long, placing them just a notch below the best hikes.

Three over the Border

King's Peak in Utah's Uintas Mountains Check this one out; it's just over Colorado's northwest border. The Uintas Mountains are the only major range in the Lower 48 US states that run east-west rather than north-south.

Wheeler Peak in New Mexico It's in the Sangre De Cristo Range and is the high point of New Mexico; check it out if you visit Taos.

Medicine Bow Peak in Wyoming Just north of the border, near the town of Saratoga Springs. It's a fun climb and a shorter drive from Fort Collins than many peaks in Colorado.

Hikes that Didn't Make the Cut

When selecting the hikes for this book, I climbed several peaks that were a lot of fun but not quite good enough to make the cut. Here's a sample of the contenders that fell short.

Hallets Peak This Rocky Mountain National Park favorite has a very long approach via its standard route—a bit too long.

Bills and Byers Peaks Two mountains in the Vasquez Mountains. Nice hikes, but they have very long approaches and aren't as scenic as Stanley Mountain and Vasquez Peak.

Milwaukee Peak Another awesome Sangre hike, but the scrambling is class 4 in brief sections.

South Arapahoe Peak An Indian Peaks classic, it's got a great snow route but a standard hiking route. Good views all around from this big boy.

Chair Mountain A very fun Elk Range hike. Unfortunately, the peak is surrounded by private land, and rangers have warned me that landowners have been less than inviting to hikers who stumble onto their property. It was a major bummer to have to omit it from the book.

North Mamm Peak Sometimes they just look better on the map then they do in person.

South Rawah Peak You'll have great views of this mountain from the top of Clarks Peak. It lacks the fun skywalk of Clark, so it only gets an honorable mention.

Appendix B

Mountain Miscellany

Colorado Mountain Trivia

Stuck in your tent? Up for 20 questions? Give these trivia questions a shot, and see how much you know about Colorado's mountains and surrounding areas.

1. What fabled 14er was originally known as James Peak in honor of the first person to climb it? *Answer: Pikes Peak, first climbed by Edwin James in 1820.*

2. Can you name all the 14ers of the Collegiate Peaks named after institutes of higher learning? *Answer: Columbia, Yale, Harvard, Princeton, and Oxford. Belford was named after James B. Belford, a territorial judge who earned the nickname "the Red-Headed Rooster of the Rockies."*

3. You may know Mount Elbert is the highest peak in Colorado. Can you name the 10 highest peaks in the lower 48 US states? *Answer (mountains are in Colorado if not specified otherwise): 1-Mount Whitney, California (14,494 ft.) 2-Mount Elbert (14,433 ft.) 3-Mount Massive (14,421 ft.) 4-Mount Harvard (14,420 ft.) 5-Mount Rainier, Washington (14,411 ft.) 6-Mount Williamson, California (14,375 ft.) 7-Blanca Peak (14,345 ft.) 8-La Plata Peak (14,336 ft.) 9-Uncompahgre Peak (14,309 ft.) 10-Crestone Peak (14,294 ft.)*

4. Which mountain in Colorado has yielded more valuable ore than any other single mountain in the US? *Answer: Mount Sneffels.*

5. What is the name of the mountain in Golden that is the burial site of "Buffalo Bill" Cody? Bonus points for naming the state William Cody was born in. *Answer: Lookout Mountain. Buffalo Bill was born in Iowa.*

6. What four Colorado Mountains are within 20 feet of 14er status? *Answer: Sunlight Spire (13,995 ft.), Grizzly Peak (13,988 ft.—not the one in this book; this one is farther south in the Sawatch Range), Stewart Peak (13,983 ft.), and Columbia Point (13,980 ft.)*

7. One would think that Summit County would have the highest peak in the state, but it doesn't; that honor goes to Lake County and Mount Elbert. Can you name the summit that tops the charts for Summit County? *Answer: Grays Peak (14,270 ft.).*

8. Culebra Peak is the "forbidden 14er." The mountain is on private land and the owners demand $100 per hiker to attempt the summit. What does the word *culebra* mean in Spanish? *Answer: Snake.*

9. Which is the only 14er that does not have mount, mountain, point, or peak in its official name? *Answer: Crestone Needle.*

10. What mountain range in Colorado has flora that is unique to it and an Arctic island where NASA tested the Mars rover equipment before launch? (This island is the second largest in the world.) Points for the range and the island. *Answer: Indian Peaks and Devon Island in the Canadian Arctic.*

11. In 1893, what mining boomtown attempted to have the capital of Colorado moved from Denver to its city limits? *Answer: Georgetown. The 2010 population of Georgetown was roughly 1,100 people.*

12. The Silverton & Durango Narrow Gauge Railroad is a great way to visit the 14ers in the Chicago Basin. The railroad has run every year since its inception. In what year did the trains first puff up the tracks? *Answer: 1881. The train has also been featured in several movies and TV shows.*

13. What is the name of Colorado's oldest military fort, which was commanded by Kit Carson in 1858? Hint: You likely drive through it on your way to Blanca Peak. *Answer: Fort Garland.*

14. Who was the first person to officially climb all of Colorado's 14ers? *Answer: Who else but Albert Ellingwood?*

15. What Colorado 14er is rumored to harbor a hidden cache of gold, jewels, and other gems buried by the Spanish in the 1700s, which has yet to be discovered? *Answer: Mount Princeton.*

16. I already mentioned in the Eureka Mountain hike that redundancy is sometimes lost in translation, such as Rito Alto Creek, which translates to High Creek Creek (though in today's Spanish, the word *creek* is *cara*). What Colorado town name means "hot springs springs" when translated back into the Ute language? *Answer: Pagosa Springs.*

17. Colorado's mountain birds are among the most regal and beautiful on Earth. Can you name Colorado's state bird? Bonus points if you know Colorado's state flower and animal. *Answer: The rather plain prairie lark, also known as lark bunting, is the state bird. Columbine is the state flower, and Rocky Mountain bighorn sheep is our state animal.*

18. In the winter of 1956–57, pilots were shocked to see a horse trapped in the saddle between Mount Harvard and Mount Yale at 12,500 feet. A massive effort was made to save the animal; he was finally rescued before he froze to death. What was the name of the program to save the horse, and for bonus points, what was the horse's name? *Answer: This bizarre but true story had a happy ending for the animal, which turned out to be a local Buena Vista bay horse named Bugs. The program instituted to save Bugs was called Operation Haylift and involved planes actually dropping tons of*

hay from their crafts to the animal. The horse was fed by the "haylift" until ranchers on foot were able to rescue it when conditions improved.

19. What climber joined John W. Powell on his historic first ascent of Longs Peak? (Hint: The route they took was later named in his honor.) *Answer: L. W. Keplinger was the first of Powell's group to reach the summit; he almost summited solo the previous day while scouting a route to the top. Keplinger's Couloir is a class 3 alternative to the famous Keyhole Route.*

20. In the Geissler Mountain Rimwalk chapter, I mention that Unnamed Peak 13,001 (visible from the route) is the lowest ranked 13er in Colorado. What is the lowest officially named 13er? *Answer: Ruffner Mountain in the San Juans, 13,003 feet above sea level.*

Appendix C

Colorado's 100 Highest Peaks

Thanks to Summitpost.org for this chart. Peaks not listed with a rank are considered unofficial, meaning they are too close to a neighboring summit to be considered a ranked mountain. Highlighted mountains are featured in this book as standard or optional hikes.

Peak Name	Rank	Elevation	Range
Mount Elbert	1	14,433	Sawatch
Mount Massive	2	14,421	Sawatch
Mount Harvard	3	14,420	Sawatch
Blanca Peak	4	14,345	Sangre De Cristo
North Massive		14,340	Sawatch
La Plata Peak	5	14,336	Sawatch
Uncompahgre Peak	6	14,309	San Juan
Crestone Peak	7	14,294	Sangre De Cristo
Mount Lincoln	8	14,286	Mosquito
Grays Peak	9	14,270	Front
Mount Antero	10	14,269	Sawatch
Torreys Peak	11	14,267	Front
Castle Peak	12	14,265	Elk
Quandary Peak	13	14,265	Tenmile
Mount Evans	14	14,264	Front
Longs Peak	15	14,255	Front
Mount Wilson	16	14,246	San Juan
Mount Cameron		14,238	Mosquito
Mount Shavano	17	14,229	Sawatch
Mount Belford	18	14,197	Sawatch
Crestone Needle	19	14,197	Sangre De Cristo
Mount Princeton	20	14,197	Sawatch
Mount Yale	21	14,196	Sawatch
Mount Bross	22	14,172	Mosquito
Kit Carson Peak	23	14,165	Sangre De Cristo
El Diente		14,159	San Juan

Peak Name	Rank	Elevation	Range
Maroon Peak	24	14,156	Elk
Tabeguache Peak	25	14,155	Sawatch
Mount Oxford	26	14,153	Sawatch
Mount Sneffels	27	14,150	San Juan
Mount Democrat	28	14,148	Mosquito
Capitol Peak	29	14,130	Elk
Pikes Peak	30	14,110	Front
Snowmass Mountain	31	14,092	Elk
Mount Eolus	32	14,083	San Juan
Windom Peak	33	14,082	San Juan
Challenger Point	34	14,081	Sangre De Cristo
Mount Columbia	35	14,073	Sawatch
Missouri Mountain	36	14,067	Sawatch
Humboldt Peak	37	14,064	Sangre De Cristo
Mount Bierstadt	38	14,060	Front
Conundrum Peak		14,060	Elk
Sunlight Peak	39	14,059	San Juan
Handies Peak	40	14,048	San Juan
Culebra Peak	41	14,047	Sangre De Cristo
Ellingwood Point	42	14,042	Sangre De Cristo
Mount Lindsey	43	14,042	Sangre De Cristo
North Eolus		14,039	San Juan
Little Bear Peak	44	14,037	Sangre De Cristo
Mount Sherman	45	14,036	Mosquito
Redcloud Peak	46	14,034	San Juan
North Maroon Peak		14,019	Elk
Pyramid Peak	47	14,018	Elk
Wilson Peak	48	14,017	San Juan
Wetterhorn Peak	49	14,015	San Juan
San Luis Peak	50	14,014	San Juan
Mount of the Holy Cross	51	14,005	Sawatch
Huron Peak	52	14,003	Sawatch

Peak Name	Rank	Elevation	Range
Sunshine Peak	53	14,001	San Juan
"Sunlight Spire"		13,995	San Juan
Grizzly Peak A	54	13,988	Sawatch
Stewart Peak	55	13,983	San Juan
Columbia Point	56	13,980	Sangre De Cristo
Pigeon Peak	57	13,972	San Juan
Mount Ouray	58	13,971	Sawatch
Fletcher Mountain	59	13,951	Tenmile
Ice Mountain	60	13,951	Sawatch
Gemini Peak		13,951	Mosquito
Pacific Peak	61	13,950	Tenmile
Cathedral Peak	62	13943	Elk
French Mountain	63	13,940	Sawatch
Mount Hope	64	13,933	Sawatch
"Thunder Pyramid"	65	13,932	Elk
Mount Adams	66	13,931	Sangre De Cristo
Gladstone Peak	67	13,913	San Juan
Mount Meeker	68	13,911	Front
Casco Peak	69	13,908	Sawatch
Red Mountain A	70	13,908	Sangre De Cristo
Emerald Peak	71	13,904	Sawatch
Drift Peak		13,900	Tenmile
Horseshoe Mountain	72	13,898	Mosquito
"Phoenix Peak"	73	13,895	San Juan
Vermilion Peak	74	13,894	San Juan
Frasco Benchmark		13,876	Sawatch
Cronin Peak	75	13,870	Sawatch
Mount Buckskin	76	13,865	Mosquito
Vestal Peak	77	13,864	San Juan
Jones Mountain A	78	13,860	San Juan
North Apostle	79	13,860	Sawatch
Meeker Ridge		13,860	Front
Clinton Peak	80	13,857	Mosquito

Peak Name	Rank	Elevation	Range
Dyer Mountain	81	13,855	Mosquito
Crystal Peak	82	13,852	Tenmile
Traver Peak		13,852	Mosquito
Mount Edwards	83	13,850	Front
California Peak	84	13,849	Sangre De Cristo
Mount Oklahoma	85	13,845	Sawatch
Mount Spalding		13,842	Front
Atlantic Peak	86	13,841	Tenmile
Hagerman Peak	87	13,841	Elk
Half Peak	88	13,841	San Juan
Turret Peak	89	13,835	San Juan
Unnamed Peak 13,832	90	13,832	San Juan
Holy Cross Ridge	91	13,831	Sawatch
Iowa Peak		13,831	Sawatch
Jupiter Mountain	92	13,830	San Juan
"Huerfano Peak"	93	13,828	Sangre De Cristo
Jagged Mountain	94	13,824	San Juan
"Lackawanna Peak"	95	13,823	Sawatch
Mount Silverheels	96	13,822	Front
Rio Grande Pyramid	97	13,821	San Juan
Teakettle Mountain	98	13,819	San Juan
Unnamed Peak 13,811	99	13,811	San Juan
Dallas Peak	100	13,809	San Juan

Appendix D

Works Consulted/Recommended Reading

Arps, Louisa Ward and Elinor Eppich Kingery. *Rocky Mountain National Park High Country Names.* Boulder, Colorado: Johnson Publishing Company, 1972.

Benson, Maxine. *1001 Colorado Place Names.* Kansas City: University of Kansas Press, 1994.

Bright, Wiliam, *Colorado Place Names.* Boulder, Colorado: Johnson Publishing Company, 2004.

Eberhart, Perry and Philip Schmuck. *The Fourteeners: Colorado's Great Mountains.* Chicago: The Swallow Press Inc, 1970.

Gebhardt, Dennis. *A Backpacking Guide to the Weminuche Wilderness.* Durango, Colorado: Basin Printing Company, 1976.

Graydon, Don and Kurt Hanson, eds. *Mountaineering: The Freedom of the Hills.* Seattle: The Mountaineers Books, 1998.

Houston, Charles. *Going Higher: Oxygen, Man and Mountains.* Seattle: The Mountaineers Books, 2005.

Johnson, Kirk R. and Robert G. Raynolds. *Ancient Denvers: Scenes from the Past 300 Million Years of the Colorado Front Range.* Denver: Denver Museum of Nature and Science, 2006.

Schimelpfenig, Todd and Linda Lindsey. *NOLS Wilderness First Aid.* Lander, Wyoming: Stackpole Books, 2000.

Wilkerson, James A. *Medicine for Mountaineering and Other Wilderness Activities.* Seattle: The Mountaineers Books, 2001.

Online Sites Consulted

14ers.com
A thorough and active community all about Colorado's 14,000-foot peaks. Maps, route descriptions, and thousands of trip accounts, not to mention lively message boards (I post there from time to time as well).

Mountainous Words
mountainouswords.com
My personal writing site that features additional hikes, trip reports, and more.

Summitpost
summitpost.org
This website is made up of user-contributed information about mountains, hikes, routes, and trailheads. Most of it is very reliable, though there are occasional inaccuracies and misinformation.

Wikipedia
wikipedia.org
Another user-contributed site, I found it useful as a starting point for a lot of information on the natural world, such as wildlife, the Laramide Orogeny, plant life, the Colorado Mineral Belt, and mining history. It's not perfect, but it's a great place to begin your research.

National Park Service
nps.gov
This is the official (if rather dry) source for websites for America's national parks.

Index

Your car-camping guide to scenic beauty, the sounds of nature, and an escape from civilization

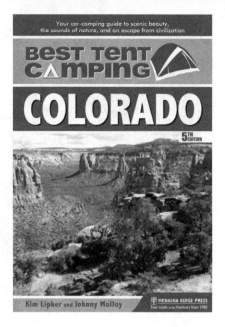

MENASHA RIDGE PRESS
Your Guide to the Outdoors Since 1982

Best Tent Camping:

Colorado

By Kim Lipker and Johnny Molloy
ISBN: 978-0-89732-990-3
5th Edition

6x9, 176 pages
maps, photos
$15.95

The Colorado landscape is rich with opportunities for tent camping. Millions of acres of public lands are dotted with hundreds of campgrounds—but you probably only have a precious amount of limited time. Which campgrounds do you choose? Where should you go? When should you go? That's what this book is for—to help you make the wisest use of your time in the wilds of the Centennial State.

Whether it's a large family looking to get away for the weekend, a scout troop that wants to try something new, or a serious outdoors enthusiast searching for a place to adventure for the day and crash for the night, *Best Tent Camping: Colorado* has done all the work in finding those special, out-of-the-way campgrounds and gives campers the tools to plan an amazing, unforgettable camping trip.

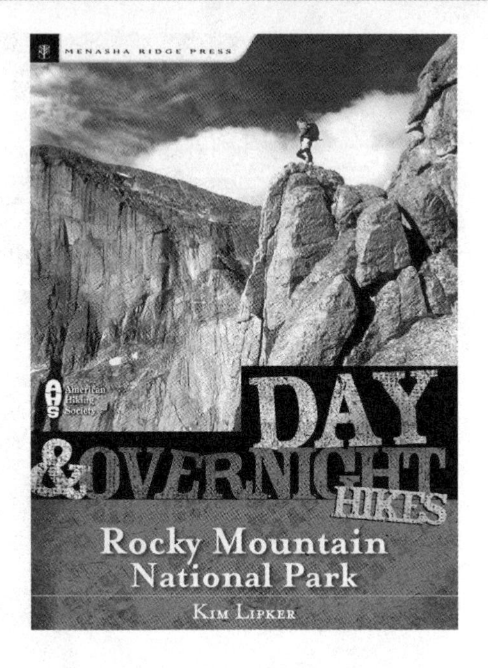

Day & Overnight Hikes:

Rocky Mountain National Park

By Kim Lipker	5x7, 190 pages
ISBN: 978-0-89732-655-1	maps, photos
1st Edition	$15.95

Choosing the best day and overnight hikes from the 359 miles of hiking trails and 200 backcountry sites is a major mission. Get on the trail faster with the confidence that you've made the right choice by referencing *Day & Overnight Hikes: Rocky Mountain National Park*. This guide includes original GPS-based trail maps, detailed trail descriptions, overnight camping recommendations, trail guides suitable for different experience levels, and more.

This guide is perfect for those wanting to get out on the trail for some much needed solitude or for those with families looking for something to do together. So hit the trails and have some fun.

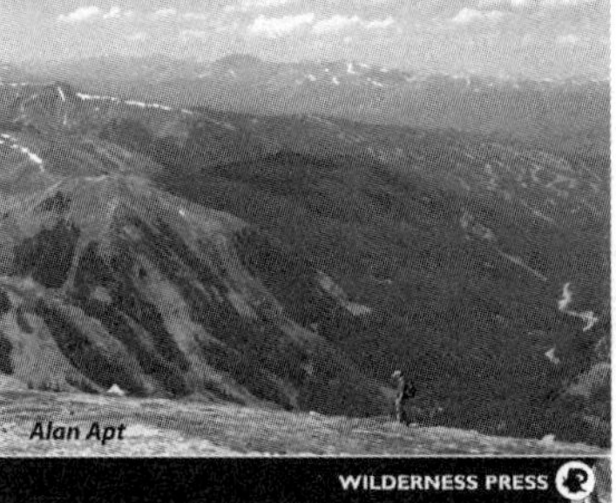

Afoot & Afield: Denver/Boulder & Colorado's Front Range

By Alan Apt	6x9, 360 pages
ISBN: 978-0-89997-406-4	maps, photos
1st Edition	$19.95

Afoot & Afield: Denver/Boulder & Colorado's Front Range takes hikers throughout the Colorado Rocky Mountains and their foothills, rivers, and plains. Featuring more than 200 trips, from trails near the state's Wyoming border to Pikes Peak near Colorado Springs, author Alan Apt maps out hikes both long and short, exploring trails accessible from Denver, Boulder, and other Front Range communities.

- Highlights summarize the best features of each trip, which range from convenient day hikes to weekend excursions. Easy-to-read maps, plus complete trip descriptions and hiking directions, make sure that hikers find their way.
- More than 200 hikes, ranging from short day hikes to long weekend treks, are each featured on a trail map.
- Each trip includes at-a-glance essential information—distance, time, elevation change, and difficulty rating.
- Additional trail-use information, such as which trails are suitable for children, dogs, horseback riding, and mountain bikes, is included.

A Pilgrim in Chinese Culture

Faith Meets Faith

An Orbis Series in Interreligious Dialogue
Paul F. Knitter, General Editor

In the contemporary world, the many religions and spiritualities stand in need of greater communication and cooperation. More than ever before, they must speak to, learn from, and work with each other in order both to maintain their vital identities and to contribute to fashioning a better world.

FAITH MEETS FAITH seeks to promote interreligious dialogue by providing an open forum for exchanges among followers of different religious paths. While the Series wants to encourage creative and bold responses to questions arising from contemporary appreciations of religious plurality, it also recognizes the multiplicity of basic perspectives concerning the methods and content of interreligious dialogue.

Although rooted in a Christian theological perspective, the Series does not endorse any single school of thought or approach. By making available to both the scholarly community and the general public works that represent a variety of religious and methodological viewpoints, FAITH MEETS FAITH seeks to foster an encounter among followers of the religions of the world on matters of common concern.

FAITH MEETS FAITH SERIES

近鄰

A Pilgrim in Chinese Culture

Negotiating Religious Diversity

JUDITH A. BERLING

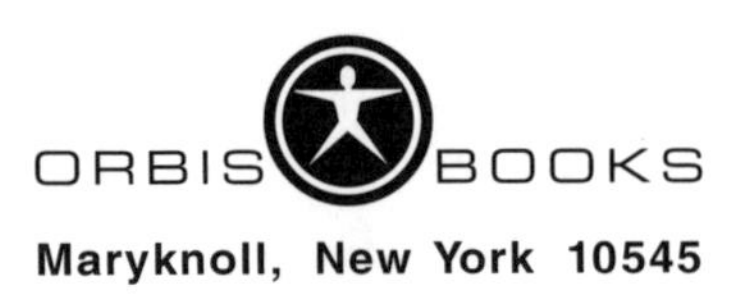

Maryknoll, New York 10545

The Catholic Foreign Mission Society of America (Maryknoll) recruits and trains people for overseas missionary service. Through Orbis Books, Maryknoll aims to foster the international dialogue that is essential to mission. The books published, however, reflect the opinions of their authors and are not meant to represent the official position of the society.

Published by Orbis Books, Maryknoll, NY 10545-0308

Manufactured in the United States of America

Library of Congress Cataloging-in-Publication Data

Berling, Judith A.
A Pilgrim in Chinese culture : [Chin lin] : negotiating religious diversity / Judith A. Berling.
p. cm. — (Faith meets faith series)
Includes index.
Parallel title in Chinese characters.
ISBN 1-57075-152-8 (alk. paper)
1. China—Religion. 2. China—Religious life and customs.
I. Title. II. Series: Faith meets faith.
BL1802.B47 1997
299'.51—dc21 97-30863
CIP

Contents

Prologue

In 1987 after twelve years of teaching Chinese religions in the Religious Studies department of Indiana University, I assumed the position of Dean and Vice President for Academic Affairs of the Graduate Theological Union (GTU).[1] This was more than a change of jobs; it was in several respects a fundamental move in my life.

The most obvious move was institutional—from a state university to a consortium of theological schools. The GTU (sometimes known informally as God Talk Unlimited) is comprised of nine theological schools (three Roman Catholic, one Episcopalian, one Unitarian-Universalist, four Protestant), with centers and institutes adding Jewish, Eastern Orthodox, and Buddhist voices, as well as those of Pacific and Asian Christians. The GTU is ecumenically structured, following the lines of religious diversity; each school or center is an autonomous institution which represents a particular voice or viewpoint. The GTU has a firm commitment to maintaining the independence and particular mission of each of the member institutions. The GTU is founded on the conviction that bringing diverse religious perspectives into dialogue in denominationally based curricula creates extraordinary theological education. In our daily life together we also come to know intimately the challenges of religious difference. Through our experience, we become adept at what I have termed "daily ecumenism," the sensitivities, mutual understanding, and skills required to negotiate religious difference as part of our common life.

The move to the GTU was also geographic, a shift from the Midwest to Northern California, from the Bible Belt to the Pacific Rim. Although every corner of U.S. culture is increasingly marked by cultural diversity, such diversity is particularly vibrant in Northern California. As many have noted, California's demography is a window on the American future, for the coming century will be increasingly dominated by Pacific economies and cultures. As Europe was once the world's center of gravity, in the next century we will increasingly look to Asia. As a scholar of Chinese religions, the promise of a Pacific century fascinates me—the implications for our culture are myriad. The diversity of Northern California is not simply cultural or ethnic; it is also religious. Its religious landscape goes far beyond Jews and Christians to include Hindus, Muslims, Sikhs, Buddhists, Afro-Brazilian cults, new

age groups, Druids, and a host of others. Living in Northern California brings the issue of diversity—both cultural and religious—very close to home. Californians are beginning to realize the implications of the world into which we are moving.

The move was also a move from religious studies to theological education. The shift of context from university to theological school entailed a serious reconsideration of the focus of my teaching and writing. The theological world demanded that I locate myself and my commitments and that I address the religious issues vital to theological studies. My thirty-year pilgrimage in Chinese studies could no longer be cast as study *about* Chinese religions, as many in religious studies would have it[2]; I was now faced with the implications of the study of Chinese religions for my own faith and for other persons of faith. I was asked not only what I knew *about* China, but also what I as a person of faith had learned *from* China.

As a teacher I have always sought to bring Chinese religions alive for my students. My twelve years at Indiana University convinced me that teaching Asian religions was a fundamental contribution to helping Americans learn to live in a pluralistic world.[3] My move to theological education, however, challenged me to articulate the implications of my work for those studying and working within the context of religious communities.

It has taken me some time to find my *theological* voice as a scholar of Chinese religions. First, I had to be clear that I am not a spokesperson for Chinese religions. As deeply as I have been enriched by my encounters with Chinese religions on all levels, I am neither Chinese nor a follower of any Chinese tradition. I have gained much in the way of wisdom and spiritual insight from Chinese teachers, living and dead, to whom I defer for faithful interpretations of the spiritual core of their traditions. My role is to assist others to understand Chinese religions, serving as a cultural bridge by invoking the authoritative voices of Chinese masters and explaining the context in which they taught and practiced.[4] My community and my audience is that of North American Christians; I want to help them to understand and appreciate the spiritual practices of the Chinese with "joy and equality."[5]

Second, as one who has learned the languages, struggled with the texts, and considered the complexities of Chinese history, I aim to provide textured accounts of how practices, ideas, or institutions functioned in their cultural settings. Ideas or practices lifted from a cultural setting may seem more accessible, but they can seriously mislead and compound misunderstandings. Although I want to help theological colleagues learn *from* and not just *about* Chinese religions, I am aware of the dangers of not attending carefully to the distinctively Chinese. One must look and listen carefully, seeking to understand the Chinese as much as possible on their own terms, before jumping to

the stage of drawing lessons for oneself. Learning from another cultural and religious tradition requires respect and a willingness to stretch the horizons of understanding, to seek to imagine how their world and their faith looks to them.

Not wanting to speak for the Chinese but wanting to honor the rich cultural context, I have chosen in this book, and in my teaching and writing generally, to rely heavily on stories, both historical and based on personal experience. Stories have the advantage of creating a narrative world, a context.[6] A tale, like a biography, "forms a kind of looking-glass which enables readers to peer into—and step through into—another world."[7]

My tales are deliberately chosen to represent different times and places, to offer a range of perspectives on the diversity and richness of traditional Chinese religious practices. They include tales of my own experience (in which I am both a participant and the narrator) and tales told from the viewpoint of some particular person, event, or period in Chinese history. The book is structured thematically rather than historically, suggesting the development of my insights into Chinese religious life, as I have reconstructed them ex post facto. I have deliberately juxtaposed figures and events from different historical settings when they seem to speak to a common theme. On the other hand, tales are told with some attempt to convey their location and specificity. I do not attempt an encompassing narrative which would convey "Chinese religions" or the relationship of Chinese religiosity and Christianity.[8] The tales are intentionally fragmentary and specific, glimpses into another religious world, but not a comprehensive portrait.

My use of stories is, at least implicitly, a dialogical method for imparting information—a story assumes an audience. It invites the audience into the narrative world, inviting them to imaginatively "try on" an aspect of Chinese culture, and empowering them as observers and interpreters of that world. Through the use of stories I seek both to engage the readers' interest and also to invite them to draw their own interpretations, particularly as to how the Chinese stories might relate to their own lives.

The development of these stories and this manuscript has also been dialogical in practice; without the aid of valued colleagues, who kindly acted as my audience and my critics, this book would never have been written.

My primary dialogue partner has been Margaret McLean, who has worked with me as a Newhall fellow[9] for five years, developing this and other manuscripts. Margaret is a specialist in health care ethics, not a scholar of Chinese studies. That choice was intentional, since the audience for this book was to be outside of the Chinese field. Margaret has pushed me to identify and address my new audience. She has been an extraordinary critic and collaborator, muse and drill sergeant

(keeping me on track and marching to cadence). Margaret's role in this project has been central; she is a full partner.

Jim Emerson, a friend and colleague from the GTU Board of Trustees, offered thoughtful comments on an early draft. Kevin Cheng, a GTU doctoral student from Hong Kong, served as a research assistant on an early draft, tracking down additional references and sources.

Thanks to Kevin Koczela for producing the models of the Chinese religious field in chapter 2.

In January 1994, Margaret and I took the manuscript formally to an "audience" by convening a Round Table of GTU faculty and doctoral students: Michael Aune, Dwight Hopkins, Mary Beth Lamb, Kenan Osborne, Kathryn Poethig, and Susan Smith. These stalwart colleagues discussed the manuscript for an entire day, offering extraordinary insights and encouragement for the work. Their comments sharpened the focus of this book.

During the fall semester of 1995, as the Ann Potter Wilson Distinguished Visiting Professor at the Divinity School at Vanderbilt University, I offered a doctoral seminar on the book manuscript. Six outstanding students—Emily Askew, Judith Bishop, Laurel Cassidy, Melissa Stewart, Minette Watkins, and Zhao Zuo—took this course, offering lively and insightful reactions to the manuscript.

In the spring semester of 1996, the manuscript was one of the texts for a reading course on Chinese religious practice taken by Geoff Foy and Denis Thalson at GTU. Their comments and responses were also immensely helpful.

I have shaped the stories to the responses of these audiences throughout the text and have sought to include their voices, particularly in the last chapter of reflections, in order to help to open up the tales to the readers' thoughts and interpretations.

The book is a collection of tales brought back from China by a pilgrim whose life has been profoundly enriched by her journey. Some of the tales are direct reports of my adventures in Taiwan; others are adventures I had in texts or in the course of study. All pertain, directly or indirectly, to the issue of living with religious diversity. They recount the examples which helped me appreciate Chinese strategies for living with religious neighbors, beginning from a premise of religious inclusivity (many Ways are valid) rather than exclusivity (there is only one true faith).

The book is organized in three sections. The first introduces the origins of my engagement with the issue of religious diversity and inclusivity, the shape of my pilgrimage in China, and my particular stance as an author. Chapter 1 introduces the concept of religious diversity and why it has become a central issue for me. Chapter 2 introduces my pilgrimage and how its meaning is shaped by Chinese notions of religious journey. Chapter 3 identifies my particular interpretive

stance and distinguishes it from that of others who have sought to include interfaith views within Christian ecumenism.

The second section contains key tales from Chinese culture. Chapter 4 offers the notion of "religious field" as a way of modeling the dynamics of religious pluralism in Chinese culture. Chapter 5 explores the tensions between government and local communities over who governs the rules of play on the Chinese religious field. Chapter 6 speaks of how the myriad gods and deities in China are related to a transcendent spiritual unity. Chapter 7 discusses the distinctive Chinese notion of Truth as having many different embodiments. Chapter 8 discusses the patterns of hospitality which sustain a fragile balance of diverse religious communities in Chinese life.

The third section (chapter 9) invites readers to join in some reflections, to consider what insights the Chinese tales may offer us about living with religious diversity. This section begins the process of opening the stories from China to a range of reactions and interpretations from the cultural standpoint of North American Christians, seeing whether the alternative model presented by China does indeed help us to see with fresh eyes new possibilities for our own traditions.

Explanations for the Chinese characters that accompany each chapter appear at the foot of the first page of the chapter.

Time Line

Note on Chinese Romanization: This book uses the Wade-Giles system of Romanization of Chinese rather than the Pinyin system currently used in newspapers and periodicals because the bulk of research on traditional Chinese religions is still in Wade-Giles.

Shang Dynasty **c. 1523-1122 B.C.E.**	System of priest-kings preserved on oracle bones
Chou Dynasty **1122-256 B.C.E.** **(Warring States)** **(403-221 B.C.E.)**	Confucius, 551-479 B.C.E. Mencius, 372?-289? B.C.E. Chuang Tzu, 369?-286? B.C.E. Lao Tzu, Sixth century, or Third century B.C.E.
Ch'in Dynasty **221-209 B.C.E.**	Burning of the books
Former and Later Han **206 B.C.E. - 8 C.E.** **23-202 C.E.**	Han historians, First century B.C.E.; First century C.E. Tung Chung-shu, 179?-104? B.C.E. Chang Tao-ling, Second century C.E.
Period of Disunity **202-589 C.E.**	Hsü Sun, 239-292 Monk Hui-yüan, 334-417 Neo-Taoists
Sui Dynasty **589-618**	Emperor Yang-ti, r. 605-616
T'ang Dynasty **618-907**	Monk Yüan-chien Monk Hsüan-tsang (Tripitika), ca. 596-664

	Veneration of Hsü Sun Han Yü, 786-824 Monk Ennin, 798-864 Edict on Persecution of Buddhism, 845
Sung Dynasty 960-1279	Emperor Chen-tsung, r. 998-1022 Su Shih, 1037-1101 Liu Yi-chih, 1078-1160 Emperor Hui-tsung, r. 1102-1125 Chu Hsi, 1130-1200 Pai Yü-ch'an, 1194-1229 Li Ch'en, 1144-1218 Ch'iao Li-hsien, 1155-1222 Ch'en Nan (Ni-wan), 1171?-1213
Chin (Jurchen) Dynasty 1115-1234	
Yüan (Mongol) Dynasty 1260-1368	
Ming Dynasty 1368-1644	Emperor Ming T'ai-tsu, r. 1368-1398 Wang Yang-ming, 1472-1529 Wu Ch'eng-en, c. 1500-1582 Lin Chao-en, 1517-1598 Cho Wan-ch'un, Sixteenth century Li Chih, 1527-1602 White Lotus movements strong
Ch'ing (Manchu) Dynasty 1644-1912	
Republican Period 1912-1949	
People's Republic of China 1949-present	

A Pilgrim in Chinese Culture

CHAPTER 1

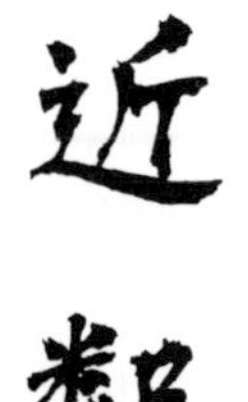

Living with Religious Neighbors

But the lawyer, desiring to justify himself, said to Jesus, "And who is my neighbor?"

(Luke 10:29)

Over the past few years I have heard three stories which touched a deep vein of hope all too often obscured by the contention of the 1990s.

Catholics and Buddhists

> A Portuguese Catholic friend told me of a special Portuguese saints' day at a Bay Area parish during which the faithful deck the saints in flowers and carry them in the procession through the neighborhoods around the church. Vietnamese Buddhists who had settled in the community saw this festival, and it reminded them of their Buddhist festivals wherein they deck the Buddha-images with flowers and parade them through the neighborhood. Seeing a familiar religious practice, the Buddhists joined in the Catholic festival, and an interfaith friendship was begun.

"Close Neighbor"
Literally, nearby village, and by extension, neighbors. The term would include those with whom one had regular encounters (at markets, etc.), but were the members of one's own clan.

近鄰

Tlingits and Russian Orthodox

> On a visit to Sitka, Alaska, I learned that when the Russian settlers married into native Tlingit clans, they devised an ingenious way to honor both native and Russian Orthodox traditions for funerals: the funeral would begin in the Tlingit long-house with traditional ceremonies and then would solemnly process to the Orthodox church for a funeral. A shared tradition of funerary processions helped to tie together the long-house ceremonies and the Orthodox funeral.

Evangelical Christians and the Chinese Moon Festival

> After a lecture I gave at Western Illinois University, an evangelical Christian shared with me that their church had opened a center for international students, including students from China. In order to make the Chinese students feel more welcome, she told me, the church had invited the Chinese to celebrate their Moon Festival with the members of the local congregation.

These three stories represent relatively rare successes at bridging religious boundaries, opening communities in our increasingly diverse society to the richness of living with religious neighbors. The troubling question is, why are such stories so rare?

One answer is that the scope of religious diversity in our society has expanded. Where U.S. society could once be appropriately analyzed in terms of *Protestant, Catholic, Jew,*[1] such a depiction would now not only be simplistic, it would be downright inaccurate. As Diana Eck has noted, "By the 1990s, there were Hindus, Sikhs, Buddhists, and Jains. There were more Muslims than Episcopalians, more Muslims than Presbyterians, perhaps soon more Muslims than Jews." In her Harvard classes in the 1990s, she was struck that the representatives of "Asian" religions were now American citizens. "There were Muslims from Providence, Hindus from Baltimore, Sikhs from Chicago, Jains from New Jersey. They represented the emergence in America of a new cultural and religious reality."[2] Our communities, our schools, our workplaces, our hospitals, and even our families are increasingly interreligious.[3] Moreover, as Eck's article points out, we can no longer neatly relegate those "other religions" to other parts of the world.

> Today, the Islamic world is no longer somewhere else, in some other part of the world; instead, Chicago with its 50 mosques and nearly half a million Muslims is part of the Islamic world.

> America today is part of the Islamic, the Hindu, the Confucian world. It is precisely the interpenetration of ancient civilizations and cultures that is the hallmark of the late twentieth century. *This* is our new georeligious reality. The map of the world in which we now live cannot be color-coded as to its Christian, Muslim, or Hindu identity, but each part of the world is marbled with the colors and textures of the whole.[4]

近鄰

More clearly than ever before in history, these folks are indeed our religious neighbors, not only globally, but also locally. Yet Christians and Jews have developed few positive resources for understanding and developing positive relationships with religious neighbors; we still carry the weight of centuries (if not millennia) of exclusivistic attitudes and patterns of association.

One has only to open a daily newspaper to grasp that religious difference is a volatile—even a deadly—force in our contemporary world: in Rwanda, Bosnia-Herzegovina, the former Soviet Union, the Arab states, and Israel. In the United States, tensions between Native American religious groups and the courts, between African-Americans and Jews, and between pro-life and pro-choice forces all have religious undercurrents. Too often we see religion as a force which divides us into hostile camps. The response is either to pull back into our own community and raise the fences higher, or to leave religion behind altogether. Neither strategy will help us to negotiate religious diversity. We need to find some ground of mutual respect and genuine conversation with neighbors from many traditions and cultural backgrounds, a ground from which we can join in the effort to face the deep ethical and spiritual issues confronting humankind.[5]

In his book *Race Matters*, Cornel West has commented on the racial and religious strains between American blacks and Jews:

> The present impasse in black-Jewish relations will be overcome only when self-critical exchanges take place within and across black and Jewish communities not simply about their own group interest but also, and, more importantly, about what being black or Jewish means in *ethical terms*. This kind of reflection should not be so naive as to ignore group interest, but it should take us to a higher moral ground where serious discussions about democracy and justice determine how we define ourselves and our politics and help us formulate strategies and tactics to sidestep the traps of tribalism and chauvinism.[6]

West argues that the ethical identity of blacks is rooted in religion and music. He writes: "The best of black culture, as manifested, for example, in jazz or the prophetic black church, refuses to put whites or

近鄰

Jews on a pedestal or in the gutter" (114). West's book is important for many reasons, but one of them is that he articulates the moral, religious, and cultural dimensions of tensions too often dismissed as merely racial or political. Moreover, he notes that religion can be a key part of the solution, and not simply a part of the problem. Religion contains the best of our cultures, even if we do not always act upon the best in our religions.

We must learn to live with religious difference, or else the fabric of our society will be rent asunder; the rich tapestry of U.S. culture will fray into a mass of tangled threads. This is an issue about which I care, worry, and pray, and to which I dedicate my work, including this book.

Several formative encounters with "difference" led me to the study of traditional Chinese religions, where I discovered a rich alternative model for understanding religious diversity.

Encounters with Difference and Discovery of China

When I was ten years old, my family moved from the northern Midwest to the boot heel of Missouri in the deep South. The year was 1955, the year of *Brown vs. the Board of Education.* At the turbulent beginning of the Civil Rights Movement, we were Yankees in the South. I was just old enough to experience this as a severe culture shock. If I ever had views of a single "American" culture, my experience in the South undermined them. I was deeply attracted to parts of Southern culture and profoundly confused by or resistant to others; but through it all, I knew I was a Yankee and did not belong.

After a year in Missouri, my family moved to Dubuque, Iowa. As Presbyterians in Roman Catholic Dubuque (75 percent Catholic and known as "little Rome"), we were members of a religious minority. In Dubuque, church and church-related activities mattered: pre-Vatican II Dubuque was still fighting the Reformation; everyone in town could identify Protestant and Catholic properties and businesses; and there were street fights between Catholic and Protestant youth.[7] If you were a Dubuque Protestant, you knew the doctrinal and liturgical reasons why. Church and church-related activities were the nexus of social as well as religious life, since the Protestant leaders wanted to keep the youth not only in the church, but in the right church! Accordingly, I was deeply involved in church activities, concerned to locate myself in this world of religious competition, so that I could maintain my heritage, which I, of course, was convinced was the right one.

Caught up in the ecumenical fervor surrounding Vatican II, I majored in religion at Carleton College in Northfield, Minnesota. For two years, I belonged to a student team ministry which served as the collective (unordained) pastor of a tiny United Church of Christ parish in

Zumbrota, Minnesota. I was headed for Union Theological Seminary in New York, and ordination. However, two experiences transformed my tidy world. First, one Sunday in 1966, I took a close college friend with me to the church in Zumbrota. My friend was Japanese. Takashi was an articulate, gentle Christian, and I was completely unprepared for how he would be received in Zumbrota.

I brought him to the church to meet the parishioners and to share something of his faith journey and his cultural background. The parishioners, however, were stiff and uncomfortable with him, and one began a question with, "Why do you Japs . . . ?" To my shock and chagrin, these good Christian folk unabashedly laid on him their angry stereotypes of Asians. Both he and I came away more than a little shaken. I had become increasingly aware of racism as a cancer in our society, but it had never shoved its face so forcefully into mine; this experience taught me profoundly about our culture's fear and ignorance of Asians.

Shortly thereafter, a course on Chinese religions dramatically opened up my world, putting me literally in awe of the depth and richness of this culture so little known and understood in the West. Here was an entire stream of cultural and spiritual heritage of which I had no inkling; my former vision of what it meant to be well learned and "cosmopolitan" was stretched until it burst like a bubble.[8] "Asia" was not absent from cultural parlance in the 1960s; at times it seemed that "Asia" was everywhere. There were at least three contending views of Asia in the U.S. culture of the 1960s, not one of them remotely accurate: not the stereotypes of Asians in the context of the Vietnam War; not the denunciations of experimentation with Eastern religions as "a loss of values"; and not the claims of pop culture to be "into" Eastern religions.

Perhaps because of my Dubuque experience, with its emphasis on religious identity and tradition as defining the boundaries of the "right" and "the normal," I became convinced that Americans needed a broader cultural and religious horizon in order to negotiate an increasingly diverse world. I was no longer comfortable in the worlds of Dubuque or Zumbrota. Because in Dubuque and Zumbrota, Asia was not really part of the world, it followed all too readily that Asians were not fully human, and Asian religions were construed either as exoticized rebellion or dangerous heresy. My experience of middle-America was that it was far from ready for what some now speak of as the "Pacific century," but even in the mid-1960s the Pacific was on the horizon, either as a promise or as a threat.

In that semester, in that course, my deepening sense of the injustice and ignorance of racism was dramatically juxtaposed to the broadening of my cultural and ethicospiritual horizons in the course on China. I had discovered a vocation, a significant lifetime undertaking. It be-

近鄰

came clear to me that through learning and teaching about China I could seek to perform a ministry which would work at eroding the foundations of racism and building the foundations of cross-cultural understanding.

As a junior, I dropped my plans for seminary and opted instead to study Chinese language, culture, and religion in a doctoral program at Columbia University in New York. I wanted to learn the language, immerse myself in the literature and history, live among the people, visit temples and experience the worship, in order to understand more fully the richness of the heritage; and then I wanted to interpret what I had learned for those who had not had such experiences first-hand. I sought to become a cultural bridge, one who could translate and interpret Chinese cultural values and beliefs in ways that would help others see their value and appreciate their contributions to the global heritage. In her writings Carter Heyward has linked the notion of a bridge to the ideal of transcendence. She writes, "To transcend means, literally, to cross over. To bridge. To make connections. To burst free of particular locations."[9] By becoming a bridge, I hoped to transcend and help others to transcend limited horizons, thereby advancing the cause of multicultural understanding, since mutual ignorance and suspicion seemed to be at the root of so much of the world's pain and injustice.

My sojourn into the depth and richness of Chinese culture did not uproot me from Western culture, but it put Western culture and its achievements into a fuller, more global context. It taught me at a deep level that the story of the West is not *the* font of human achievement, but is rather *one* story and source of human achievement. Seen in a global perspective, not only could the great achievements of Western culture be celebrated as *not inevitable*, and therefore remarkable, but also the failures or inadequacies of Western cultural history could be also seen as *not inevitable*, and therefore as examples of human fallibility from which humankind might learn.

China and Religious Diversity

My discovery of China was at first a simple but dramatic broadening of my cultural horizons, a call to a broader and more inclusive vision of the rich human heritage. However, as I experienced more of Chinese culture and religion, I began to understand my deeper attraction, what I sought in this foreign land. Traditional Chinese religion compelled my attention because of one striking characteristic: that while the Christian history of Europe and North America had been shaped by exclusivist and sectarian forces, the traditional history of Chinese religions had been based on the opposite, inclusivist, premise.

This premise was stated succinctly by the early student of Chinese religions, W. E. Soothill:

> While a few of the laity devote themselves, some solely to Buddhism, some solely to Taoism, the great mass of the people have no prejudices and make no embarrassing distinctions; they belong to none of the three religions [Buddhism, Taoism, or Confucianism], or, more correctly, they belong to all three. In other words, they are eclectic, and use whichever form best responds to the requirement of the occasion for which they use religion.[10]

This striking contrast to the patterns of the monotheistic cults of Christianity and Judaism created a very different cultural dynamic of religious diversity. Traditional Chinese life entailed a rich pattern of religious diversity. As Valerie Hansen has written:

> Temples dedicated to popular deities studded the medieval Chinese landscape. Contemporary writers pointed out that even the smallest villages contained more than one temple, while temples in the large cities numbered in the hundreds. The laity asked the gods to bring rain, to clear the skies, to drive out locusts, to expel bandits, to suppress uprisings, to cure illnesses, to enable them to conceive, to prevent epidemics, and to help them pass the civil service examinations.[11]

The diversity of religious groups and practices in every Chinese community constituted a rich religious field in which to pursue both worldly and other-worldly goals. Over the centuries, the Chinese developed strategies for living with religious diversity, and these strategies offer a suggestive alternative to the exclusivistic model for a religiously plural society, a hypothetical case that can help us to see new options and possibilities. The Chinese case invites us to ask a series of questions:

- What happens if a society starts from the premise of inclusivity, that religions are not mutually contradictory, and that multiple religious affiliation is not dangerous, but is perhaps the norm?
- What happens if religious organizations are hospitable to one another in order to create and sustain the larger community?
- What happens if a culture develops patterns to create and sustain mutual familiarity and regular interaction among members of various religious groups?

Traditional China does not hold all the answers to the challenge of religious diversity, but it provides a useful model for understanding what would be entailed in an inclusivist approach to religious difference.

This book shares what I have learned as a pilgrim in Chinese culture around the issues of religious diversity. Although my initial visit to East Asia was long ago, the pilgrimage has continued as I have pur-

近鄰

sued my studies. China is a rich and complex land with many faces; the stories of my pilgrimage and the tales of China will not all focus narrowly on diversity, but they will provide the context for understanding something of how and why the Chinese negotiated the religious differences in their culture. I hope that this book will open up horizons for those seeking to negotiate cultural and religious diversity more effectively.

The other two chapters in this section will help to situate this book and my stance as author. Chapter 2 will articulate how my nearly thirty years of study and travel have been a pilgrimage of self-discovery and broadening horizons. It will begin to identify the theological dimensions of the enterprise. Chapter 3 will locate my particular approach in this book among other approaches to interfaith understanding.

CHAPTER 2

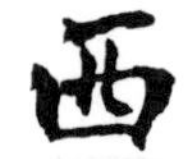

遊記

The Pilgrimage and the Pilgrim

She who would valiant be 'gainst all disaster,
let her in constancy follow the Master.
There's no discouragement
shall make her once relent
her first avowed intent
to be a pilgrim.

Who so beset her round with dismal stories,
do but themselves confound, her strength the more is.
No foes shall stay her might,
though she with giants fight;
she will make good her right
to be a pilgrim.

Since, Lord, thou dost defend us with thy Spirit,
we know we at the end shall life inherit.
Then fancies flee away;
I'll fear not what they say,
I'll labor night and day
to be a pilgrim.

—Percy Dearmer, after John Bunyan
Hymn #564, Episcopal Hymnal
(adapted for female "pilgrim")

"Journey to the West"
Journey to the West is the name of a popular Chinese novel, about a famous pilgrim's search for Buddhist truth on a trip to India, to be discussed in this chapter.

Pilgrimage to Lion's Head Mountain

In December 1971, I had been living in Taipei for three months, honing my spoken Chinese, studying calligraphy, visiting temples, observing traditional rituals, and collecting books on Chinese religion and culture. Just before Christmas, I asked my Taipei colleague Cynthia McLean to join me on a visit to Lion's Head Mountain (Shih T'ou Shan), a Buddhist pilgrimage site in central Taiwan. What started as a pleasant outing turned into an extraordinary adventure, a pilgrimage which provided a frame of meaning for my studies in Chinese culture.[1]

Taipei in the 1970s was brimming with traditional Chinese religious practices, but these were tucked into the corners and back alleys of a rapidly modernizing city. The journey to Shih T'ou Shan was, symbolically, a journey back to more traditional times. This was marked in part by our modes of transportation. We set out from Taipei on a rapid modern train, transferred to a nice bus, then transferred again to an old, rickety bus that carried almost as many chickens as people. The town at the base of Lion's Head Mountain still offered pedicabs as its primary mode of public transportation, and the town store (which catered mainly to pilgrims) lacked the amenities common to urban shops. The ladies room, for instance, was a privy adjacent to the pigsty, down a ladder below the shop, a clear signal that we were entering a different world.

As we left the town and started up the mountain, vestiges of the modern world faded, save for the watches and cameras of the pilgrims. The only paths were footpaths, and supplies were delivered by the traditional Chinese mode of slinging items from a long pole balanced across the shoulders. As the modern world receded, the world of traditional Buddhism and Chinese religions appeared before us. The mountain displayed a comprehensive vision of Chinese religious life, with multiple levels of faith, many streams of practice. As the pilgrims climbed, we advanced through layers of religious imagination, spiritual discipline, and symbolism. After devoting five years to the study of Chinese religions, I finally came to understand on this mountain that, for the Chinese, the many forms of religious expression were all aspects of a single Way.

At the first stop on the climb, easily accessible to all visitors, there were attractions for the children. Most striking, in 1971, was a tiny coin-operated carousel of flags of the United Nations,[2] and another carousel depicting the Eight Immortals of "Taoist" folk religion.[3] At this stop, grannies, aunts, or big sisters were left to mind the small children, while others continued up the path. But even at this "children's corner" the carousels taught basic principles of Chinese religion: patriotic virtue—in this case as Chinese citizens of the world

—and belief in spirits who can grant boons such as long life. They may not have come far, but all pilgrims who made it to this first stop had "entered the way," and would receive religious merit for their journey.

The subsequent gradual climb featured scenic views and eventually offered a vision of a temple ornately decorated with colored carved glass. The hips of the roof and every inch of eaves, pillars, and rafters pulsed with colorful carvings, statues, and paintings of popular Chinese folk deities. Closer inspection revealed walls covered with grisly scenes of sinners' torments in hell. Pilgrims could contemplate all this from comfortable benches while enjoying a snack blessed by a deity.

This temple displayed the basic premise of Chinese folk traditions: moral retribution for sins and reward for good deeds. The deities of the temple could assist the faithful in their struggle to defeat the powers of evil and ally themselves with the powers of good. The elaborate decorations caught the attention of the pilgrims, and the entire temple functioned as a text, a pedagogical tool. The illustrated myths and tales served as mnemonic or pedagogical devices for Chinese folk beliefs; even the illiterate (and they were legion in traditional China) could "read" this temple, provided they had at some time heard the tales from a family member or priest or seen them performed in a temple or village drama. They learned their religion by "reading" the text of temple paintings to reinforce what they had heard in story or drama. Such illustrated tales were the primary form of religious and moral education in traditional China.[4] Pilgrims at this temple imbibed the lessons of basic Chinese religious belief and were invited to make or renew a fundamental commitment to do good deeds. Thus they would seek the help of the gods to avoid the torments of hell so graphically depicted on the walls of this temple, and to win rebirth in heaven, as depicted on the main altars.

As we left this temple and ascended the steep path along increasingly dramatic mountain vistas, the crowd of pilgrims began to thin. Each new temple was less colorful and folksy; the number and density of illustrations waned; interiors grew dim; and deities represented higher ranks in the Buddhist pantheon. Taoist and folk deities had by and large disappeared. Gilt images of Buddhas and Bodhisattvas shone mysteriously in the dim light of rooms redolent of generations of incense. The long vistas and the silent temples drew pilgrims symbolically into the dual cultivation of Buddhist wisdom. Buddhist practice produces both insight or vision (*kuan*) and stillness or quiescence (*chih*). The sweeping scenic expanses on the way up the mountain symbolized the development of broader insight or vision, while the silent dimness of the temples evoked stillness. These well-placed mountain shrines offered a foretaste of the fruits of this religious path, in which adepts cultivate insight and quiescence through the discipline of meditation.

After a rigorous climb to a spot near the peak of the mountain, the few remaining pilgrims reached an active monastery where pilgrims could stay, for a modest offering, as long as we observed the monastic schedule of the monks during the visit (bath, vegetarian meal, vespers, early bed, predawn worship, vegetarian breakfast). My friend and I gladly accepted the hospitality offered. During meals we had opportunity to chat with the monks and the abbot about Buddhist teachings and life. An overnight stay in the monastery gave us a taste of the monastic path: the order and ascetic simplicity of daily life; the monotonous vegetarian meals, which gradually weaned monks from the delights of the world; the quiet pleasures of regular worship; the steady focus on spiritual formation through every activity. The abbot was a delightful host who emanated great joy and peace. His warmth and gentle instruction made us wish for a longer visit, even though we were not sure that we could long sustain the rigors of monastic life.

I was thrilled when, as I made ready to depart, the abbot offered me a parting gift of Buddhist scriptures hand-copied by the monks. His gift not only honored my willingness to learn about his faith, but also made me a "real" Buddhist pilgrim. In historical times, the Chinese emperors commissioned famous monks (like Hsüan-tsang [c. 596-664], immortalized in the novel *Journey to the West*) to undertake pilgrimages to India to collect and bring back to China Buddhist scriptures. Later Japanese Buddhist monks such as Ennin (798-864) came to China seeking Buddhist scriptures to take to Japan. More than a thousand years later, this abbot offered me hand-copied Buddhist scriptures as a token of my pilgrimage, assimilating me into a long line of pilgrims who had sought truth in faraway Buddhist monasteries.

After we bid our reluctant farewells, Cynthia and I chose to descend the mountain by the back way, and so experienced yet another dimension of Buddhist life and practice. Although it looked equal on the pilgrim's map we had purchased in town, the back way was in fact longer and more arduous, dotted with lonely hermitages of monks who had withdrawn into solitude for a period of silent contemplation and prayer. Several hermits had carved stone or wooden images of Buddhas in the walls of their caves or huts to provide them with spiritual companionship. If the front mountain path represented the way of communal and organized Buddhism, the rear path represented the solitary quest for realization of the Buddhist Way.

The Buddhists, in their distinctive fashion, did not explain the different levels of practice and iconography depicted on the various paths and by-ways of the mountain.[5] Yet the lessons were not lost on us or other pilgrims. The visual contrasts created strikingly different atmospheres of Chinese folk religion, Taoist worship, and Buddhist piety, which combined to depict a religious path with many layers of symbolism and practice, all of which, however, advanced one on the Way.

The Buddhists on this mountain, like many other schools or centers of Chinese religion, had absorbed into their religious vision a version of the entire Chinese religious field; all paths, they suggested, help the faithful in their spiritual progress.

西遊記

This journey helped me understand Chinese religious life; such was the major purpose of my stay in Taiwan. Yet for many years after that visit to Lion's Head Mountain, my thoughts returned to the days on that mountain with a persistent question: What had been the meaning of my pilgrimage? Why did I take it? Why, in fact, had I undertaken the study of Chinese religions? The journey to Shih T'ou Shan brought home to me that I was in Chinese culture as a pilgrim. What was I seeking there? What did I hope to bring back?

To Be a Pilgrim

The story of how I came to study Chinese religions provides a context of meaning for my pilgrimage to Lion's Head Mountain and in Chinese culture. This pilgrimage was first and foremost an intellectual sojourn, the project of a historian of Chinese religions. I had devoted myself to the study of Chinese religions and cultures. After four years of language study and course work at Columbia, I went to East Asia to write my dissertation, but also to experience and observe first-hand everything I could of Chinese religious life and practice. I frequented temples, festivals, and rituals, knowing that first-hand observation of religion would flesh out the picture I had gleaned from formal study. This was particularly important, since my classes at Columbia had focused on Chinese thought and history, not on the practices of Chinese religious life.[6] In Taiwan I had wonderful opportunities to observe the living practice of Chinese religions, to put the ideas and texts into the context of actual human behavior.

The pilgrimage was also, in a somewhat larger sense, a broadening of my cultural horizons, an extension of my experience and vision of the richness of the human heritage. My nearly three years in Asia during the research and writing of my dissertation offered an opportunity to steep myself in the art, literature, food, social patterns, and religions of East Asia: Taiwan, Japan, Korea, and Hong Kong. The experience of living in Taiwan stretched me in many ways. After some difficult adjustments, I began to feel comfortable—almost at home—in many aspects of East Asian culture. The pilgrimage to Lion's Head Mountain was an important piece of opening myself to the horizons of Chinese culture; never before or after did I immerse myself so completely in a traditional Chinese context. There were, for example, no modern amenities nor any English speakers, except Cynthia and myself, on Lion's Head Mountain. For this period, at least, I entered

fully into a traditional Chinese setting. Thus my assimilation into the traditional pattern of the Buddhist pilgrim through the gift of the scriptures from the abbot was a kind of seal of this crossing of boundaries. Accepted into the company of Chinese Buddhist pilgrims, even temporarily, I had tangible confirmation that my cultural horizons had expanded. My world had grown to encompass realities from long ago and across the great waters.[7]

But if my pilgrimage had yielded intellectual understanding and expansion of my cultural horizons, it also had deeper implications. As I learned about Chinese religions, I also came to understand the deeper implications of my wanderings, for the notions of journey, wandering, path, and pilgrimage are central to Chinese metaphors for the religious life.

Chinese Notions of Religious Life as Pilgrimage

The notions of pilgrimage and wandering are central to the Chinese image and practice of the religious life. In this section, I will discuss the Chinese concept of Tao (path, way, and hence journey) as a basic metaphor for all of religious life. Then I will discuss the image of "wandering" as the means by which a person's soul or spirit matures and grows spiritually. Finally, I will relate the extraordinary religious pilgrimages of two Chinese thinkers who wandered beyond the bounds of their known world in order to discover a deeper religious vision.

Tao as Path—A Basic Metaphor

No term comes closer to conveying the Chinese equivalent of "religion" than "Tao." Tao, at base, means a footpath. The written character combines the pictorial elements of a foot and a leader—"a 'head' topped with the two plumes that were used in ancient days to signify the rank of general"[8] (see figure 2.1). Thus, Tao is a footpath going in a definite direction, or a path of action. From the notion of path or path of action, the character came to mean an art or skill, as in the Tao of archery. From this notion of art or skill, it further came to have connotations of the principles underlying the art or skill, hence a teaching, a way, an approach to either a specific arena of action or to life in general.

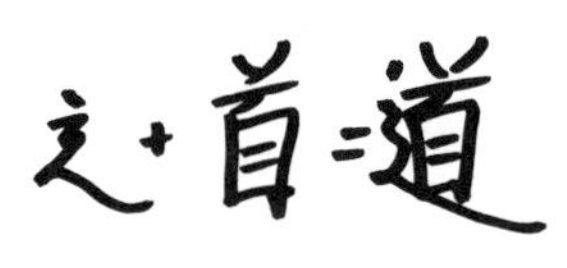

Figure 2.1

Very early in Chinese history, various religious groups used the term "Tao" as a label for the religious path, the practices and approach to life which their particular community advocated and lived. By exten-

sion, it stood for the truth or core of their teachings. Thus it was that the term came to be virtually synonymous with truth or source of truth; that which is and underlies all that is sacred and authentic.

The concept of Tao is an important common term in Chinese religious life. Different teachers or communities had their own distinctive definitions of it. Some, like Lao Tzu (dates unclear; some say sixth century B.C.E.; others fourth or even third century B.C.E.), saw Tao as the ultimate, beyond which nothing existed.

> There is a thing confusedly formed,
> Born before heaven and earth.
> Silent and void
> It stands alone and does not change,
> Goes round and does not weary.
> It is capable of being the mother of the world.
> I know not its name
> So I style it "the way."[9]

For him, Tao was also the source of all that is, the origin of the cosmos. He wrote,

> The way begets one; one begets two; two begets three; three begets the myriad creatures.
> The myriad creatures carry on their backs the *yin* and embrace in their arms the *yang* and are the blending of the generative forces of the two. (XLII, p. 103)

For Buddhists or Confucians, Tao was the teachings, path, truth, or principles of Buddha or of the sages, an ultimate reality and approach to religious life expounded by the great masters. In all cases, however, Tao was the Way, the path of religious life with its appropriate teachings, principles, and arts.

The many layers of meaning of Tao—as path, as principle or truth, as skill or art—all shaped the Chinese image of religious life: as a path, as a way to be followed, as a pilgrimage. The pilgrims on Lion's Head Mountain were not simply performing a discrete act of travel to a sacred site. Because of the comprehensive vision of Chinese religious life on the mountain, they were also in effect retracing the whole of Chinese religious life. The outward journey to the mountain made visible the day-to-day sojourn of their own religious faith and practice.

The Chinese notion of religion as path, and of religious life as a pilgrimage through many layers and levels of spirituality, revealed to me the spiritual dimensions of the broadening of my cultural horizons. My pilgrimage in China was not only of body and intellect, but also of the soul or spirit. In Chinese religious life, the soul's progress came

西遊記

about through some form of "wandering"—either guided by ritual or meditative discipline or a roaming triggered by one's moral state and concerns.

Wanderings of the Spirit: Internal and "External"

In traditional China, there were rich traditions of travel of the soul (*shen*).[10] In many forms of Chinese ritual and meditation, the spirit of the practitioner might travel to the spirit world. In other rituals or meditations, a segment of the spirit world—for example a mandala or a set of deities—was introjected into the self.[11] In either case the distance between the practitioner's individual soul and the world of the spirits was bridged, causing the soul to make progress on its journey of realization of the Way. As the soul expanded in experience and command of the spirit world, it gained health and strength and perfected its skills and powers. Thus these travels of the soul were essential to the spiritual growth of the individual.

In some practices, the sojourn of the soul was charted step by step, as depicted in the symbolism and iconography of religious texts, art, and discourse. In Taoist Inner Alchemy (*nei-tan*) meditation, for instance, this internal pilgrimage led the spirit back to the very beginning of creation, when the Tao was unified and undifferentiated, before one begat two. Following the structures and symbols of the alchemical laboratory, various aspects of the physical vitality and spiritual-cognitive powers of the adept were gradually withdrawn from their dissipating entanglements with the external world of desires; quieted, cleansed, and purified; centered; and reunited to recover the original undifferentiated unity of Tao. This reunification was also a form of "intercourse," which "conceived" a new spiritual Self. The "spirit embryo" was carefully gestated and nurtured, until ready for its "birth" up channels along the spine and through the tiny anterior fontanelle, a hole at the top of the skull which is open at birth. This spiritual Self, at first weak and unstable like a new infant, learned gradually to wander, accumulating skills and strength, and to expand until it filled heaven and earth. When the spiritual Self was congruent with the universe, the practitioner had fully embodied the Way.[12]

The elaborate internal pilgrimage of Inner Alchemy Taoism was a complex process of meditative withdrawal, quiescence, reunification, rebirth, and the nurturing of a spiritual Self which had the capacity to embody the Tao completely. It was perhaps the most complex and fully developed of all of the techniques of Chinese meditation. The metaphor of pilgrimage was reinforced by the very gradualism and complexity of the process. It also covered vast—indeed cosmic—ground.

In popular culture, spirit travel functioned on two levels. First, Chinese popular religion offered a highly elaborated notion of the

postmortem journey of the spirit through the courts of hell. Chinese rituals surrounding death attempted to call back the soul, which was believed to have departed the body. If the soul could be retrieved, the individual would recover from the death.[13] Once it was clear that the individual was irrevocably dead, the family sought through rituals, often accompanied by elaborate religious dramas, to provide various forms of assistance to the soul in its sojourn to the realms of the dead. These would include money to bribe officials and bridge keepers; horses, carriages, food, and servants[14]; spiritual escorts who knew the roads and could help the traveler negotiate pitfalls; spiritual merits of the living transferred or donated to the benefit of the deceased in order to balance off any outstanding sins; the intercession of deities, Buddhas, and Bodhisattvas who had clout with the judges of hell. Thus, in the minds of many Chinese, the longest and most dangerous religious journey was the posthumous search for a final resting place.

A second form of spirit travel in the popular imagination was the wandering of the soul or spirit during dreams. The Chinese understood dreams as the roaming of the spirit outside of the body. During these excursions the spirit could meet the souls of dead ancestors, run into ghosts or spirits, visit strange lands, and have a variety of adventures which could be terrifying or reassuring portents, or simply edifying experiences.

The Chinese soul traveled frequently, either in dreams or guided by meditation or ritual practice. The wanderings of the soul, guided or not, were paralleled by the spiritual-ethical journey of the individual in his or her lifetime. Those who followed the Way nurtured a healthy and strong spirit prepared for the afterlife. Those who did not would encounter difficulties and suffering in this life, or in the spirit world. The spiritual sojourn was not separate from the rest of the individual's life; it gave shape to all aspects of a person's life, now and in the hereafter. Likewise, the physical wanderings of persons in search of spiritual Truth nurtured the strength and powers of their soul.

Wanderers beyond the Bounds: Two Extraordinary Religious Journeys

The path of traditional Chinese religion incorporated the values and practices of Chinese religious life. Many people did not venture far along the path, sticking to a basic this-worldly religion of spiritual boons. There were those, however, whose experiences, gifts, and temperaments sent them on a long religious quest for a defining reality. They sought an authentic Way, a fresh vision of their distinctive place in the religious culture.

Such a one was Pai Yü-ch'an (1194-1229). The teachings he espoused, the rituals he practiced, and the traditions of the religious community whose history he recorded represented very different

forms of Chinese religious life; yet in his pilgrimage, Pai was touched by them all.

When Pai Yü-ch'an's father died in his youth, he left home to follow the Taoist master Ch'en Nan (Ni-wan) (1171?-1213) for nine years and to learn from him the arts of Inner Alchemy meditation and Taoist thunder rites.[15] Pai's early life story suggests that the Taoistic[16] notion of living *fang-wai* (outside the bounds of normal society) sometimes—perhaps often—had real social roots; some Taoists left home, but others were left rootless by circumstances beyond their control. The cultural trope of the Taoist wandering beyond the bounds provided a mode by which to resolve an anomalous social status.

Pai became the formal disciple of Ch'en Nan in 1205. In 1213, when he realized the Way for himself (*te-tao*), he was formally initiated by Ch'en. From that time on, students and scholars from the four directions gathered around Pai Yü-ch'an "like the hairs on a bull."[17] Pai drew deeply from the common pool of Chinese religious practices and teachings, appropriating many ideas from them alongside those he had acquired from Ch'en Nan. He established a permanent retreat on Mt. Wu-i, on the border of Kiangsi and Fukien. There he gathered disciples and was visited by scholars and religious personalities; on his travels he met many priests and scholars. He was active in the religious discourse of his day, exchanging letters, poems, inscriptions, and other occasional writings with a wide range of colleagues and acquaintances, although not with persons of particularly great renown.[18]

At the age of ten or eleven, this bright young man had found himself fatherless and hence quite literally rootless. It is not surprising, then, that he left home to follow a Taoist master. Pai's journey began with a sense of loss, a literal uprooting from the foundations of his world. Although he established his own center, he continued to travel and to make connections with multiple religious streams and practices.

Another wanderer was Lin Chao-en (1517-1598), second son of an eminent and learned family from P'u-t'ien, Fukien. Lin Chao-en's family pedigree seemed to augur a life of enormous success and influence in the world of Chinese scholar-officials and the Fukien local elite. However, in his twenties, he lost his wife, his grandfather, and his father, all in the space of five years. At the age of thirty, he also lost his uncle, the rising star of the family and Lin's hope of sponsorship for making his way in the world. All of this precipitated a crisis for the young man, who abandoned studies for the official examinations and set off in search of the Way, spending several years in the rather dubious company of one Cho Wan-ch'un (flourished sixteenth century), a "disheveled Taoist" type. In this period, he visited a number of religious sites and masters, and in 1551 met an enlightened master (probably in a dream or a vision) who taught him the true Way. From this point on, he began to gather disciples and to function as a religious teacher, although his teachings and practices continued to evolve.[19]

Lin's journey into the religious life, like Pai Yü-ch'an's, was impelled by the loss of loved ones and also of those who could help him establish a foothold in Chinese elite society. Like Pai, he journeyed beyond the bounds (*fang-wai*) to find answers and meaning, and—having found them—began to gather around himself a community of disciples with whom he could establish a practice and curriculum which would help them to embody the principles of the Way.

Lin Chao-en did not remain separated from the world or his family. His relatives helped to edit and publish his writings and were involved in his religious organization. Lin Chao-en himself was justly famous in his home town for philanthropic work on behalf of the victims, living and dead, of Japanese pirate raids. His spiritual journey inspired him to offer a new teaching, a combination of what he considered to be the authentic aspects of the Three Teachings in a single religious movement (*san-chiao ho-i,* lit. Three Teachings combined in one). In Lin's system, Confucian, Buddhist, or Taoist groups would follow their distinctive teachings and practices and yet understand their underlying unity. Lin's vision embraced something from various paths or streams, and he brought them together and justified them with his distinctive rhetoric. His Way of the Three Teachings was a creative union of elements from many paths of the Chinese religious field into an ethical, meditative, and curative practice in Nine Stages.[20]

The stories of these two men illustrate important aspects of the religious path or journey. Both were moved to wander beyond the bounds by a personal loss or reversal. As they wandered beyond the bounds, their horizons were expanded and they were touched by multiple streams of Chinese religious tradition. It was in unlikely locations and from unlikely sources that they found their answers. Their journeys were marked by loss, followed by wandering in new and uncharted territory in the hopes of finding a sure foothold on the Way.

My own pilgrimage also had begun with loss: the loss of my cultural and religious center as my horizons expanded. In addition, my father had died unexpectedly while I was a freshman in college. An American who had come of age during the Second World War, my father had rather traditional expectations of my life as a woman; his death both freed and challenged me to chart a bolder course for my life. To find that course, I too wandered beyond the bounds, embracing exile from my Western culture in order to explore uncharted territories. In my pilgrimage in Chinese culture, I was touched by many streams of religious life and practice. Like the two men in these tales, I too found insights in unlikely places. And, like them, I learned the benefits of wandering, of being a pilgrim or seeker.

I identified with both of these stories, but most especially with the most famous story of Chinese pilgrimage, captured in the novel *Journey to the West.*

Journey to the West

西遊記

All of the themes of Chinese religious journey are brilliantly and entertainingly presented in Wu Ch'eng-en's (c. 1500-1582) novel *Journey to the West*, skillfully and perceptively translated by Anthony Yü.[21] This novel, first published in the late sixteenth century and immensely popular in traditional China, is a tale of religious quest and pilgrimage. Paralleling the Chinese genius for developing layers and levels of religious symbolism, the journey takes place at many levels.

At one level, the tale is a fictionalized account of the journey of the historical pilgrim Hsüan-tsang (c. 596-664), commissioned by the T'ang emperor to travel to India and return to China with the full range of Buddhist writings. Hsüan-tsang undertook a long and arduous overland journey along the silk route, the steppes, and the mountains to India and back, passing through many cultures and realms along the way. Although an emissary of the T'ang emperor, Hsüan-tsang was also a pilgrim in his own right; the novel is an account of his spiritual growth.

In the novel, Hsüan-tsang (or Tripitika, as he is more frequently called) is accompanied by three companions who act as his guardians or champions—Old Monkey, Pa-chieh, and Sha Monk—each of whom has a monstrous or beastly appearance, symbolizing their need for spiritual refinement.[22] Like Dorothy's companions on her journey to Oz, these were unlikely, albeit endearing, champions. Despite their attainment of considerable spiritual powers, they had committed grievous sins which they sought to expiate through this pilgrimage, thereby purging their monstrous aspects. Thus the tale also recounts the pilgrimage of the three guardians or disciples. The tales of these three are raucous; their foibles are so apparent that readers laugh and at the same time recognize them as all too human. As each of these three makes progress on the journey, readers are comforted with the thought that even such obvious character flaws might be transcended by means of a commitment to the Way.

Along the physical journey, the four pilgrims encounter a stunning array of cultures and strange, sometimes hilarious, obstacles; they meet every kind of monster and demon imaginable and fight scores of battles. On the most external level, their successes in these battles chronicle their progress on the road. Yet in each of the battles, one or more of the pilgrims learn a deeper, inner lesson; thus inner progress and spiritual insight always accompany external victory.

On another level, the pilgrimage takes these characters through virtually every sort of Chinese religious practice. Along the way, they have ample opportunity to test the rules and boundaries of the religious field. Thus although at a very superficial level the structure of the pil-

grimage is "Buddhist" (after all, it is a Buddhist monk commissioned by the emperor to seek Buddhist scriptures), it is fundamentally a journey through the entire Chinese religious landscape.

As the pilgrims progress, each achievement is challenged by a new danger and obstacle. As they grow in strength, faith, courage, and discernment, they are called upon to face greater challenges and to advance even further in the Way. Even after they finally reach their goal and request the scriptures, the Buddha's disciples give them wordless scriptures.[23] The Buddha of the Past recognizes,

> Most of the priests in the land of the East are so stupid and blind that they will not recognize the value of these wordless scriptures. When that happens, won't it have made this long trek of our sage monk completely worthless? (391)

In order not to discourage the "stupid and blind priests," the Buddha of the Past arranges for the four pilgrims to discover that the scriptures are empty and to trade the wordless scriptures for more conventional scriptures. Nonetheless, the point has been made: the true "dharma" is wordless, and the scriptures were not the ultimate prize. Thus this tale of religious quest serves as a brilliant depiction of the open-ended, never-final Way of Chinese religious life.

The novel is beloved by the Chinese as a witty, raucous story; the story is often depicted in popular forms (opera, cinema, even cartoons) for sheer entertainment, especially for children. At that level it functions as a kind of religious fairy tale, where the "good guys" finally win after overcoming all of the dangers. But the novel, like Lion's Head Mountain and Chinese religious teaching, offers layer upon layer of meaning, and one could wander through its pages numerous times, never failing to discover new insights.

An important meaning is that Tripitika had to leave the bounds of Chinese culture to make his pilgrimage; he had to wander beyond the bounds (*fang-wai*) in order to seek the Truth. Like Dorothy in *The Wizard of Oz,* he too ultimately returned home transformed.

Characteristically, his sojourn encompassed many levels:

- it was a historical pilgrimage from China to India and back;
- it could be read as an allegory of either Buddhist or Taoist practice;
- it incorporated myriad elements of the Chinese religious field and its many lessons;
- it embraced, interiorized, and then shed various levels of religious belief and practice;
- it was an interior journey toward self-awareness and self-transcendence;
- it related the conquest of various demonic and beastly powers within each person;

西遊記

- it satirized both religion and culture and simultaneously affirmed their deepest values.

Perhaps most importantly, however, it was a lesson about religious life *as* journey, for every time the pilgrims passed through one part of the journey, another opened before them, and what they believed they had obtained always turned out not to be the prize. It was the journey, and what each of the pilgrims learned on it, that comprised the Way. As it was for Dorothy and her companions, the journey was all.

Journey to the West adds significant dimensions to the Chinese concept of journey and to my understanding of my pilgrimage on Lion's Head Mountain. It teaches that even ordinary, fallible folk profit from the journey; those who undertake the journey learn from their experiences, from their failures as well as their triumphs. It underscores the profound notion that the point of the journey is not to achieve some goal or gain a prize. The journey *is* the pilgrim's progress. As I achieved one insight in my study of China, new vistas opened before me, promising further spiritual growth. Most profoundly, it encompasses all of the aspects of an intentional life (even the ridiculous and embarrassing) under the umbrella of the pilgrimage, or the Way. Spiritual progress is not always smooth and dignified; it is, however, the adventure of life.

Final Thoughts

Having learned from the Chinese something about their understanding of religious journey, I could discern more clearly the meaning of my own sojourn in Chinese culture. It was intellectual and cultural, yes; but it was much more. It was a pilgrimage which broadened my spiritual as well as cultural horizons. It was a journey of the spirit, which strengthened my spiritual life and health. It was a wandering beyond the bounds, a quest for a broader vision of my specific place in the spiritual landscape.

I sought in Chinese culture a remedy to my own former narrow cultural and religious vision, expiation for the sins of cultural and religious chauvinism and the attendant distrust and hatred of "the other." Seeking this remedy entailed the spiritual discipline of becoming an outsider,[24] an "other," as I had been in the South in 1955. I became an "other," both to learn from Chinese culture as a guest, and to learn an appropriate global humility, recognizing that my natal culture is not the norm of the entire world. Broadened cultural horizons required recognizing many centers in the human community, and broadened religious horizons required recognizing many vital religious communities. This spiritual discipline cultivated a healthier horizon. This form of spiritual journey has roots in my own heritage; in the images of the

people of Israel wandering forty years in the wilderness before they reached the promised land or of Jesus' spending forty days in the wilderness in prayer. In my tradition, as in the Chinese, one is sometimes called to wander beyond the bounds in preparation for renewed vision or commitment.

Along the way, I was touched by many forms of religious life which enriched me or gave me new perspectives on my Christian heritage. The embracing of many levels of Chinese religion in the single path up Lion's Head Mountain and the stunning affirmation of many layers and levels of religiosity in *Journey to the West* presented a strikingly different approach to the many paths and practices of religion. I was inspired to learn from the Chinese an alternative way of understanding religious neighbors.

CHAPTER 3

道

Forging a New Path

Beyond the Dilemma of the Wider Ecumenism

[Hsüan-tsang] toured throughout the Western World for fourteen years, going to all the foreign nations in quest of the proper doctrines. He led the life of an ascetic beneath the twin sâla trees and by the eight rivers of India. At the Deer Park and on the Vulture Peak he attained strange visions. He received ultimate truths from the senior sages and was taught true doctrines by the highest worthies. . . . The multitudes, once full of sins, are now brought back to blessing. Like that which quenches the fire in a burning house, the power of Buddhism works to save humanity lost on its way to perdition. Like a golden beam shining on darkened waters, it leads the voyagers to climb the other shore safely.

—*Wu Ch'eng-en*
Journey to the West

The Buddhist pilgrim Hsüan-tsang traveled fourteen years to India and back to bring the full panoply of Buddhist teachings to China. The benefits of Hsüan-tsang's pilgrimage went beyond his own spiritual maturity and that of his disciples; he also brought back to his native land religious ideas, practices, and writings which benefited his people and his community. Similarly, I write this book in the spirit of a pilgrim, bringing tales from my sojourn in China to my community.

"Entering the Path"
Entering the path or embarking on a journey or religious practice. In Chinese religious life, the most significant point is the beginning, as in the folk saying, "A journey of 10,000 miles begins with a single step."

I am by no means the first Christian writer to seek wisdom from other traditions. Many have gone before me, and I have learned from them. Popular writers like Alan Watts and Thomas Merton have long inspired Christian readers with the potential of combining or bringing into dialogue Asian and Christian spiritualities; that work is being continued today by scholars like Ruben Habito.[1] Scholars such as John Cobb and Abe Masao, not to mention a number of ongoing groups and societies, have been advancing inter-religious dialogues.[2] Robert Neville and Thomas Kasulis, among others, are pursuing comparative philosophy.[3] Alan Race, John Hick, Paul Knitter, and Francis Clooney are seeking to develop global theologies or comparative theologies.[4] I have profited from these colleagues, and deeply respect what they have achieved.

In this book I am addressing related but different issues. I am not asking about theological warrants or making arguments for openness to beliefs and practices of other religions; rather I am looking for attitudes and strategies by which Christians could live and interact more fruitfully with the members and institutions of other religious communities. I am joining in the conversation from my particular perspective and with my particular expertise. I do not intend to supplant what others have accomplished, but rather to open up a fresh approach to learning from our Asian neighbors, particularly with regard to the challenges and opportunities of living with religious diversity.

Religious diversity has been a particular nemesis for Christians because of the long historical habit of Christian exclusivism. Christian claims of universal and exclusive salvation create a set of dilemmas for those who seek to be open to their religious neighbors. In this chapter, I briefly recount those dilemmas and present my particular approach to them.

Christian Exclusivity

The Christian tradition of exclusivity is ancient and has been supported by passages from the Gospels, such as John 14:6: "I am the way, and the truth, and the life; no one comes to the Father, but by me." For the early church, a fragile movement struggling to establish itself among a plethora of religious options in the ancient Near East, insisting on a firm commitment to the community of faith was no doubt an important survival strategy, even more so in periods of persecution.

As the church became established and state-sponsored, however, claims of exclusivity became a justification for enforcing conformity (orthodoxy) as opposed to allowing nonconformity (heresy or apostasy),[5] or for conquering and converting "heathen" lands, thereby saving the souls of the inhabitants.

入道

Challenges to Exclusivity

Assumptions of exclusivity began to be challenged as Western Christians from the mid-nineteenth century on developed fuller knowledge of world religions and cultures. Such knowledge helped "erode the plausibility of the old Christian exclusivism."[6] As the European colonial system crumbled after World War II, Christian and non-Christian groups throughout the world raised their voices to challenge the assumptions and parochialism of Western Christians and their complicity in colonialism.[7]

These challenges to assumptions of Christian exclusivism have sparked a debate within Christianity about its relationship to other religions. The debate currently rages under the rubric of the "wider ecumenism."[8] Alan Race has grouped current Christian stances toward other religions into three categories: exclusivist, inclusivist, and pluralist.[9]

In Race's typology, exclusivists argue for the uniqueness and superiority of the Christian path to salvation and basically affirm that "outside of the Christian faith, there is no salvation." Although the dominance of this position is eroding, it has had a long history and still colors the attitudes of many Christians.

Inclusivists concede that adherents of other religions experience the grace of God and may find salvation outside of the Christian faith, but still maintain the superiority of the Christian way to salvation. Those who find God in other traditions are "anonymous Christians" (Rahner) or have experienced a vestige of Christian revelation through some other form. Ultimately, in this life or the next, those practicing other faiths will find their full salvation *as Christians*. Critics have noted the condescension of this view toward the adherents of other traditions who would not welcome seeing themselves as anonymous Christians, any more than Christians would welcome being seen as, say, anonymous Muslims.

Pluralists affirm that there are a diversity of legitimate religious faiths and paths to salvation. Some, like John Hick, argue that the many faiths are all responses to one Ultimately Real, and that the differences among them reflect not only the limitations of human language and cultural constructions of faith, but also the specific historical conditions in which those faiths have emerged.[10] Hick challenges Christians to rethink their fundamental theological categories in such areas as Christology and atonement in order to open Christianity to the truths and ways of other religious traditions.[11] He proposes a philosophy of religion and a reading of Christian theology which can embrace the full range of religious diversity.

In general terms, exclusivists fortify and protect the boundaries of Christianity, upholding its distinctive message as the only viable way

to salvation. Inclusivists provide a cautious opening to other traditions, embracing them under the Christian umbrella, while preserving the unique saving power of the gospel message. Pluralists push hardest at the boundaries, seeking a way to re-envision Christianity as one religion among many peer religions.

入道

All three positions imply a strategy for living with religious neighbors. The exclusivists would opt at best for peaceful coexistence, arguing that "good fences make good neighbors." They pray for and work towards the conversion of all peoples to the gospel of Christianity. The inclusivists affirm other religions as disguised forms of Christianity; they cautiously welcome neighbors from other religious communities, seeing their distinctive practices as underdeveloped forms of Christianity.[12] The pluralist approach is genuinely open to interacting with other religious communities as neighbors and equals, and thus would seem to have some promise for the issues discussed in this volume. This approach merits a closer look.

The Pluralist Approach

Two recent volumes capture fairly well the current discussions in pluralist theology. *The Myth of Christian Uniqueness: Toward a Pluralistic Theology of Religions*,[13] edited by John Hick and Paul Knitter, is derived from a conference at the School of Theology at Claremont in 1986. *Christianity and the Wider Ecumenism*,[14] edited by Peter Phan, is based on papers from a 1988 conference sponsored by the Council for the World's Religions in Istanbul, Turkey. Both conferences were conversations about Christian attitudes toward world religions among Christians who had devoted considerable time and energy to interfaith dialogue. North American voices dominated, although both conferences included representatives from other continents, including Europe, Africa, and Asia. These two volumes push steadily at the boundaries of Christian parochialism. They make a number of claims about why the issue of pluralism must engage contemporary Christians.

Langdon Gilkey argues that a pluralist approach to Christianity is a necessary adjustment to the end of the unquestioned dominance of Western culture and the Christian religion. [15]

Stanley Samartha argues that Christians must attend to the negative impact of exclusivist attitudes on non-Western cultures. He admonishes:

> Theological claims have political consequences. This is particularly true in contemporary India where the exclusive claims made by any one particular community of faith affects its relationships with members of other communities of faith. . . .

> Such claims, open or hidden, also raise basic theological questions concerning God's relationship to the whole of humanity, not just to one stream of it.[16]

If Christians hope to establish a presence in cultures like India's, they will have to watch their attitudes toward other religions and send messages consistent with the gospel to which they witness.

In these volumes, Christians who have discovered "elements of openness [which] pulsate throughout the biblical witness, contending with contrary impulses of ethno-centrism and religious imperialism,"[17] seek to explore and correct the errors of exclusivistic readings of the Bible, and to point to what can be learned from inter-religious scriptural interpretation.[18] Some follow Hick in attempting to revalorize traditional Christian theological categories in ways more open to the pluralism of religions.[19] Others look to modern theological writings to find a theological base in the church for openness.[20] Seiichi Yagi turns to a Buddhist theologian/philosopher for constructive help in understanding the relation of divine and human in the person of Jesus.[21] Others revisit the history of the Christian church to understand the intentions and limitations of attacks on "those outside the faith."[22] The liberationists find in the search for justice a possible common ground among the world's religions, or at least an opening for such a ground.[23]

One sees in these writers an emergent vision of Christianity, continuous with tradition, but open to the religious diversity of the world in which we live. One also sees an unfinished struggle with the still-dominant exclusivistic attitudes within Christianity. Even the pluralists themselves are not entirely comfortable with all moves proposed, fearing that some may threaten the integrity of Christian faith.

Peter Phan, who edited one of these volumes, criticizes the pluralists for being a bit too open in their Christology.

> This imperceptible slippage from Christianity to Jesus, whether intentional or not, is, in my opinion, the Achilles' heel of the pluralist stance, for, and this is my contention, while it is not possible to claim that Christianity is unique in the sense of definitive, absolute, normative, and superior to other religions, it is legitimate to claim that Jesus is the only Christ and savior.[24]

Phan is thus implicitly critical of John Hick's celebration of a "metaphorical Christology," where Jesus' divinity is not ontological, but inspirational.[25]

Mary Ann Stenger has captured the dilemma that many in the pluralist camp experience.

入道

> Many of us grew up with [an exclusivistic] "Christian" outlook, but today we are uncomfortable with the imperialism of such an approach which often went hand in hand with economic and political imperialism. From a popular, liberal standpoint, some resolve this discomfort by rejecting all efforts at conversion and saying, "To each, his/her own." But if we look at this stance more deeply, we are also dissatisfied with an unthought-out pure relativism.[26]

Thus many Christians who seek openness to other religions and who engage in inter-religious dialogue fear that the theological moves of the pluralists go too far, undermining the very heart of what it means to be Christian. Paul Knitter perceptively comments:

> All of these reservations, which come not from the Falwells and Ratzingers but from some of the more liberal thinkers in our communities, are based on the perceived clash between the new nonabsolute views of Christ and the *sensus fidelium*. So, if these new christologies [nonabsolute views of Christ] have any future within Christian theology, they need a better *ecclesial mediation* in order that they might be "received" by the faithful.[27]

The pluralist position is in an early process of development and is still sorting through debates about the dangers and limits of its various moves. Some of the reservations concern the preservation of the distinctive integrity of Christianity and building an ecclesial foundation for the new openness; others concern the potentially unhappy implications of relativism or pluralism as ends in themselves.

Mark Heim has raised another level of concern about the pluralist position, exposing a potentially profound contradiction in the arguments of pluralists who insist that all religions are "fundamentally" the same. He wonders whether their rush to affirm the compatability of religions masks a worry about conversion, about genuine and significant change in religious affiliation. He writes, "We could consider another possibility. Perhaps it is not difference that is the primary source of tension but the dynamic of religious change itself. Does the core difficulty rest not in the recognition of differences among the traditions but in the life option of migration among them?"[28] As Heim points out, in the contemporary world more and more people "are born into cultures that contain multiple religious options."[29] Thus one's religious affiliation is less a given, less a certainty, than in premodern times. The pluralists, by denying the "real" or "significant" differences among religions, he argues, render the significance of conversion null, and thus make it less attractive. Genuine pluralism, he argues, would recognize the significant differences among religions, recognizing fully that each considers itself the only true way. In other words, it would develop a theology of multiple religious truths or alternatives.

Francis Clooney's important book *Seeing through Texts* argues for close, detailed, multifaceted, linguistically informed theological studies of other traditions to lay a groundwork for sober, careful comparison. Acknowledging that similarities unearthed will tempt one to make comparisons, he sounds a note of caution:

> From the very beginnings of such comparisons, though, we need to recognize that much will have already been done to make them plausible, likely to succeed, just by the prior decisions made in the identification of such possibilities. Any such comparison must be moderated by a lively sense of how each side of the comparison fits—theologically, textually, culturally, etc.—with its entire context, and where we are standing when we observe these materials together. It is helpful to undertake such comparisons with the expectation of always doing more of them, trying other kinds of comparisons as well: of concepts, poetic texts, excerpts from treatises, ethical norms, ritual enactments, festivals, etc. If one crosses the religious boundary intelligently, no single comparison can be decisive, even if one determines with a rare degree of certitude that in this or that instance either similarities or differences are preponderant.[30]

Clooney argues for deferring the move to creating a comparative theology, in order both to continue correcting one's understanding through further scholarship, and also to examine more deeply the agenda one brings to the endeavor and the appropriate resistances representatives of the other tradition might have to that agenda. He notes that the building of a meaningful encompassing narrative which included both traditions would require the establishment of a new religious community, committed to both, for whom that narrative would be meaningful.[31] The cautions raised in this book merit thoughtful attention, as does the groundbreaking scholarship which deepens the foundation for the possibility of a comparative theology.

Affirming Particularity and Openness

As a historian of religions, I bring another level of analysis to the debates within the pluralist movement. Seen from the standpoint of comparative religious patterns, pluralists, as they seek to redress the exclusivistic excesses of Christian history, run the danger of neglecting a vital aspect of religious affiliation and identity: its particularizing role in establishing identity and social location.

入道

Anthropologists and historians of religion have long noted that religion is one means—along with language, dress, dietary habits, social customs, music, dance, and others—by which human groups situate themselves among a range of possibilities in the world; religion is one of the ways communities define a home base, a center, a distinctive identity and location. In some societies all of these markers define the social boundaries between one community and a neighboring one; in modern societies, these markers locate one's "own" in the complex social landscape.

Alice Walker, a leading African-American woman novelist, writes movingly of her discovery of a religious and communal bond while reading the stories of Zora Neale Hurston, a pioneer African-American author:

> I will never forget, reading Zora, and seeing for the first time, written down, the prayer that my father, and all the old elders before him, prayed in church. The one that thanked God that the cover on his bed the night before was not his winding sheet, nor his bed itself his cooling board. . . . Reading her, I saw for the first time, my own specific culture, and recognized it as such, with its humor always striving to be equal to its pain, and I felt as if, indeed, I had been given a map that led to the remains of my literary country.[32]

It is striking that the "literary country" was marked as hers by the prayer her father prayed; religion establishes powerful markers of identity, and sustains and transmits the distinctive traditions of the community. It is part of the map of each community's distinctive territory of meaning and practice.

While the history of humankind makes it abundantly clear that this role of religion in establishing social location and boundaries can give rise to the horrific abuses of religious persecution, oppression, and violence against "the other," denying the importance of this aspect of religion creates other problems. If the human world were simply a vast marketplace of ideas, practices, beliefs, and mores with no boundaries and no identifiable communities of meaning, we would all be adrift in a sea of anomie and would have no place from which to establish relationships. The Catholic Theological Union in Chicago, committed to nurturing a global perspective in theology and ministry, sees a secure Christian identity as the indispensable foundation of the "global person":

入
道

> [A] global person is understood as someone who is secure in personal, cultural, and religious identity. Freed by this security, a global person does not need to prejudice or dismiss others because of their identity. A global person shows qualities of being humble and of open-minded disposition, has empathy and the ability to show solidarity with the oppressed and the marginalized. A global person is able to enter into relations of mutuality and interdependence with the oppressed and marginalized as well as building bridges with systems and members of the dominant society.[33]

The particularizing aspect of religion locates persons among the world of possibilities. Religion also has a counterbalancing aspect which pulls toward relationship with other communities and opens us to new experiences. Anthropologists, folklorists, and historians of religion thrive on tracing the diffusions, cultural influences, and adaptations of motifs, practices, and tales which cross the lines of religions and cultures. Religious communities absorb and adapt images, tales, and practices from their neighbors as a way of enriching and developing their community life: whether it is Babylonian myths finding their way into the book of Genesis; the influence of early mystery cults and other religions on the Christian practice of baptism and the celebrations of Christmas and Easter; or the absorption of local practices and motifs in the "universal" religions of Buddhism, Christianity, and Islam as they spread and take root in diverse cultures around the world. Often the external elements are absorbed in a friendly way without impacting central teachings and practices, as in the cases cited above. At other times, the external element is seen as a challenge to religious beliefs and practices of the community, and it must be incorporated into a revised and expanded sense of religious life in order to safeguard the future of the community. Not only do religious communities and cultures establish ways to mark themselves off from one another, they also interact and borrow from their neighbors.

Moreover, religious communities establish transcendent spiritual and ethical ideals which point beyond the current practices and achievements of the community to a more demanding, holier ideal. This spiritual idealism can open the community to new experiences and realizations, to discovering a limitation or even an error in some previous "given" of the community. For example, if John 14:6 is frequently cited by Christians in favor of exclusivist views, an equally strong biblical case can be made for openness to the stranger and love for the neighbor. Durwood Foster has written an essay in *Christianity and the Wider Ecumenism* articulating sound biblical warrants for ecumenical and interfaith openness.[34] Christianity, like most religions, has

both a boundary-setting, exclusivist side, and a broader, more open aspect.

入道

The interplay of the opening and boundary-setting dimensions of religious life is of crucial importance to the flourishing of human civilization. Without a clear sense of identity and a community of identification, we can find no place to stand in a vast and challenging world. We lose our center, and the world slips from a meaning-filled cosmos into a demonic chaos.[35] Without an openness to our neighbors, on the other hand, we are cut off from vast reserves of human creativity for the nurture of human life. The exclusivists stress the particularizing side, the pluralists the open aspects of Christianity. As a historian of religions, I would argue that both aspects will have to be honored if Christianity is going to continue to flourish in the global and multireligious world. The issue is, how to find the balance.

A New Path

The pluralist theologians have recovered in the Bible, and in Christian history and doctrine, foundations for a less exclusive and more open version of Christianity. They have done important work, but have frequently run up against long-standing patterns of Christian interpretation, history, and thinking dominated by exclusivist assumptions. Progress toward a less exclusive and more open version of Christianity will inevitably be very slow, because of the need for ecclesial mediation.

Diana Eck has opened a new and very promising path in her excellent book *Encountering God: A Spiritual Journey from Bozeman to Banaras.*[36] Eck is an Indologist and historian of religions by training, and a church woman with extensive experience in interfaith work. Her book, like mine, recounts tales from her spiritual and intellectual journey, bringing the voices and views of her Hindu and other non-Christian friends and colleagues to her readers, and also sharing her conversations with fellow Christians about the potential for Christian openness.

Eck's book centers around the notion of God as having many forms and levels, encountered by following many paths. The theme is aptly chosen, for it represents brilliantly the Indian/Hindu approach to religious diversity. She creates with and for her readers a profound respect for the genuine religious faith and life of others, and for their extraordinary vision of the multiplicity of God. I warmly commend this book to those who have not already read it.

My approach is closer to Eck's than to the pluralist theologians, but it follows yet another path. I do not seek to forge an ecumenical theol-

入道

ogy, nor to find biblical, ecclesial, or doctrinal warrants for openness to Asian religions. I do not seek to persuade the North American Christian community of any compatibility of belief, doctrine, or approach, or even that "God" can be found in Chinese religions, although that is certainly my experience.

As one who has sojourned extensively along the paths of Chinese religions, it is my observation and experience that relations with other religions are more readily built upon practice and symbols than on doctrine and scripture.[37] In saying this I do not denigrate the importance of engaging doctrinal and scriptural issues; I simply acknowledge that such a path is long and rocky, best traversed by specialists willing to invest considerable time in studying the scriptures, traditions, and theologies of other religions.

If doctrine and scripture are stumbling blocks to our interactions with other religions, symbol and practice can bypass some of these road blocks. The inter-religious accessibility of symbols is evidenced in the power of religious art to inspire persons from outside of the faith. Art has long been an important proselytizing and inspirational tool of religious communities. In addition, the mutual accessibility of spiritual practice may rest on one of several grounds. Practices of different faiths may seem familiar, and thus draw the interest of another group. One example is the case of Vietnamese Buddhists joining the Portuguese Catholics' saints day celebration, cited at the beginning of chapter 1.[38]

The practices of another community can also provide a new avenue for expressing spirituality.[39] Thus some Christians have studied Zen meditation techniques as a way of nurturing their Christian contemplative life; Protestant groups have held retreats with leaders specializing in Benedictine spirituality.[40] Finally, practices of another community can open one's vistas to new horizons of spiritual expression in a particular dimension of life. I, for instance, was deeply moved by the Chinese practice of reporting to the ancestors events and decisions in the life of the family, maintaining the communication link with deceased loved ones. This practice gave me a spiritual venue for extending into my adult life the relationship with my deceased father.

Such spiritual practices can be relatively easily assimilated into one's religious life without requiring that all of the attendant theological and ecclesial issues be addressed or even acknowledged, although they do raise such issues as they are entered into more deeply.[41] Such accommodations simply reflect our ability to learn from others and to adapt our behavior. They are, at least at the outset, a path of little resistance and few obstacles. The problem is that, until such practices come to be understood in their full context, the authentic interfaith

issues have not been addressed; it is at this moment that the more difficult (yet more promising) issues come to the fore.

This book, then, takes another path. From traditional China I bring accounts of religious patterns and practices, of strategies for living with religious diversity day by day. These are not offered as a model for North American Christian life, since the accounts represent cultural patterns from a distant time and place, a context which no longer exists. These accounts do, however, function as a mirror; they pose a fascinating alternative to the Western story of religious exclusivity and sectarianism. In recounting the tales from traditional China, I use the tools and perspectives of the historian of Chinese religions, recounting ways in which another culture has met these issues and addressed them quite differently than in the West.

The historian of religions begins with observation of religious life and behavior in a variety of cultures. She notes patterns of religious behavior, commonalities and differences, and noteworthy strategies. She places similar examples in juxtaposition, to allow for comparison and contrast. Comparative analysis brings out aspects of all examples which are not obvious when they are viewed in isolation. It challenges and stretches culturally embedded assumptions and categories of analysis, highlighting both the distinctiveness of each example and what each neglects or suppresses. Comparisons of patterns of religious life refine powers of observation and analysis, so that one begins to see more clearly how members of a religious community shape their traditions through selective observance.

In this book, I assume the voice of a pilgrim. No mere observer, I seek to bring out, in the stories which I select and the way in which I recount them, those aspects of Chinese religious life that strike me as edifying. I deliberately intersperse stories in which I recount from first-hand experience—narrating events through my distinctive interpretive lens—with stories which surprised me or challenged me to see things in a very different Chinese way. In these latter, I seek to convey faithfully the perspectives and lenses of the Chinese narrators, even though (and because) this stretches both my horizons and those of my readers. I find in China a remarkably textured pattern of religious life which offers striking alternative approaches to religious diversity.

The strategies and attitudes of traditional China are not a panacea; the remarkable patterns which are noted here began to break down as internal and external pressures crumbled the very foundations of traditional Chinese culture. The Chinese cannot go back to those lost days, and the West certainly cannot model itself on the Chinese imperial system. Although Chinese culture does not have all the answers to the challenge of religious diversity, these stories offer a fascinating

alternative scenario to the history of religious sectarianism and competition in Western countries.

The stories I tell of China pose the following questions, and more.

- What happens if a society starts from the premise that multiple religious affiliations are *normal*?
- What happens if religious organizations are hospitable to one another in order to create and sustain the larger community?
- What happens if a culture develops patterns to create and sustain mutual familiarity and regular interaction among members of various religious groups?

These stories have given me a fresh perspective on the history and patterns of religious life in my culture; I hope they may do so for others. I also hope that they will help us to recognize and recover in our own cultural heritage traditions of hospitality, generosity, and mutual respect. These may become the foundations for exhibiting more open attitudes toward religious neighbors, while at the same time building vital communities of faith and practice which can serve as effective spiritual centers for persons and families in our richly diverse society.

Part 2

Tales of Chinese Religious Diversity

CHAPTER 4

井

Diversity and Competition in the Chinese Religious Field

Filial piety can dissolve all the calamities of life.
If we practice filial piety toward our aged parents,
This is the equivalent of opening (and reading) the sutras all day. . . .
If we wish to emulate the upright characteristics of the Buddha, then there is nothing that can surpass filial piety.

—*Yüan-chien*
Erh-shih-ssu-hsiao ya-tso-wen

As a pilgrim on Lion's Head Mountain, I saw clearly that the Chinese envisioned their diverse religious traditions as part of a single Way. However, given my long-ingrained habits of exclusivist thinking about religion, I found myself repeatedly surprised and confused by Chinese inclusivism. While I could celebrate the general idea as an alternative to Western religious sectarianism and intolerance, I could not grasp the implications of shifting to an inclusivist perspective; I just couldn't "get it" at first, as much as I wanted to. I was, in the initial stages of my pilgrimage, considerably slowed by my difficulties in grasping the inclusivist perspective.

Take the epigraph to this chapter. What is Yüan-chien, a T'ang dynasty (618-907) Buddhist monk, doing claiming that filial piety (a cardinal Confucian value) is the best way to practice Buddhism? Yüan-chien's Buddhist paean to filial piety is an excellent example of

---

"Well"
The character for well is the symbol of the well-field system, which is one image used in the chapter to represent the Chinese religious field.

crossover and mutual borrowing among various religious groups in China. Yüan-chien, as we shall see later in the chapter, is not simply combining elements from two traditions important in his religious life; he is defending the place of Buddhism in Chinese religious life. He is pledging his allegiance, as it were, to the inclusive religious system of China.

This Chinese cultural practice of religious crossover is the antithesis of historical Christian patterns of exclusivity. It is grounded in a history of religious interaction very different from that which characterized Christianity in Europe and North America. That real and significant difference, that "otherness," held the promise of my pilgrimage, but also raised serious obstacles of understanding which I would have to overcome.

For instance, like virtually all Western scholars of Chinese religion (until very recently), my exclusivistic lenses distorted my perceptions so that I seriously misread the Chinese categories of the Three Teachings (Confucianism, Buddhism, and Taoism). Viewing the Three Teachings through Western lenses, we Western scholars saw the Three Teachings as independent, competing religions.[1] We were blind to the actual dynamics of the Chinese religious system.

This chapter will begin with the story of religious pluralism in China as we have gradually come to understand it. It is a story which challenges exclusivistic biases and assumptions.

As I became more and more aware of the inclusivistic patterns of religious pluralism in China, I was moved to develop a heuristic model which would help me and others from my culture to establish a framework on which to envision and understand the inclusive dynamics of religious pluralism. The second part of the chapter will develop that heuristic model.

As I became more familiar with the patterns and strategies that characterized religious pluralism, I also had to grow beyond my initial idealism, my delight in discovering "inclusivity." I learned that the patterns of Chinese inclusivity were intricately embedded in the patterns and dynamics of the culture. Like the religious history of the West, Chinese religious history was embroiled in politics, patronage, and power. If religion is to be part of "real life," it is inevitably implicated in the webs of social interaction and competition. The third part of the chapter recounts the entry and assimilation of a foreign religion, namely Buddhism, into Chinese culture. This tale illustrates well the dynamics of inclusivity, and the forces shaping and constraining it.

The Story of Religious Pluralism in China

From the earliest traces of human civilization, the territory which came to be China yielded a wealth of religious beliefs and practices:

mythological images, symbols, and stories; divination arts; elaborate burial and funerary practices; shamanistic and demon-exorcising rites; schema for understanding and ordering the cosmos. As religious ideas evolved, they also developed into multiple streams which later came to be labeled "Confucian," "Taoist," and "Buddhist." In reality, however, there were numerous currents within each of those larger rivers, and some tributaries which flowed beyond them; the banks between the streams and tributaries were porous and changeable.

There were, from the outset, religious tensions in China: genuine philosophical differences, rival rituals and pantheons, jockeying for patronage of the wealthy and powerful, attempts by local and national officials to domesticate the religious impulse.[2] Yet despite these very real tensions and rivalries, the dominant story of religious pluralism in China was one of tolerance of all teachings in the realm under Heaven (*T'ien-hsia*). Like modern-day Japanese whose religious affiliations in the 1983 census added up to nearly twice the total population,[3] virtually all Chinese participated in more than one religion in the course of their lifetimes, sometimes sequentially and sometimes simultaneously. The Chinese state affirmed the multiplicity of religious groups and practices. Chinese imperial governments, like European monarchies, reserved to themselves the right to establish religious orthodoxy and orthopraxy, and to declare any religious book or practice illegal on the grounds that it threatened morals or state security. Although the state had a strong bias for establishmentarian religious beliefs and practices, it primarily sought to control religious life by bringing it under the patronage, sponsorship, and support of local and national officials. The Chinese state did not adopt a single official religious teaching, but rather cast itself as the patron and protector of all legitimate forms of religion.

The Many Streams of Chinese Religious Life

In an attempt to impose some order in the Chinese religious world, the labels "Confucian," "Buddhist," and "Taoist" were adopted by Han dynasty (206 B.C.E.-202 C.E.) historians as classifications for writings, biographies, and temples or shrines. Leaders of religious movements came to use these labels polemically as each sought to differentiate his movement from key contemporaries. Government authorities used the labels to classify religious movements and practices for the purposes of patronage and control.

Traditionally, the label "Confucian" was applied to those who took as their canonical writings the *Four Books* ("The Great Learning," "The Doctrine of the Mean," and the writings of Confucius [551-479 B.C.E.] and Mencius [372?-289? B.C.E.]), as well as the *Thirteen Classics*.[4] Confucian thinkers focused on ethical and political issues, seek-

ing to identify the learning and practices which were the basis of a moral life and harmonious society.

"Taoist" was applied to four classes of writers: 1) philosophers who looked back to the writings of Lao Tzu (6th or 3rd c. B.C.E.), Chuang Tzu (369? - 286? B.C.E.), or the "Neo-Taoists"[5]; 2) thinkers in one of many ritual lineages of Taoism[6]; 3) specialists in forms of Taoist meditation (particularly Inner Alchemy) or in the arts of nurturing long life[7]; 4) and persons associated with temples designated as Taoist *kuan*. Taoist philosophers (both classical and Neo-Taoist) reflected on the Way of nature, and on the principle of the natural or spontaneous (*tzu-jan*) as an approach to human life. Ritual Taoists learned to introject spirits in order to heal, exorcise, or comfort souls. Meditative Taoists taught the reintegration of the fragmented self through a process of returning to original unity. Practitioners of the arts of long life practiced medicine, *t'ai-ch'i*, alchemy, or other occult arts.

"Buddhists" based their teachings on Buddhist scriptures and practices, originally transmitted from various Buddhist schools in India or Tibet, but later refined and developed in China. The Chinese ultimately developed their own distinctive forms of Buddhism in the Pure Land and Ch'an traditions. Buddhists taught enlightenment or salvation through cultivation of insight (*kuan*) and quiescence (*chih*) by means of a variety of ritual and meditative practices or by faith in Buddhas and Bodhisattvas who would aid the faithful in their cultivation of the Buddhist Way.[8]

Published lineages of religious texts (which identified certain schools of thought), lineages of masters or teachers, esoteric ritual practices performed only by certain lineages of priests, and schools of interpretation of classical texts—all of these served as markers of distinct religious movements or schools in China. These divisions, while significant, also evolved over time, and as they did religious boundaries were redrawn and traditions reconfigured, as reshapers of one tradition borrowed liberally from others motifs, symbols, practices, and even deities.[9] Often this borrowing honored the teachings of other traditions in a friendly spirit; in other cases it was a form of competition through co-optation and expansion into a rival's religious terrain. The borders between groups were by no means absolute, and—most significantly—their devotees, patrons, and even occasionally their religious professionals overlapped and crossed boundaries. As C. K. Yang has noted,

> In popular religious life it was the moral and magical functions of the cults, and not the delineation of the boundary of religious faiths, that dominated people's consciousness. Even priests in some country temples were unable to reveal the identity of the religion to which they belonged. Centuries of

> mixing gods from different faiths into a common pantheon had produced a functionally oriented religious view that relegated the questions of religious identify to a secondary place.[10]

In addition, the plethora of local and popular traditions do not neatly fall under any of the three labels, Confucian, Buddhist, or Taoist. As such practices grew they were sometimes classified or misclassified as belonging to one of the three teachings, but the fact remains that a vast portion of Chinese religious life was centered around local deities or practices; the labels "Confucian," "Buddhist," or "Taoist" are simply not helpful in these cases.[11]

An Alternative Model for Conceptualizing Chinese Religious Life

For these reasons, it is inadequate to think of Chinese religious life and practice as comprised of three separate, distinct, and competing religions called Confucianism, Buddhism, and Taoism. We need to take into account that religious communities both overlapped and competed with each other, drawing from a common pool of religious images, texts, symbols, and practices.

In order to facilitate such understanding, I employ the notion of Chinese religious field as a heuristic device to convey the patterns, interactivity, and permeability of Chinese religious practices and communities. The concept of religious field helped me to grasp the realities of Chinese religious pluralism in a number of ways.

First, it reminds me of the common pool of elements from which religious communities were free to draw. The Chinese religious field can be depicted in a number of ways: one is in terms of the idealized system of the agricultural "well-field" (*ching-t'ien*), described in the *Classic of Rites* (*Li Chi*), and invoked by Chinese reformers over the centuries as a remedy against the evils of excessive government centralization and taxation. The idea is based on the "tic-tac-toe" structure of the character *ching* (well) (see figure 4.1).

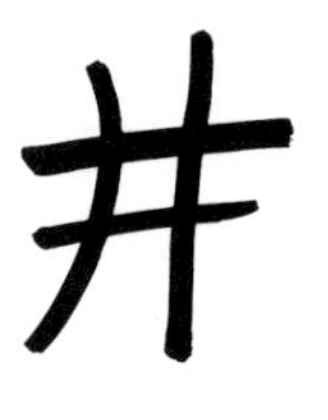

Figure 4.1

Mencius describes the system:

> Each well-field unit is one *li* square and contains nine hundred *mu* of land. The center lot is the public field. The eight households each own a hundred-*mu* farm and collaborate on cultivating the public field. When the public field has been properly attended, then they may attend to their own work.[12]

井

The well-field system, although it may never have been implemented in China, was invoked as an ideal because 1) it gave each family a plot of land for their support, and 2) it provided a localized system of self-help in lieu of central government taxation. It represented a utopian society where everyone had sufficient land and strong central government was superfluous.

I invoke this notion of field for the Chinese religious system because it metaphorically equalizes the various religious groups which surround the public field or common pool. At the center of the religious field, in my use of the metaphor, is a public or common pool of religious elements and motifs from which local institutions may draw (see figure 4.2). This field functioned primarily locally, for each locality had its distinctive set of temples and practices honoring local deities and teachers.[13] They might import elements of neighboring regions, be visited by teachers from afar, or collect texts which represented broader teachings. If these external elements were to have lasting impact, however, they would be incorporated into the local religious field.

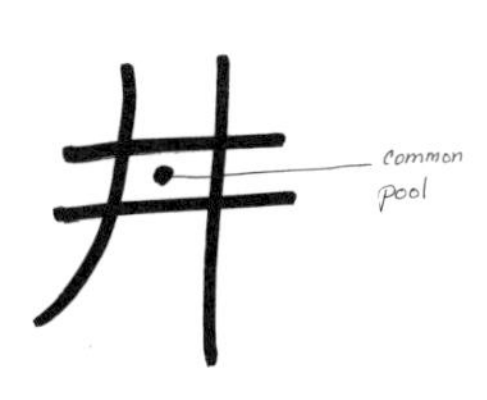

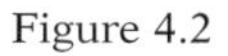
Figure 4.2

At a second level, the metaphor of religious field can be depicted as a grid in which each local religious temple or shrine finds its appropriate niche (see figure 4.3). Chinese temples and deities in any given locale tend to sort themselves into complementary functions and ritual specializations, each developing a particular niche or location in the religious field. Moreover, the round of community festivals, rotating among the established religious temples and groups, creates a complementarity of religious patronage in the community. Local residents learn the powers and specializations of each shrine or deity, and approach them accordingly. Local elites develop patterns of religious patronage which express their leadership role in the community. Thus the field of local religious institutions has two distinct dimensions: 1) it reflects the social hierarchy of the community through the patterns of patronage, and 2) it establishes a range of complementary religious powers to protect and sustain the community. The grid aspect of the Chinese religious field is similar to the notion of religious field developed by Stanley Tambiah to analyze the relationship of Buddhism to Thai spirit cults.[14]

If the notion of Chinese religious field embraces the notion of the public field or common pool of religious elements, and of field as a grid in which each religious group finds its appropriate niche, the Chinese religious field must also have a dynamic or active aspect, for it is a field of religious interaction. Here religious leaders vie for patronage, seeking to strengthen their position on the local religious field. Here the laity seek instruction, boons, and ritual succor from

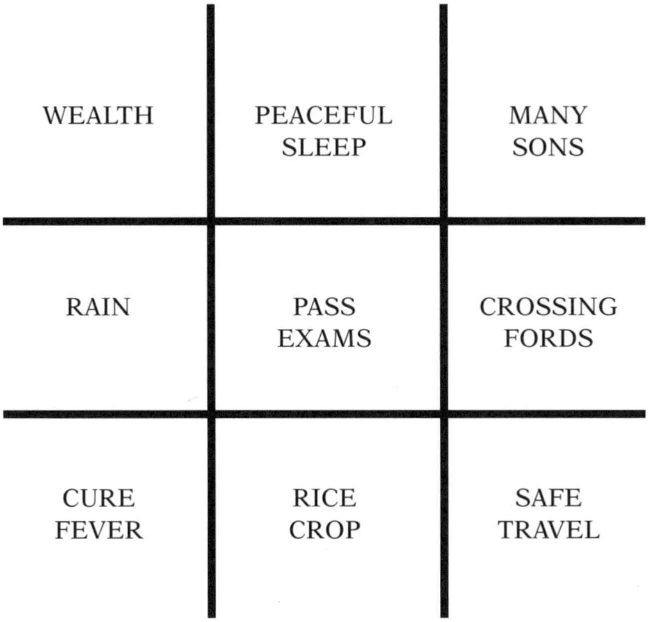

WEALTH	PEACEFUL SLEEP	MANY SONS
RAIN	PASS EXAMS	CROSSING FORDS
CURE FEVER	RICE CROP	SAFE TRAVEL

Figure 4.3

local religious resources, flocking to those deities or teachers who could deliver spiritual boons. People look to religion to further their fortunes, secular (health and wealth) and sacred (progress on the Way).

The Chinese religious field is a field of action, a playing field (or, if you will, a religious treasure hunt)[15] or a field of socio-economic competition. The latter builds on the notions of Pierre Bourdieu, who sought to reconcile the ideas of Durkheim, Marx, and Weber in an original theoretical model which could: 1) describe the contribution of religious institutions and practices to the perpetuation of social structure; 2) articulate the various pressures on religious institutions and leaders to compete as effective producers and distributors of religious goods; and 3) identify the role of socio-economic circumstances in shaping the views and needs of the groups to whom religious goods are delivered.[16] The play on the Chinese religious field takes place in the complex socio-economic web which Bourdieu seeks to model. In the analysis of this book, however, I will concentrate on four levels of interaction: 1) attempts by the state, both local and national, to control religious activity; 2) activities of local groups and leadership to assert their own interests in the religious field; 3) the role of religious leadership in developing and shaping religious traditions; and 4) the mechanisms through which the faithful learn about and take advantage of religious resources.

井

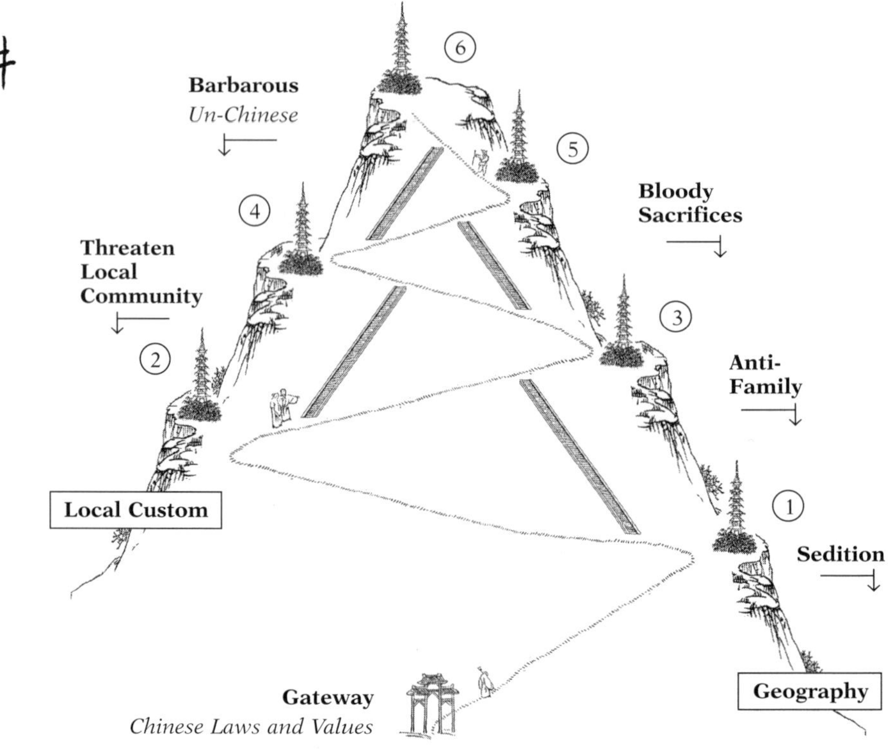

Figure 4.4

Since the Chinese have no tradition of competitive games on playing fields (unless one counts mahjong or chess), the dynamic aspect of the Chinese religious field is best visualized as a path on a mountain (See figure 4.4). Most local religious fields had a pilgrimage site (a mountain where available), and so this visualization builds on a solid Chinese tradition of representing a comprehensive vision of the religious field. Pilgrimage sites or major temples display a vision of the religious field which includes many religious groups and deities, each in the proper place accorded to them by the host temple. For some religious groups, the best pilgrimage site is a steep mountain, as they would portray the religious field as demanding and their own tradition as offering the best way to complete the challenge journey. For others, the mountain would have to be much more level, more accessible, for they offer a version of the Way that is easy and open to all. Thus their version of the mountain would be a small hill, or even a level plain. Those of us living in the information age might want to think of figure 4.4 as a computer model in which the steepness of the mountain can be adjusted, according to which group is presenting the religious field.

Figure 4.4 suggests a path up a mountain representing the local religious field. The path is long and winding, wending its way through the variety of traditions represented in the local field (depicted as shrines 1-6). The narrow bridges between paths are ritual or meditative short-cuts advocated by some particular leader or group. These bridges can speed one along the Way but, like all short-cuts, have attendant dangers, and thus require spiritual assistance. (For those schools offering an easier path, these bridges might be elevators, or they would become easy strolls across a small stream.)

Although the path through the religious field encompasses considerable diversity, it does have its boundaries. The gate at the bottom represents Chinese (state) law and Chinese values (embodied in the classics). Without accepting these, one cannot enter the field. One can fall from the path into danger (heresy) by means of religious acts or beliefs which go beyond the bounds of the religious field: those that threaten the local community or are viewed as seditious by the state; those which are religiously offensive (bloody sacrifice or cannibalism); those practices which are outside the purview of Chinese civilization (i.e., barbarous); those which destroy the fabric of society (anti-family practices).

What complicates the visualization of the religious field is that in many locales, where more than one religious group competed for dominance, these strong groups each had their own picture of the shape of the whole, or the place of each shrine on the path and the location of effective short-cuts. What they shared was a notion that the religious field embraced the religious diversity of the community.[17]

The metaphor of the religious field is not intended to suggest that Chinese religion is merely a game; instead, it highlights certain aspects of the dynamics of Chinese religious life:

1. There are rules of play.

   These are established by cultural patterns and values, and encoded in laws and social customs, which are enforced by the government and the local elites.

2. The field is marked by obstacles which must be negotiated.

   Chinese cultural practices as well as social and economic forces shape the needs of the populace, and the ways in which religion can function.

3. There are traditional sets of moves or plays.

   The Chinese religious field contains a common pool of elements which are adapted by various religious groups; the pool can be extended through variation or acceptable forms of innovation.

4. There are at least two sets of players:

- Religious leaders and institutions vie for patronage, devotees, and religious or cultural influence.
- Religious persons and families vie for blessings or boons (health,

wealth, and progeny are perennial favorites), social status or influence, and spiritual fulfillment.

Religious persons must learn not only to negotiate the path, but also to discern the appropriate goals and means to achieve them. Since the various temples offer not only transcendent, ultimate goals but also worldly boons and blessings as proof of the spiritual efficacy of their deities and practices, players have both short- and long-term goals in negotiating the course of the religious field.

I developed the notion of religious field to help me understand how various practices or groups complemented each other within the wholistic social fabric. It highlights the dynamics of religious activity on that common ground. I will invoke it often throughout the book to help the reader visualize the dynamics of religious diversity in China.

Now let us turn to the tale of the accommodation of Buddhism to Chinese culture to illustrate the dynamics of the Chinese religious field within the web of patronage, politics, and power.

Pluralism in the Chinese Religious Field: The Assimilation of Buddhism

When, as a pilgrim, I encountered the story of the introduction and assimilation of Buddhism into China, beginning in the early centuries C.E., I began to appreciate the complex real-life dynamics of Chinese religious inclusivity. Buddhism was a very foreign religion; the challenges facing its entry into China were daunting. The Indian sub-continent had produced a rich culture, a sophisticated philosophical heritage, and institutions based on distinctive cultural patterns; China had also produced a rich literature and sophisticated culture based on very different patterns. These two cultures had radically different cosmological views, conceptions of time and space, and attitudes toward the oral and written word. The Buddhists started from a position well outside of all of the boundaries of the Chinese religious field. Neither in accord with Chinese values nor recognized by Chinese law, Buddhism had not entered the gate of the religious field. Moreover, it represented non-Chinese ("barbarous") beliefs and values, and thus posed the threat of heresy to its followers.

Both distance and geography (the Himalayas, vast deserts and steppes roamed by various tribal peoples, and treacherous seas) had separated these two seats of ancient culture and kept contacts to a minimum. Thus translation of Buddhist teachings from Sanskrit to Chinese was a formidable challenge, not merely because of the considerable philosophical differences, but also on purely linguistic grounds. There was no pool of persons adept in both languages. Because there were no ready-made cultural categories adequate to express Buddhist

views, early Chinese Buddhist texts made lavish use of Taoist vocabulary. It was the closest match in Chinese culture, but it added an exaggerated Taoistic coloration to the Buddhist teachings. As a result, from the Later Han (23-202 C.E.) through the T'ang (618-907) dynasties, Buddhist and Taoist discourses met and melded into each other. If this meant that the Chinese at first saw Buddhism through a distinctively Taoistic lens, it was equally true that the injection of Buddhist ideas and practices dramatically affected the course of Taoist metaphysical speculation and opened hitherto unforeseen vistas of Taoist philosophy. The Buddhists profited from this translation strategy, because Buddhist deities, ideas, and practices gained currency in *Chinese* terms, thus finding their way onto the local religious fields; they began to blend with local customs and local cults. The Taoists benefited by having their pantheons, myths, rituals, and practices enriched by the store of Buddhist teachings and practices; they adapted these Buddhist enrichments to strengthen their own positions and moves on the Chinese religious field. Over centuries, Buddhists and Taoists borrowed liberally from each other's ritual and meditation techniques, adapting them to their own distinctive terms and practices. The introduction of Buddhism dramatically broadened the range and depth of Taoist thought and practice, and the Buddhist route through Taoistic terminology and religious sensibilities laid the groundwork for the adaptation of Buddhism into distinctively East Asian cults.[18]

Religious borrowing helped Buddhists establish footholds in the local religious fields throughout China. Buddhists also faced a major challenge in accommodating themselves to the Chinese values which the state was committed to uphold. Early Buddhist missionaries felt keenly the Chinese resistance to a religion which did not seem to uphold these traditional values; an early apologist for Buddhism sought to answer the various cultural objections to Buddhist teachings, asserting (as his translators point out) "that it is possible to be a good Chinese and a good Buddhist at the same time, that there is no fundamental conflict between the two ways of life, and that the great truths preached by Buddhism are preached, if in somewhat different language, by Confucianism and Taoism as well."[19]

The Buddhists went well beyond apologetics, adapting themselves centrally to Chinese religious life by offering themselves as religious functionaries for funeral and memorial services. No cultural values were more distinctively Chinese than the obligation to continue the family line through the birth of sons and to venerate the souls of the ancestors. The Chinese initially saw Buddhism as in conflict with these sacred familial duties: 1) because the highest path of Buddhism was leaving one's family to join a religious community, a practice which the Chinese initially saw as in conflict with their strong obligation to continue the family line; and 2) because a core teaching of

Buddhism is that there is no soul, no eternal substratum of the True Self, which seemed to argue against the veneration of ancestors. By establishing themselves as specialists in memorial services, the Buddhists not only found a way to cultivate the support and faith of the Chinese *through their commitment to Chinese family values*, but also succeeded in allaying the fear that Buddhism was un-Chinese.[20] The Buddhist adaptation to Chinese family values required some fancy theological footwork—the Buddhists had to justify commemorating the souls of ancestors who, according to Buddhist theology, had no souls—but it was worth it. By establishing their role in the memorial and funerary rites, the Buddhists purposefully insinuated themselves into an active and advantageous position on the Chinese religious field, where they worked to assimilate local deities and practices to make Buddhism ever more Chinese.

Chinese Buddhist monks naturally stressed passages in traditional Buddhist scriptures which taught filial respect for ancestors:

> We should be filial, obedient, and compassionate toward our parents, our brothers, and other relatives.
> If we are children of the Buddha, we should constantly entertain the earnest wish of being filial and obedient to our parents, teachers, monks, and the Three Jewels [of Buddhist practice].[21]

Moreover, the monk Yüan-chien wrote a Buddhist paean to twenty-four models of filial love.

> Filial heart is the true bodhisattva,
> Filial conduct is the great arena of the *Tao*.
> Filial conduct is the sun or moon shining on a dark street,
> Filial heart is the ship crossing over the sea of misery. . . .
> In Buddhism, piety is the basis for becoming the Buddha,
> In all matters, one must be filial toward one's parents.
> By being in accord with piety in our present life, we can avoid rebirth in the future.
> Filial piety can dissolve all the calamities of life.
> If we practice filial piety toward our aged parents,
> This is the equivalent of opening (and reading) the sutras all day. . . .
> If we wish to emulate the upright characteristics of the Buddha, then there is nothing that can surpass filial piety.[22]

Until the Buddhist persecutions of the ninth century C.E., the traditional Indian Buddhist sects flourished in China, establishing vast centers of Buddhist learning. However, these traditional centers and sects

were virtually destroyed in the mid-ninth century during a great persecution of Buddhism, in which thousands of monks, priests, and nuns were defrocked, temples razed, and images melted. This would seem to belie the image of openness and tolerance in the Chinese religious field. However, the persecution was not designed to wipe out Buddhism as a religion or to force conversion to other faiths; rather it curbed the *economic* power of certain schools of Buddhism which had not been fully successful at accommodating to the Chinese religious field.

In the polemical literature of the T'ang dynasty there was, to be sure, an intensification of anti-Buddhist polemic. And yet this polemic was not against Buddhist doctrine as such, but rather against its foreignness, its inadequate assimilation into the Chinese religious field. Han Yü (786-824), an uncompromising public official and trenchant satirist, delivered the most scathing attack on Buddhism in a famous memorial criticizing the emperor's decision to permit a procession of a famous Buddhist relic (the finger bone of the Buddha) in the Chinese capital.

> Now Buddha was a man of the barbarians who did not speak the language of China and wore clothes of a different fashion. ... If he were still alive today and came to our court by order of his ruler, Your Majesty might condescend to receive him, but it would amount to no more than one audience ... and he would then be escorted to the borders of the nation, dismissed, and not allowed to delude the masses. How then, when he has long been dead, could his rotten bones, the foul and unlucky remains of his body, be rightly admitted to the palace? Confucius said: "Respect ghosts and spirits, but keep them at a distance!" So when the princes of ancient times went to pay their condolences at a funeral within the state, they sent exorcists in advance with peach wands to drive out evil, and only then would they advance. Now without reason Your Majesty has caused this loathsome thing to be brought in and would personally go to view it. No exorcists have been sent ahead, no peach wands employed.[23]

There are three noteworthy motifs in Han Yü's rhetoric: 1) the Buddha is a mere barbarian (read, foreigner) and should be treated as such; 2) these are the rotten remains of a corpse, and thus inauspicious (no concession to their status as a sacred relic); 3) if they were to be received, it should be with traditional Chinese funerary rituals (the exorcists with the peach wands), thus following the customs of the Chinese religious field. Han Yü's rhetoric reflects the distaste of some Chinese scholars for the residual foreignness of Buddhism. It was attitudes such as Han Yü's that Yüan-chien's Buddhist paean on filial

piety sought to counter. Han Yü's essay demonstrates that Buddhism had its ideological enemies, but the persecution of Buddhism was motivated primarily by politics, not by ideology.

The government acted because Buddhism had become too *economically* powerful, threatening the revenue base of the imperial state. Wealthy families had built lavish temples and donated their lands for the support of temples as a form of tax shelter with accompanying religious merit. To make matters worse (from the government's standpoint), monks and nuns were exempt from the tax registers. Thus each son or daughter sent into monastery or convent was removed from the tax rolls as well as from the labor pool.[24] The government became increasingly alarmed at its shrinking tax base and the removal of young men from the labor pool. Emperor Wu-tsung issued an edict in 845:

> Each day finds its monks and followers growing more numerous and its temples more lofty. It wears out the strength of the people with constructions of earth and wood, pilfers their wealth for ornaments of gold and precious objects, causes men to abandon their lords and parents for the company of teachers, and severs man and wife with its monastic decrees. In destroying law and injuring mankind indeed nothing surpasses this doctrine! Now if even one man fails to work the fields, someone must go hungry; if one woman does not tend her silkworms, someone will go cold. At present there are an inestimable number of monks and nuns in the empire, each of them waiting for the farmers to feed him and the silkworms to clothe him, while the public temples and private chapels have reached boundless numbers, all with soaring towers and elegant ornamentation sufficient to outshine the imperial palace itself.[25]

The last line may be said to hold the key: not only had the wealth of Buddhist establishments threatened the tax base; it also threatened to overshadow the imperial palace and its monuments and thus had become in effect a seditious force. The vast Buddhist temples had become overly strong players in the Chinese religious field and were threatening the power of the state to control them.

The persecution of Buddhism, while it destroyed many wonderful temples and works of art, did not wipe out the practice of Buddhism. The most successfully assimilated forms of Buddhism (various forms of Ch'an and Pure Land Buddhism) re-absorbed many aspects of broader Buddhist teachings and practice, creating popular Buddhist movements which continue to this day. The persecution of Buddhism shifted dominance away from Indian-based schools of Buddhism to

the forms which had arisen in China, and thus were the most fully assimilated.

The story of the entry, assimilation, persecution, and survival of Buddhism in China is a revealing illustration of how a foreign teaching might fare in the Chinese religious field. The Buddhists had to acquaint themselves with the common pool of religious elements so that they could play on the Chinese religious field. They had to accommodate to basic Chinese values, particularly family values. They had to learn the rules of the game both in dealing with governmental authorities and in attracting patrons and devotees. They had to identify a distinctive role or position (funerary rites) which would give them a strong niche, overcoming their outsider status. They learned that on this field a player can be too successful, and can thus lose his/her place; it was, ironically, the economic success of the great Buddhist cults that was ultimately their downfall.

The Buddhist players who accommodated most fully to the rules of the Chinese religious field (Ch'an and Pure Land) established strong and lasting positions. It was they who borrowed most extensively from the common pool of deities and practices, who emulated native genres of writing, and who cast Buddhist teachings in the practical this-worldly vein so attractive to the Chinese. It was they who made Buddhism genuinely accessible to the Chinese people.

A striking aspect of this tale is the long, slow process of Buddhist assimilation. It was nearly a millennium before the process of identifying the enduring forms of Chinese Buddhism was complete. The moral of the tale is that playing on the Chinese religious field is a complex and subtle art. The Buddhists were successful in gaining access and finding a foothold, but it took them many centuries to establish themselves securely in the hearts of the Chinese.

Final Thoughts

The tale of assimilation of Chinese Buddhism was of immense value to me as a pilgrim in Chinese culture, for it helped me to understand the real-life, on-the-ground dynamics of religious diversity. It spoke eloquently of cultural resistance to foreign religious values and patterns, and how these must be patiently interpreted and accommodated for any mutual understanding to emerge. Thus I came to see that my pilgrimage would be a long one, and that patience and persistence would be required of me if I were to make progress in genuine interfaith understanding.

It exposed the many dimensions of potential religious misunderstandings (linguistic, familial, political, economic, customary). Every religious tradition is embedded in a nest of cultural patterns, each one

of which must be integrated into a new cultural setting. Understanding another religion would require focus on more than religion by itself; it demanded an understanding of the embeddedness of religion, of what was at stake on many levels in each belief or practice.

It illustrated the ingenious adaptations which religious groups make as they adapt to new cultural settings. Presumably such adaptations are also required of Christianity, not only as it enters cultures originally dominated by other religions, but also as it adapts to the new global religious pluralism in what have been seen as Christian cultures.

Most of all, it exposed (by contrast) the marked impatience of North Americans to have changes effected and issues settled within a remarkably brief time frame. Granting that post-modern culture moves at lightning speed compared to traditional Chinese culture, nonetheless we as Americans profoundly underestimate the complexity and overestimate the pace of cultural change.

The conceptual model of the Chinese religious field helped me to make sense of this tale and to visualize its dynamics. This heuristic model will also help illuminate other tales to be related in the following chapters.

CHAPTER 5

王

Cultural Unity and Local Variation

Vying for Control on the Chinese Religious Field

The Sages of the Three Teachings are heroes who stand firmly on earth and reach to heaven. Clearly there is no room for differences. Therefore it is said, "There are not two Ways under heaven; the sage or worthy does not have two minds."

—Hsün Tzu

Our eminent Founder [the first Ming emperor] united the world and established the domain. He respected Confucius, Lao Tzu, and Sâkyamuni [Buddha] as though they were one person. Therefore in the Collection of Imperial Writings, *he often speaks of the Sages of the Three Teachings. And he often uses these two statements [i.e., the above two-part quotation] to judge them in order to show that they are not different. Now the Way is identical with the mind, so how can there be any differences? Not even ignorant men and women, not even insects and plants, go outside the purview of this Way and this mind. How much less the Sages of the Three Teachings? Even if one wished to have two Ways or two minds, one would not be able to do so.*

—Li Chih
San-chiao p'in

"King"
The character for king symbolized, in ancient Chinese thought, the role of the ruler (represented by the vertical line) to hold in harmony the realms of heaven, the human, and the earth (the three horizontal lines from top to bottom).

The model of the Chinese religious field was a major breakthrough in my pilgrimage. I now had a useful tool for understanding the examples of Chinese religious life which I encountered, so that I could move ahead with more confidence and less trepidation. The tale of the assimilation of Chinese Buddhism brought me to a higher plateau, for I had begun to face the real-life embeddedness of religious life and practice; I had left behind my romantic and overly idealistic portrait of Chinese inclusivism. The Chinese had not transcended all competitive tendencies or power struggles; they had simply developed a different set of strategies, strategies that evaded the ills of religious exclusivism. Having climbed to this plateau and accustomed myself to the elevation, I was now ready to confront more directly the issues of power and competition. Who controlled (or vied for control of) the Chinese religious field? What was at stake for the various competing parties? How did competition and control play themselves out?

As I continued my journey with questions of power in the forefront, I found myself facing another challenge to understanding. I noticed striking discrepancies between the portraits of Chinese religious life portrayed by the normative texts, particularly those endorsed by the imperial government and its representatives, and reports on Chinese belief and practice based on the field reports of anthropologists. In the 1970s, while I was in graduate school, scholars trained in textual work were just beginning to read anthropological reports seriously, and anthropologists were reading (and challenging) work based solely on texts. This occurred both because Chinese studies as a whole was flourishing, producing a stream of provocative and important scholarship; and also because, with the development of social history, the study of Taoism and vernacular literature, and the opening of research on sub-elites and local elites, the vast territory between the normative texts and field reports was being entered by many, including this pilgrim. Both textual and field-work based models for understanding Chinese society were gaining nuances as our knowledge of Chinese history and culture grew. The issues of power had to be viewed in two directions: from the top down, and from the bottom up. In this chapter, I first discuss the origins and implications of the Chinese myth of cosmological unity and its implications for the religious field. I then explore the motivations of the imperial government in embracing, celebrating, and controlling religion. Turning to the bottom-up view, I explore the room for local variation or dissent within the unity of Chinese culture. I conclude with the tale of Ching-ming Tao (Way of the Pure and Perspicacious) to illustrate the interplay of the unifying and local forces in the Chinese religious field.

In the last chapter, I recounted the tale of the slow assimilation of Buddhism to Chinese culture through its accommodation to mainstream Chinese values of filial piety and ancestor veneration. The foreign Buddhists gained entree to the Chinese religious field by aligning

themselves with the values and practices of Chinese law and custom. As a foreign pilgrim in Chinese culture, I too was acutely aware of my outsider status, of the many cultural patterns and codes I would have to master to enter this amazing world. The Chinese have a long-standing and proud sense of their civilization, encoded in practice, recorded in the classics, interpreted by the literate elite, and enforced by the imperial government. Outsiders had to bow to the values which represented this civilization before they could enter the gate of the Chinese religious field.

The Chinese imperial government, supported by the scholarly elite, sustained the sense of values and of Chinese cultural unity. In the epigraph to this chapter, Neo-Confucian writer Li Chih (1527-1602) praised the Ming dynasty founder T'ai-tsu (r. 1368-1398) for uniting the realm both politically and religiously; T'ai-tsu accomplished this by respecting "Confucius, Lao Tzu, and Sâkyamuni [Buddha] as though they were one person." T'ai-tsu, in other words, understood that political unity, cultural unity, and religious unity were of a piece, and that his role as emperor was to sustain unity on all three levels. As Li Chih remarked, if even plants and insects are included in the Way, how could any of the Three Teachings stand outside its purview? The unity of the cosmos was the foundation and base for the unity of civilization and of religion.

The State and the Myth[1] of Cultural Unity

The distinctive relation of the state to religion was shaped by the early history of China.

The Ancient System of Priestly Governance

From the beginnings of Chinese civilization, earthly rule was founded on Heavenly authority; the ruler was also a priest. The rulers regularly consulted Heaven by means of prayer and divination, seeking counsel for everything from hunts to auspicious days for government ceremonies.[2] The ruler's priestly role, his connection to the ancestral or autochthonous nature deities in Heaven, gave him the power to rule; he was but the medium for the deities who exercised sovereign authority.

In the period known as the Warring States (403-221 B.C.E.), a number of leaders vied for supremacy in China by means of military and political strategies, directly challenging the traditional power of the ruler as priest. It was a period marked by political intrigue, alliances and counter-alliances, plots, battles, assassinations, and coups. Stronger states conquered, absorbed, or dominated weaker neighbors. China

was moving toward unification by force, and the issue was only which state would survive the struggle.

The period of the Warring States precipitated a *religious* crisis for ancient Chinese culture, for the premise that the authority of the ruler, of government itself, rested on divine guidance of the gods and ancestors was now challenged. Antireligious positions asserted that strong laws and effective statecraft were the true basis of sovereign authority. This challenge stimulated traditionalists to reinterpret and elaborate ancient models of ancestor and nature worship as alternatives to the antireligious position; these elaborations became the cores of the Confucian and Taoist traditions. Thus an intense socio-political struggle laid the intellectual foundations of the Chinese religious field. In this formative period of Chinese history, religious thought was deeply enmeshed in brutal worldly issues.

The victor among the Warring States was the Ch'in dynasty (221-209 B.C.E.), the champion of the most secular of all the contending ideologies, that of the "statecrafters." The statecrafters scoffed at the ancient beliefs that sovereignty was morally and ritually grounded in Heaven, as much sacerdotal as it was political. The statecrafters advocated authoritarian government, sustained by strict laws, military power, and efficient governmental institutions. The Ch'in dynasty, in its brief reign of twelve years, accomplished a great deal toward building a unified state, but it also imposed a strict police state, ruthlessly destroying all writings which opposed its official views. The strain of massive public works and political repression took its toll on the people and eroded their support of the government. The Ch'in dynasty fell at the death of its first ruler, and became the "evil empire" of traditional Chinese historiography.

Some of the achievements of the Ch'in were highly beneficial, but traditional historiography gave most of the credit for creating the unified culture of China to the successor Han dynasty (206 B.C.E. - 202 C.E.). The Han built on the positive efforts at centralization while developing an ideology and cosmological/religious foundation for cultural unity that became definitive for the remaining two millennia of Chinese imperial history.

The Han System of Cultural Unity

According to Han ideology, the Chinese ruler was the pivot which held in harmony and balance the three tiers of cosmology[3]: the heavens, the earth, and the human realm. This image or metaphor is built on the visual form of the character for ruler (*wang*) (see figure 5.1). The ideogram has three horizontal lines, representing heaven, earth, and the human, with a single vertical stroke in the center as

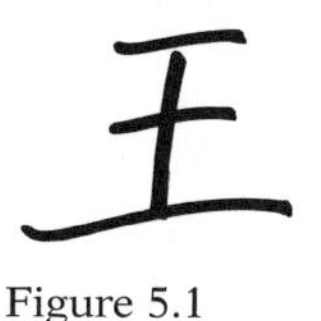

Figure 5.1

the connecting link; the vertical stroke represents the ruler, who connects the three tiers.[4] How were these three tiers held in balance? Cosmological balance was sutained by the ruler through acts of governance, moral propriety, observance of ritual duties, and divination. Thus the Han thinkers transformed and expanded ancient motifs of the ruler's priestly duties in the service of a unified imperial state.

王

In order for the new religious ideology to become effective, the Han thinkers also had to reconcile the cosmological systems and religious practices which had previously developed in the various states. The Han government gathered and correlated diverse cosmological principles of the various religious specialists into a single system, based on an elaborate series of *correspondences*.[5] Having learned its lesson from the resistance to strict laws and ruthless enforcement which had led to the fall of the Ch'in, the Han did not impose only one out of the many competing options; instead it created an ingenious *overarching system* which could accommodate already existing systems through a system of correspondences. By intentionally combining many systems, the Han thinkers established a central feature of the relatively inclusive Chinese religious field: a mechanism to accommodate local practices into a religious system which expressed China's cultural unity, and thus sustained the sovereign authority of the imperial state. This move completed the unification of many feudal states, for it gave the unity a cultural basis and an integrating mechanism.

The success of this system and the ideology which surrounded it was remarkable. From the Han dynasty onward the Chinese had an unshakable belief in the *normative unity* of Chinese culture; Chinese civilization was to embrace all under heaven (*T'ien-hsia*). Although China was often politically divided into two or more states, and although premodern communications systems made the whole of China nearly impossible to govern from one center, the Chinese elite steadfastly maintained that cosmological, cultural, and political unity were normative. The three levels of unity could not be disentangled. The role of China's ruler was to unite and harmonize the entire cosmos—the civilized world. The religious field was also structured to embrace "all under Heaven," as Li Chih insisted in the epigraph to this chapter. That such an ideology would last over two millennia and be adopted by foreign rulers of China such as Mongols, Jurchens, and Manchus, is testimony to the power of the cultural system and its religious underpinnings.

Official Patronage as a Strategy for Affirming and Controlling Multiplicity

We noted above that the Chinese cosmological system was developed in large part so that the government could extend its mantle over the

whole of the Chinese civilized world. For two thousand years of imperial history, the Chinese state cult retained a significant ritual role for the ruler, symbolizing his (very rarely, her) role in unifying and maintaining the cosmos. This ritual role also extended to the obligation of the ruler and governmental officials at all levels to provide patronage and official guidance for religion in the realm. As noted in chapter 4, the Chinese state reserved to itself the authority to establish the appropriate bounds of religious belief, writing, and practice; there was no notion of separation of church and state. From the T'ang dynasty (618-907) onward, the government sought to make official patronage of religion at least as powerful as the patronage of local families and notables; in other words, it sought to extend the imperial government's role in the sponsorship (and control) of religion.[6]

Government Mechanisms for Control of Religion

In the T'ang dynasty, the government established imperial bureaus of Buddhism and Taoism and sponsored bibliographic projects to publish great compendia of Confucian, Taoist, and Buddhist writings, as well as encyclopedias on history and other matters. The state bureaus kept records, published books, and administered government regulations about the classifications of priests, books, and rituals.[7] There were no state bureaus for folk religion, so that any imperially recorded and approved religious item had to be classified as Buddhist, Taoist, or Confucian.[8]

The T'ang government also developed and controlled the state examination system to award Confucian degrees, which qualified candidates for government service.[9] The state established an official Confucian cult, building temples to honor Confucian worthies in seats of government throughout the realm, and officially bestowing the title of "worthy" on selected persons.

The government's management of the Chinese religious world was exercised both through legal control (including persecution) and through patronage. Government laws and edicts outlawed various sects and groups, prohibited specific religious practices, burned texts as heretical, and banned public assemblies.[10] The motive was two-fold: 1) to maintain the value base of Chinese culture, and 2) to ensure that religion continued to support rather than threaten the status quo.

In late imperial China (fifteenth century-1912), the status quo was fragile, threatened by external and internal forces. In this period, the government tended to see any large-scale popular activity as a threat. Modern scholars have studied "folk Buddhist" (millenarian or White Lotus) groups, which arose sometime around the twelfth century and became a powerful cultural phenomenon in the fifteenth century. The

government at times saw folk Buddhist movements as potentially or actually seditious (and hence heretical, in legal terms), although the research suggests that neither the beliefs nor the practices were intended to be seditious or threatening.[11] These folk Buddhist sects were carefully watched and sometimes vigorously persecuted by the state. Some of these groups hastened to accommodate their writings more carefully to mainstream religious ideas, thereby protecting themselves against suspicion.

Government Patronage

Although a major motivation of the government was control, its sponsorship and patronage of religious practices also condoned a broad pattern of religious multiplicity. Each county seat not only had its official academy and Confucian hall of worthies, but also had a number of imperially sponsored temples, labeled as Buddhist or Taoist. These official temples were listed in county and prefectural gazetteers, along with tidbits of their history and their official and imperial patronage. Government sponsorship authorized the tonsure of monks and nuns, and provided stipends in support of the temples. Local officials were expected to attend major rituals at the official temples as representatives of the government; their presence as a representative of the emperor replicated locally the ritual role of the emperor at the capital. The officials paid respects to the deities on behalf of the state and asked for the support of the deities in maintaining order, thus sustaining the harmony of the cosmos.

The government also asserted its patronage and control of local religion by appointing (i.e., giving a title to) the deity of the city wall temple (*ch'eng-huang miao*). Generally a local hero around whom stories of religious protection had posthumously collected, the city wall deity became a spirit general with an assignment to protect the city and its surrounding countryside.[12] In appointing the city-wall gods, the government paid public homage to a local hero and coopted his powers into a heavenly hierarchy which sustained the unity of the empire. The government embraced all significant religious communities so that they would form part of the religious support of imperial power and order. I will recount one such instance in the tale which ends this chapter.

Unity and Diversity: Strategies Which Leave Room for Variation

The paternalistic controlling impulse of the government was only one side of the dynamic of the Chinese religious field. China is a vast coun-

try, geographically larger and embracing more languages and dialects than Europe, a patchwork quilt comprised of many subcultures and minority peoples who have lived under the cultural and political dominance of "Han" (Chinese) culture.

Because of the striking diversities among regions and linguistic groups, local communities had to exercise considerable ingenuity to mask from themselves and from the authorities in the capital the extent of their deviation from the standard norm, as defined in law and in the governmentally sanctioned classics. For some years scholars who read both studies based on official documents and the work of anthropologists in regions far from the capital marveled at the discrepancies between these two pictures of Chinese religious life.

The Chinese empire, at least by the time of the T'ang dynasty (618-907), was vast and diverse. Lacking modern communications, there was no way for the central government to be fully informed about activities in the provinces, nor could it fully control them. This was not for lack of interest, but rather a reflection of the limitations of central control over vast areas in the premodern world.

This section deals with the role of regional dialect and local moral consensus in allowing some room for variation within standard orthodoxy. This space for variation affords freedom for varieties in both the rules and style of play in local or regional versions of the Chinese religious field.

The Chinese Language as a Vehicle for Expressing Diversity

Chinese culture is a patchwork of subcultures, dialect groups, and minority peoples, and the myth of cultural unity is to some degree a myth in both senses of the word: a mistaken assertion, and an attempt to create reality by representing it as a story invested with meaning which can be sustained through ritual practice. One of the primary bonds sustaining the unity of Chinese culture was its written language, a *lingua franca* for the educated elite which could be read in a variety of diverse spoken dialects.

Chinese is not an alphabetical language. That is, there is not a limited number of letters or symbols representing the sounds of the spoken language, which can then be transcribed into writing. Rather it is an ideographic language, with tens of thousands of characters or ideograms developed to represent individual words. Some of the characters started as a pictograph or ideogram, a representation of the thing to which the spoken word referred. The pictorial hint worked as a mnemonic device, helping the reader to recognize the word indicated. Many words, however, could not be easily pictured, and so a character was built by combining a classifier (indicating the kind of thing it

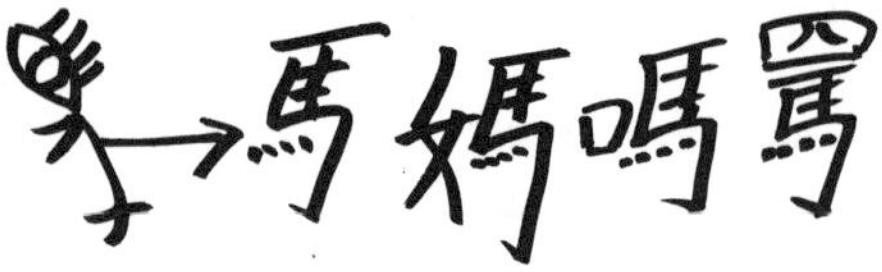

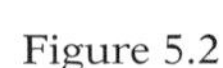

Figure 5.2

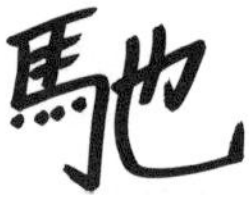

Figure 5.3

is) with a homophonic picture. Thus the word for horse (*ma*) was originally a picture of a horse, but combined with the classifier for "woman," it became mother (*ma*); with the classifier for "mouth," it became a question indicator (*ma?*); with the classifier for "blood," it became a curse (*ma*) (see figure 5.2). Or, horse can itself be a classifier to indicate "horsy things" so that with the phonic *ch'i*, it means to gallop (see figure 5.3). Other markers were added to other characters until a vast vocabulary had been built up.[13]

The characters did give some indication of a sound, but could not be read easily, since the phonic element was both hard to identify and might have evolved over time; the pronunciation of each character had to be memorized individually.

While Chinese is not the easiest language to learn to read and write, the writing system has one aspect of genius for maintaining Chinese cultural unity: speakers of the scores of Chinese dialects could each learn the written language (*wen-yen*), pronouncing it in their own local language. This contrasts sharply with Latin, which served as a *lingua franca* in medieval Europe, and was always and clearly distinct from spoken languages. One could read *wen-yen* in and through the lens of one's mother tongue.[14]

Thus the canonical and normative texts which defined Chinese-ness were in this pan-Chinese written language, which was pronounceable in, but not the same as, the spoken language of the particular region; *wen-yen* could be read by literate persons in their local dialectical pronunciation, but it did not transcribe the local dialect itself. This allowed an opening for two levels of discourse: the more universal, which took place in the written language and followed the norms and mores of a unified Chinese culture, and the local dialect, incomprehensible to outsiders, in which the locals could sustain their linguistic and cultural distinctiveness.

The two-tiered language system also allowed for stories told or written[15] in the local vernacular to reflect regional perceptions of reality, including their distinctive interpretations of the imperial Sacred Edicts.[16] Even novels could reflect a view of the Chinese way which stretched the boundaries and sensibilities of the imperial orthodoxy.[17] The Chinese people and local communities often acceded to the political authority of the imperial government, but reserved to themselves

some moral authority based on their own experience. If the local community and the representatives of the imperial government judged that a practice was normative and supportive of moral values and the social order, then it was accepted as canonical or orthodox even if it seemed to clash with what was written in the classics or the legal code. Thus, a local practice regarding burial or mourning might differ significantly from that prescribed in the classical texts, but as long as the local practice reflected "the way things are done" the discrepancy was simply ignored. Barbara Ward has called this ingenious stratagem "varieties of the conscious model."[18] Outsiders who served as government officials in the district often noted the distinctive local customs, but if they seemed to reflect cultural normalcy (to reinforce rather than undercut social order and harmony), this was not seen to be in conflict with the Chinese Way.

Thus we have seen that although the government sought to control and co-opt religion, it did so in the spirit of embracing all forms of religious life which sustained the social order, and hence strengthened the sovereignty of the state. Local deviations from the norm were tolerated, so long as they were, at bottom, establishmentarian. The Chinese religious field was, with the support of the government officials, both capacious and sufficiently flexible about rules of play to embrace a broad diversity of religious life and practice.

The specific role of the government in embracing religious diversity and supporting emergent religious movements can be well illustrated with the case of Ching-ming Tao.

The Tale of Ching-ming Tao (Way of the Pure and Perspicacious)

In many periods of Chinese history, emperors realized that the best way to deal with the variety of local religions and powerful temples was to embrace them by means of imperial patronage, thereby pulling them into the orbit of religious support of imperial power. Such temples became official temples and regularly offered prayers and ceremonies for the health of the state, with local magistrates and other officials in attendance. The temples in turn received financial support, authorization for more clergy, and funds to hold visible and dignified ritual ceremonies which might attract the patronage of local gentry families.

Once a temple became a major Buddhist or Taoist monastery (which trained and housed ordained priests or monks), official recognition was more or less assured; in such cases recognition followed upon success. The more complex and fascinating story, however, is how a local religious group functioning outside of the bounds of either

Buddhism or Taoism, came to be enfolded into the system of imperial patronage during the Sung dynasty (960-1279). This tale shows both government authorities and local believers maximizing their positions on the religious field.

What came to be known as Ching-ming Tao was originally a local popular religion, founded by Wu Meng (flourished, third century, C.E.). Wu Meng performed magic, exorcised demons and monsters, and taught some rudimentary forms of ritual and self-cultivation from the common Chinese religious field.[19] Between 644 and 670, Hsü Sun (239-292), who had originally been Wu Meng's disciple, came to be venerated as the primary deity of the movement. Devotion to Hsü Sun was well established at the group's center on Hsi-shan, and shrines to him appeared all over southeast China from the Sung dynasty onward.

Hsü Sun was lionized as a local magistrate who used religious arts to battle demons, monsters, and plagues. Over the centuries he also developed a reputation as a deity who helped besieged communities defend themselves against bandits. His effectiveness as a protector positioned his religious movement as a defender of the state, and thus attracted elite patronage.[20]

Sung imperial interest in the cult began when early Sung emperors adapted a divination system devised by Hsü Sun, which had reportedly been very helpful to the Sui Emperor Yang-ti (r. 605-616). Sung emperor Chen-tsung (r. 998-1022) named Hsü's temple Yü-lung kuan (The Abbey of Jade Beneficence).

Sung imperial patronage entered a new phase under emperor Hui-tsung (r. 1102-1125). Hui-tsung once fell asleep reading and dreamed he saw a Taoist master holding a cup decorated with a nine-flower pattern, attended by two men dressed as priests and holding swords. The Taoist master informed the emperor that he was Hsü Sun, an official in Heaven, whom the gods had dispatched to aid the Sung government in its present difficulties with the Jurchen.[21] Hsü reported that during his tenure as a magistrate in the third century, he had defeated demons and malicious spiritual forces (*yao-ch'i*) in his domain. Since the incursion of barbarian forces once again threatened the region he had once governed, he was coming to the aid of the throne.[22] This account of spiritual prowess caught Hui-tsung's interest, for the emperor sought help in warding off the threats of the Jurchen invaders and in controlling monsters and demons, whose worship he believed threatened the stability of the Chinese religious field.

On waking from his dream, the emperor ordered his attendants to locate Hsü Sun's temple.[23] He had a portrait painted from his description of the deity in his dream. This portrait he circulated to temples throughout the land, asking them if this deity resided in their temple. The circulation of the portrait gave local temple leaders a chance to promote their causes. When the temple had been located, the emperor

sent a young Taoist to convey his respects to the deity Hsü Sun. In 1112, Hui-tsung sent jade tablets to announce his patronage of the temple and ordered an elaborate seven-day *chiao* ritual with thirty-seven Taoist masters and ritual masters in attendance; the banquet on the last day of ritual fed 360 guests.[24]

A few months later, Hsü Sun once again appeared in Hui-tsung's dreams to thank him for his efforts on his behalf. He lamented that his main temple, Yü-lung kuan, was in a state of disrepair and asked the emperor to restore it. (One wonders if the temple leaders had not made the same case to the imperial envoys who brought the emperor's messages of respect.) The emperor immediately ordered the restoration; he had six major halls and twelve minor halls restored, installed new images, repainted the murals, sent new bronze incense burners, vases, and other ritual equipment, and personally penned couplets and inscriptions for the temple, which credited Hsü Sun with saving the region from a Jurchen invasion.[25]

In 1118 Hui-tsung incorporated this temple into the system of imperially sponsored official temples by naming it a *kung*, an official Taoist temple. Imperial recognition brought with it a new layer of religious duties, representing ritual traditions and practices extraneous to the internal and local history of Ching-ming Tao. Priests would now regularly perform rituals in the service of the state. The religious leaders of Ching-ming Tao would not originally have been trained in such elaborate rituals.[26] Imperial rituals, such as the *chiao*, required the temporary or permanent assignment to the temples of formally trained Taoist priests. The assignments of these priests in itself changed the character of the temple, and brought it into the mainstream of imperially recognized forms of religion. This was the price of the considerable benefit of the lavish restoration paid for by the emperor.

The local traditions of the group were not, however, entirely eclipsed by their entry into the mainstream of official temples. The author of Hsü's biography describes in some detail a pilgrimage at the shrine.[27] The pilgrimage path was believed to retrace routes which Hsü had traveled as a magistrate. Each twist and turn of the path, each ford of a river, had a story or tradition connected with Hsü's life—his battle with a white snake, or his conquering of an evil force. The account of the pilgrimage, which is local and popular, suggests that the group maintained its local traditions and practices alongside the new Taoist ones. Thus two levels of ritual, one official and one local, existed side by side. The character and stature of the religious institution had been expanded, but at least during the Sung, the community maintained its local traditions while honoring the official boons and duties of becoming an imperially sponsored temple. Two distinct religious traditions were practiced at the same temple.

The story of Ching-ming Tao helps us to understand the role of the government and of local tradition in the Chinese religious field. Imperial patronage and recognition had clear advantages for a religious institution: restoration of temples, financial support, the residence of priests trained for formal and impressive rites, the nearly mandatory participation of local officials and elites in ritual activities designed to support the state. On the other hand, there was room for local tradition and the continuation of some of the older practices alongside the official ritual roles of a recognized temple. The government had its view of the role and responsibilities of the temple; the local adepts had their view of its history, traditions, and practices.

The Chinese religious field supported both the myth of cultural unity and the richness of local variation. The local cult, in order to attract imperial patronage, had to accommodate to the nationally recognized categories for religion; the imperial government, in order to co-opt the support of the local religious movement, had to honor and support the local deity and his temple. Both Ching-ming Tao and the Sung government benefited from their relationship, but each side tacitly acknowledged the discrepancy between local and national perceptions and made room for both local and imperial customs and practices.

Final Thoughts

In my early days as a pilgrim in China, I had a tendency to idealize or romanticize Chinese practices, seeing them as somehow more idealistic and less compromised than the religious history of Christianity. Still a young woman, I shared with many young Christians disillusionment at the imperfections of the Christian churches and the contradictions between ideals and practices. The messy and compromised history of the church, often enmeshed in power struggles within its ranks and with secular authorities, seemed to sully true Christianity.

However, anything beyond the most superficial acquaintance with Chinese religion insists that there is no division between the sacred and secular, between religion and politics: religion is central to society at all levels, and is thus deeply embedded in political, social, and cultural struggles.

It was an important lesson for me to realize that Chinese religious inclusivity did not arise from some transcendent idealism, but rather was embedded in the commitments of both the ruling classes and the local populations to their own religious visions and paths. The Chinese negotiated religious diversity shrewdly, and they allowed space for others in order to ensure their mutual survival and flourishing.

The story of Ching-ming Tao helped me grasp more concretely how

王

the Chinese accommodated the pressures for cultural unity while honoring the local. Different embodiments of this movement could coexist as different parties made room for the other view, while holding to their own.

One the other hand, the role of Taoist priest Pai Yü-ch'an illustrated to me how readily the boundaries between the government version of Ching-ming Tao and the local version could be crossed. Pai was invited to Yü-lung kung to officiate at specialized Taoist rituals, the new rituals required by the recognition of the temple. He stayed on to write a detailed record of Hsü's life and the development of the religious movement. Although Pai came to the temple to represent mainstream Taoist rituals, he was so moved by the religious vitality of the local movement that he left a vivid record of their story and local practices. Pai did not join Ching-ming Tao; his own practice followed another school. Yet he celebrated Ching-ming Tao's contributions to the Chinese religious field. Pai had no personal agenda with regard to Ching-ming Tao. He simply saw both Ching-ming Tao and his own practices as part of the Chinese religious field; he might well cite the saying of Hsün Tzu invoked by Li Chih in the epigraph to this chapter: "There are not two Ways under heaven; the sage or worthy does not have two minds." Pai's celebration of Ching-ming Tao is eloquent testimony to the genuine cultural pattern of religious inclusivity sustained by the Han system of cultural unity.

Pai Yü-ch'an's role as the chronicler of Ching-ming Tao, author of a vibrant account of its history and its spiritual legacy, helped me to discern my role as a scholar of other religions. Pai initially came in a formal priestly capacity on a temporary visit, but stayed on as a guest, accepting the hospitality of the tradition in order to learn about it and to share that knowledge with others. He honored the history and the religious values of the tradition, recording them faithfully in his account along with original sources. As it happened, his work became the most vibrant record of and witness to the religious vitality of this movement; he became, in a sense, an unwitting theologian, or authoritative commentator, of the tradition.

More than twelve years after my original visit to Chinese territory, I found myself in a similar position. I had gone to China to do dissertation research on Lin Chao-en, on whom I would later publish the only full-length book available in any language. In the 1980s, Lin Chao-en's religious movement was being revived in Fukien and southeast China, and I was invited to a conference as the major authority (i.e, essentially a theologian) of the movement. It was a strange sensation.

Like Pai Yü-ch'an, I had sought to honor the integrity of Lin's life and teaching, and to convey in my work the religious vitality of the movement which he founded. Both Pai and I no doubt benefited from our sustained and respectful attention to the values and virtues of the

traditions which we chronicled. Yet in neither of our cases did this mean a conversion or even a dramatic change of direction in our own spiritual developments and affiliation. We were both honoring religious communities whose teachings deserved broader attention, and seeking to discern and learn from virtues and values which might enrich our own lives and those of our communities.

Too often scholars of religion have claimed to be only "learning about" or "teaching about" the religions they study; that is disingenuous, since it ignores the ways in which all genuine learning enriches the self and contributes to growth. On the other hand, too many Christians have assumed that all exposure to another religion in effect opens one to the competition and weakens one's loyalty to one's own community. Such an attitude is overly defensive, and it overlooks the fact that a religious person may be well positioned to appreciate the religious values and qualities of other religious persons' lives, enhancing one's own religious sensibilities in the process. The middle ground is to be a respectful guest, to honor another tradition as far as possible on its own terms, and to be open to benefiting from the exchange, while at the same time being clear about who I am and how my identity and location shape my experience as a learner of the other tradition. If I can do both of those, I will be able to learn well and also recount what I have learned effectively to those in my own community.

CHAPTER 6

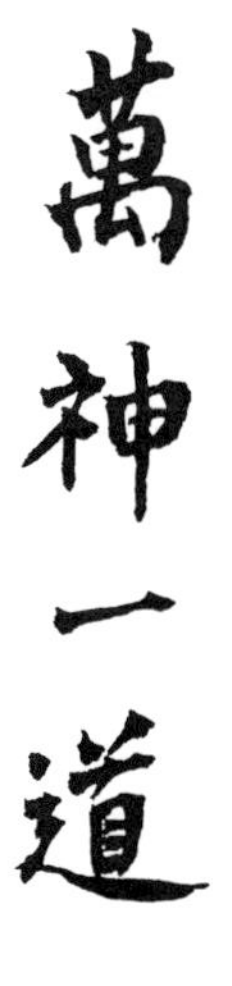

Myriad Spirits and the Transcendent in the Religious Field

*[Liu Yi-chih (1078-1160)] said, "The sentient beings are the essence of things (*t'i-pen*) and the fulfillment of enlightenment (*yüan-ch'eng*). So we and the bodhisattva [Kuan-yin] are the same, and there is no difference between us and her. Because of this non-duality (*wu-erh*) and non-differentiation (*wu-pieh*), the faith in the hearts of the sentient beings extends everywhere without physical trace. The bodhisattva not only has no fixed identity but also no fixed dwelling. Yet, you put up a statue in a designated place for them to seek refuge. Are you not creating a false distinction?"*

Chiu replied, "Not so. The goddess's manifestations are limitless. Because she has no one place of her own, but is worshipped in the hearts of believers, she thus has a place. I see that monks and lay people go in front of the statue, gather their robes and bow, burn incense and pray on their knees, and tell her of all their illnesses and troubles, and ask for help. Full of sincere emotion, sweat dripping down their faces, they tell her their inner thoughts. The bodhisattva responded to their faith by appearing in a dream.

"Ultimately, they [the bodhisattva and sentient beings] are as one. I admire the place she is worshipped and make it imposing in order to augment their faith. If they believe, in one instant they view matter, and they understand emptiness. Then they will attain enlightenment. They will know that the

---

"Many Spirits, One Way"
These characters represent the Chinese affirmation of both a plethora of deities and the transcendent unity of the Tao.

bodhisattva does not arise from her image. She is everywhere, in all directions. Every place is her place of worship. And this place of worship is nowhere specific."

—Liu Yi-chih

temple inscription from T'iao-hsi chi

By this point in my journey, I was well on the way to developing powers for apprehending the dynamics of the Chinese religious field. I had confronted the role of power and patronage, of political motivations both at the national and local levels. I had begun to appreciate the interplay between the myth of cultural unity and the realities of local variation, as government authorities and local communities vied to promote their interests in controlling a religious place or tradition. However, more challenges were ahead for this pilgrim.

My next challenge was to deal with the stunning and vast array of gods worshipped by the Chinese. I began to wonder how such rich diversity could maintain any unity whatsoever—wasn't this simply a case of "anything goes"? How did the tens of thousands of gods and spirits relate to the Way of Heaven which encompassed all in the Chinese religious field? Did the many competing deities offering worldly boons suggest, as early Western observers tended to believe, that Chinese religion was merely pragmatic and this-worldly and had no impulse toward the transcendent?

The temple inscription of Liu Yi-chih, which formed the epigraph to this chapter, raised a related question: if the Bodhisattva Kuan-yin was omnipresent and could take many forms, how did one justify building a statue, which occupied only one place and only one form of the bodhisattva, for her worship?

In this chapter I deal with the issues surrounding this relationship of the multiplicity of deities and images to the transcendent unity of the Way. In it, I explore: the relationship of deities to their images, the importance of a deity's demonstration of power to sustain worship (and vice versa), the multiplicity of spirits in any local religious field, the moral continuum of humans and spirits, and the theology of transcendence. I conclude with a tale of how a single Taoist religious ritual simultaneously honored the transcendental aspects of the holy and the particularistic worldly or popular expressions.

The Relations of Gods to Their Images

A foreign visitor to a Chinese temple or shrine is immediately struck by the plethora of images: crude and elaborate, small and large. Some are little more than carved dolls; others are larger than life-size, decorated with gilt, paint, lacquer, and/or elaborately embroidered garments. Many images boast beards made of human hair. If the temple

萬神一道

is too poor to have a carved image, it may have a drawing, painting, or wood-block print to portray the deity. These deities are offered incense, food and drink, and money; they may be feted with music and dance, or taken in a sedan chair to visit their territory or to attend a rite or festival at another temple. They are approached in prayer by individuals and asked by priests and shamans to lend their power to rituals. There is no question that these images are the focus of piety and worship.[1]

There is a tendency among Christians, particularly Protestants, to assume that such worship involving images or pictures of deities is necessarily idolatry, a confusion of the nontranscendent with the transcendent. There are, however, indications in Chinese ritual practice that this charge of idolatry is misplaced; these images are not confused with the higher spiritual powers which they represent.

There is, for example, the ceremony of opening the eyes, the ritual for installing an image in a Chinese temple. Anyone can purchase an image of a particular deity, but such figures are merely statues until they are ritually invested in a temple (or at a home altar) by means of the *k'ai-yen* (opening the eyes) ceremony.[2] The *k'ai-yen* ritual invites the heavenly deity (of which the statue is a depiction) to descend and inhabit the image with its luminosity (*ling*), thus animating it with spiritual power. In traditional times, the ceremony also included the insertion of paper drawings of organs into an opening in the rear of the statue, vivifying the hollow wooden body with symbolic organs. Only so long as the image was inhabited by the *ling* of the deity was it considered holy.[3] The presence of *ling* meant that the deity inhabited its image and could perform miracles in answer to prayers. If the image was not in good condition, the deity would not have a "healthy body" to inhabit, and its power to perform miracles would be harmed.[4] A natural disaster, such as flood or fire, could injure the *ling* of the image; in that case, the image might either be discarded, replaced with a new image, or ritually revived with another *k'ai-yen* ceremony.

Another practice for revivifying images can be seen in the phenomenon of branch temples of a famous deity, such as Ma Tsu.[5] Such temples are formal branches of an original temple, extending the spiritual grace and prowess of the deity to outlying locations. The branch temples periodically send representatives to the main temple, carrying their local image or their incense censor to the main temple to be reinvested with the spiritual power (*ling*) of the main image. This practice suggests that images are important but fragile loci for the spiritual power and presence of the deity; the concentration of *ling* in the locus of the image enables worshippers to pray to the deity, from whom they expect protection and miracles.[6]

Judged by Their Power

The Chinese attitude toward spirits is a matter of faith frequently confirmed by the demonstrated power of the spirits. As Laurence Thompson has written,

> *The gods are alive because they have manifested themselves through their works.* Their spiritual power, called *ling* in Chinese, is the evidence of their existence. . . . Any claim or attribution of *ling* that gains a certain public currency may result in deification of a person. Rumors having spread and credibility having been established through confirmation that the spirit responds to prayers, a temple will be put up through public subscription. From then on the growth or decline of the cult is a matter of god's efficacy. This means that the death of the gods is also commonplace. When public confidence in the power of a deity has waned, he will be neglected and eventually forgotten.[7]

The continual judging of deities according to their demonstrated power is the distinguishing mark of the Chinese worship of spirits. This accountability is not confined to illiterate worshippers. Valerie Hansen recounts an example of a Sung dynasty magistrate using the principle in his attempts to recruit spiritual support for ending a drought.

> An 1107 inscription from Liyang county, Jiangsu, reports that a district magistrate unsuccessfully prayed for rain at each of the nearby temples during a long drought. Upon consulting a local history, he learned about a temple twenty li to the northeast where the resident deity had always responded to entreaties. He prayed there, and rain followed.[8]

The magistrate consulted a local history, while the illiterate populace depended on word-of-mouth reports on which deities were able to deliver each boon. The principle was the same.

Chinese worshippers expected accountability on the part of a deity, or at least ongoing evidence of active spiritual presence. They understood that deities whose images or temples were in disrepair, or whose offerings were too meager, required more active worship and support in order to produce miracles. However, if the worshippers were doing their part and the deity still did not respond, it was assumed that the deity had lost its powers or was no longer present. For instance, a deity who did not respond to prayers to end a drought might first be

萬神一道

exposed in the noonday sun of the marketplace to get a taste of the drought and then summarily dumped into the river for having lost her or his power to protect the people.[9]

The people relied on the deities to deal with serious life disasters. As Hansen has written,

> Whenever illness befell individuals or epidemics struck entire towns, whenever drought, locusts, or torrential rain hit agricultural communities, and whenever marauding troops or bandits threatened settlements, Chinese people who had no other means of tackling these problems looked to the gods for protection.[10]

A large-scale or serious disaster for which prayers did not bring immediate solace might cause the local community to pull out the stops and consult every specialist or deity they could think of, sometimes simultaneously.

> A drought occurred in Fuchou (Fukien), and a respected member of the gentry led a procession of Buddhist monks, Taoist practitioners, spirit mediums, and three hundred peasants to pray for rain at a well thought to be the residence of the local dragon.[11]

If the purpose of the gods was to protect people from the ailments of life and the afterlife, then major ills might require multiple protection.

The Western observer of these practices is often curious about how seriously the Chinese believed in these deities. Valerie Hansen, in dealing with this issue, cites a number of incidents of authors or storytellers who express a certain skepticism, cynicism, or detachment about the gods, but she notes of one of these skeptics, "Once he himself is in danger, he, like the sailors [about whose practices he was skeptical], begs the gods for help."[12] Having few tools at their disposal to deal with life's challenges, the traditional Chinese relied heavily on their gods.

The Need for Many Gods in the Local Religious Field

For the vast majority of traditional Chinese, the world thronged with ghosts or demons (*kuei*) and spirits or deities (*shen*), who—if properly propitiated—could assist them through the vicissitudes of human life. Even educated persons, who might harbor skepticism about the stories and powers attributed to deities, seldom dismissed the gods entirely. As Hansen comments about two skeptics, "For both, however,

the hazards of life—be they in the course of an official's daily routine or on a perilous ocean voyage—were so great that they could not pray to just one god."[13]

The Chinese religious field pulsated with spiritual forces. At one level were the ghosts and spirits, the souls of all who had lived, inhabiting graves, spirit-tablets in ancestral shrines, the fields and glens, the heavens and the hells. Particularly worthy spirits might become deities in the heavenly pantheon. A person's spirit (*shen*) was the imaginative, transcendent aspect of the human mind-and-heart, which—if properly cultivated—could develop considerable intelligence, wisdom, and prowess. Every human being had multiple connections to spirits and ghosts: they were one's ancestors or the ancestors of the community; they were powerful or malevolent deities or demons from human history; they were the spiritual and demonic aspects of one's self. The great Confucian thinkers even liked to depict the terms "spirits" (*shen*) and "ghosts/demons" (*kuei*) as the expansive or contractive aspects of the human mind, or even the expansive and contractive breaths of the cosmos as a whole.[14]

Add to this throng of spiritual beings an ancient belief that the land of China itself was animated by veins of auspicious and malevolent energy which might attract the habitation of positive spirits or malevolent demons. Human use or domestication of the land (particularly for homes or graves) had to be respectful of the spiritual forces of the land. Understanding and tapping the positive benefits of the spiritual forces of the land was the domain of geomancy (*feng-shui*), a proto-science for planning the location and orientation of graves, homes, and other buildings to accord with the forces of the land. Depending on the appropriateness of their gravesites, the honor accorded them by the memorials of their descendants, and the cumulative deeds of their human lives, the spirits of the dead could become benevolent protectors, hungry ghosts, or angry demons who threatened all living beings.

To manage this crowded and complex world of spiritual forces one needed an array of effective rituals. It was not unusual for participants in the Chinese religious field to combine more than one level of "spiritual management" in caring for the welfare of the living, the newly dead, and the ancestors. Given the myriad religious practices and traditions open to the Chinese, and the lack of an obligation to choose among them, the religious location of a person or community in the Chinese religious field was remarkably fluid and functional, shifting with needs and circumstances. One assumed multiple religious locations and roamed the field at will. The multiple locations reflected the multiple roles and responsibilities of a particular person or family. As the place of the family and the individual in Chinese society became more complex, so did the religious and ritual obligations attendant upon them.

The spirit world and human approaches to it were extensions of the human world; religious patterns of behavior sustained and reinforced social patterns of behavior in the culture. In a famous article, anthropologist Arthur Wolf deftly captured the general pattern of worship and offering which encoded the practices of Chinese religious life. According to Wolf, three classes of spirits were worshipped in different places, under different circumstances, with different offerings, and by different officiants. An analysis of the differences among the three classes of spirits suggests a clear cultural code: gods were approached with the deference, courtesies, and offerings appropriate to public officials and rulers; ghosts were treated like bandits, beggars, and bullies, kept at bay through bribes offered out the back gate; ancestors were treated like honored family elders, included in family banquets and celebrations.[15] Thus the vast range of deities and of styles of rituals reflected and maintained the structures of Chinese society.

A Moral Continuum

Chinese popular deities were very often former human beings. These could be moral exemplars who had attained a spiritual appointment after death or they could be locals whose lives had been cut off prematurely. After death, their tombs gave off auras or they would appear in dreams to announce their powers.[16] The careers of these deities depended on their powers in answering prayers and on their moral attainments. Gods, like human beings, remained on the continuum of moral retribution which was basic to Chinese folk beliefs.

Chinese plays and folk tales abound with stories of deities being promoted or demoted because of their deeds.[17] Chinese deities were not viewed as eternally existent beings, but rather as spirits of the dead who have achieved divine status because of their virtue and their development of spiritual powers.[18] In their careers as deities, they continue to be held accountable to a higher power, depicted in fiction as a heavenly bureaucracy under the rule of the Jade Emperor, but also—since the Jade Emperor himself was not a font of perfect wisdom—accountable ultimately to a power higher than all deities: Tao in itself, or the Cosmic Buddha (all reality as Buddhahood), or the will of Heaven. Thus empowering each image is the spiritual efficacy (*ling*) of a deity, a being on a spiritual journey who is seeking, like the faithful who worship him, to embody as fully as possible the Tao in itself.

If the gods were subject to the same moral principles as humans, then tales of the gods also had a moral dimension. The best of the gods modeled for the faithful the virtues of generosity and public-spiritedness; ghosts and demons represented vengeful and selfish forms of behavior.

Transcendence and Immanence

The fortunes of deities, as of human beings, rise and fall. The rapidly changing landscape of deities led thoughtful religious persons to posit a source of spiritual power beyond the multiplicity of the gods.[19] Ordinary people did not care about the theological subtleties of the source beyond; they simply judged the gods by their abilities to answer prayers and perform miracles. Seeking evidence of power, they were content to move from god to god to have their needs addressed. The theologians, however, sought to articulate a continuous source from which emanated the myriad spirits.

The Chinese accepted the reality that it would be impossible for human beings to pray to, relate to, or depict Tao, Buddha, Heaven, the Way, the Truth as they were in themselves, because any such attempt would inappropriately limit and constrain the vast cosmic reality within a specific set of terms and categories. This is most famously stated in chapter 1 of the *Tao te ching*:

> The way that can be spoken of
> Is not the constant way;
> The name that can be named
> Is not the constant name.
> The nameless was the beginning of heaven and earth;
> The named was the mother of the myriad creatures.[20]

Even in this statement, Lao Tzu acknowledges that the named (the embodied) is necessary as a connection with the myriad creatures; yet it is not the thing in itself.

Alongside this notion of the transcendent Tao beyond all human depictions, categories, and names—indeed beyond all attributes of personality—is a conviction that the Tao is both utterly transcendent and ineffable and at the same time is *everywhere*. The latter point is graphically captured by the great "Taoist" writer Chuang Tzu in his famous exchange with Master Tung-kuo:

> Master Tung-kuo asked Chuang Tzu, "This thing called the Way—where does it exist?
> Chuang Tzu said, "There's no place it doesn't exist."
> "Come," said Master Tung-kuo, "you must be more specific!"
> "It is in the ant."
> "As low a thing as that?"
> "It is in the panic grass."
> "But that's lower still!"
> "It is in the tiles and shards."

萬神一道

"How can it be so low?"
"It is in the piss and shit!"
Master Tung-kuo made no reply.[21]

Between the ineffable, transcendent, and unapproachable Tao, and the radical ubiquity of Tao's presence in even what seems most vile and least sacred, is the world of humans and of spirits. The myriad deities are like us humans when compared to the Tao in itself; they are like us in many ways, and thus are approachable with our hopes, fears, praise, and petitions. As in the case of the images discussed in the beginning of the chapter, personified deities were concentrations or loci of spiritual power accessible to worship and petition.

The plethora of spirits and divinities creates a complex religious cosmology, a picture of heaven and hell. If the Chinese religious field were to be negotiated by the faithful, this multiform spiritual world had to be mapped so that ordinary people could find their way. This was done in temple paintings or wood-block prints, in temple or ritual iconography, in religious drama and local stories, and in various teachings and rituals.

One of the most common ways for people to see the representations of the religious cosmology was to visit any significant temple in the community. Such temples displayed not only the major deities whom the temples honored, but also a host of minor deities (local deities, gods of nearby temples, gods of other religions), arranged in a clearly subordinate role, but nonetheless honored and the object of active veneration. These arrangements offered the temple's interpretation of the local religious field and of the religious cosmology.

Religious leaders were aware that popular religious piety and imagination looked for signs of the power and miracles of the gods, and that people cared little for the theological fine points and the sectarian distinctions between deities. Thus even deities with long-standing ties to one religion or a particular school of a religion were also seen as popular deities in a more general sense. Religious leaders encouraged such devotions, because it met the needs of the faithful.

For instance, the epigraph to this chapter cites a monk's justification for encouraging the popular worship of Kuan-yin, even though, theologically speaking, "there is no difference between us and her." He cites the people who "pray on their knees, and tell her of all their illnesses and troubles, and ask for help. Full of sincere emotion, sweat dripping down their faces, they tell her their inner thoughts. The bodhisattva responded to their faith by appearing in a dream." Valerie Hansen comments,

> However undesirable an image of Kuan-yin might be from a doctrinal standpoint, if the monastery is to attract followers, it cannot adhere to traditional doctrine. It must offer the poten-

> tial followers a deity in terms familiar to them. . . . Buddhist monks increasingly used the discourse of popular religion, by encouraging the worship of gods like Kuan-yin.[22]

萬神一道

Thus the theological affirmation of transcendence had to be balanced with the popular demand for immanence so that gods would hear prayers and address the ills which beset believers.

The tale of the Taoist *chiao* ritual is a splendid example of this balance between the transcendent and immanent aspects of spiritual presence. It is an outstanding example of how the many gods are united by the Way in a common religious field.

Transcendent Tao and Immanent Deities in the *Chiao* Ritual

Every so many years or to mark a significant turning point, such as the end of an epidemic or the defeat and repulsion of invaders, a Taoist temple and its community sponsored a *chiao* ritual. Readers may recall that Sung emperor Hui-tsung sponsored a seven-day *chiao* ritual at Yü-lung kuan to celebrate the god Hsü Sun's help in repulsing the Jurchen invaders. The *chiao* was the highest Taoist rite, performed to ritually cleanse a community or other site of threatening, corrosive, and debilitating spiritual forces and to renew and reforge its connections to the cosmic source of spiritual wholeness and renewal.

This tale recounts a community *chiao* in Chunan City, northern Taiwan, in 1970.[23] Because of the cumulative grievances of angry ghosts or demons, every community needed a thorough ritual cleansing from time to time; such was the basis of cyclical or regular *chiao*. The survival of a major disaster (such as epidemic or invasion) could leave behind residual negative forces from those whose lives had been prematurely ended by the disaster, and thus also required a ritual cleansing to ensure that the community was thoroughly cleansed of the pestilence.

Since the purpose of the *chiao* was to cleanse and restore the community, the entire community joined in sponsoring it. Every family in the community was invited to participate and to put out its offerings for public display. Participation in this gala ritual event brought the people together around a mutually beneficial common cause; all contributed to its success and all enjoyed the celebration. Deities and special guests from neighboring communities were invited, as were the souls of the dead. Visiting deities were even provided housing in temporary shelters.[24] Souls of the dead were important guests and had to be treated delicately. Their invitation sought to comfort or appease any recently dead who were aggrieved or angry because of ritual neglect; such neglected ghosts could wreak havoc in the community. By inviting and feasting these souls, the ritual integrated them into the posi-

tive spiritual forces who sustain rather than threaten community health and welfare. However, the community did not want such souls or ghosts hanging around indefinitely, so they were given a special ritual send-off toward the end of the *chiao*.[25]

The *chiao* was sponsored by a temple of some distinction, which usually had both major deities (seated in the position of honor on the main altar, facing south) and minor deities (around the sides and the back of the temple). On normal days, the faithful and priests of the temple prayed to these deities for help and succor in meeting the challenges of life. The high ritual of the *chiao*, during which renewal of the cosmos itself was at stake, looked beyond the myriad deities to the Tao in itself as the source of all spiritual power.

In preparation for this ceremony, normally performed by a highly trained Taoist priest,[26] the deities to whom the temple was dedicated and who occupied the seats of honor, were removed to the other end of the temple (facing north) to become observers and worshippers alongside the human participants. As the deities were ritually invited to become observers and worshippers in the *chiao*, the vacated worship space was ritually reconstructed for the special service. In the place of the deities were ritually installed abstract scrolls invoking the Three Pure Ones, three aspects of Tao in itself. The Three Pure Ones were not depicted in embodied form; they pointed beyond the specific and particularized deities of the Chinese pantheon to the cosmic unity of the Tao.[27] In normal everyday worship, the specific embodied deities were the most effective link with specific spiritual benefactions of the Taoist Way, but for returning to the source for cosmic renewal, the ritual turned to the Tao itself, which transcended all particular embodiments.

The *chiao* rituals, performed by the Taoist high priest in the sanctuary of the temple, represented Taoist ritual practice at its most subtle and internalized. The *chiao* consisted almost entirely of an internally visualized set of ritual encounters guided by the disciplined meditation of the priest. These rituals were witnessed by other priests and a select set of temple elders and community leaders. The high priest's external actions provided only minimal markers of the different portions of the rite. There was almost nothing to watch in the temple, and the ritual would make little or no sense unless the witness was already familiar with the structure of the rite and could thus provide the content for different sections from her/his own knowledge and imagination.

The ritual structure of the *chiao* included:

- purification of the temple
- announcement to the Three Pure Ones
- invitations to the Three Pure Ones
- an audience with the Three Pure Ones at which offerings were presented along with petitions

- renewal of contract for cosmic order
- ritual send-off for the Three Pure Ones.

萬神一道

Watching the rite performed in the sanctuary was somewhat akin to watching (without the aid of a prayer book) a pre-Vatican II Latin Mass performed *sotto voce* by a priest facing the altar at the back of the sanctuary! Only worshippers with a solid familiarity with the structure of the Mass would be able to follow in any detail.

If the rite in the sanctuary had been the only ritual aspect of the *chiao*, there would have been little incentive for the community to attend the ceremonies, and interest would have waned. The priestly rite, however, was not the whole picture.

A second set of *chiao* rituals was simultaneously performed in the open-air courtyard of the temple, and viewed by the people of the village. These rituals followed precisely the same structures as the restrained and internalized rituals in the sanctuary but at a different level:

- purification of the community and of people's homes
- announcements to ghosts and spirits
- invitations to ghosts, spirits, and human guests
- a banquet for human guests as well as ghosts and spirits
- presentation of the community's petition to ghosts and spirits with the signatures of all sponsors of the ritual
- ritual send-off for ghosts and spirits.

The public rites were, by contrast with the meditative, internalized rituals performed in the sanctuary, highly dramatic and popular, crowd-pleasing performances full of color and light, drama and prowess, and good feasting. The outer rituals were as accessible and obvious as the inner rituals were mysterious and internalized. Yet they both followed the same structure and enacted the self-same rite.[28] The two levels of the rite functioned both at the level of many spirits and at the level of the transcendent One. Appropriate liturgical forces were invoked in the most powerful and theologically sophisticated manner, and yet the drama of the rite was offered in a form accessible to the entire community.

The cosmic renewal was *effected* by the Tao in a manner invisible to all, but understood by the theologically sophisticated; the ritual was *dramatized or enacted* by the theatrical rites featuring the myriad deities to whom the ordinary believer could relate.

Final Thoughts

The two levels of the *chiao* ritual helped me as a pilgrim in Chinese culture understand more deeply how the rich diversity of the complex religious field held together. The Chinese, I learned again and again, had a genius for letting multiple levels or layers of spirituality function

萬神一道

side by side. The many levels of spiritual practice were all welcomed into one path on Lion's Head Mountain. The followers of Hsü Sun at Yü-lung kung were able to maintain their local religious practices alongside the rituals of the imperially sponsored Taoist rites. In the *chiao* the subtle theological structures of Taoist ritual are externalized into a multi-day popular festival so that the faithful can visualize and celebrate the renewal of the cosmos.

As monk Chiu, in the epigraph to this chapter, defended the cultivation of the popular worship of Kuan-yin at his temple, so all leaders of the Chinese religious field encouraged popular devotion while they developed their theological insights. As Chiu said, "I admire the place she is worshipped and make it imposing in order to augment their faith." He goes on to say that each instant of faith moves the people closer to enlightenment.

My deepening appreciation of the many layers and levels of Chinese worship made me increasingly aware of how awkward I and many Christians have been at acknowledging these many layers and levels in our own lives. How can we affirm our need for more popular, accessible forms of religious symbol and worship, as well as remember that God in Godself transcends all of the symbols and layers? Too often we scoff at "popular culture" religious images as silly or superficial, even as we fail to see the limits of whatever symbols and language we use to envision or approach God.

The interplay of particular deities and the transcendent One demonstrated the tension between the needs of popular devotion and theological speculation. This is a remarkable strategy of the Chinese religious field, and it was sustained by an equally remarkable concept of open-ended or nonabsolute truth, which will be discussed in the next chapter.

CHAPTER 7

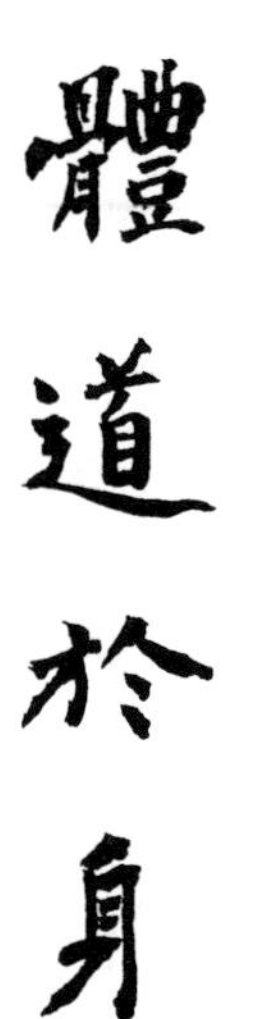

Many Embodiments of the Way

The Tao that can be spoken is not the eternal Tao [the Tao in itself].
The name that can be named is not the eternal name.
—*Lao Tzu*

At fifteen, I set my heart on learning. At thirty, I was firmly established. At forty, I had no more doubts. At fifty, I knew the will of Heaven. At sixty, I was ready to listen to it. At seventy, I could follow my heart's desire without transgressing what was right.
—*Confucius*

As a pilgrim in Chinese culture, I was profoundly impressed by the Chinese genius for bringing stunning religious diversity into a single vision: for weaving the many paths of the Chinese religious field into a single Way (on Lion's Head Mountain, or in any community) or for bringing the myriad deities to whom believers might turn for succor and protection into the all-encompassing Tao or Heaven.

But I was still a stranger, a pilgrim in this foreign land. The more I

"Embodying the Way in Oneself"
These characters (literally in one's body) represent the goal of Chinese religious practice. The Way must be realized in the living practice of each individual.

體道於身

came to know and celebrate the rich multiplicity of the Chinese religious field, the more I began to wonder about issues of truth, or as Westerners tend to construct it, *the* Truth. How did the Chinese respond to the fact that these various deities and religious groups had different teachings? Did not the reality of doctrinal difference destroy the unity of the Chinese religious field? How could the Chinese live with the doctrinal differences without great qualms about lack of consistency? Did they not want to know what, in the end, was Truth? What was the highest or final teaching of the Way?

The Hindus of the Indian subcontinent, particularly those who espoused the school of nonduality (*Vedânta*), argued that the plurality of deities and of realities were illusory projections of ignorance; only the One was real.[1] In China this answer did not suffice. Although the many spirits pointed to the one Tao and the many practices and insights of the pilgrimage were part of one Way, the multiplicity within the Chinese religious field was not taken to be error or illusion. In the Chinese religious field, the many gods, ghosts, and ancestors *were* vivified by Spirit or Tao, and the myriad practices and insights *were* stepping stones of the Way. Multiplicity and unity were *both* real. Reality was both/and, not either/or.

My next challenge as a pilgrim was to understand that the Chinese religious field offered a distinctive notion of the relation of the One and the many, of the relations of the Tao/Way of Heaven/Great Ultimate/Buddha[2] to its concrete manifestations. This notion is key to understanding the affirmation of diverse religious practices in the Chinese religious field.

In this chapter, I explore the significant tension in the Chinese religious field between the One and the many. Philosophically, pedagogically, and in spiritual practices, the players in the Chinese religious field maintained this tension, affirming multiple concretizations of the Tao without either absolutizing the particular or falling into a vicious relativism. One way of understanding this Chinese affirmation of many truths is through the image of *embodiment*.

I begin the chapter with an exploration of the embodiment of the Way through emulating human models, seeking enlightened teachers in books, and following learning strategies of moral practice, recitation of texts, and face-to-face dialogues. I then discuss strategies of teachers which allowed them to point beyond themselves to the Way, and music as a metaphor for the Tao and its concretizations. Finally, I recount strategies for embodying the Way as taught by three great sages of the Warring States period: Confucius, Lao Tzu, and Chuang Tzu. I follow myriad Chinese in looking to the tales of these remarkable teachers to grasp what it would mean to embody the Way.

Embodying the Way

體道於身

Looking to Human Models

One of the most striking aspects of Chinese religious practice is its reliance on human models, living exemplars of the Way. In the Sung (960-1279), Ming (1368-1644), and Ch'ing (1644-1912) dynasties, the imperial governments invoked this ancient tradition to sustain the moral fabric of the society by sponsoring village assemblies which included not only moral lectures but public rewards for local moral exemplars.[3] Carved stone memorial inscriptions honored chaste and virtuous widows, shrines commemorated filial sons and daughters, and popular genres such as illustrated penny-books lionized moral exemplars. The Chinese looked not only to literary and historical exemplars, but also to living teachers who embodied the Tao and its principles in their way of living in the world.

Although theological articulations differed, belief in the living embodiment of enlightenment, sagehood, the Way, spiritual prowess (the terms differ) was pervasive throughout the Chinese religious field. The notion that one might glimpse living sagehood in the person of an enlightened teacher was well grounded in Confucian understandings of human nature and the Way. Following the teachings of Mencius (372?-289? B.C.E.), most later Confucians agreed that human beings were essentially good; they possessed from birth the seeds of virtue and enlightenment. Study and practice cultivated and nurtured those seeds so that the innate positive potential of human nature could be fulfilled in the life of the student. The sage did not represent something wholly other. There was no radical gap between ordinary humanity and the wisdom and virtue of the sage. Achieving sagehood, however, entailed a long process of study, self-cultivation, discipline, and practice.

The forms and schools of Buddhism which flourished in China insisted that enlightenment or Buddhahood was embodied in living human beings: a central teaching of Mahayana Buddhism was "This very body is the Buddha!" In later Buddhism the recorded sayings of enlightened masters had the authority of the Buddhist Truth (dharma) taught by the Buddha in the canonical scriptures.[4] This genre made it explicit that the living masters embodied the same enlightenment as the Buddha. Thus it was crucial to find and interact with an enlightened teacher.

The best way to develop one's spiritual potential was to find a teacher who embodied spiritual values. Such a teacher offered a model for living, as well as guidance and admonition for the student. Lacking a master, one could only turn to books.

體道於身

Capturing the Teacher in Books

Chu Hsi (1130-1200), a great reformer of the Sung dynasty who articulated a renewed Confucian vision, collaborated with another scholar to produce an anthology of writings of the greatest teachers of his day in order to attract persons to serious study. Chu Hsi wrote in his preface,

> Thus if a young man in an isolated village who has the will to learn, but no enlightened teacher or good friend to guide him, obtains this volume and explores and broods over its material in his own mind, he will be able to find the gate to enter. He can then read the complete works of the four masters (anthologized in this collection), deeply sift their meanings and repeatedly recite their words, and absorb them at leisure, so as to achieve an extensive learning and return to the simple truth. . . . Someone may shrink from effort and be contented with the simple and convenient, thinking that all he needs is to be found here, but this is not the purpose of the present anthology.[5]

Chu Hsi was careful in this statement. He designed the book as "a gate" for those without a teacher, but it was only a gate. Genuine study would involve extensive effort, which was best pursued under the guidance of an enlightened teacher.

The use of books to capture the presence of a great teacher was the foundation of the genre of *yü-lu* (recorded sayings). The first *yü-lu* from within the Buddhist community were collections of *kung-an* (Jap., *koan*, lit. public case), which formed a distinctive portion of training in the Lin-chi (Rinzai) sect of Ch'an (Zen) Buddhism. However, the genre of recorded sayings took hold and spread far beyond that single Buddhist school into lineages which identified themselves as Taoist or Confucian in heritage.[6]

The style of these recorded sayings varied according to theological content and philosophies of practice. Some collections were fashioned into battles pitting famous teachers against challengers from many schools or traditions. The battle texts were probably not so much records of actual exchanges, as they were highly stylized presentations of the distinctive doctrinal or pedagogical position of the teacher in question. What these collections had in common was an attempt to capture the presence of a great teacher. The preface of an anthology of Chu Hsi's sayings remarks,

> When you read this book, it is like being in attendance when the master is at leisure, receiving the tone of his voice. A thou-

> sand years could pass, and yet it would be like meeting in the hall, and with the crowd hearing and returning with them to one [mind]. The transmission of this book, how could it be a small contribution?[7]

According to the preface, this collection brings readers into the presence of the master, attending him at leisure, hearing the tone of his voice, experiencing his teachings as though the readers were with the crowd in the hall. Being in the presence of the enlightened teacher provides the atmosphere in which one hears, sees, feels, experiences, and absorbs ideas—embodies them.

Embodying the Way in Oneself

It is one thing, though not a small one, to believe that living enlightened teachers embodied the substance of the Way and could model it for students. It is another to understand how believers were to embody the Way in themselves. Three aspects of the Chinese religious life illumine the process of embodiment.

First, in Confucian lineages study always meant *practice* (application in living) as well as clarification of cognitive understanding. Confucius said,

> A young person's duty is to be filial to parents at home and respectful to elders abroad, to be circumspect and truthful, and, while overflowing with love for all people, to associate oneself with humanity (*jen*). If, when all that is done, young persons have any energy to spare, let them study the polite arts.[8]

Since the polite arts (literature, poetry, philosophy, ethics, music, and calligraphy) were the core of Confucius's curriculum, he insisted in this saying that the active practice of virtue took primacy over formal study.

Nearly two millennia later, neo-Confucian Wang Yang-ming (1472-1529) took this teaching to its logical conclusion by insisting that knowledge and action (practice) were in fact inseparable, two aspects of one effort. He said,

> Suppose we say that so-and-so knows filial piety and so-and-so knows brotherly respect. They must have actually practiced filial piety and brotherly respect before they can be said to know them. It will not do to say that they know filial piety and brotherly respect simply because they show them in words. Or take one's knowledge of pain. Only after one has experienced pain can one know pain. The same is true of cold and hunger.

體道於身

> How can knowledge and action be separated? This is the original substance of knowledge and action, which have not been separated by selfish desires. In teaching people, the Sage insisted that only this can be called knowledge.[9]

Thus to know the Way was to practice it. Until one could embody the Way in one's life, one did not know it. To practice was to embody, internalize, and act out the principles of the Way in one's very being, to become a living sage.

The second aspect of study which helps to illumine strategies for embodiment was the *memorization and recitation of texts*. Chu Hsi noted in the preface to his Confucian anthology (discussed above) that the isolated student who used this text as a gateway should proceed in the following manner:

> He can then read the complete works of the four masters, deeply sift their meanings and repeatedly recite their words, and absorb them at leisure, so as to achieve an extensive learning and return to the simple truth.[10]

This statement suggests that recitation was important because it allowed students to absorb the words. In Chinese, the word *nien* means memorization, recitation, and study. Chinese students read and copied texts, annotated them, and wrote essays and commentaries, but the basic approach to mastering a text was to *nien* it, that is, to memorize and recite it repeatedly.

A recited text was in a very palpable sense absorbed into the voice, mind, and body of the reciter. In part because of the practice of recitation, Chinese writing was full of allusions and unattributed citations; the lines, language, and images of texts became internalized as part of the student's imagination and discourse, his pool of ideas. The text was no longer bound by its written form, fixed on a page; it became a sound and image in the mind-and-heart of the student.[11]

Significantly, the word *nien* was also used in various forms of meditation in China which involved invoking the name of a Buddha, a sage, or a sutra. Pure Land Buddhists practiced *nien-fo*, calling on the name of Amitabha Buddha; this *nien* or invocation was both a continuous prayer for the aid of the Buddha and a visualization, a holding of the Buddha or of an image of the Pure Land in one's mind through repetition of the name.

Ming dynasty thinker Lin Chao-en, who expounded the unity of Confucianism, Buddhism, and Taoism, taught the practice of reciting (*nien*) the phrase "Masters of the Three Teachings." As he wrote, "It will be as though the reciters were standing in attendance on them [the masters]; they will not dare to be lax even for a moment."[12] Recitation absorbed into the self the presence of what was recited; it

held that image (Masters of the Three Teachings, Amitabha Buddha, the Pure Land) in the mind and focused attention on it. In the Chinese religious field, recitation was a simple form of meditation (concentrated attention) which helped students to absorb their objects of study and emulation.

體道於身

A third dimension of study in the Chinese religious field was the dominant image of learning as a one-on-one conversation or *dialogue between an enlightened teacher and a student.* There is ample evidence that other forms of learning were also practiced,[13] but the dominance of the genre of recorded sayings (*yü-lu*) in late traditional China sustained the notion of the learnèd dialogue as a cultural ideal of true learning. By presenting the thought of the masters primarily as one-on-one exchanges, the recorded sayings modeled an approach to learning in which each student's internalization of the Way was tested with and against the teacher.

The three techniques of practice, recitation-and-internalization, and face-to-face dialogue were patterns followed widely in the Chinese religious field with appropriate variations for differences among groups or teachers.

The Chinese did not see the body as an obstacle to spiritual fulfillment; it was rather the medium of its own transformation. The human self as embodied could, through appropriate practice, realize its link with the structures of reality, the powers of the cosmos, and the innate virtues of Heaven. The goal of religious learning and practice was to understand arts for the embodiment of the Way as taught by one's enlightened master and one's lineage.

Pointing beyond Any Single Concretization of Tao

The Chinese were not unaware of the dangers of confusing the immanent, embodied Way with the Tao in itself. They were also well aware that the stress on human models could lead to rigidity and formalism, to thoughtless imitation of others instead of embodying the Way in one's self. Chinese teachers and masters from all of the streams in the religious field, aware of these dangers, used a variety of techniques to point beyond themselves, even as they served as models by means of the distinctive patterns of their traditions.

One way that masters pointed beyond themselves was through their humility, meticulously refusing to ascribe to themselves any title which suggested final enlightenment: sage, Buddha, immortal, perfected one, etc. Masters evaded honors by pointing their students back to ancient masters as well as to the texts, rituals, and spiritual practices which were the core of the curriculum.

A second means by which masters pointed beyond themselves was to avoid making a definitive statement of their teaching. What they

體道於身

offered instead was a series of nuanced statements which spoke to specific circumstances, powerfully adapting the Tao to the particular person with whom they were speaking.

This point can be illustrated by the vast anthology of Chu Hsi's sayings by categories (*Chu-tzu yü-lei*). This collection was immense: thirteen large, Western-style volumes, with sections containing long strings of sayings on a given doctrinal issue. Modern scholars have sought to distill and to summarize the essential teachings of Chu Hsi, since the long strings of sayings impede a general understanding of Chu's thought. Yet the collection was extremely important among traditional students of Chu Hsi precisely because it contained the nuances of his remarks on the same subject in a variety of circumstances to a variety of interlocutors. The sayings were not dated, so they were not studied in order to understand the evolution of Chu Hsi's ideas. They demonstrated rather the *adaptation* of his thought in many contexts, the shades and nuances which made the understanding of his teachings more complex rather than simpler. They showed a teacher who did not simply repeat a set of ideas in a parrot-like manner, but rather adapted them to a range of dialogical contexts.

There was no definitive single statement of Chu Hsi's position in his own writings because *such a summative statement would separate his vision from its embodiment in particular contexts*. His capacity to speak to myriad circumstances demonstrated his masterful understanding of the Way. The question was not simply "What did Chu Hsi say about x?" but rather "what would Chu Hsi say about x in this circumstance?"

The Chinese sought and depicted the Way by means of living exemplars and concrete instances of exchange between teacher and pupil. However, if teachers were incarnate in their expression of the Way, they did not constrain it with all the limitations of a particular embodiment. A given situation, saying, or master embodied the Way, *but not the whole Way*. The Way was concretized only in a particular circumstance or for a particular human personality.

The Multidimensional, Multilayered Way

All human embodiments of the Way were important as models. Yet they were partial in the sense of being neither final nor definitive, but rather limited by particularity and circumstance. The Way, as it unfolded, could and would be embodied in myriad circumstances, but never finally or completely so.

This aspect of Tao was discussed in chapter 6, where the myriad spirits were seen to be concretization of Tao, Spirit, or Heaven, *but with limited functions and influence*. It was also discussed in chapter 2, where the many paths of the Chinese religious field were seen to be part of the Tao, yet each needed to be sloughed off as its limited func-

tions were realized and transcended. The pattern is consistent: *multiple concretizations or embodiments of Tao actualize it in the world, but each of these actualizations is particular and therefore partial.* The Way is open-ended.

體道於身

Five hundred years before Wan Yong-ming and Lin Chao-en and a century before Chu Hsi, the Chinese poet Su Shih (1037-1101) suggested music as a metaphor for the Tao. This is an intriguing and useful image. The Tao is comprised of a structured set of forces or principles which form the normative grid of reality, like the tones, rhythms, and harmonies of music. Yet the possibilities for expression of music (or the Tao) are infinite; even the greatest musician in the world cannot exhaust them. A great musician may set new standards and inspire many with the potentiality and beauty of music; yet, inevitably, others will both build on and surpass what that musician did as well as honor it by emulating the genius of his or her achievement.

Music is also an apt metaphor because it is only an empty structure *except as performed,* as captured in a particular instance with its distinctive subtleties and interpretations. The structure exists to be performed by others, but the music is manifested or actualized only in performance. Su Shih wrote that the Tao is like music and practicing it is like playing the flute.

> Cut bamboo to make a flute. Hollow it out and blow into it. Even [the great musician] Shih K'uang was unable to fully realize the variations of harmony and descant, the measures of tone and rhythm. Now go back and seek it [i.e., the origin]. There are only five notes and twelve tones [in Chinese music]. At the origin of the five notes and twelve tones there is only whistling. At the origin of the whistling there is only silence. Did not those who made music in antiquity necessarily stand in the midst of silence?[14]

Su Shih's poetic evocation of the nature of the Tao suggests its open-endedness while maintaining its role as the source and structure of all being.

Tales of Embodying the Way: Advice from the Sages

This chapter has discussed a number of ways in which teachers and students sought to embody the Tao. The most venerable models for such embodiment were found in the great teachers of the Warring States period of religious debate: Confucius and the two Taoist philosophers, Lao Tzu and Chuang Tzu. While all three were important models in Chinese religious history, the primary sources of their writings do not offer a narrative of the lives of these great sages. Rather, they

record the sayings of Confucius, the poetry of Lao Tzu, and the witty stories told by Chuang Tzu. Confucius's sayings describe him and his disciples in very brief vignettes. Lao Tzu's poetry is sometimes in the voice of the first person ("I"), and sometimes the third. Chuang Tzu's stories make use of a range of colorful characters. All of these sources suggest strategies for embodying the Way. Because of the lack of narrative lives, my tales about these three sages are perhaps best thought of as sketches. They are my impressionistic renderings, drawn from my encounters with these texts and traditions as a pilgrim.

Confucius the Sage

Perhaps the most famous and most honored of all teachers in Chinese history was Confucius. He was revered for his general approach to life and for his wise interactions with his pupils and disciples.

The book which centrally honored Confucius the teacher was the *Lun-yü* (Analects or Sayings of Confucius). The one thread which ran through all of his teachings was declared by one disciple to be "loyalty and reciprocity,"[15] general moral principles which were illustrated in myriad ways throughout the book, but not central to any development or plot. The *Analects* offered brief glimpses of Confucius as a teacher and as a man.

As a teacher, Confucius insisted that learning was primarily about refining character and practicing morality. He expected his students to participate actively in this quest for learning and wisdom. He said,

> I won't teach someone who is not anxious to learn, and will not explain to one who is not trying to make things clear to him-/herself. If I hold up one corner of a square and the person cannot come back to me with the other three, I won't bother to go over the point again.[16]

His students looked to him for instruction and encouragement, and also as a human standard, a model to which to aspire. His disciple Yen Hui said,

> The Master is very good at leading a person along and teaching him or her. He has broadened me with culture, restrained me with ritual (*li*). I just could not stop myself. But after I have exhausted every resource, there still remains something distinct and apart from me. Do what I can to reach his position, I cannot find the way.[17]

The glimpses of Confucius's personality portray him as a gentle and humane person.

體道於身

> In his leisure hours, Confucius was easy in his manner and cheerful in his expression. . . .
>
> Confucius was gentle yet firm, dignified but not harsh, respectful yet well at ease.[18]

Confucius took as his mission the returning of the misguided rulers of his day to a path of virtue, but he was not successful in that endeavor. Nonetheless he remained steadfast in his faith in Heaven as the moral source of the Way of the ancestors, which he believed was the basis of a sound society. After failing as a political advisor, he devoted his life to learning and to teaching, never claiming the wisdom or stature of a sage, but coming to represent it not only to his disciples, but also to many generations throughout Chinese history. Confucius claimed no unique or new teaching ("I am a transmitter and not a creator. I believe in and have a passion for the ancients"[19]), but merely to be a lover of learning and of the Way ("Having heard the Way [*Tao*] in the morning, one may die content in the evening"[20]).

The learning to which Confucius devoted his life was not simply the mastery of a body of knowledge, nor a set of intellectual skills, but the refinement of character through the perfection of human wisdom and behavior. The character of a person, Confucius believed, was slowly carved and polished like a jade stone until its inner luminescence shone through.[21] This was a life-long process, even for Confucius, who was regarded as the finest exemplar of his teaching. This is best illustrated in his famous saying on lifelong cultivation, which served as the epigraph to this chapter. No other single comment so aptly captures the Confucian vision of the Tao as the fine art of living authentically.

The Taoist Sages

Lao Tzu and Chuang Tzu, the great ancient authors whose teachings have inspired and shaped the Taoist streams in the Chinese religious field, disagreed with the specific content of Confucian teachings about the sage, but agreed that some extraordinary individuals embodied the Tao. Chuang Tzu wrote,

> The sage penetrates bafflement and complication, rounding all into a single body, yet does not know why it is inborn nature. The sage returns to fate and acts accordingly, using Heaven as a teacher, and people follow after, pinning labels [like 'sage'] on him or her.
>
> The sage has never begun to think of Heaven, has never begun to think of human beings, has never begun to think of a begin-

體道於身

> ning, has never begun to think of things. The sage moves in company with the age, never halting; wherever he or she moves there is completion and no impediment. Others try to keep up with the sage, but what can they do?[22]

If the sage or teacher modeling him- or herself on Confucius devoted a lifetime to learning and to refining and polishing character, Chuang Tzu's sage devoted him/herself to forgetting and simplifying until the self became invisible or simply united with the world and things. One of the most famous tales illustrating this is Chuang Tzu's story of Woodworker Ch'ing.

> Woodworker Ch'ing carved a piece of wood and made a bell stand, and when it was finished, everyone who saw it marveled, for it seemed to be the work of gods or spirits. When the marquis of Lu saw it, he asked, "What art is it you have?"
>
> Ch'ing replied, "I am only a craftsman—how could I have any art? There is one thing, however. When I am going to make a bell stand, I never let it wear out my energy. I always fast in order to still my mind. When I have fasted for three days, I no longer have any thought of congratulations or rewards, of titles or stipends. When I have fasted for five days, I no longer have any thought of praise or blame, of skill or clumsiness. And when I have fasted for seven days, I am so still that I forget I have four limbs and a form and body. By that time, the ruler and his court no longer exist for me. My skill is concentrated and all outside distractions fade away. After that I go into the mountain forest and examine the Heavenly nature of the trees. If I find one of superlative form, and I can see a bell stand there, I put my hand to the job of carving; if not, I let it go. This way I am simply matching up 'Heaven' with 'Heaven.' That's probably the reason that people wonder if the results were not made by spirits."[23]

Ch'ing, as an artisan, would be an unlikely Confucian sage, for he lacked training in the polite arts; but his Taoist wisdom is based on stilling himself, forgetting, and becoming an agent of matching "Heaven" with "Heaven." Lao Tzu went so far as to depict the sage as an infant, or a fool:

> The multitude are joyous
> As though feasting after the Great Sacrifice
> Or going up to the Spring Carnival.
> I alone am inactive and reveal no signs,
> Like a baby that has not yet learned to smile,

Listless as though with no home to go back to.
The multitude all have more than enough.
I alone seem to be in want.
My mind is that of a fool — how blank!
Vulgar people are clear.
I alone am drowsy.
Vulgar people are alert.
I alone am muddled.
Calm like the sea;
Like a high wind that never ceases.
The multitude all have a purpose.
I alone am foolish and uncouth.
I alone am different from others
And value being fed by the mother.[24]

體道於身

The wisdom, freedom, and behavior of the Taoist sage transcend conventional wisdom; the Taoist sage appears murky and indistinct. If the Confucian enlightened teacher served as a clear glimpse of or window on the Tao, the Taoist sage fogged the window; the Taoist teacher undercut expectations and withdrew from clear view to keep students from seeking a premature handle on what requires extensive unlearning to achieve. The teacher or the sage became invisible so that things could unfold naturally. Lao Tzu wrote,

The best of all rulers is but a shadowy presence to his subjects. . . .
When his task is accomplished and his work done
The people all say, "It happened to us naturally."[25]

The Taoist student learned to still, forget, or strip away all sorts of conventional wisdom, views, and values so that the Tao within could be manifest. He or she had to penetrate surface appearances to uncover a deeply internal reality.

Confucius, Lao Tzu, and Chuang Tzu did not agree on how best to embody the Way, but they did agree that embodying it in oneself was the goal of life. This principle they shared with all members of the Chinese religious field.

Final Thoughts

The notion of truth as embodied, of the Tao as the art of living authentically, provided the opening to allow for the co-existence of many versions of the Way. The Way as embodied is always particular and limited; yet the embodied Way participates in the Way in itself.

體道於身

The Chinese approach to truth entailed humility about the limitations of any single articulation of doctrine and an openness to the fact that truth will never be exhausted as long as human beings live in a world of changing circumstances. As Lao Tzu said in the epigraph to this chapter, "The Tao that can be spoken is not the eternal Tao." Religious persons could disagree strongly and fundamentally on how best to embody the Way in a particular circumstance, but none could claim to articulate a final and definitive statement of the Tao.

The Chinese approach to truth also underscored the life-long art of religious cultivation, so eloquently described in Confucius's epigraph to this chapter. Like the skill of the musician, there is no absolute endpoint to the artistry of spiritual practice.

The Chinese approach to truth as embodied or performed was one of the most profound boons I received as a pilgrim in Chinese culture. It stretched my mind and my patterns of religious thinking more than anything else I encountered in the Chinese religious field. The Chinese had devised a remarkable passage between the Scylla of absolutism and the Charybdis of relativism. Too many Western Christians were opting for one or the other, and creating a profound rift between those who held the positions.

The Chinese approach suggests that the choice many Christians see between exclusivism and pluralism is based on a false or avoidable dichotomy, and that the "anonymous Christian" inclusivity of thinkers like Rahner is not the only alternative.

In the Chinese religious field, particular statements and practices could be judged against the circumstances in which they were pronounced—did they further the faithful on the Way? Such was the substance of the liveliest Chinese religious debates. However, even the liveliest debates were tempered by the conviction that the proof was in embodiment: there would be other faithful and other teachers who (like great musicians) would further refine and perfect the Way in their lives.

The Chinese way suggested that we could judge other religions by their fruits (do their teachings and practices give rise to genuine spiritual qualities in persons?), and that we must be humble about the nonfinality of our understanding of God vis-à-vis competing forms of Christianity and other religions. It also suggests that certain beliefs or practices might be grounded in, and suited to, specific circumstances; that different teachings need not always be seen in competition with one another.

To my delight my pilgrimage in China was beginning to give rise to insights about my own religious community.

CHAPTER 8

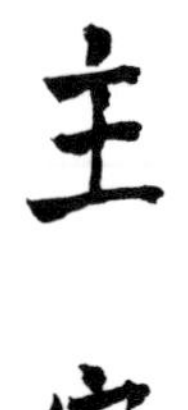

Hospitality and the Chinese Religious Field

Respectfully on high we invite
The Green Emperor of the East
Wood official who dissolves impurities;
Lord messengers, nine men.
The Red Emperor of the South,
Fire official, dissolver of impurities,
Lord messengers, three men.
The White Emperor of the West,
Metal official, dissolver of impurities,
Lord messengers, seven men.
Black Emperor of the North,
Water official, dissolver of impurities,
Lord messengers, five men.
Yellow Emperor of the Center,
Earth official, dissolver of impurities,
Lord messengers, twelve men.
Ye who bear on high the talisman
That dissolves impurities, Lord messengers;
Ye who carry below the talisman
That dissolves impurities, Lord messengers;
Ye who this year, this month,
This day, this moment bear the talismans
To dissolve impurities, messenger troops,

"Host and Guest"
Host and guest are the key roles within the structures of Chinese hospitality. Each role carries a distinctive set of social and cultural expectations, as well as different connotations of power and status. In ancient times, the terms "host" and "guests" also denoted feudal "lord" and "vassal."

主

客

Young men, Jade girls, 120 in all,
Altogether, come down to this sacred T'an!
—*An invitation of the spirits of the cosmos to purify the sacred precincts of the temple in preparation for the* Chiao *ritual*

In the last three chapters I recounted how I as a pilgrim came to understand the structures for affirming diversity within the Chinese religious field: 1) how the manifold deities, rituals, practices, symbols, teachers, and pedagogical approaches of the Chinese religious field concretized the Way and pointed beyond such specific manifestations to the unity of the Tao; and 2) how the plethora of religious options were held in creative relationship with the notion of a transcendent source and unity, a ground of the sacred. I was deeply moved by the Chinese genius for holding unity and multiplicity in creative and balanced tension.

As I continued my journey, my attention returned to practical issues. How did the Chinese come to know and to negotiate diverse religious options in the religious field? As a pilgrim in China, I was repeatedly warmed by the welcome that I or any other stranger received in a temple or at a ritual. I had first experienced that remarkable sense of welcome during the pilgrimage on Lion's Head Mountain and in the gracious hospitality of its abbot. The sense of welcome was repeated many times at many temples. Instead of enclaves of self-enclosed religious groups, the patterns of religious life created a network of hospitality which sustained mutual knowledge and relationships. How did these patterns work? How did the Chinese come to know about and negotiate the diversity of the religious field?

In this chapter, I explore those patterns of mutual knowledge and relationship, arguing that the social structures of hospitality were key to this pattern of religious interaction. As I recounted in chapter 6, Chinese deities were entertained in the manner of important officials, and ancestral spirits were included in family celebrations and feasts.[1] In the epigraph to this chapter, a Taoist priest invites the emperors of the five quadrants of the cosmos and their attendant spirits to a temple to help celebrate a ritual. The structures of religious practice are shot through with the practices of hospitality, which sustain relationships between religious groups.

I begin the chapter by examining the general structures of Chinese hospitality and illustrating its dynamics at the communal and individual levels. On the communal level, I show how religious hospitality fostered a sense of community, nurtured local leadership, and balanced tensions through cycles of reciprocity. On the individual level, I illustrate the functions and textures of religious pluralism: how persons became acquainted with other traditions and how temples hosted many guests. I conclude with a brief tale of hospitality to many deities and rituals in a temple in Tainan.

The Chinese Structures of Hospitality

主
客

Chinese religious organizations and persons used the structures of hospitality to accommodate diverse religious deities and adherents within their celebrations. They embraced or included their neighbors—divine and human—as guests in their appropriate places and roles. This is, of course, an ancient and virtually universal human strategy for embracing the stranger. The rituals of hospitality and commensality are at the very center of the human mechanisms for establishing relationships across lines of family, community, culture, and nation. And, almost universally, human cultures have accepted the principle that one honors as far as possible the mores of the host: "When in Rome, do as the Romans do." Thus the sensitive guest would not wear street shoes into a traditional Japanese home or refuse hospitality and refreshment from a Bedouin. Moreover, while Euro-American hosts would be offended if their guests were to slurp their soup ostentatiously or belch loudly after the meal, such behaviors would be courteous, if not mandatory, in other cultural settings.

In traditional Chinese society, the rounds of hosting in community festivals exposed everyone to the practices and mores of a range of religious groups and taught them how to handle themselves appropriately in those worlds. They were feted as guests, provided the best that the religious hosts had to offer, and given a chance to reciprocate. The structures of hospitality made the visitors comfortable in their role as outsiders, since they were formally welcomed *as guests or outsiders*. Thus they could ask questions, listen, observe, investigate, and enjoy; no commitment was asked of them, only their participation as guests.

If the guests were invited as observers and recipients, the hosts took responsibility for defining the terms of the affair. The Chinese term for host is revealing, for it also means "master" or "ruler," the one at the center. Chinese language suggests that the structures of hospitality are hierarchical, with the host above the guest; the host is in control, and the guest is subordinate. In ancient feudal China, the host (*chu*) was the lord, and the guest (*k'o*) the retainer or vassal; as in all feudal systems, while the relation was hierarchical, lord and vassal had mutual obligations. In Chinese society guests looked up to hosts, while hosts bore the responsibility for generosity and providing favors.[2]

What injected a note of equality in the host-guest relationship in the traditional Chinese setting was the principle of reciprocity underlying all Chinese relationships. Any relationship in Chinese society, although hierarchical, entailed *reciprocal* obligations, and none more so than host and guest. The principle of reciprocity promised to reverse the roles, and to place the host in the position of guest, and the guest in the position of host. Host and guest were expected to reciprocate with

skill to develop an ongoing connection. Such was the ideal structure of hospitality, and it was one to which the major families, religious functionaries, and officials of a community aspired in the round of festivals. Only through a network of reciprocity could the full potential of community unity and harmony be achieved.

Community Festivals: Reaffirming Cultural Unity

Building on cultural norms of hospitality, the openness to diversity in the Chinese religious field was sustained within a complex web of behavior and practice grounded in the structures of hospitality.

In the long spectrum of Chinese history until the twentieth century, festivals were community-wide events that had as one of their chief aims reaffirming the sense of commonality and unity which transcended tensions, feuds, and conflicts. As each temple celebrated the festivals that were key to its religious calendar, it became the host for a community celebration. The patterns of worship, the deities accorded central honor, and the major patrons of the festival were those of that particular religious institution. If a (Buddhist) Kuan-yin temple hosted one event, a major Kuan Kung (Taoist) temple would host the next. In the cycle of community festivals, each of the major groups had a chance to represent the unity of Chinese religion in its own distinctive way. Each invited the entire community to its celebration, and all members of the community were expected to participate and to contribute to the effort. Since all of the traditional Chinese religious streams accepted this premise of participating in the whole, the system worked well both to sustain community solidarity and to maintain the patterns of openness and reciprocity in the Chinese religious field even in the face of considerable competitiveness.[3]

The emperor or his representative (an official of the imperial bureaucracy) attended significant community religious festivals and visited important shrines or temples in order to incorporate the festival, shrine, or practice into the religious mainstream by virtue of imperial patronage; this presence reminded all religious groups of the emperor's role as the patron of all orthodox religious practice.

The Rounds of Temple Hospitality

As noted above, the rounds of the religious calendar included a variety of festivals, holidays, and birthdays of deities, each of which was the occasion for a community-wide celebration hosted and organized by the most appropriate temple or shrine. The festivals provided the organizing temple with a number of opportunities. The great festival of the temple, with its processions, rituals, and performances, was the key

opportunity to present in concrete and dramatic form the Chinese religious field as that group saw it, to depict the religious cosmos with their concerns and their deities in the central roles. To the celebration were invited members of the community, religious neighbors, local worthies, and even other deities and spirits, as depicted in the epigraph to this chapter. However, as is always true in a carefully designed party or banquet, each guest (human or divine) was carefully assigned his or her rightful place in the social and spiritual structure of that particular event.

This carefully modulated hospitality to other spirits and cults was also reflected in the everyday arrangement of temple or shrine compound. Chinese temples lodged not only images and altars to the primary deities (which were seated in the place of honor in the main hall, facing south), but also images of and altars to a host of other deities. Some of these other deities were assigned places as guardians or attendants to the main deities. These guardian and attendant figures were sometimes assimilated through a process of remythologization, in which what may have been earlier an independent religious group was absorbed into the religious movement or temple as faithful servants of the more powerful deity and its institution.[4] Subordinate deities were enshrined around the sides and back of the temple, or in smaller sub-shrines or buildings. The exact position of each in the pantheon was indicated by its spatial placement, its size and decoration, and the size and degree of ornamentation in its ritual apparatus. The presence of multiple deities established alliances with small religious movements or simply provided broader religious options for those who visited the temple. Thus the temple itself played host to selected deities who were seated in their appropriate places. On the temple's turf, their deity was the host and thus at the pinnacle of the structure of the event.

Patronage and Leadership

Each temple or shrine not only represented distinctive practices, deities, priests, and adepts, but also was supported by a group of local patrons, families who had related themselves to the temples as "members of the register."[5] Such families made contributions of land, clothing, food, or money, and also were active on temple committees. The planning for a festival or celebration involved the major temple patrons in many ways, and thus provided them an opportunity to develop their role as community leaders.[6] The introduction of a new temple or cult into a community often served as a vehicle for families new to the region or rising in their fortunes to establish their status by exercising visible patronage. Given the plethora of religious practices and deities, religious patronage was central to the survival of a partic-

主客

ular group; religious patronage was also important to families in establishing their status in a community.

In addition to providing the temple and its deities with their moment at the center, festival planning also provided an opportunity for the major patrons of the temple or shrine to play the host to their neighbors, temporarily stepping into the center of community attention. Temple festivals, like weddings and funerals, offered families a chance to express their largesse, assert their status, and establish their generosity as pillars of the community. Also, as in the case of weddings and funerals, this display had elements not only of generosity, but also of a curiously Chinese form of "conspicuous consumption," a public display of hospitality and celebration meant to keep up with or surpass "the Joneses" or, in this case, the "Wangs."[7]

Tensions and Competition

The hospitality and generosity of Chinese community festivals had competitive as well as innocently generous elements. Such was always the case in Chinese society, indeed in any human society. The flip side of ostentatious patronage or generosity is jockeying for position as the most generous patron. In the Chinese religious field, families might jockey for social position by vying to offer the most lavish festival, and temples would jockey for standing in the community by having the most elaborate processions, rituals, and performances. As we shall see in the next section, there was community pressure both to include all facets of the community (including one's rivals) in the festival, and to attend the celebrations of rival temples or groups. In this sort of environment, competition was played out through the subtle social codes of mutual generosity. Since the donations of all parties were made public when offered to the gods, there was plenty of opportunity for conspicuous generosity.

The Chinese ritual structures of enforced generosity and of reciprocity in hospitality were key to containing the tensions and smoothing the ruffled feathers of community discord for many, many centuries. Reciprocity was a key because it meant that other temples and other patrons would have their turn in playing host, being at the center, having a chance to shine or outshine on their own turf and on their own terms.

Universal Participation

One of the factors which vitiated the competitive aspect of community festivals by means of the mores of hospitality and generosity was the deep Chinese instinct to maintain cultural unity against all odds: their

strong inclination, reinforced by the watchfulness of the government, to make all community festivals inclusive of the entire community. The temple organizers were enjoined by tradition and the sense of fair play (the rules of the Chinese religious field) to invite to their celebrations the entire community and to participate in turn in the celebrations of their neighbors. As hosts, they provided the feast and entertainment. Guests were asked to make a small contribution as a gesture of affirming the importance of the celebration as a community event, as an act of participation.[8] Contributor's names were written on public placards or sheets which were displayed to the participants in the festival before being "sent to the gods" as a report. As Donald DeGlopper has written of festivals in Lukang, "A family that refused to contribute would offend the god, and, perhaps more to the point, would be mocked and scorned by their neighbors."[9]

Participation in these affairs embodied community spirit. The refusal of a sub-group to participate on the grounds of having been maltreated or insulted by the organizers was tantamount to withdrawal from the community, a very hostile act. Community festivals were times to mend differences, not to display them.

The introduction into the Chinese religious field of Christianity and Islam, which did not share the nonexclusive assumptions about religion, challenged these time-honored patterns of mutual hospitality. Christians or Muslims who exempted themselves from the festivals on the grounds of religious difference were perceived as also exempting themselves from the community. Moreover, in the late eighteenth and nineteenth centuries, the movement of large and relatively diverse populations into Chinese urban areas undercut traditional patterns of mutual participation and disrupted the traditional rounds and reciprocities of hospitality.[10] Thus as China began slowly to move into the modern world, the tenuous balance of religious diversity was strained both by external intrusions and by population moves.

In traditional China, however, community-wide festivals quite literally broke down boundaries between religious streams and groups, encouraging visitations between temples and devotees. They provided some basic information as well, since the rituals, performances, art, and honorary inscriptions of the festival presented succinctly the special powers, messages, and practices of the deities and groups represented by the shrine or temple. The round of participation featured each temple in turn, while enacting the myth of cultural unity which held together the Chinese religious field.

Courtesy Calls: Hospitality Accorded to Visitors

If the round of festivals within a community created a structure for various competing groups and social forces both to express their social

positions and to be each other's guests, other patterns of behavior in the Chinese religious field created opportunities for individuals or families to learn about and become familiar with the practices and sites of a broad range of religious groups.

主
客

Petitioners or Supplicants

Chinese temples and shrines had relatively few periods of formal worship, but were open for visits by worshippers or passers-by. Some, indeed many, visitors to a shrine or temple came to avail themselves of the spiritual services for which the temple was known. Since many deities, not to mention shrines and temples, had established their niches in the religious field by dint of their specialization in a particular sort of religious boon or ritual, visitors often came because of their need for the particular boon which a temple offered. They might have heard of its reputation through a relative or acquaintance, through conversation or gossip at the market place or a tea house, through reference in a story or play, through a performance or ritual at a community festival. In whatever way they came by the knowledge, their visit sustained the temple or shrine's connection to the specific religious boon sought.[11]

Such visitors were supplicants, callers seeking a specific favor from the deity. Like other Chinese supplicants cultivating the largesse of a patron, they observed the general norms and mores of a courtesy call in traditional Chinese culture, in which the deity is understood as the host, the one with the greater power, the master. First, they came with a gift in hand. The appropriate religious gift was an offering, generally some cooked food or drink appropriate for a deity (*shen*).[12] Second, visitors introduced themselves, paid formal respects, presented their problems or special circumstances, sought assistance, and thanked the deity/host in an appropriate manner. If their problems were particularly delicate or grave, visitors might need a well-placed patron to provide an effective introduction, character reference, and sponsorship. In the religious setting, this generally entailed enlisting the services of a priest or other religious functionary who could appropriately represent one's case to the deity or who would perform the appropriate ritual to invoke the god's help. Important petitions to very highly placed deities might well be presented in writing, as formal petitions were presented to high government officials.[13] Thus in the case of petitionary worship, the god or temple played host for courtesy callers seeking boons or favors which the deity had in his or her power to bestow.

During their visits the temple decorations (wall paintings, statuary, inscriptions, and the like), temple literature, the ritual itself, and any interactions with the priests or religious functionaries offered visitors

further information about the temple and its distinctive version of religious mythology and practice.[14] Although on one level the visit was a functional and focused spiritual petition, on another level it was a brief exposure to a particular depiction of the spirit world in the Chinese religious field. Moreover, if the boon was granted (if the ritual was effective or the prayer answered), the supplicant became indebted to the deity and to the temple; he/she was obligated to repay the kindness. This indebtedness established an ongoing relationship which might be more or less demanding. The supplicants may have made a vow to the deity, a promise which they would fulfill if their prayer were answered or the ritual achieved its purpose. Even if this obligation were slight, the successful granting of the boon enlisted the visitors as members of the company of those who maintained the reputation and fame of the temple by affirming the efficacy of its deity and its practices.

Courtesy in Casual Visits: Making Acquaintances

While the most common visits to a temple or shrine were petitionary, others were more casual. Urban or village temples in China were, because of their location and their ample grounds, frequently the sites of markets, theatricals, or other community events. These events were as much commercial, social, and entertaining as they were religious, and thus we must assume that the motivations of those attending were as mixed as the characters of the events themselves. Yet these events drew visitors into the temple or shrine compound, exposing them to the art, the ambiance, the sights, sounds, and smells of temple life. Fundamentally, however, it reinforced the sense that these temples were part of the community and part of the fabric of life. It established their place not only in the religious field, but in the cultural rhythms of the community.

Some temples and shrines were located outside the walls of the city, "beyond the bounds" (*fang-wai*) in the mountains or other places more remote from the everyday cares of the world. Such outlying temples provided an atmosphere suitable for meditation, study, ritual practice, and monastic routine; thus they were appropriate for the training of monks, nuns, and priests. They were often, if the landscape allowed, located high up in the hills or mountains, literally as well as symbolically above it all; even the effort to get there expressed the aspiration for transcendence and progress in the Way.

The spatial remove of these temples and shrines, however, did not totally isolate them from each other or from contacts with those within the bounds of society. In addition to crowds which might appear for festival days or petitioners seeking the special boons of a temple or its

主
客

religious adepts, casual visitors found their way to the temples or shrines in their remote and beautiful settings. Scholars on outings, travelers, or families enjoying a day in the countryside visited temples renowned for scenic beauty, following roads or paths to temples, also traveled by pilgrims, monks and priests, petitioners, and those who had regular business with the temples. Temples established tea houses or pavilions for the rest and refreshment of travelers. Merchants and local families also established wayside stands.[15] In modern-day Taiwan or China, for example, shops or stands near the base of pilgrimage routes often do a brisk business in refreshments, maps of the temple site, walking sticks, and cold drinks for the road-weary traveler. Such businesses have a long history in China.[16]

The temples and the mountains on which they were often located offered attractions beyond the scenery: historical sites commemorated by stone inscriptions or pavilions, remembrances of famous visitors, statues or religious paintings, ancient buildings or ruins, hermitages or studios of famous contemporary or recent scholars. Thus many temples had a religious, literary, and artistic history, in addition to a number of sites of scenic interest. Temples were foci of a premodern form of tourism, and remain tourist or Sunday outing sites to this day.

Visits to temples were made even more memorable for those with literary interests by the Chinese tradition of presenting commemorative poems on such occasions to friends or to the temple. Poems were sometimes penned directly on the walls of temples or of tea houses, but often the group carried paper and ink with them with the intention of a friendly poetry contest. Chinese poetry anthologies and travel books abound with examples of such poems. While these poems might simply commemorate the scenery, they were often laced with more specific allusions about the temple itself and its practices.

Scholars visiting a temple were accorded generous hospitality. During my visit to Taiwan in 1972, I had occasion to experience the modern version of such a visit at a lovely Ch'an temple, where I was invited to tea with the abbot. Naively expecting to have a chance to ask my specific questions about Buddhist life, I was inexorably drawn into the traditional ritual of conversation, in which the questions one asked and the answers received were structured and stylized to reflect a Buddhist notion of courteous discourse about the basics. Thus I learned that such visits were governed by a formal ritual structure of hospitality. In exchange for the tea and hospitality, visitors would inquire politely about the history, traditions, and teachings of the temple. The abbot or priest would do his best both to entertain and enlighten visitors, making use of a brief opportunity for instruction. Occasionally, the conversation would "strike home" for one of the visitors, who might return or strike up a correspondence with the master.

Such outings were primarily pleasure trips, but they were also a

medium for introducing travelers, particularly the educated elite, to the range of traditions and practices in the Chinese religious field. They fostered familiarity and general knowledge, as well as human relationships. Even if visitors were not tempted to seek the Way through the particular form of religion practiced at the temple, they came away with a pleasant and friendly impression. Such encounters oiled the mechanisms of mutual openness in the Chinese religious field.

Hosting Adepts from Other Traditions

There was another significant category of visitation that was key to the interconnections and development of mutual familiarity in the Chinese religious field. Religious masters, monks, and disciples regularly visited shrines, temples, monasteries, and masters from other religious streams or communities. This pattern of behavior runs deep in Chinese religious history. In the *Analects* and other classical Confucian writings, there are numerous stories of one teacher's students visiting other teachers to question them and test their understanding of the Way. Such students challenged their teacher's rivals, hoping to test and reaffirm the superiority of their own master's practices and teachings.

Many streams of Taoist practice encouraged wandering outside of the bounds (*fang-wai*), removing oneself from the city and society in search of a more natural and free mode of living. These wandering Taoists often came upon teachers of various sorts, and not infrequently set up hermitages in mountains where they were visited by other seekers of the way.

Buddhists, given their cultural roots in India, went so far as to institutionalize the wandering of monks and their visits to other temples. In India, holy "renouncers" wandered completely beyond the bounds of society and community. While Buddhism taught the middle way of monastic community outside the normal bounds of family and society, they institutionalized the wandering of monks during certain seasons both to ensure that life did not become too comfortable and also to encourage the exposure of monks to other teachings and practices. There was an established ritual at temples and monasteries to welcome and assimilate monks and priests from other temples and traditions.[17] Such monks and priests were assimilated into monastic practice and entered into conversations with resident monks and priests about the practices and teachings of the host temple.

The above discussion has perhaps given the misleading impression that a monastery would represent a single and consistent stream of practice. That *might* be true if one were referring to the monastery in a narrow way, that is, to the meditation hall and monks who lived in the

主客

dormitories surrounding it under the direction of the abbot. However, monasteries were located on mountains (or at least on a substantial tract of lands) and the paths to and from the monastery were dotted with temples and shrines representing various levels and dimensions of Chinese piety as well as hermitages of monks and priests in their solitary practices.

Historically, the mountains which housed active monasteries were even more religiously diverse. Mount Wu-i, where Pai Yü-ch'an had his hermitage, for instance, had a long and rich religious history, and the path up and down was dotted with temples, shrines, studios, and hermitages bearing a diversity of Taoist, Buddhist, and Confucian religious streams as well as a host of folk traditions.[18] Thus practitioners of many religious streams lived and practiced side by side. Visitors to one shrine, temple, or studio passed by and sometimes dropped in on others.[19] Each religious mountain, then, became a version of the diversity and complementarity of the Chinese religious field. Such places offered many opportunities for exchanges between the representatives of more than one religious discipline; diverse practices and pedagogical approaches did not evolve in isolation from each other. Some of these exchanges were depicted in collections of recorded sayings, thus capturing the group's perception of their position vis à vis their religious neighbors in the Chinese religious field.

If community festivals brought together all who lived in a single community or region to celebrate the traditions of a particular religious group, the patterns of visitation to temples or shrines provided ample opportunity to cross religious boundaries and learn from many religious groups. Temples and shrines played host to petitioners, casual visitors, pilgrims, and devotees of other religious streams, and their devotees in turn paid courtesy calls on other temples. These rounds of visitation encouraged mutual familiarity, provided opportunities to take advantage of the specific boons or arts of a religious group, and offered a context for exchanges of traditions, histories, practices, and ideas.

Tales of Hospitality in the Chinese Religious Field

Several of the tales I have told earlier in this book witnessed to the hospitality in the Chinese religious field.

The tale of the *chiao* in chapter 6 is an excellent example of a temple festival fostering unity in the community through hospitality. Not only were all of the families of the community invited to join, but also local and regional deities and the ghosts of the dead. Moreover, in the epigraph to this chapter, the deities of the five directions of the cosmos and their attendants were invited to remake the sacred space in which the ritual renewal of the cosmos was to occur. All facets of the commu-

nity (living, gods, ghosts, and ancestors) were gathered for a major feast of reconciliation.

The tale of Pai Yü-ch'an in chapter 2 recounted how an individual could come to know and to be connected with many strands of the Chinese religious field. In his wanderings, Pai studied with a number of teachers, mastered a range of Taoist rituals, and became the chronicler of the Way of the Pure and Perspicacious (Ching-ming Tao). Moreover, at his retreat on Mount Wu-i, he hosted many visitors from a variety of traditions. Pai negotiated the Chinese religious field with skill, taking advantage of his patterns of hospitality.

For an understanding of how hospitality to many deities functioned within a major temple, I now share an adventure from my visit to Tainan in November 1971. A friend and I went to Tainan for five days to study as many shrines and temples as we could fit into a brief visit. As we approached a large Yü-huang miao (Temple to the Jade Emperor), we heard traditional Chinese instruments and chanting—sure signs that a ritual was underway. The music drew us behind the main altar in the central hall to the rear courtyard of the temple, dotted with perhaps a dozen deities less than two feet in height. By contrast the image of the Jade Emperor and his attendants on the main altar were significantly larger than life size, seated on an imposing throne.

In front of one of the tiny deities in the back was a large table piled with offerings (tangerines, Coca-Cola, sweet rice cakes, dumplings) and nearby were a red-head priest[20] and two assistants, plus a couple of musicians, undertaking a ritual before what appeared to be an extended family of twenty or so people.

Since the ritual promised to be lively, my friend and I hovered inquisitively around the corners with our camera and tape recorder, exuding friendly interest in the ritual. After a few minutes, we received the blessing of senior family members to record the rite.

The family had suffered a series of economic and health misfortunes. They had been advised by a priest that these ills were signs that a recently deceased relative was in distress in the afterlife. They gathered at this temple to ask the priest to learn from their deceased relative what was amiss so that they could correct it. They were thus sponsoring a rather elaborate spirit-possession ritual which would bring them a direct message from their dead relative, so that the family (living and dead) could be brought to peace.

The first part of the rite, into which my friend and I had stumbled, made an offering and initial prayers to the black-faced deity Chang Tao-ling (a Taoist leader in the second century, C.E.), who would guide the priest in his journey to the world of the shades. After the family had laid out their offerings, the priest offered prayers of invitation and petition, inviting the deity and his attendants to assist him in his journey to the land of the dead.

主
客

After the deity, who had a subordinate role in Yü-huang's temple, had been put on alert, as it were, the priest and his entourage moved into the main sanctuary and made a full report of the day's happenings to the Jade Emperor, who was, after all, the master of the temple. In Chinese popular mythology, the Jade Emperor is also the ruler of heaven and, as such, dispatches the deities of the pantheon as spirit marshals to undertake various assignments. Thus the ceremony in the main sanctuary politely asked the Jade Emperor to delegate his officer for this journey and sought assistance of various spirit attendants to protect the god and the priests on their quest.

The third and most dramatic part of the ceremony, again in the back courtyard, enacted the priest's crossing over the bridge from the land of the living to the haunts of the dead. The bridge was depicted by a small bench covered with a charm painted on blue cloth. Under the bench burned a series of candles to light the way. After the priest had achieved the appropriate level of trance he dramatically danced or leaped over the bridge to the other side, after which his behavior became quite unworldly. He battled with demons and monsters, performing martial steps as he negotiated his way along the dangerous roads of death. He carried with him a T-shirt which had belonged to the deceased relative as a way of "keeping him on the scent." When he finally met and was possessed by the soul of the dead relative, his body convulsed violently and then he slumped forward, twitching involuntarily. His assistants supported him as he began to speak in the voice of the spirit, a combination of mumbles, pants, and gasps which had to be interpreted by one of the assistants.

The message from the departed one advised the family what they must do to correct the situation to bring comfort both to the departed and to the living. At the end of the ritual, the family were visibly relieved and relaxed, for they now knew what was wrong and had a plan of action.

This tale illustrates the patterns of hospitality in a number of ways. First, the family had arranged and paid for what was an essentially private ritual to deal with a family problem. They had engaged the priest and his assistants for the day to make contact with their dead relative and heal the situation. They knew through their local contacts that these Taoists and this deity had successfully brought messages back from the world of the dead. They had chosen this specific deity and the priests of this temple to solve this religious problem on the basis of their established reputations. The success of their ritual reinforced the perception in the Tainanese religious field that such spirit possessions were indeed a specialty of the god and the temple.

Second, they did not directly approach the Jade Emperor, the main deity of the temple. The temple had installed a number of other deities in subordinate positions to the Jade Emperor, and each—like Chang

Tao-ling—had her or his reputation for a specific religious power. The temple had successfully expanded its sphere of cooperation by inviting the lesser deities to have their place.

Third, the central portion of the rite announcing the ritual intentions to the Jade Emperor had the dual function of acknowledging the host/master status of the main deity of the temple and of educating the family (and me and my friend) about the worship of the Jade Emperor. Although the ritual was assisted by the deity Chang Tao-ling, the Jade Emperor was invoked as a higher and authorizing spiritual power.

Finally, despite the private nature of the ritual, two strangers and outsiders (American women armed with cameras and tape recorders) were invited to observe and record the rite. This level of openness educated us about the practices and beliefs of the temple, as it might have any observer who happened to wander in. Except for very esoteric rituals, most celebrations in the Chinese religious field were open to the onlooker. There were numerous chances to observe the panoply of religious options.

Final Thoughts

In this chapter we have explored how the structures of hospitality shaped the practices of the Chinese religious field. The skills and obligations of hospitality enabled the Chinese to use religious festivals as a means of sustaining the cultural/community unity which was such an important Chinese ideal. They also established various mechanisms through which individuals would become familiar with a range of religious deities and temples, so that she or he could negotiate the religious field to her or his maximal spiritual advantage.

Throughout my pilgrimage in Chinese culture, I was deeply touched by the hospitality of Chinese religions. I visited scores of temples and was able to observe and enter into any ongoing activities almost instantly. I frequently walked in on rituals "off the street." I kept my ears cocked for the distinctive music of a Chinese funeral, often following it many blocks out of my way to observe another example.[21] I followed announcements in local papers and word-of-mouth information through the networks of the *Kuo-yü chung-hsin* language school about unusual rites and festivals, including a spellbinding fire-walking ceremony in the suburbs of Taipei. No doubt my methods for familiarizing myself with the religious field bore some resemblance to those of Chinese throughout history, although the local academy, the marketplace, or tea houses would have been the traditional venue for exchange of oral information.

Never was I more moved by the power of Chinese religious hospi-

主客

tality than on my pilgrimage to Lion's Head Mountain, recounted in chapter 2. The mountain was inviting to all who came, and it offered something of interest for virtually anyone. Above all, the hospitality at the monastery atop the mountain welcomed all seekers as honored guests. For many centuries, countless Chinese had learned about religion and advanced their religious journey through pilgrimage. My pilgrimage on Lion's Head Mountain and my stay in the monastery planted in my heart a firm faith in the ability of religious persons to welcome each other across the lines of religion and culture. The welcome of my Buddhist hosts inspired me to return with the tales of a pilgrim, exploring the possibilities for hospitality to the pilgrim in our religious world.

Part 3

Bringing the Tales Home

CHAPTER 9

歸根

Christians and Religious Neighbors

"Wu-k'ung," said the T'ang monk, "tell us when we shall be able to reach our destination."
Pilgrim said, "You can walk from the time of your youth till the time you grow old, and after that, till you become youthful again; and even after going through such a cycle a thousand times, you may still find it difficult to reach the place where you want to go to. But when you perceive, by the resoluteness of your will, the Buddha-nature in all things, and when every one of your thoughts goes back to its very source in your memory, that will be the time you arrive at the Spirit Mountain."

—*Wu Ch'eng-en,*
Journey to the West

Through many dangers, toils, and snares
I have already come.
'Tis grace that brought me safe this far
And grace will lead me home.

—*Traditional Hymn 671,*
Episcopal Hymnal

As I have recounted in this book, my pilgrimage in Chinese culture was a journey of discovery and delight, of opening to new learnings, of

---

"Returning to the Roots"
This phrase carries a double meaning: it symbolizes the return to the original unity or source in Chinese practices of meditation, and it also represents the "homecoming" of the pilgrim to share tales of the journey with her own community.

近鄰

deep personal and spiritual growth. I encountered moments of awe and reverence, of trepidation and anxiety, of confusion, of discovery, of hard-won insight. At times the journey seemed endless; I was a long, long way from home, cut off from the familiar, encountering the strange and the new. Although this remove from my familiar texts, symbols, and ways of thinking was precisely what freed me to experience the world of Chinese culture and religion, I sometimes felt a stab of fear about when I would be able to return and act as the cultural bridge I had set out to become. Like the T'ang monk in the epigraph to this chapter, I wanted to know what further challenges I would have to face, how far it was to my destination.

In chapter 24 of *Journey to the West,* just prior to the epigraph, the pilgrims realize that they have covered not even one-tenth of the 108,000-mile journey to the West. One of the companions asks, "How many years do we have to travel before we get there?" Taking into account the spiritual powers developed by the three companions in their previous lives, Pilgrim (Old Monkey) replies, "If we were talking about you two, my worthy brothers, this journey would take some ten days. If we were talking about me, I could probably make about fifty round trips in a day and there would still be sunlight. But if we are talking about Master, then don't even think about it!"

This passage, about a quarter of the way through the novel, is the first indication that the journey is not to be measured in miles, but in insights. If the T'ang monk persists in believing that the goal of his pilgrimage is to arrive at some external destination, then a thousand lives will not suffice for him to complete the journey. It is when he realizes the Buddha-nature in his own mind that he will arrive: his destination is within himself, not "out there."

So it was with my pilgrimage. I would never exhaust the study of Chinese culture; there would always be more to learn, more to read, more to understand. My insights would continually be chastened and refined, nuanced and corrected. But as a writer and a teacher, as a Christian and a North American, the time came to go home. If I had not achieved anything like the enlightenment which would be the end of the T'ang monk's journey, I had at least attained a level of insight and understanding which would allow me to teach and write, to share my tales with others. Perhaps because my journey was not capped with an enlightenment experience, the process of coming home was an extension of the pilgrimage, for now I had to integrate and translate my fragmentary insights into forms that I could share with my students and my church community.

Part of the adjustment was cultural re-entry. I returned home expecting to feel at home and instead felt strange in my own land. My sojourn in Chinese culture had left a deep imprint of experiences, sensibilities, and perspectives that those at home did not immediately

understand or appreciate, since they had not shared my experiences. In their eyes I had "gone native" in some respects; I had changed in unaccountable ways. My extended stay in another cultural world also made me see my home with new eyes, the eyes of an outsider in some ways. I had to adjust to the strangeness of the familiar and reorient myself on my home turf. I was betwixt and between cultures as I went through the re-entry process, and nowhere entirely at home. These discomforts passed with time.

近鄰

My first major step into the role of cultural bridge came when a student on the very first day of my very first course at Indiana University asked from the back row: "Is this course being taught by a Christian?" For a Religious Studies professor at Indiana University in 1974 this was a delicate question, for our mandate was to teach *about* religion and keep any trace of our own religious affiliations outside of the classroom. Without any time to deliberate, I replied:

> I have just returned from three years in East Asia, and I feel as though I have a foot on each side of the Pacific. It's not exactly a comfortable position, but it's the one I find myself in. What that means in response to your question is that my experience in Asia led me to profound respect for its traditions, although I have the humility not to claim to belong to any of them. I also maintain profound respect for the Christian tradition in which I was raised.

Teaching at Indiana University, I became an interpreter of East Asian cultures and religions. Because in order to teach them well I had to convey the coherence of its world view, its beliefs, and its practices, I developed "skillful means"[1] to convey Chinese religious thought and practice to Indiana students. However, because of the ethos of the state university, until I moved to the GTU I was able to dodge the harder issue of the implications of the pilgrimage for my Christian life and faith. This twelve years of grace gave me time to ponder what I as a Christian have learned from my pilgrimage in China.

My theological[2] voice developed slowly and in dialogue with many friends and colleagues. I spoke in theological environments on why Christians should know something about Asian religions. I led retreats on Chinese spirituality for my church. I sought to articulate to a range of faculty and students how I saw my role in the theological curriculum. I stretched the sensibilities of some fellow Christians by using Chinese examples or texts to shed light on a Christian issue. I learned that my responses to the stories and examples I encountered in China were shaped by my personal experiences and history; by no means do I stand for all Christians. However, I also came to appreciate that sharing my Christian reflections on the Chinese experience invited dia-

近
鄰

logue and conversation; it stimulated others to respond to the Chinese examples on their own terms.

In the spirit of opening a conversation, I assume in this chapter a more overtly theological voice. I do not offer a definitive interpretation of the lessons of Chinese religious inclusivism for our culture, for such a move would be itself profoundly inconsistent with Chinese notions of truth. Rather, I share insights and ideas which have arisen from my pilgrimage, inviting others to respond in terms of their own journeys.

Living with Religious Neighbors

"Which of these three, do you think proved neighbor to the man who fell among the robbers?"
He said, "The one who showed mercy on him."
And Jesus said to him, "Go and do likewise."
(Luke 10:36-37)

In chapters 1 and 3, I rehearsed the historical and contemporary difficulties which Christians face in developing affirmative stances toward other religions. Because of our history of exclusivism and religious intolerance, and the doctrinal and Biblical warrants which have been used to justify that history, openness toward other faiths has been seen as a difficult if not intractable issue. Its intractability is reinforced by the two major ways in which we have tended to construct the problem.

One major way in which the problem has been understood is to ask whether the beliefs and doctrines of the other religions can be reconciled with those of Christianity. Can one remain faithful to central Christian tenets (i.e., have a genuinely Christian Christology) and also affirm the truth of other faiths? When constructed in this way, the only route to a genuine openness to the truth of all faiths is to interpret Christianity in such a general way that it is no longer recognizably Christian to many. Such was the criticism of John Hick's "metaphorical Christology" in chapter 3.

Another major model of interfaith relations has been drawn from international relations. In this model, representatives of traditions enter into conversations seeking to negotiate some limited common ground while defending their own territories. The saga of the Council on Church Union, while limited to Christianity, is an excellent illustration of how the idealism which inspires such discussions can become mired in a plethora of hard details. It is perhaps not surprising that if historical disagreements have led groups to segment off from one another, it will be no easy task to reverse such divisions through nego-

tiation. The issues which caused the divisions have become the defining marks of each community.

Many thoughtful persons have engaged in interfaith dialogues which fall into neither of these self-defeating models, but the history of such dialogue has been slow to create for the Christian community an acknowledged foundation for relationships with other faiths.[3]

My encounters with Chinese religions opened up for me an entirely different approach to interfaith understanding: the simple, pragmatic issue of living with religious neighbors. I did not focus on Chinese religious polemic or borrowing, although there is a rich literature on both. I did not remain focused on how individual thinkers understood and reconciled the multiple religious strands of their lives, although that was the focus of much of my early research.[4] I sought instead to understand the patterns of behavior, the strategies, the diverse motivations, and the cultural incentives the Chinese had for negotiating religious diversity by means of multiple religious participation. The local, community dynamic of the Chinese religious field impressed upon me that the religious field was comprised of face-to-face human interactions; it was a set of strategies for living with one's religious neighbors.

In our increasingly religiously diverse society, this issue of religious neighbors is by no means abstract; it does not affect only scholars and political and religious leaders. Christianity is beset with internal differences, some of which have created ugly rifts in our society. Moreover, neighbors of other faiths are all around us: in our communities, our schools, our workplaces, and even our families. Living with religious neighbors, negotiating genuine religious diversity, is an issue for all Christians, an immediate and daily issue for many.

Living with religious neighbors, then, is an inescapable issue. One can seek to ignore one's neighbors, but that is in itself a way of living with them, though a distinctly unneighborly way. The pragmatic issue of living with one's neighbors encompasses many layers and levels. It begins on a detached, passive level: staying out of the neighbor's way, seeking to commit no actively offensive acts (live and let live). It includes basic courtesy (do unto others as you would have them do unto you). It extends to proactive, neighborly initiatives: welcoming, greeting, small acts of kindness or thoughtfulness, cooperation, favors, or friendship. Ultimately, for Christians, it would entail "loving your neighbor as yourself."

Christian teaching acknowledges that love of neighbor is not always easy or convenient. The tale of the Good Samaritan eloquently conveys this point. In the parable, the priest and the Levite are so caught up in their own religious obligations and notions of purity that they pass by the wounded man, not wishing to impede their own religious agenda. However, a Samaritan, a distrusted foreigner and non-Jew, goes way out of his way to show kindness to the victim. Jesus' parable forces the

近鄰

lawyer who had asked "who is my neighbor?" to admit that it was the non-Jew, the foreigner, who in the story fulfilled the deepest obligation of all: to love God and one's neighbor. Despite their religious and cultural differences, despite the history of antipathy between Jews and Samaritans, it was the Samaritan who became the model for loving God and neighbor.

The parable of the Good Samaritan offers an important caution for Christians who contend that only those who profess the Christian Way can follow the teachings of Jesus. In this parable, Jesus goes out of his way to remind us that those who profess the Way may not live it, and those who do not profess it may live it.

I believe that Christians are called to develop their skills for living with religious neighbors by accepting and loving them as neighbors. As we become more skilled in doing so, we will develop with our neighbors a level of daily ecumenism in which mutual knowledge and familiarity help us to grow in mutual sensitivity and respect.

The Religious Field: Seeking Common Ground

"In my Father's house are many rooms."

(John 14:2)

The Chinese notion of religious field, so central to my appreciation of the dynamics of Chinese religious inclusivity, is not a model which is readily transferable to our cultural context. In the first place our notion of "field" has to do with tilled land which is owned, which is some individual's or corporation's private property. While our culture has a well-developed sense of philanthropy and generosity, it is no longer tied to the land; there is in current Western practice no "charitable field."

Second, insofar as the Chinese religious field is a playing field, it does not fit our cultural models of the playing field. Our fields (for football or soccer) are arenas in which two teams fight to defend their goals; they are battlegrounds. Throughout Western history, the image of battleground has been all too apt as an image of the exclusivist religious field. The notion of field, alas, does not provide an image of common ground for our culture.

Our primary term for common ground is "community" (its very root suggests commonality, or unity), and an important image is the public square, the center of the community in which public events occur. The public square is, in the tradition of the town meeting, also the ground on which different viewpoints are expressed, where they encounter one another. Community is still an important ideal, but it is increasingly a nostalgic, utopian ideal.

The growth of urban centers has strained traditional ideals of com-

munity. The modern city is simply too large for town meetings or one central place of assembly. Neighborhood associations and a host of interest groups have replaced "community" as the gathering point of civic concern and discussion. This patchwork of groups creates a chorus of competing interests which are hard to reconcile in the traditional patterns of building community consensus. Cities are comprised of many competing communities.

The globalization of cities and towns throughout America has also strained the traditional sense of community and common ground. The global diversity brings much richness to a community in terms of cultural traditions, art forms, cuisines, and festivals, but the downside is that the cultural common ground becomes less clear. The traditional religious and cultural classics which served as the common heritage of "Americans" must now be supplemented by the many cultural traditions represented by all of our citizens. Globalization has its consequences.

Still, the community is a primary locus for finding common ground for living with religious neighbors. Many communities celebrate the festivals of diverse cultures and ethnic groups, holding a round of civic events not unlike the traditional rounds of temple festivals in China. Civic leaders are expected to "make the rounds" in order to symbolize and affirm the inclusion of diverse groups in the larger community. In many areas, it is becoming a custom for folks to visit each other's cultural festivals.

In some communities, neighbors join across the lines of faith in interfaith councils to work collaboratively on issues of concern to the community. In Sacramento, California, for instance, an interfaith network of congregations operating a program for youth at risk includes not only churches and synagogues, but also mosques.[5] In other communities, people join hands across lines of faith to fight against the evils of hatred and intolerance. A Presbyterian member of an interfaith council in Dallas reported that her reason for becoming involved in such work was that "Skinheads are vandalizing synagogues in Dallas, and we need to band together to stop these acts of violence."[6] Such alliances against intolerance echo alliances of white and African-American churches to rebuild burned churches and work to prevent further destruction.

In Chicago, a Jewish congregation lost its synagogue and found itself without a meeting place. The leadership made an agreement with a local church to share the church's worship space. The cross is installed for Christian worship, and replaced by the ark of the covenant for Jewish worship. The two congregations worship jointly once a year, after which they meet to discuss maintenance of their shared space. By sharing the space, both Christians and Jews have grown in respect for each other's traditions of worship.

These examples each grew out of specific relationships and events

近鄰

in a local community and were enabled by the relationships developed between persons of different faiths. The parties involved were creative in discerning the openings for developing common ground. They are small but path-breaking examples, concrete steps in developing a network of interfaith relationships in these communities.

The work of these persons is all the more impressive because we lack cultural images or metaphors to envision the common ground on which we might meet persons of other faiths. The lack of such images or models impoverishes our imaginations and makes it harder to recognize openings for meeting points.

One possible image, though not without its difficulties, is the image of God's house with many rooms, in John 14:2. The potential of this image as a Christian model for negotiating religious diversity was brought home to me (if you will forgive the pun) in a book by Linda Moody. Moody invoked the image of a house from the writing of a secular feminist theorist, Rosemarie Tong. Tong developed her image as an attempt to transcend the bitter divisions within the feminist camp. She wrote,

> It is a major challenge to contemporary feminism to reconcile the pressures for diversity and difference with those for integration and commonality. We need a home in which everyone has a room of her own, but one in which the walls are thin enough to permit a conversation, a community of friends in virtue, and partners in action.[7]

Tong's image builds on Virginia Woolf's famous notion that some private space, a room of her own, is a necessity for the development of woman's consciousness and voice.

It is a fitting image for religious communities as well. For the vast majority of religious folk, the distinctive space of their community provides a much-needed venue of worship, prayer, reflection, and conversation which develops their religious identity and sense of a place in the world. While we seek common ground on which to meet and to celebrate one another, we also need to know who we are and to affirm our communities of choice.

The image of the house can, I believe, be enriched by linking it to the biblical image of the "Father's house with many rooms." However, this would entail an expanded reading of this biblical passage. All too often our reading of John 14:2 is solely individualistic, seeing the Father's house as full of rooms for individuals, and the saying as assurance that we, in effect, won't have missed the housing deadline—there will be a room available for us personally. In the gospel context, Jesus is assuring his disciples that, although he is going away, he will come again for them, and there will be a place for them.

The question, however, is: How wide is God's love? How capacious is God's house? Is it possible that the many rooms in God's house will also have places for those who have found paths to God different from our own? They may be in another wing of the house, but do those who have sought God in many paths ultimately end up under God's roof, in the vastness of God's embrace? We cannot know for certain, but as a Christian, what I have glimpsed of the steadfastness and vastness of God's love assures me that it is always beyond my comprehension, far vaster than my heart or my imagination can reach.

Assuming that God's house has many rooms, there will be room for my particular Episcopalian sense and sensibility, but also rooms for many others. And we as Christians have sound warrant to believe that the reach of God's love will be very great indeed. We are all likely to meet, in God's capacious house, folks we did not expect to see there.

Moody's development of the image of the house of many rooms moves beyond the size of the house to note that the image of a house suggests common spaces: spaces which run up against white middle-class need for privacy. Such folks are a bit cautious about mixing it up. Moody warns,

> It is not necessary for us to have our room completely decorated and pictures hung on the wall before venturing out [into the common spaces]; in fact, it is critical that we move back and forth from our room to common living spaces even as we deepen our own wellspring.[8]

U.S. white middle-class assumptions of privacy in the home have been developed to an unusual point in the second half of this century. In most cultures and classes, indeed in most times in U.S. history, homes were multigenerational and included large groups of family and even nonfamily members. Privacy was minimal; spaces were shared, doors remained open. Moody suggests in a very thought-provoking way that the development of spacious nuclear family homes with a wealth of private spaces has compromised the development of our skills for sharing and opening ourselves to others. We have become intensely private people, and the development of computer technologies may be exacerbating this trend despite their vaunted interconnectedness. God's love not only loves us as we are and invites us to be our authentic selves (and thus provides us a room of our own) but also invites us to ever broader love in the common rooms of this divine complex.

Consider the common spaces of a house: they serve multiple purposes. In the kitchen and dining room, we prepare food either for our families or to invite others to eat with us. The dining room of God's capacious house is extremely important, since commensality, the invitation to share food, is the most ancient and venerated form of hospi-

tality, of entering into relationship with the stranger. In living rooms or parlors, we entertain, converse, or hold meetings. In sewing rooms, computer rooms, or game rooms we come together for common purpose or activities. We meet informally daily in the hall, the kitchen, and the backyard. In attics and basement are items stored from the past, not often used or perhaps forgotten, that nonetheless may be recovered for our own group or lent to another. The common spaces of the house are meeting grounds, places of interaction, or mutual hosting. They can provide chance encounters (for those who happen to be in or pass through the same space at the same time) or intentional meetings or celebrations.

The image of a house with many rooms has some promise as a Western, Christian, biblically rooted model for understanding and negotiating religious diversity in our context. It offers some common ground, but also the assurance of private spaces in which to preserve the particular identities of our various traditions. It does not challenge us to become one or transcend our particularities, only to meet one another in God's love.

The image of the house, however, makes clear that our own rooms are connected to the common spaces under one roof (in the Biblical sense, the roof is God's love); it challenges our instincts to see *only* the private and particular and to refuse to envision or enter the common ground. This model may have some potential to open up our Western Christian imaginations to see new possibilities for living with religious neighbors.

Embodiment

> *"And the Word became flesh and dwelt among us, full of grace and truth."*
>
> *(John 1:14)*

The Chinese notion of truth as embodied, of the inseparability of knowledge and action, of the Way as not only the highest truth but also a way of life or an art of living, struck a deep, resonant chord in me as a Christian and as a woman.

Although much of church teaching has focused on doctrines or statements about God and creation, the central content of that teaching has to do with Christology and incarnation. The fundamental truth and paradox of Christian teaching is that "The Word became flesh and dwelt among us," was crucified, died, and buried, and rose again from the dead, in accordance with the scriptures. It begins with and grows out of the incarnation, the embodiment of the Word of God in human form.

The doctrine of Word made flesh, God in human form, puts the embodiment of truth, its living out in an actual human life, at the very center of Christianity. There is, to be sure, a fundamental divide between Christianity and Chinese (and Indian) traditions over the Christian claim of the uniqueness of the incarnation. That is, and will long remain, a stumbling block for those seeking to reconcile Christian beliefs with those of other religions. However, the affirmation of the incarnation also opens a broad avenue to appreciating the Chinese approach to truth.

Embodiment of truth goes beyond the incarnation itself, although the incarnation creates a theological foundation for such embodiment. Christians, like the Chinese, look to human models for inspiration about how to live out their faith. They look not only to Jesus, but also to other models: the disciples, famous teachers and theologians, pastors, saints of the church, and other religious figures—Mother Theresa, Martin Luther King.

Moreover, despite our Western Christian proclivities to focus excessively on doctrinal ways of understanding God as opposed to contemplative ways of apprehending the mystery,[9] the history of Christian spirituality provides many techniques and images for internalizing or embodying the sacred. A striking example of an embodied spirituality comes from Hadewijch, of thirteenth-century Flanders, who wrote "The Allegory of Love's Growth." This poem portrays the growth of love in the Christian soul as gestation within the womb. The first month is faithful fear; the second, joyful suffering; the third "raises the number/As the soul thus can carry all,/And it knows that it carries Love"; the fourth is the state of sweetness; the fifth month "brings to effect the most sweet burden that the soul has received"; the sixth month is confidence; the seventh, justice; the eighth the wisdom of Love.

> The ninth month is as if wisdom engulfs
> All that is love in love.
> Then love's moment of power comes
> And continually assaults wisdom.
> As man with all that man is
> Contents Love and is conformed to Love,
> So in the ninth month is born
> The Child that lowliness has chosen.[10]

Gestation is perhaps the most explicit of all images of embodiment, for it suggests that Love grows from the very body and being of the worshipper.

Embodied spiritualities are not always as dramatic as Hadewijch's gestation imagery, and—in the view of feminists—they place the locus

of Christian faith and life squarely in everyday, ordinary lives. Linda Moody has studied the feminist theologies of white, African-American, Caribbean, and Hispanic and Latino women, finding many important and ineradicable differences among these authors. Among the few commonalities was that they all profess an embodied spirituality. She comments:

> In part, this effort stems from a rejection of the abstract theologizing of the past that excluded women's lives. Theological reflection is built upon the concrete, everyday experience of women in each of these theologies. God, too, is seen as embodied, with real concern for the material, physical welfare of women and their families.[11]

The feminist theologians' assertion that the locus of spirituality is in everyday life is consistent with what we have seen in the Chinese religious field, where the particular deities function to assist human beings in dealing with daily and this-worldly troubles. Spirituality for the Chinese, as well as for feminists, begins in the concrete concerns of the everyday, and builds from there to more transcendent dimensions and levels. The Way is rooted and grounded in the body and in the real lives of human beings; it includes the experiences of family and household, of daily life and illness, the struggles and joys of everyday living as its root or base.

One of the contributions of feminist theology has been to recover for Christians the importance of embodiment, the practice or living out of the Christian life. This resonates well with the contemporary (and often unchurched) interest in spirituality: spiritual practices, values, and beliefs. While the popular forms of spirituality are sometimes—in the eyes of those steeped in a particular tradition—fragmentary, rootless, and superficial, the interest in spirituality becomes a potential meeting point between the churched and the unchurched, a common ground on which to open conversation. This is important because living with religious neighbors successfully also means reaching out to the unchurched and the nonobservant, who in some areas are becoming the religious majority.

One of the great potentials of the notion of embodiment for living with religious neighbors is that embodiment is done individual by individual (although often supported, informed, and influenced by participation in a religious community). Because each of us must practice religion for him/herself, we can each speak out of our own experience of practice. We can meet other faithful persons, either from our own tradition or from another, and learn from one another.

In a fascinating development of the late twentieth century, much of the encounter with other traditions through reading, retreats, and

workshops is precisely in the area of spiritual practice. There seems to be a strong impulse to find ways to bring faith alive, to revitalize prayer or contemplation, to learn from and about the practices of other religious traditions. Perhaps this is simply another form of self-help, but the pattern does provide an opening or meeting ground for many to become acquainted with other faiths.

近鄰

Another level of embodiment from which we can all learn are specific examples of interfaith partnerships: marriages, projects, or ministries. Our culture is replete with specific experiments such as these, and we would benefit from attending to them and learning from their experiences, good and bad, about the promise and challenges of living with religious neighbors.

Hospitality

"I was a stranger, and you welcomed me."
(Matthew 25:35)

As I recounted in chapter 8, the structures of hospitality were key to the dynamics of the Chinese religious field. Members of various temples and shrines in a given community played host and guest to each other in a round of religious festivals and celebrations. Visitors were welcomed at temples and pilgrimage sites, entertained and instructed. It was customary to pay courtesy calls to temples and shrines, not only because of their historical and cultural interest, but to learn about and honor their traditions and their contributions to the religious field.

The metaphor of hospitality to one's religious neighbors is very promising, for hospitality is a venerable tradition in our culture and religious history. The structures of hospitality define civilized behavior and govern one's relation to strangers. While in the informal ethos of contemporary American life, we often play fast and loose with traditional rituals and codes of hospitality, nonetheless hospitality remains an important means of establishing, defining, and sustaining relationships.

Thomas Ogletree has argued that the Christian notion of hospitality to the stranger is a fundamental metaphor for the Christian moral life.

> To offer hospitality to the stranger is to welcome something new, unfamiliar, and unknown into our life-world. On the one hand, hospitality requires a recognition of the stranger's vulnerability in an alien social world. Strangers need shelter and sustenance in their travels, especially when they are moving through a hostile environment. On the other hand hospitality designates occasions of potential discovery which can open up

近鄰

> our narrow provincial worlds. Strangers have stories to tell which we have never heard before, stories which can redirect our seeing and stimulate our imaginations. The stories invite us to view the world from a novel perspective.[12]

Ogletree's analysis goes far beyond simply being neighborly, acknowledging the existence or propinquity of the neighbor through an act of hospitality. It includes sensitivity to the power dynamic of the encounter: if the other is a stranger in the sense of being in an alien social world (i.e, represents a minority culture or tradition not well understood), then he or she is vulnerable and needs our support and protection. He also notes that the stranger has gifts to contribute to our world, "stories to tell which we have never heard before." The stranger will contribute to, enrich, and expand our life-world in fundamental ways. Thus this hospitality opens us and our world to transformation and enrichment.

Ogletree notes that the stranger represents otherness in all of its manifestations:

> wonder and awe in the presence of the holy, receptivity to unconscious impulses arising from our being as bodied selves, openness to the unfamiliar and unexpected even in the midst of our most intimate relationships, regard for characteristic differences in the experiences of males and females, recognition of the role social location plays in molding perceptions and value orientations, efforts to transcend barriers generated by racial oppression.[13]

Ogletree here suggests that hospitality to the stranger and attentiveness to the other in many forms can accomplish the sorts of goals for which I undertook my long pilgrimage in Chinese culture. We all, he argues, have manifold opportunities to encounter the other, to expand our horizons, to develop our sensibilities to the richness of being in relation to our specific location.

He also notes that in order to realize the moral fruits of hospitality we cannot only play the generous host, putting ourselves thereby in a position of privilege and power.

> My readiness to welcome the other into my world must be balanced by my readiness to enter the world of the other. My delight in the stories of the other as enrichment for my orientation to meaning must be matched by my willingness to allow my own stories to be incorporated into the values and thought modes of the other.[14]

Ogletree's theological understanding of hospitality to the stranger provides a wonderful foundation for Christian hospitality toward the religious neighbor.

近
鄰

Hospitality implies face-to-face relations; it cannot be accomplished simply by talking or reading about neighbors. One must meet them. Through meeting, a relationship is established. If all goes well, trust may be built and may even flower into friendship.

Hospitality need not imply any attempt to convert or co-opt the other. Too often in Christian churches we have seen our welcome to the visitor simply as a strategy for recruitment. Interfaith hospitality needs to be structured so as to allow the guest to be simply a guest, true to his/her values, identity, and commitments.

In my local parish, we are on the verge of establishing interfaith biblical study groups with a local Jewish congregation. We have agreed that what we seek is small groups meeting over food (using commensality as a hospitality structure, with due regard for the dietary observances of our Jewish colleagues), and in groups of equal numbers of Christians and Jews. The numerical equity is intended to keep either side from feeling overwhelmed or tokenized. We will discuss texts from the Hebrew Bible with an eye to understanding our very different readings. We hope that the Christians will become more aware of the Jewish roots of these texts, and that Jews will experience the genuine openness and regard of Christians for the richness of their heritage.

Issues of Truth

> *"A sound tree cannot bear evil fruit, nor can a bad tree bear good fruit. Every tree that does not bear good fruit is cut down and thrown into the fire. Thus you will know them by their fruits."*
>
> *(Matthew 7:18-20)*

Jesus' metaphor for helping his followers to recognize false prophets is a useful biblical teaching for considering the issues of truth in interfaith relations. Living with and even loving one's religious neighbors does not mean that one condones that which is against one's deepest convictions and values. But it does require more than looking for total agreement on all points of belief and interpretation. The Chinese would agree with Jesus' metaphor: you will know them by their fruits.

The beliefs and practices of others might be very different from one's own, but what sort of persons do they produce? Can we discern genuine spiritual qualities, authentic moral values, true holiness in the

近鄰

followers of other traditions? It is impossible to articulate a clear principle of what each of these would look like, but—although this is not a simple matter—we are capable of recognizing the holy when we encounter it, even in a new form. As Diana Eck has written,

> Each of us brings religious or ethical criteria to our understanding of the new worlds we encounter. When I "recognize" God's presence in a Hindu temple or in the life of a Hindu, it is because, through this complex of God, Christ, and Spirit, I have a sense of what God's presence is like. Recognition means that we have seen it somewhere before. I would even say that it is Christ who enables Christians—in fact, challenges us—to recognize God especially where we don't expect to do so and where it is not easy to do so.[15]

Eck's point is eloquent. If we have developed our Christian faith in God, that faith will help us to recognize God and God-like teachings in other venues and forms. It is not a simple test, but one rooted in our faith and spirituality.

The other important aspect of the Chinese understanding of truth is its affirmation of humility, of the incompleteness of *any* statement or articulation of the truth. Theologically, this statement affirms the freedom of God to continue revealing new understandings to us, and the freedom—indeed the mandate—of Christians to continually reappropriate the Christian gospel in the light of new contexts and situations. The gospel is not a fixed, dead letter, but the Word of God. If we believe that God loves the world and that the Holy Spirit continues to infuse the church with vitality, then new understandings of Christian faith and life will continue to unfold, and our present understanding is not the final word.

Such appropriate humility leaves open the door to learn from other faiths insofar as God is present in and through them.

Conclusion

In this final chapter I have cited a number of examples that suggest that Christians in our culture are beginning to develop creative strategies for living more affirmatively with their religious neighbors. I celebrate these initiatives and pray that we will build on them.

The three stories I cited in the opening of chapter 1 also illustrate the sorts of strategies which I have lifted up in this chapter.

The Catholic and Buddhist friendship in a Bay Area suburb illustrates two of my points. It started with a similarity of practice: process-

ing with saints/Buddhas on a feast day. Despite considerable theological differences, the similar form of veneration was the opening which allowed Vietnamese Buddhists and Portuguese Catholics to recognize some common ground. Second, the Catholics recognized a gesture of friendship and extended the hand of hospitality to their Buddhist neighbors, thereby creating an ongoing pattern of interaction.

近鄰

The Tlingit and Orthodox accommodation in funerals, bridging the long-house ceremony to a church funeral by a solemn procession, is important because it is a historical example of neighborly accommodation across religious lines. This is an issue of contextualization, of Christians being willing to make space for the traditions of peoples adapting to Christianity. For many Native Americans and for Christians from cultural backgrounds where religious and cultural identity and practices have been densely interwoven, the openness of Christians to such observances is a vital issue. How open are we as Christians to the rich global identities within our churches? Do we ask folk to shed their roots in order to belong to the church? In this case, the issue of hospitality is not in relation to other faiths and communities, but the willingness of our own churches to welcome the cultural and global richness of its members.

The story of an evangelical church celebrating the moon festival with Chinese international students illustrates an unusually generous hospitality. This church did not simply invite the Chinese students into their space on the church's own terms, but also sought a way to become guests as well as hosts by celebrating a tradition of the Chinese students. The church presumably became comfortable about celebrating the moon festival by seeing it as merely a festival (i.e., not a pagan religious belief). In China the moon festival is a secular festival, but it is also rooted in the religious and cultural values of the Chinese. This raises a fascinating point. The line between secular and sacred is drawn very differently in other cultures. The border around religious issues in contemporary U.S. society is, in the perspective of global world history, a very narrow line, designating only formally professed beliefs, membership, and participation in a specific religious institution. Many cultural observances, such as Thanksgiving, are viewed as secular, although they are profoundly shaped by religious beliefs and traditions.

On the one hand, we need to recognize that what may look to us like secular matters (such as whether a Muslim woman or a Christian Scientist will accept certain medical treatments) may be not only influenced but also mandated by religion. On the other hand, the narrow line we draw around "the religious" opens the door for various forms of interaction with religious neighbors which are not seen as in conflict with our faith commitments.

近鄰

Living with religious neighbors requires that we honor the religious sensibilities of our neighbors and of ourselves. We will not be able to honor them until and unless: 1) we are each well rooted in our own faith; 2) we come to know more about one another; and 3) we begin to talk face-to-face. May we all grow in the art of being good religious neighbors.

Notes

Prologue

1. I left the Deanship in June 1996, but stayed on to teach and write at the GTU.

2. In the early years of establishing religious studies departments at state universities, the general principle applied by the courts was that departments could teach *about* religion, but they could not *teach religion*. This distinction is still used by some in religious studies.

3. See my "Religious Studies and the Exposure to Multiple Worlds," in *Beyond the Classics? Essays in Religious Studies and Liberal Education,* ed. Frank E. Reynolds and Sheryl L. Burkhalter (Atlanta: Scholars Press, 1990), pp. 179-202.

4. It is not uncommon in theological studies for schools to prefer having "other religions" represented directly by spokespersons for their faith; only then, it is argued, do we treat these religions as equals. While there is merit in this approach, there is also an important difficulty: given the linguistic, symbolic, and cultural gaps between religious traditions, on whose shoulders is the weight of translation? Do we require that Buddhists and Hindus know not only their own language and context, but also our own? Can Christian scholars of other religions who have learned the languages, lived in the cultures, and come to know well representatives of the traditions, be translators from our side? The role of persons like me is not to replace direct voices from other traditions, but to help North American Christians to do our part in building the bridge, in reaching out to other traditions by setting foot, so to speak, on their territory.

5. This phrase evokes the self-understanding of Elsa Tamez, a United Methodist Mexican of mixed heritage, who understands her task as helping those who are not Indian or Black to receive the spiritual practices of others with equality and joy. Elsa Tamez, "Quetzalcoatl Challenges the Christian Bible," paper presented at the annual meeting of the American Academy of Religion, November 1992, San Francisco. Cited in Linda Moody, *Women Encounter God: Theology across the Boundaries of Difference* (Maryknoll, NY: Orbis Books, 1996), p. 123.

6. I acknowledge that every storyteller, whether a Chinese master, a Chinese historian, or myself, selects and reshapes the material through his or her particular lens. It is not possible to convey fully and objectively another context. Although the contexts of the story are filtered both by Chinese tradition and by my retelling, they nonetheless provide some texture, some grounding, for the religious practices or ideas portrayed.

7. The phrase was used by Vivian-Lee Nyitray to characterize the biographies of the *Shih chi,* an early Chinese history. See her *Mirrors of Virtue: Lives of Four Lords in Ssu-ma Ch'ien's Shih Chi* (Stanford: Stanford University Press, forthcoming), MS. p. 11.

8. Thus, like Francis Clooney, I step back from any claim of an encompassing, comprehensive narrative, much less an interpretation which would embrace the realities or truth of both Chinese religions and Christianity. I aspire only to small insights and fruitful suggestions. Francis X. Clooney, S.J., *Seeing through Texts: Doing Theology among Srîvaisnavas of South India* (Albany: State University of New York Press, 1996), pp. 299-304. Clooney's work and his distinctive methodology will be discussed in chapter 3.

9. Newhall fellowships are a GTU program which invites collaboration between faculty and doctoral students in the fields of research or teaching.

1. Religious Diversity and the Pilgrimage to China

1. As in Will Herberg's classic, *Protestant, Catholic, Jew: An Essay in American Religious Sociology* (Garden City, NY: Doubleday, 1955). This neat picture left out Native American traditions and a number of small religious minorities, but it represented public perception in the 1950s. Even the perception has changed. Martin Marty, in the June 15, 1995 edition of *Context: A Commentary on the Interaction of Religion and Culture* (vol. 27, no. 14), noted that at a recent Senate Finance Committee meeting, senators were struggling with how to characterize our national religious ethos. At one point Senator Moynihan commented, "It's now official. Ours is a *Judeo-Christian-Islamic* heritage. If anybody feels left out, we've got some more hyphens" (p. 1). It is in fact not easy to describe the religious ethos of the nation.

2. Diana L. Eck, "Neighboring," *Harvard Magazine* (September–October 1996), p. 40.

3. As we discussed in the doctoral seminar at Vanderbilt, the acknowledgment of diversity in key institutions varies according to the part of the country in which one lives. Laurel Cassidy, a student in the seminar, had worked in Nashville hospitals, where examples of cultural and religious diversity continued to be seen as exceptions for which no general policies were necessary. Laurel's paper sought to develop case studies of actual examples which could be used with health professsionals to help alert them to the ways in which cultural and religious difference could affect their relations with patients.

4. Eck, "Neighboring," p. 44.

5. I want to thank Denis Thalson for pushing me beyond the much-invoked but less than specific notion of "common ground" to specify more clearly the challenge facing us.

6. Cornel West, *Race Matters* (New York: Vintage Books, 1994), p. 109.

7. After Vatican II, this situation changed dramatically, and Dubuque became a

leading center of ecumenical dialogue and cooperation. By the time of Vatican II, however, I was away at college. The Dubuque I knew was pre-Vatican II, a time when Catholics and Protestants perpetuated the religious competition which had long marked the community.

8. In college I had developed a profound interest in Greek mythology and its resonances through Western literature. Having discovered the richness of cultural allusion woven through Western art and literature, I developed a notion of what it was "to be educated"—I would be a person who could appreciate these allusions! The Chinese course brought home dramatically that there were voices and images of which I had not dreamed. This discovery paralleled the resurgence of many voices (women, nonelite, ethnic, dissenters, gays, and lesbians) which have challenged our notion of canon. The course on China was simply the gate through which I happened upon this discovery, but because of the enormous depth and richness of the Chinese literary and artistic heritage, the challenge to my previous notion of "culture" was resounding.

9. Carter Heyward, *Our Passion for Justice: Images of Power, Sexuality, and Liberation* (New York: Pilgrim Press, 1984), p. 245.

10. William E. Soothill, *Three Religions of China: Lectures Delivered at Oxford* (London: Oxford University Press, H. Milford, 1923), p. 13.

11. Valerie Hansen, *Changing Gods in Medieval China, 1127-1276* (Princeton: Princeton University Press, 1990), p. 3.

2. The Pilgrimage and the Pilgrim

1. Denis Thalson has reminded me that "a pilgrimage" is marked by the intention—generally religious—of the pilgrim. This is an important point. However, pilgrimages can creep up on you, so to speak, especially in East Asia. Scattered throughout China and Japan are famous historic pilgrimage routes. These routes are followed by groups of devout and committed pilgrims, true pilgrims in Denis's sense, in that they undertake their journey with a religious intent. However, the routes are also followed by tourists and visitors like Cynthia and myself, who may not have, or may not be aware of, the religious intent and shape of the journey. However, some, like myself, are taken by surprise (and grace) when the journey does in fact turn out to have a deeper meaning, and their motivations turn out to be deeper than they knew. As is also made clear in Wu Ch'eng-en's great novel of Chinese pilgrimage, *Journey to the West,* even committed pilgrims are likely to discover levels of meanings and intentions of the pilgrimage which are quite distinct from those they began with. As they travel, their understanding and insights grow.

2. This was an example of patriotism or national pride, since the Republic of Taiwan was proud of its membership in the United Nations and its permanent seat on the Security Council representing "China." However, close to the time of this pilgrimage, the U.N. voted to replace Taiwan with the People's Republic of China as the representative of China. That vote was traumatic for the Taiwan government. Since I have not returned to Shih T'ou Shan, I have not been able to determine whether this carousel remains. I suspect that it was removed in the period after the U.N. vote.

3. The Eight Immortals were colorful characters each reputed to offer a distinctive boon, such as long life, many sons, success in business, to devotees. They

represent the most pragmatic and this-worldly version of the Chinese religious imagination: religion offers specific blessings to enhance one's lot in this life. See Kwok Man Ho and Joanne O'Brien, trans. and ed., *The Eight Immortals of Taoism: Legends and Fables of Popular Taoism* (New York: Meridian, 1987).

It has long been a practice of scholars, both Chinese and Western, to label most religious practices or ideas under one of the so-called Three Teachings: Confucianism, Buddhism, and Taoism. The writings of anthropologists have added a fourth or "folk" label, recognizing that many practices cannot be included under the other three. As we will discuss in chapter 4, scholarship has increasingly questioned the boundaries between the Three Teachings and the accuracy of the labels. However, for the sake of clarity, I am sometimes compelled to use the labels. The use of quotation marks in this sentence indicates that although the Eight Immortals were conventionally labeled Taoist, they can equally be seen in the province of the amorphous folk traditions of China.

4. See Wolfram Eberhard, *The Local Cultures of South and East China* (Leiden: E.J. Brill, 1968).

5. It is a basic principle of Buddhist pedagogy that each seeker must learn for him- or herself. The skillful Buddhist teacher seeks to expose seekers to experiences or stories which will help them to find the truth, but does not offer truth on a platter.

6. I was fortunate to do a tutorial with William Theodore de Bary on Taoism and folk religions which greatly extended the boundaries of Columbia's core courses. This tutorial gave me a context of knowledge in which to place my observations of religious life.

7. In the *I Ching* (Book of Changes), the phrase "to cross the great waters" signifies an undertaking of significance and challenge.

8. See Barbara Aria with Russell Eng Gon, *The Spirit of the Chinese Character: Gifts from the Heart* (San Francisco: Chronicle Books, 1992), p. 19.

9. D. C. Lau, trans., *Lao Tzu, Tao te ching* (Middlesex, Eng.: Penguin Books, 1963), XXV, p. 82.

10. The Chinese divide the soul into an earthly and a heavenly component. The earthly component resides in the body, and—after death—in the grave until it is reabsorbed into the earth from which it came. The heavenly or spiritual portion carries the intellectual and spiritual powers of the human being; it is this spirit (*shen*) which travels to other realms and which hears the prayers of the filial descendants.

11. See, for instance, Yü Ying-shih, "'O Soul, Come Back!' A Study in Changing Conceptions of the Soul and Afterlife in Pre-Buddhist China," *Harvard Journal of Asiatic Studies* 47: 2 (Dec 84): 391; and C. Stevan Harrell, "The Concept of Soul in Chinese Folk Religion," *Journal of the Association of Asian Studies* 38:1 (May 79): 519-528. I thank Kevin Cheng for suggesting these references.

12. See Lu Kuan Yu, *Taoist Yoga, Alchemy and Immortality* (New York: Samuel Weiser, Inc., 1973), esp. xii-xvii and p. 68.

13. See Amy Tan, *Joy Luck Club* (New York: Putnam's, 1989), p. 240. Traditional Chinese society did not distinguish between fainting, coma, and death. It was just that some deaths became permanent. They were all "deaths" because the soul had left the body.

14. Many readers may have seen in museums versions of the Han ceramic models of horses, food, servants, and even barns and homes meant to supply the dead with the accoutrements of the living.

15. Different schools or lineages of Taoism developed and specialized in specific

rituals which teachers handed on to worthy disciples. Thunder rituals represented one of the many streams of Taoist rites. See Judith M. Boltz, *A Survey of Taoist Literature: Tenth to Seventeenth Centuries*, Chinese Research Monograph Series, no. 32 (Berkeley: Institute of East Asian Studies, 1987), pp. 47-49, 69-70, 176-179, and 263 n. 54.

16. The use of "Taoistic" in this case indicates that although *fang-wai* has been primarily associated with Taoism, it is a general pattern of Chinese religious life, and should not be considered Taoist in any clear sense.

17. Miyakawa Hisayuki, "Nansô no Dôshi Haku Gyozen no jiseki" (On the life of Southern Sung Taoist Master Pai Yü-ch'an), in *Uchida Gimpu hakushi shôju kinen tôyôshi ronshû* (A festschrift commemorating the sixtieth birthday of Professor Uchida Gimpu) (Kyoto: Dôhôsha, 1978), p. 502.

18. Miyakawa has documented examples of correspondence with members of the middle-level officialdom, notably Li Ch'en (1144-1218) and Ch'iao Li-hsien (1155-1222) (Miyakawa, "On the Life of Pai Yü-ch'an," 512), and there are a few disciples who have left some writings. My attempts to identify upwards of eighty persons named in poems and occasional writings proved fruitless. Pai's activities were primarily local and mostly among the subelite, although his contacts with abbots on Lung-hu shan and at Hsi-shan are reasonably well documented.

19. See Judith A. Berling, *The Syncretic Religion of Lin Chao-en* (New York: Columbia University Press, 1980), chapter 4.

20. See ibid., chapters 6 and 7.

21. Wu Ch'eng-en, *Journey to the West*, 4 vols., trans. Anthony Yü (Chicago: University of Chicago Press, 1977-1981).

22. See Christian Jochim, *Chinese Religions: A Cultural Perspective* (New Jersey: Prentice Hall, 1986), p. 106, for an explanation of the names.

23. *Journey to the West*, vol. 4, p. 391. In Buddhist teaching, all reality is "empty" of permanent existence; the wordless scriptures perfectly represent "reality as it is."

24. Chinese call foreigners *wai-kuo-jen*, literally, people of outside countries.

3. Forging a New Path

1. Ruben L. F. Habito, *Total Liberation: Zen Spirituality and the Social Dimension* (Maryknoll, NY: Orbis Books, 1989). See also Alan W. Watts, *The Art of Contemplation: A Facsimile Manuscript with Doodles by Alan Watts* (New York: Pantheon, 1972), and *The Spirit of Zen: A Way of Life, Work, and Art in the Far East* (New York: Grove Press, 1960); Thomas Merton, *Mystics and Zen Masters* (New York: Strauss and Giroux, 1967), and *Zen and the Birds of Appetite* (New York: New Directions, 1968).

2. John B. Cobb, *Beyond Dialogue: Toward a Mutual Transformation of Christianity and Buddhism* (Philadelphia: Fortress Press, 1982); Abe Masao, *Zen and Western Thought*, ed. William R. LaFleur (Honolulu: University of Hawaii Press, 1985).

3. Robert C. Neville, *The Tao and the Daimon: Segments of a Religious Inquiry* (Albany: State University of New York Press, 1982); Thomas P. Kasulis, *Self and Body in Asian Theory and Practice*, ed. Thomas P. Kasulis, with Roger T. Ames and Wimal Dissanayake (Albany: State University of New York Press, 1993).

4. Alan Race, *Christians and Religious Pluralism: Patterns in the Christian Theology of Religions* (London: SMC Press, 1982); John Hick and Paul F. Knitter,

eds., *The Myth of Christian Uniqueness: Toward a Pluralistic Theology of Religions* (Maryknoll, NY: Orbis Books, 1988); Francis X. Clooney, S.J., *Seeing through Texts: Doing Theology among Srîvaisnavas of South India* (Albany: State University of New York Press, 1996).

5. See Jaroslav Pelikan, *The Christian Tradition: A History of the Development of Doctrine*, vol. 1, *The Emergence of the Catholic Tradition (100-600)* (Chicago: University of Chicago Press, 1971), esp. chapter 2, "Outside the Mainstream," pp. 67-120.

6. John Hick, "The Non-Absoluteness of Christianity," in *The Myth of Christian Uniqueness*, p. 17.

7. See Mark Heim, "Mapping Globalization for Theological Education," *Theological Education* 26, Supplement 1 (Spring, 1990): 9-10.

8. Traditionally, Christians have used the term "ecumenism" primarily to refer to their relations with other Christian groups and—in some cases—with the Jewish communities. However, the term *oecumene* refers to the "house," and has been historically used to refer to the whole world. Thus the term "wider ecumenism" has been coined as a way of extending the ecumenical attitude toward interfaith relations. See Peter Phan, "Introduction," in *Christianity and the Wider Ecumenism*, ed. Peter Phan (New York: Paragon House, 1990), pp. ix-x.

9. Alan Race, *Christians and Religious Pluralism*, chapter 2, pp. 10-37.

10. See, for example, his volume *Problems of Religious Pluralism* (New York: St. Martin's Press, 1985).

11. John Hick, "Rethinking Christian Doctrine in the Light of Religious Pluralism," in *Christianity and the Wider Ecumenism*, pp. 89-102.

12. This bears a striking resemblance to the much-criticized assimilationist approach to U.S. culture, which assumes that in the "melting pot," cultural differences could be melted away until groups became "American." What this means, in actuality, is that the cultural minorities are expected to conform to the mores and sensibilities of groups which had assumed the role of "mainstream cultural elite."

13. (Maryknoll, NY: Orbis Books, 1988).

14. (New York: Paragon House, 1990).

15. Langdon Gilkey, "Plurality and Its Theological Implications," in *The Myth of Christian Uniqueness*, p. 39.

16. Stanley J. Samartha, "The Cross and the Rainbow," in *The Myth of Christian Uniqueness*, p. 69.

17. Durwood Foster, "Christian Motives for Interfaith Dialogue," *Christianity and the Wider Ecumenism*, p. 24.

18. Ibid.; and Martin Forward, "How Do you Read?: The Scriptures in Interfaith Dialogue," in *Christianity and the Wider Ecumenism*, pp. 103-115.

19. Monika Hellwig, "The Wider Ecumenism: Some Theological Questions," in *Christianity and the Wider Ecumenism*, pp. 75-88; and M. Darrol Bryant, "Interfaith Encounter and Dialogue in a Trinitarian Perspective," in *Christianity and the Wider Ecumenism*, pp. 3-20.

20. Mary Ann Stenger, "The Understanding of Christ as Final Revelation," in *Christianity and the Wider Ecumenism*, pp. 191-206; Donald W. Dayton, "Karl Barth and the Wider Ecumenism," in *Christianity and the Wider Ecumenism*, pp. 181-190; and Frederick M. Jelly, "Tillich, Rahner, and Schillebeeckx on the Uniqueness and Universality of Christianity in Dialogue with the World Religions," in *Christianity and the Wider Ecumenism*, pp. 207-220.

21. Seiichi Yagi, "'I' in the Words of Jesus," in *The Myth of Christian Uniqueness*, pp. 117-134.

22. Myrtle S. Langley, "One More Step in a Journey of Many Miles: Toward a Theology of Interfaith Dialogue: Report, Reception, and Response," in *Christianity and the Wider Ecumenism*, pp. 221-232; Joseph Osei-Bonsu, "'*Extra Ecclesiam nulla Salus*': Critical Reflections from Biblical and African Perspectives," in *Christianity and the Wider Ecumenism*, pp. 131-146; Joseph H. Fichter, "Christianity as a World Minority,"in *Christianity and the Wider Ecumenism*, pp. 59-74.

23. Paul F. Knitter, "Toward a Liberation Theology," in *The Myth of Christian Uniqueness*, pp. 178-200; Rosemary Radford Ruether, "Feminism and Jewish-Christian Dialogue: Particularism and Universalism in the Search for Religious Truth," in *The Myth of Christian Uniqueness*, pp. 137-148; Marjorie Hewitt Suchocki, "Religious Pluralism from a Feminist Perspective," in *The Myth of Christian Uniqueness*, pp. 149-161.

24. Peter C. Phan, "Are There Other 'Saviors' for Other Peoples?: A Discussion of the Problem of the Universal Significance and Uniqueness of Jesus Christ," in *Christianity and the Wider Ecumenism*, p. 168.

25. John Hick, *God Has Many Names: Britain's New Religious Pluralism* (London: Macmillan, 1980), pp. 59-79.

26. Mary Ann Stenger, "The Understanding of Christ," p. 192.

27. Paul F. Knitter, "Toward a Liberation Theology."

28. S. Mark Heim, *Salvations: Truth and Difference in Religion* (Maryknoll, NY: Orbis Books, 1995), p. 187.

29. Ibid., p. 189.

30. Francis X. Clooney, *Seeing through Texts*, pp. 296-297.

31. Ibid., pp. 299-304.

32. From "Anything We Love Can Be Saved," an address by Alice Walker at the First Annual Zora Neale Hurston Festival, Eatonville, FL, January 26, 1990, cited in Playbill for "Spunk: Three Tales by Zora Neale Hurston," Berkeley Repertory Theater, November 1-December 21, 1991.

33. Anne C. Riessner, "Piece by Piece: A Mosaic of Global Theological Education," *Theological Education* 27.2 (Spring 1991): 113.

34. "Christian Motives," pp. 21-34.

35. This was one of the central insights in the theory of religions developed by Mircea Eliade, articulated in his classic, *The Sacred and the Profane: The Nature of Religion: The Significance of Religious Myth, Symbolism, and Ritual within Life and Culture* (New York: Harcourt, Brace, and World, 1959).

36. (Boston: Beacon Press, 1993).

37. In the Vanderbilt doctoral seminar, Emily Askew pointed out that my approach is pragmatic, offering a back, or at least a side door to avoid the obstacles of a more direct, head-on approach to the matter. This statement illumines how very Chinese my approach is. First, the Chinese are well-known for being profound religious pragmatists; they follow "what works" and what shows evidence of success. Second, Chinese architecture and *feng-shui* (geomancy, or the art arranging space so as to augment auspicious energies and to guard against negative forces) always argue against a straight pathway into the front door. Such a path, they believe, invites evil—human or otherwise. An obstacle needs to be erected to create bends or turns in the path, so that one goes around the side rather than entering directly.

38. Students in the Vanderbilt doctoral seminar, notably Laurel Cassidy, reminded me that there are limits to the mutual accessibility of symbols, and some are less transferable than others. The cross, for instance, is so profoundly embedded in the full Christian story that it would not appear to be easily accessible to non-Christians. My point is not the absolute, but the relative accessibility of symbols, which allow us to glimpse the views of another faith.

39. For another book starting from the premise that practice is a promising ground for interfaith understanding, see Robert Aitken and David Stendl-Rast, *The Ground We Share: Everyday Practice, Buddhist and Christian* (Boston: Shambhala, 1996), a dialogue between a Zen master and a Benedictine monk on issues of religious practice.

40. By European and North American standards, Protestants and Catholics are both Christians, but in Asia these are viewed as two different religions. Even in Europe and North America, and despite post-Vatican II developments, there is a considerable historical and traditional gap between the traditions from which Protestants and Catholics have tended to draw.

41. Peter Feldmeier of the GTU wrote his doctoral dissertation on the issue of on what grounds would a Christian be able to practice Buddhist Vipassina meditation? What was at stake in such an inter-religious form of practice? See "Interrelatedness: A Comparison of the Spiritualities of St. John of the Cross and Budhhaghosa for the Purpose of Examining the Christian Use of Buddhist Practices" (Doctoral dissertation, Graduate Theological Union, 1996).

4. Diversity and Competition in the Chinese Religious Field

1. The use of the term "religion" in regard to China is complex. There is no exact equivalent of the Western notion of religion (based on a Christian model) in classical Chinese. Tao (the Way) may be the closest equivalent. The Chinese used *chiao* (teaching) to refer to and classify philosophical, doctrinal, and spiritual ideas, writings, and practices. Sometimes, particularly in relation to Taoism, *tao-chiao* referred to religious practices and traditions, and *tao-chia* to philosophical thinkers.

Confucianism was deemed by early Christian missionaries, and thence by the Chinese themselves, not to be a religion in the Western sense. It does indeed lack certain characteristics of Western monotheistic religions (ordained clergy, rituals of membership, theistic beliefs). It was deemed a way of life or a sociomoral philosophy. Yet in the last thirty years, students of Chinese thought and religion have noted that Confucian beliefs, values, and observances are at the very heart of Chinese spiritual life, and they intersect in complex ways with the more overtly "religious" practices and beliefs of Taoism, Buddhism, and folk traditions. (See for instance Rodney L. Taylor's *The Religious Dimensions of Confucianism* [Albany: State University of New York Press, 1990].) Thus whether or not Confucianism is a religion depends on one's definition of "religion." Yet it is not possible to fully understand the dynamics of the Chinese religious world without taking Confucianism into account. (This was brilliantly illustrated in C. K. Yang's classic *Religion in Chinese Society: A Study of Contemporary Social Functions of Religion and Some of Their Historical Factors* [Berkeley: University of California Press, 1967].)

Given all this, while I acknowledge that "Confucianism" stretches one's definition of religion and that most Chinese people would not call it a religion, I nonethe-

less treat it as part of the Chinese religious field and maintain that the practices and values of Confucianism have profound religious implications.

2. Jan Jakob Maria de Groot has catalogued these sectarian and divisive elements in his rather polemical tract, *Sectarianism and Religious Persecution in the History of Chinese Religions* (Amsterdam: J. Muller, 1903-4). See also C. K. Yang, "Confucian Thought and Chinese Religion," in *Chinese Thought and Institutions*, ed. John K. Fairbank (Chicago: University of Chicago Press, 1957), pp. 587-588.

3. In 1983, 120 million Japanese citizens recorded 220 million religious affiliations. See Josef Kreiner, "Religion in Japan," in *Japan*, ed. Manfred Pohl (Stuttgart, 1986), pp. 387-392. This reference is cited from Hans Küng, "Dual Religious Citizenship: A Challenge to the West," in Hans Küng and Julia Ching, *Christianity and Chinese Religions* (New York: Doubleday, 1989), p. 274.

4. On the *Thirteen Classics* and the *Four Books*, see *Sources of Chinese Tradition*, compiled by William Theodore de Bary, Wing-tsit Chan, Burton Watson (New York: Columbia University Press, 1964) I: 1-5 and 113.

5. Ibid., I: 239-250.

6. One of the best and most accurate surveys of Taoist lineages and literatures is Judith M. Boltz, *A Survey of Taoist Literature: Tenth to Seventeenth Centuries*, China Research Monograph No. 32 (Berkeley: Institute of East Asian Studies, 1987).

7. A somewhat dated but still usable survey of the arts of nurturing life is found in Holmes Welch, *The Parting of the Way* (Boston: Beacon Press, 1966), pp. 97-112, and 130-141.

8. For a classic introduction to Chinese Buddhism, see Kenneth K. S. Ch'en, *Buddhism in China: A Historical Survey* (Princeton: Princeton University Press, 1964).

9. In the last decade scholars of Chinese religion have begun major work on tracing the reconfiguration of lineages. See, for instance, Judith Magee Boltz, "Taoist Literature: Five Dynasties to Ming," in William Nienhauser, Jr., ed., *The Indiana Companion to Traditional Chinese Literature* (Bloomington: Indiana University Press, 1986), pp. 153 ff.; and Judith M. Boltz, *A Survey of Taoist Literature*.

10. C. K. Yang, *Religion in Chinese Society*, p. 25.

11. Robert Redfield suggested dealing with this problem by referring to Confucianism, Buddhism, and Taoism as the "great traditions" of China, and to the folk religions as the "little tradition." See his *Peasant Society and Culture: An Anthropological Approach to Civilization* (Chicago: University of Chicago Press, 1956), pp. 67-104. Such an approach, however, fails to do justice to the "folk" or popular elements of "great" traditions, and to elite patronage of "folk" traditions. Christian Jochim addresses the issue by discussing the religions of China under the title "The Four Traditions." See his *Chinese Religions: A Cultural Perspective* (New Jersey: Prentice Hall, 1986), esp. pp. 12-16. His approach is preferable to Redfield's, but may suggest a coherence which folk traditions simply do not sustain. I am grateful to Kevin Cheng for pressing me to clarify this point.

12. *Mencius* 3A:3; translated in *Sources of Chinese Tradition*, I: 95.

13. Gazetteers recorded information about local shrines and temples as well as local customs to record the distinctive religious practices of the region.

14. Stanley J. Tambiah, *Buddhism and Spirit Cults in North-east Thailand* (Cambridge: Cambridge University Press, 1970), chapter 19, pp. 337-350.

15. I thank the students in the Vanderbilt seminar for this image, which helps to escape the notion of a football or soccer field where teams defend opposing goals.

The latter clearly does not work in China. The point of the Chinese game is not to vanquish an opponent, but to gain maximum treasure (religious boon or fulfillment).

16. Pierre Bourdieu, "Genèse et structure du champ religieux" (Origin and structure of the religious field) *Revue Francaise de Sociologie* 12 (1971): 295-334.

17. The computer model suggested above would help here; once you plug in the group which is depicting the religious fields, all of the temples and paths would rearrange themselves accordingly.

18. See Kenneth K. S. Ch'en, *The Chinese Transformation of Buddhism* (Princeton, NJ: Princeton University Press, 1973), pp. 46-53, and *Shih shuo hsin yü: A New Account of Tales of the World* by Liu I-ch'ing with commentary by Liu Chün, trans. with introduction and notes by Richard B. Mather (Minneapolis: University of Minnesota Press, 1976).

19. Introduction to Mou Tzu, *Li-huo lun* "The Disposition of Error," in *Sources of Chinese Tradition* I: 274.

20. Chinese fears are articulated in ibid., in which he attacks Buddhism on the grounds that: 1) it is not mentioned in the Chinese classics; 2) monks are unfilial in that they harm their bodies and do not marry; and 3) Chinese should not be influenced by the ways of barbarians.

21. From *Fan-wang ching, Taishô tripitika* 24.10006a, 1007b; cited from Kenneth K. S. Ch'en, *Transformation of Chinese Buddhism*, p. 34.

22. *Erh-shih-ssu-hsiao ya-tso-wen* (British museum, Stein 3728, P I), cited from Kenneth K. Ch'en, *Transformation of Chinese Buddhism*, pp. 35-36.

23. Han Yü, "Memorial on the Bone of the Buddha," from *Ch'ang-li hsien-sheng wen-chi* (Collected Writings of Master Han Yü), in *Sources of Chinese Tradition*, I: 373-374.

24. Kenneth K. Ch'en, *Transformation of Chinese Buddhism*, pp. 125-178.

25. From *Chiu T'ang-shu* (Older T'ang History), in *Sources of Chinese Tradition*, I: 380-381.

5. Cultural Unity and Local Variation

1. The term "myth" is used here not in the colloquial sense of something which is not true, but in the religious sense of a story which seeks to define a community's sense of reality in such a way as to ground it in a central ideal. As we shall see, the Chinese had as much trouble living up to their myths or ideals as any people, but the myths nonetheless had formative and defining power.

2. See David N. Keightley, "The Religious Commitment: Shang Theology and the Genesis of Chinese Political Culture," *History of Religions* 17:3,4 (Feb-May, 1978): 211-225.

3. Cosmology is the science of the cosmos, beliefs about the entire order of being. A cosmological system, then, is a view about the order and structure of all that is.

4. Tung Chung-shu, *Ch'un-ch'iu fan-lu*, Sec. 43, 11:5a-b; in William Theodore de Bary, Wing-tsit Chan, Burton Watson, *Sources of Chinese Tradition* (New York: Columbia University Press, 1960), vol. 1, pp. 163-164.

5. See Kenneth Scott Latourette, *The Chinese: Their History and Culture*, 4th ed. (New York: Macmillan, 1964), pp. 78-87; and Wolfram Eberhard, *A History of China*, 4th ed. (Berkeley: University of California Press, 1987), pp. 47-59.

6. Valerie Hansen, for instance, has studied the government practice of granting titles to gods in a symbolic effort to express the emperor's patronage of and control over the divine realm. See *Changing Gods in Medieval China, 1127-1276* (Princeton: Princeton University Press, 1990), pp. 79-104.

7. See, for instance, Chün-fang Yü, *The Renewal of Buddhism in China: Chu-hung and the Late Ming Synthesis* (New York: Columbia University Press, 1981), pp. 144-170; and Arthur F. Wright, "T'ang T'ai-tsung and Buddhism," in *Perspectives on the T'ang*, ed. Arthur F. Wright and Denis Twitchett (New Haven: Yale University Press, 1973), pp. 261-263.

8. Local gazetteers, by contrast, contained sections on "local customs" and "shrines and temples" which recorded these traditions in some specificity.

9. See William Theodore de Bary, "Chinese Despotism and the Confucian Ideal: A Seventeenth-Century View" (pp. 178-180) and E.A. Kracke, Jr., "Region, Family, and Individual in the Chinese Examination System" (pp. 251-268), in John K. Fairbank, ed., *Chinese Thought and Institutions* (Chicago: University of Chicago Press, 1957).

10. Jan Jakob Maria de Groot, *Sectarianism and Religious Persecution in the History of Chinese Religions* (Amsterdam: J. Muller, 1903-1904); T'ao Hsi-sheng, *Ming-tai tsung-chiao* (Ming dynasty religion) (Taipei: Tai-wan hsüeh-sheng shu-chü, 1968); Mano Senryû, *Mindai bunkashi kenkyû* (The cultural history of the Ming dynasty) (Kyoto: Dôhôsha, 1979).

11. The Ch'ang-sheng chiao of the eighteenth century is a case in point. See Daniel L. Overmyer, *Folk Buddhist Religion: Dissenting Sects in Late Traditional China* (Cambridge, MA: Harvard University Press, 1976), pp. 7-11. See also, Susan Naquin, *Millenarian Rebellion in China: The Eight Trigrams Uprising of 1813* (New Haven: Yale University Press, 1976) and *Shantung Rebellion: The Wang Lun Uprising of 1774* (New Haven: Yale University Press, 1981).

12. See David Johnson, "The City-God Cults of T'ang and Sung China," *Harvard Journal of Asiatic Studies* 45:2 (Dec 1985): 363-457; and Stephan Feuchtwang, "School-Temple and City God," in G. William Skinner, ed., *The City in Late Imperial China* (Stanford: Stanford University Press, 1977), pp. 581-608. The origins of Chinese local deities are not unlike the processes by which local saints come to be venerated within folk Catholicism.

13. The historical process of the development of the Chinese language was vastly more complex than this statement suggests. These examples are meant only to convey some of the distinctive characteristics of this nonalphabetic language system.

14. Alert readers will wonder how educated officials from various parts of the realm communicated with each other. They did so partly in writing, but they also developed a spoken language for the court (*kuan-hua*, lit. language of officials), which was a somewhat stilted and literary form of Peking dialect.

15. In late imperial China, some writers began experimenting with writing stories or fiction in language at least strongly colored by local dialect. The style was sometimes known as *pan-wen pan-pai* (half classical, half vernacular). As more authors sought to write in the vernacular language, local language and perceptions were more and more clearly reflected in literature. Only in the twentieth century did written vernacular fully develop, so that literature could be written in something like the spoken language. Once vernacular writing took hold, however, Peking dialect had to be promoted as a standard language, or else the plethora of dialects would have fragmented Chinese literature.

16. Victor H. Mair, "Language and Ideology in the Written Popularizations of the *Sacred Edict*," in David Johnson, Andrew Nathan, and Evelyn S. Rawski, eds., *Popular Culture in Late Imperial China* (Berkeley: University of California Press, 1985), pp. 325-359.

17. See, for example, Robert H. Hegel's analysis of *The Water Margin* in *The Novel in Seventeenth-Century China* (New York: Columbia University Press, 1981), pp. 67-84; and Paul S. Ropp, *Dissent in Early Modern China: Ju-lin wai-shih and Ch'ing Social Criticism* (Ann Arbor: University of Michigan Press, 1981).

18. Barbara E. Ward, "Varieties of the Conscious Model," in Michael P. Banton, ed., *The Relevance of Models for Social Anthropology* (London: Tavistock Publications, 1968), pp. 113-137.

19. The rituals associated with the early cult appear to have been "an early regional variation deeply rooted in the 'Taoist' Ling-pao heritage." See Judith M. Boltz, *A Survey of Taoist Literature: Tenth to Seventeenth Centuries*, China Research Monograph Series, Number 32 (Berkeley: Institute of East Asian Studies of the University of California, 1987), p. 71.

20. See Pai Yü-ch'an, "Ching-yang Hsü chen-chün chuan" (Biography of Realized Gentleman Hsü Ching-yang) in *Yü-lung chi* (Record of Yü-lung), ch. 33, preserved in *Hsiu-chen shih-shu*, in the *Tao-tsang*, Harvard Yenching #263.

21. Jurchen invaders from Central Asia, who ruled North China from 1115-1234. The remnant Sung government in the South was waging a battle to expel the invaders and to keep them from invading South China as well.

22. Note the similarity in reasoning to that behind the deity of the city-wall temple; his concern is to protect the local region, but this is presented as loyal aid to the throne.

23. The reader may be wondering why the emperor did not make the connection to Hsü Sun's divination system and the temple Sung emperors had previously patronized. The account does not explain, but it is noteworthy that deities could be known by several names or titles. For some reason (either faulty memory or an alternate name), the emperor did not make the connection and had to order a search for the temple.

24. The ritual document of the feast was preserved and published in Pai Yü-ch'an's life of Hsü Sun. "Ching-yang Hsü chen-chün."

25. "Ching-yang Hsü chen-chün chuan," 34.1a-5b.

26. The *chiao* was the highest ritual of organized Taoism, and could only be performed by Taoist priests with specialized training. See Michael R. Saso, *Taoism and the Rite of Cosmic Renewal* (Pullman: Washington State University Press, 1972), pp. 84-94.

27. "Ching-yang Hsü chen-chün chuan," 34.8b-10a.

6. Myriad Spirits and the Transcendent

1. I saw the same sort of authentic faith and spirituality in the Chinese worship of images that Diana Eck observed in the religious practices of Hindus in India. See Diana L. Eck, *Encountering God: A Spiritual Journey from Bozeman to Banaras* (Boston: Beacon, 1993). There are also striking similarities between Chinese veneration of their deities and popular Roman Catholic veneration of Our Lady of Guadalupe. These similarities merit scholarly study to advance our understanding of popular spiritualities.

2. Note the similarity between this and the animal carvings of native groups available for sale in the United States which, when prepared and blessed in the proper ritual environment, would become fetishes rather than mere carvings.

3. This belief in ritual vivification contrasts with Roman Catholic views of images, which are understood to be holy, but not inhabited by the saint.

4. Valerie Hansen, *Changing Gods in Medieval China 1127-1276* (Princeton: Princeton University Press, 1990), pp. 52-59.

5. A goddess who protects, among others, those who travel on water. Her main temple is in Fukien province in China, but she was very popular throughout southeast China and in Taiwan.

6. The example of the branch temple clearly illustrates that the deity is not fully or exclusively present in any one image; there may be thousands of such images around China. It also points out that each deity has a sacred site at which he or she is most effectively present. This main temple of a deity is the locus at which one can have fullest access to the spiritual power of the deity.

7. Laurence G. Thompson, *Chinese Religion: An Introduction,* 2d ed. (Encino, CA: Dickenson Publishing, 1975), p. 57.

8. *Chiang-su chin-shih*, 10:22a, cited in Hansen, *Changing Gods*, p. 24. There is a temporal gap of some eight hundred years between Hansen's examples and those from anthropological field observation. In juxtaposing these examples, I do not mean to ignore the fact that there were changes in the Chinese religious field over eight centuries. Nonetheless, the mutual illumination of these temporally distant sources testifies to powerful continuities in the basic dynamics of the Chinese religious field.

9. See Alvin P. Cohen, "Coercing the Rain Deities in Ancient China," *History of Religions* 17:3,4 (Feb-May, 1978): 244-265. See also Stephen Feuchtwang, "School-Temple and City God," in G. William Skinner, ed., *The City in Late Imperial China*, (Stanford: Stanford University Press, 1977), p. 603; and C. K. Yang, *Religion in Chinese Society: A Study of Contemporary Social Functions of Religion and Some of Their Historical Factors* (Berkeley and Los Angeles: University of California Press, 1967), p. 25.

10. Hansen, *Changing Gods,* p. 29.

11. Ibid., p. 47. Romanization system adapted for consistency with this text.

12. Ibid., p. 33. This is, roughly, the Chinese equivalent of "There are no atheists in fox holes."

13. Ibid., p. 34.

14. See *Reflections on Things at Hand: The Neo-Confucian Anthology Compiled by Chu Hsi and Lü Tsu-ch'ien*, trans. with notes by Wing-tsit Chan (New York: Columbia University Press, 1967), #33 (p. 26) and #46 (p. 32).

15. Arthur P. Wolf, "Gods, Ghosts, and Ancestors," in Arthur P. Wolf, ed., *Religion and Ritual in Chinese Society* (Stanford: Stanford University Press, 1974), pp. 131-182.

16. Hansen, *Changing Gods*, p. 9.

17. This is a major motif, for instance, in Wu Ch'eng-en's famous *Hsi-yu chi* (Journey to the West). The three guardians were promoted or (more frequently) demoted in the heavenly ranks because of their good or bad deeds; having slipped badly, they are assigned to guard Tripitika to expiate their faults and begin to regain their standing in the heavenly ranks.

18. C. Stevan Harrell, "When a Ghost Becomes a God," in *Religion and Ritual in Chinese Society*, pp. 193-206.

19. The term "posit" here reflects the fact that the human conceptualization of Tao or the ultimate source was required in part by the multiplicity. The Tao or source pre-exists and transcends human conceptualization, but the Chinese are quite clear about the distinction between their conceptualizations and the Tao in itself.

20. *Lao Tzu, Tao te ching,* trans. D. C. Lau (Middlesex: Penguin, 1963), I, p. 57.

21. *Chuang Tzu,* chapt. 22; in *The Complete Works of Chuang Tzu,* trans. Burton Watson (New York: Columbia University Press, 1968), p. 241.

22. Hansen, *Changing Gods,* p. 36. Romanization of Kuan-yin adapted to be consistent with this book's style.

23. Based on the field observation and scholarly analysis of Michael R. Saso in *Taoism and the Rite of Cosmic Renewal* (Pullman: Washington State University Press, 1972).

24. Ibid., p. 32.

25. Ibid., pp. 43-44.

26. Valerie Hansen notes that because of the sale of ordination certificates in the Sung dynasty (as opposed to the examination system for certifying ordination), there was considerable slippage in the training of priests for particular ceremonies, even the *chiao*. *Changing Gods,* p. 44.

27. See Michael R. Saso, *Taoism and the Rite of Cosmic Renewal,* pp. 38-41 and 51-52.

28. Ibid., chapters 2 and 4.

7. Many Embodiments of the Way

1. See Ainslee T. Embree, ed., *The Hindu Tradition* (New York: Modern Library, 1966), pp. 197-205.

2. These represent various names for the ultimate, the Sacred, in various Chinese religious streams.

3. See William Theodore de Bary, *The Liberal Tradition in China* (New York: Columbia University Press, 1982), pp. 32-37; Monika Ubelhor, "The Community Compact (Hsiang-yüeh) of the Sung and its Educational Significance," in William Theodore de Bary and John W. Chaffee, eds., *Neo-Confucian Education: The Formative Stage* (Berkeley: University of California Press, 1989), pp. 371-388; Chu Hsi, *Tseng-sun Lü-shih hsiang-yüeh* (Amended community compact of Mr. Lü), in *Chu tzu ta-ch'üan* (The great compendium of writings of Master Chu) (Ssu-pu pei-yao ed.) 74: 23a-29b. I thank Kevin Cheng for his assistance in developing this note.

4. See Judith Berling, "Bringing the Buddha Down to Earth: Notes on the Emergence of Yü-lu as a Buddhist Genre," *History of Religions* 27: 1 (August, 1987): 56-88.

5. Preface by Chu Hsi to *Chin-ssu lu,* in *Reflections on Things at Hand: The Neo-Confucian Anthology Compiled by Chu Hsi and Lü Tsu-ch'ien,* trans. and with notes by Wing-tsit Chan (New York: Columbia University Press, 1967), p. 2. The exclusive language may be grating to the modern reader, but in this case the kind of study indicated in the statement would have been open only to males. Yet the principle about the *intent* of the book would be applicable, in a contemporary setting, to Confucians of both genders.

6. See Berling, "Bringing the Buddha Down to Earth."

7. Preface to *Chu-tzu yü-lei* (Categorized sayings of Master Chu), ed. Li Ching-te (reprinted, Taipei: Cheng-chung shu- chü, 1962), 1: 1.

8. Analects of Confucius 1: 6; cited from *Sources of Chinese Tradition*, compiled by William Theodore de Bary, Wing-tsit-Chen, Burton Watson (New York: Columbia University Press, 1964), 1: 24. Translation adapted for inclusive language.

9. Wang Yang-ming, *Ch'uan-hsi lu* (Instructions for Practical Living), in *A Source Book for Chinese Philosophy*, trans. and comp. by Wing-tsit Chan (Princeton: Princeton University Press, 1963), p. 669; see also pp. 10-11.

10. Preface to *Chin-ssu lu*, cited in Chan, *Reflections*, p. 2.

11. There is a large literature on the differences between oral and literate cultures, and the impact of writing and books, and also an emerging literature on the different *concepts and uses* of books and writing in various cultures. Although writing was venerated in China from a very early date, the importance of recitation maintained the oral aspects of learning and reinforced the link between learning and human behavior. The Chinese throughout their history lamented learning which became too bookish and abstract and failed to bear fruit in the living of human life.

12. Lin Chao-en, *Hsin-sheng chih-chih* (Direct pointing to the Mind as Sage) II: 2.3b, translated in Judith A. Berling, *The Syncretic Religion of Lin Chao-en* (New York: Columbia University Press, 1980), p. 131.

13. See *Neo-Confucian Education: The Formative Stage*, ed. William Theodore de Bary and John Chaffee (Berkeley: University of California Press, 1989); and Tadao Sakai, "Confucianism and Popular Educational Works," in *Self and Society in Ming Thought*, William Theodore de Bary and the Conference on Ming Thought (New York: Columbia University Press, 1970), pp. 331-366.

14. *Su Shih I-chuan* (Su Shih's comments on the Book of Changes), 9.190; in Kidder Smith, Jr., Peter K. Bol, Joseph A. Adler, Don J. Wyatt, eds., *Sung Dynasty Uses of the I Ching* (Princeton: Princeton University Press, 1990), p. 89.

15. Analects of Confucius, 4: 15, in *Sources*, 1: 25.

16. Ibid., 7: 8; in *Sources,* 1: 24. Translation adapted for inclusive language.

17. Ibid., 9: 10, in *Sources* 1: 25. Adapted for inclusive language.

18. Ibid., 7: 4; 7: 38; in *Sources* 1: 20.

19. Ibid., 7: 1; in *Sources* 1: 23.

20. Ibid., 4: 8; in *Sources,* 1: 23.

21. Ibid., 7: 25; *Sources* 1: 24.

22. *The Complete Works of Chuang Tzu,* trans. Burton Watson (New York: Columbia University Press, 1968), chapter 25, p. 281, 282-283. Translation adapted for inclusive language; this is particularly apt in the *Chuang Tzu* since several of the sages or teachers depicted in the book are women.

23. Ibid., chapter 19; pp. 205-206.

24. Lao Tzu, *Tao Te Ching*, chapt. 20. Translations combined from *Lao Tzu, Tao Te Ching*, trans. with an introduction by D. C. Lau (Middlesex, Eng.: Penguin, 1963), pp. 76-77; and Arthur Waley, *The Way and Its Power: A Study of Tao Te Ching and Its Place in Chinese Thought*, Arthur Waley (New York: Grove Press, 1958) pp. 168-169.

25. Lao Tzu, *Tao Te Ching*, D. C. Lau, trans., chapt. 17; p. 73.

8. Hospitality and the Chinese Religious Field

1. Arthur P. Wolf, "Gods, Ghosts, and Ancestors," in Arthur P. Wolf, ed., *Religion and Ritual in Chinese Society* (Stanford: Stanford University Press, 1974), pp. 131-182.

2. This applies even when the guest is of higher social status than the host, although it is true that in Chinese society the rituals of entertainment would vary according to the relative social positions of host and guest. I thank Kevin Cheng for this comment.

3. See C. K. Yang, *Religion in Chinese Society: A Study of Contemporary Social Functions of Religion and Some of Their Historical Factors* (Berkeley and Los Angeles: University of California Press, 1967), pp. 81-103.

4. This story was repeated often in the history of various religious groups in China, and was also a well-established pattern in the history of Buddhism going back to India. For instance, the four kings which guard the four corners of the Buddhist altar were vanquished and assimilated deities of Hindu and other local cults.

5. See Kristofer Schipper, "Neighborhood Cult Associations in Traditional Tainan," in G. William Skinner, ed., *The City in Late Imperial China* (Stanford: Stanford University Press, 1977), pp. 651-676.

6. See James Hayes, *The Hong Kong Region, 1850-1911: Institutions and Leadership in Town and Countryside* (Hamden, CT: Archon Books, 1977), pp. 98-101.

7. Jan Jakob Maria de Groot, in his multivolumed description of the practice of religion in southeast China at the turn of the century, described in wonderful detail the conspicuous display of Chinese weddings and funerals. Anthropological studies have reconfirmed his findings in a number of other sites. Jan Jakob Maria de Groot, *The Religious System of China: Its Ancient Forms, Evolution, History and Present Aspect, Manners, Customs, and Social Institutions Connected Therewith*, 7 Vols. (Amsterdam: J. Muller, c. 1901-04; reprinted by Ch'eng-wen Publishing Company, Taipei, 1969).

8. This contribution is roughly parallel to our custom that guests should bring a gift to a wedding or party.

9. Donald DeGlopper, "Religion and Ritual in Lukang," in *Religion and Ritual in Chinese Society*, p. 54.

10. A similar occurrence in eighteenth-century England was documented in Keith Thomas's classic *Religion and the Decline of Magic* (New York: Scribner and Sons, 1971), pp. 556-569.

11. Valerie Hansen discusses the sources through which the literate and illiterate heard about gods and miracles during the Sung dynasty in her introduction to *Changing Gods in Medieval China, 1127-1276* (Princeton: Princeton University Press, 1990), pp. 3-28.

12. For the code of offerings appropriate to deities of various classes, see Arthur Wolf, "Gods, Ghosts, and Ancestors," in *Religion and Ritual in Chinese Society*, pp. 131-182.

13. Emily Ahern has explored the intriguing parallels between petitioning deities and the government in her *Chinese Ritual and Politics* (Cambridge: Cambridge University Press, 1981), esp. pp. 2-24, 95-108.

14. When I visited two Buddhist monasteries in the People's Republic of China in October 1996, I noted that the restoration of wall paintings and carvings were

still serving this purpose. Visitors asked many questions about these illustrations in an effort to educate themselves about the Buddhist heritage.

15. See Chikusa Masaaki, *Chûkoku Bukkyô shakaishi kenkyû*(On the Social History of Chinese Buddhism) (Kyoto: Dôhôsha, 1982).

16. Such shops were doing a thriving business at Lion's Head Mountain. For the historical precedents, see G. William Skinner, *The City in Late Imperial China*, pp. 3-31, 211-252, 253-351.

17. Sec Holmes Welch, *The Practice of Chinese Buddhism, 1900-1950* (Cambridge, MA: Harvard University Press, 1967), pp. 303-356.

18. These are all recorded in the mountain gazetteer: *Wu-i shan-chih* (Mount Wu-i gazetteer), 24 ch., ed. Tung T'ien-kung (1846), Reprinted in *Chung-kuo ming-shan sheng-chi ts'ung-kan* (Compendium of the Scenic and Historic Traces of Famous Chinese Mountains).

19. One of the sadder legacies of the Cultural Revolution in China today is that the reconstruction of temple complexes has lost this multireligious dimension. Since Taoist sources are paying for Taoist restorations and Buddhist for Buddhist, the restored temple complexes are more religiously homogeneous than in the past; this development erodes the traditional Chinese religious field.

20. Michael Saso identifies the "red-head" priests as follows: "Members of this class are expected to cure sickness, win blessing, expel demons, and, in general, perform rituals for the living." Michael Saso, *Taoism and the Rite of Cosmic Renewal* (Pullman: Washington State University Press, 1972), p. 84. The red-head refers to a distinctive red scarf worn by such priests, not to red hair, which would be truly rare in Chinese society.

21. Since I also tried to record the music there are several quite hilarious tapes of funeral music accompanied by the under-beat of my feet running along the pavement. I pray that these not fall into other hands, giving rise to some theory of strange Chinese drumming traditions.

9. Christians and Religious Neighbors

1. The Buddhist term for pedagogical strategies geared to the level of understanding and spiritual maturity of one's audience.

2. I mean the term "theological" in the broadest possible sense, since my reflections focused primarily on religious behavior, practice, and pedagogy. I do not aspire to systematic theology.

3. Many participants in the dialogue have developed promising principles for Christian participation in such conversations (the most common one being that one cannot be an effective partner in conversation unless one brings one's beliefs and values with one), but these principles are not well known in the Christian communities.

4. See for example my book on syncretist Lin Chao-en, for whom such reconciliation was a major concern. Judith Berling, *The Syncretic Religion of Lin Chao-en* (New York: Columbia University Press, 1980).

5. My thank to James Keddy of Sacramento for informing me about the network.

6. I met this person at the National Interfaith Network in Wichita, Kansas, 1988.

7. Rosemarie Tong, *Feminist Thought: A Comprehensive Introduction* (Boulder,

CO: Westview Press, 1989), p. 7. Cited in Linda Moody, *Women Encounter God: Theology across Boundaries of Difference* (Maryknoll, NY: Orbis Books, 1996), p. 132.

8. Linda Moody, *Women Encounter God*, pp. 124-125.

9. This case is made by Karen Armstrong in *A History of God: The 4,000 Year Quest of Judaism, Christianity, and Islam* (New York: Ballantine Books, 1993).

10. *Hadewijch: The Complete Works*, trans. and intro. by Mother Columba Hart, O.S.B. (New York: Paulist Press, 1980), pp. 346-349.

11. Linda Moody, *Women Encounter God*, p. 111.

12. Thomas W. Ogletree, *Hospitality to the Stranger: Dimensions of Moral Understanding* (Philadelphia: Fortress Press, 1985), pp. 2-3.

13. Ibid., p. 3.

14. Ibid., p. 4.

15. Diana L. Eck, *Encountering God: A Spiritual Journey from Bozeman to Banaras* (Boston: Beacon Press, 1993), p. 79.

Index

Other Titles in the Faith Meets Faith Series

Toward a Universal Theology of Religion, Leonard Swidler, Editor
The Myth of Christian Uniqueness, John Hick and Paul F. Knitter, Editors
An Asian Theology of Liberation, Aloysius Pieris, S.J.
The Dialogical Imperative, David Lochhead
Love Meets Wisdom, Aloysius Pieris, S.J.
Many Paths, Eugene Hillman, C.S.Sp.
The Silence of God, Raimundo Panikkar
The Challenge of the Scriptures, Groupe de Recherches Islamo-Chrétien
The Meaning of Christ, John P. Keenan
Hindu-Christian Dialogue, Harold Coward, Editor
The Emptying God, John B. Cobb, Jr., and Christopher Ives, Editors
Christianity through Non-Christian Eyes, Paul J. Griffiths, Editor
Christian Uniqueness Reconsidered, Gavin D'Costa, Editor
Women Speaking, Women Listening, Maura O'Neill
Bursting the Bonds?, Leonard Swidler, Lewis John Eron, Gerard Sloyan, and Lester Dean, Editors
One Christ—Many Religions, Stanley J. Samartha
The New Universalism, David J. Krieger
Jesus Christ at the Encounter of World Religions, Jacques Dupuis, S.J.
After Patriarchy, Paula M. Cooey, William R. Eakin, and Jay B. McDaniel, Editors
An Apology for Apologetics, Paul J. Griffiths
World Religions and Human Liberation, Dan Cohn-Sherbok, Editor
Uniqueness, Gabriel Moran
Leave the Temple, Felix Wilfred, Editor
The Buddha and the Christ, Leo D. Lefebure
The Divine Matrix, Joseph A. Bracken, S.J.
The Gospel of Mark: A Mahāyāna Reading, John P. Keenan
Revelation, History & the Dialogue of Religions, David A. Carpenter
Salvations, S. Mark Heim
The Intercultural Challenge of Raimon Panikkar, Joseph Prabhu, Editor
Fire and Water: Women, Society, & Sprituality in Buddhism and Christianity, Aloysius Pieris, S.J.
Piety & Power: Muslims and Christians in West Africa, Lamin Sanneh
Life after Death in World Religions, Harold Coward, Editor
The Uniqueness of Jesus, Paul Mojzes and Leonard Swidler, Editors